Deep Vein Thrombosis and Pulmonary Embolism

Deep Vein Thrombosis and Pulmonary Embolism

Edwin J.R. van Beek

Department of Radiology,
Carver College of Medicine, University of Iowa, USA
and
Department of Radiology,
Royal Infirmary, University of Edinburgh, UK

Harry R. Büller

Department of Vascular Medicine,
Academic Medical Centre, Amsterdam, The Netherlands

Matthijs Oudkerk

Department of Radiology,
Academic Medical Centre, Groningen, The Netherlands

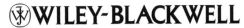

WILEY-BLACKWELL

A John Wiley & Sons, Ltd., Publication

Library of Congress Cataloging-in-Publication Data:

Deep vein thrombosis and pulmonary embolism/edited by Edwin J.R. van Beek, Harry R. Büller, Matthijs Oudkerk.
     p. ; cm.
   Rev. ed. of: Pulmonary embolism/Matthijs Oudkerk, Edwin J.R. van Beek, Jan W. ten Cate (eds.). c1999.
   Includes bibliographical references and index.
   ISBN 978-0-470-51717-8
   1. Pulmonary embolism. 2. Thrombophlebitis. I. Beek, Edwin J. R. van. II. Büller, H. R. III. Oudkerk, Matthijs.
IV. Pulmonary embolism.
   [DNLM: 1. Venous Thrombosis–diagnosis. 2. Diagnostic Imaging–methods. 3. Pulmonary Embolism–diagnosis.
4. Pulmonary Embolism–therapy. 5. Venous Thrombosis–therapy. WG 610 D311 2009]
   RC776.P85D44 2009
   616.2'49–dc22

                                                                                                2008052794

ISBN   978-0-470-51717-8(H/B)

Typeset in 10/12pt Times by Laserwords Private Limited, Chennai, India.
Printed in Great Britain by CPI Antony Rowe, Chippenham, Wiltshire.

First Impression   2009

Cover image:Hippocrates treating thrombophlebitis on a relief located at the National Archeological Museum, Athens, Greece - image courtesy of Dr van Beek.

Dedications

To Miriam, Andrew and Steven with thanks for your support and understanding. To Jan-Wouter ten Cate, who taught me the basics of and love for thrombosis and haemostasis.

Edwin J.R. van Beek

I dedicate this book to the eminent German pathologist Rudolf Virchow (1821–1902), who discovered that blood clots in the pulmonary arteries originate as venous thrombi elsewhere. To this pathogenesis Virchow bestowed the name 'Embolia'.

Matthijs Oudkerk

To my teachers.

Harry R. Büller

Contents

Preface

When we completed the first edition of this work, simply called *Pulmonary Embolism*, we could not have envisioned the many changes we would face over such a short period of time.

First, the rapid introduction of CT pulmonary angiography quickly changed the way in which imaging was involved in the diagnostic management of patients with suspected pulmonary embolism. In part, the easy accessibility of CT allowed a significant increase in tested patients, resulting in larger number of patients under evaluation for this disease. This led to a decrease in the prevalence of pulmonary embolism in the tested population, and an increasing concern regarding radiation burden as well as the burden (and costs) on healthcare.

Second, two important tests (plasma D-dimer and clinical decision rules) came of age, and this allowed for the simplification of the diagnostic assessment of many patients with either chest (PE) or leg (DVT) symptoms. The most recent guidelines all propose that with normal outcomes of these relatively simple tests, further imaging is no longer required and anticoagulant therapy can be safely withheld.

Third, the treatment went from cumbersome hospital-based approaches to a community and outpatient approach through the development of low molecular weight heparins and in the near future new oral anticoagulants. This has altered the rates of hospital admissions and also changed the way in which patients with DVT and PE are being seen and monitored. Last but not least, the role of nuclear perfusion/ventilation scanning diminished dramatically and also that of the gold standard, pulmonary angiography, became marginal with the development of multidetector CT systems which permit isotropic sub-millimetre resolution.

With all these (and other changes), it became apparent that a new edition of the book would be of potential use to the wider community, and we are grateful for the team at Wiley (which merged with our previous publisher, Blackwell), which allowed us to revisit the various chapters and produce a second edition, now also incorporating DVT. We have opted to keep to our previous sections approach, and have updated the current guidelines and various diagnostic tests completely to bring this work into the 21st century. We are extremely fortunate to have found such a wonderfully talented group of contributors from all over the world to participate in this endeavour. It is a rather thankless task to write book chapters, as the work is significant and the deadlines fairly strict in order to keep to publishing timetables. We have truly enjoyed working with such an esteemed group, who kept to time and helped create a book that is based on the literature evidence. This evidence-based approach is important as it is the only way to truly help understand the disease, perform the correct testing in the appropriate setting and treat the patient with optimal results.

Finally, Jan-Wouter ten Cate was unable to join this partnership due to health reasons, and we are grateful to Harry Büller for joining the Editors. We have been involved with many collaborative studies and projects over the years, and this work is just another example of what a dedicated team of authors, Editors and publishing team can achieve. We truly hope that this work will be of help to many practising physicians in a wide spectrum of specialities, whether based in primary care or situated in hospital-based practice, the content of this book is surely going to assist you in managing your patients.

Edwin J.R. van Beek, Iowa City, IA, USA/Edinburgh, UK
Harry Büller, Amsterdam, The Netherlands
Matthijs Oudkerk, Groningen, The Netherlands

About the Editors

Professor Edwin van Beek is a Professor of Radiology, Medicine and Biomedical Engineering at the University of Iowa and practices as a cardiothoracic radiologist. An alumnus from Erasmus University Rotterdam Medical School, he received his formal radiology education and also obtained his PhD in the field of pulmonary embolism under the guidance of Professor Jan-Wouter ten Cate (a former editor of this book) and the current co-editor Professor Harry Büller. He has just accepted the Forbes Chair of Medical Imaging at the University of Edinburgh, Scotland, UK, where he will continue his work in the field of multimodality cardiac and pulmonary imaging from June 2009.

Professor Harry Büller is a Professor of Vascular Medicine at the Academic Medical Centre, Amsterdam, and a world-renowned expert in the field of venous thromboembolism. He received his medical training at the University of Amsterdam, and subsequently underwent his training in Internal Medicine in Amsterdam, after which he spent time at McMaster University, Hamilton, for his education in clinical epidemiology. He has been a sought-after consultant, has been involved in many key studies of management and treatment and has published widely on this topic during a career spanning more than 15 years.

Professor Matthijs Oudkerk is full Professor of Radiology at the State University of Groningen and internationally known for his pioneering work in the field of CT and MRI for cardiovascular and pulmonary vascular diseases at Erasmus University Rotterdam and the University Medical Centre Groningen. He received and obtained his medical education, PhD and his radiological training at Leiden University. For his work on cardiovascular radiology he was honoured by the Russian and Polish Academies of Sciences. He was the initiator of the development of management strategies in pulmonary embolism, about which he wrote the first publications together with Professor van Beek and Professor Büller in the early 1990s. He initiated and edited the first edition of this book together with Professor van Beek and Professor ten Cate.

The three editors of this second edition have worked together on a variety of projects for more than fifteen years, ranging from multidisciplinary consensus working groups, writing of articles to collaboration in multicentre trials.

Contributors

Giancarlo Agnelli
Internal and Cardiovascular Medicine, University of Perugia, Via G. Dottori 1,
06129 Perugia, Italy

Juan I. Arcelus
Department of Surgery, University of Granada Medical School, Granada, Spain

Fabrice Guy Barral
Thrombosis Research Group: EA 3065 – CIE3, University Hospital of Saint-Etienne,
Université Jean Monnet, 42055 Saint-Etienne, France

Cecilia Becattini
Internal and Cardiovascular Medicine, University of Perugia, Via G. Dottori 1,
06129 Perugia, Italy

Henri Bounameaux
Division of Angiology and Hemostasis, Department of Internal Medicine,
Geneva University Hospital and Faculty of Medicine, 24 rue Micheli-du-Crest,
1211 Geneva 14, Switzerland

Harry R. Büller
Forbes Chair of Medical Imaging, Clinical Research Imaging Centre, University of Edinburgh,
Little France Crescent, Edinburgh EH16 4SA, Scotland, UK.

Joseph A. Caprini
Department of Surgery, Evanston Northwestern Healthcare, Glenbrook Hospital,
2100 Pfingsten Road, Glenview, IL 60025, USA

Wee Shian Chan
Department of Medicine, University of Toronto, Women's College Hospital, 76 Grenville Street,
Toronto, Ontario, Canada M5S 1B2

Heok K. Cheow
Department of Nuclear Medicine, Addenbrooke's Hospital, Cambridge, UK

Robin Condliffe
Pulmonary Vascular Disease Unit, Royal Hallamshire Hospital,
Glossop Road, Sheffield S10 2JF, UK

Hervé Decousus
Thrombosis Research Group: EA 3065 – CIE3, University Hospital of Saint-Etienne,
Université Jean Monnet, 42055 Saint-Etienne, France

Renée A. Douma
Department of Vascular Medicine, Academic Medical Centre, Meibergdreef 9,
1105 AZ Amsterdam, The Netherlands

Jane A.E. Dutton
Department of Nuclear Medicine, Addenbrooke's Hospital, Cambridge, UK

Charlie A. Elliot
Pulmonary Vascular Disease Unit, Royal Hallamshire Hospital,
Glossop Road, Sheffield S10 2JF, UK

Raimund Erbel
Universitätsklinikum Essen, Centre for Internal Medicine, Clinic for Cardiology,
Hufelandstrasse 55, 45122 Essen, Germany

Ian N. Gillespie
Department of Clinical Radiology, Royal Infirmary of Edinburgh, Little France Crescent,
Edinburgh EH16 4SA, Scotland, UK

Jeffrey S. Ginsberg
Department of Medicine, Thromboembolism Unit, McMaster Medical Centre, 1200 Main St W,
HSC-3 W15, Hamilton, Ontario, Canada L8N 3Z5

Lawrence R. Goodman
Diagnostic Radiology & Pulmonary Medicine & Critical Care, Thoracic Imaging,
Medical College of Wisconsin, 9200 West Wisconsin Avenue, Milwaukee,
WI 53226-3596, USA

Günter Görge
Klinikum Saarbrücken, Innere Medizin II, Winterberg 1, 66119 Saarbrücken, Germany

Harriet Heijboer
Emma Children's Hospital/Academic Medical Center, Department of Pediatric Hematology,
P.O. Box 22700, 1100 DE Amsterdam, The Netherlands

Stuart W. Jamieson
Division of Cardiothoracic Surgery, University of California at San Diego Medical Center,
200 West Arbor Drive, San Diego, CA 92103-8892, USA

Pieter W. Kamphuisen
Department of Vascular Medicine, F4, Academic Medical Centre, Meibergdreef 9, 1401 AG
Amsterdam, The Netherlands

Hans-Ulrich Kauczor
Department of Diagnostic Radiology, University Hospital Heidelberg, Im Neuenheimer Feld 110,
69120 Heidelberg, Germany.

David G. Kiely
Pulmonary Vascular Disease Unit, Royal Hallamshire Hospital, Glossop Road, Sheffield S10 2JF, UK

Silvy Laporte
Thrombosis Research Group: EA 3065 – CIE3, University Hospital of Saint-Etienne, Université Jean Monnet, 42055 Saint-Etienne, France

Grégoire Le Gal
Department of Internal Medicine and Chest Diseases, EA3878, Brest University Hospital, Brest, France, and Thrombosis Program, Division of Hematology, Department of Medicine, University of Ottawa, Ottawa, Ontario, Canada

Willem M. Lijfering
Division of Haemostasis, Thrombosis and Rheology, Department of Haematology, University Medical Centre Groningen, Hanzeplein 1, 9713 GZ Groningen, The Netherlands.

Michael M. Madani
Division of Cardiothoracic Surgery, University of California at San Diego Medical Center, 200 West Arbor Drive, San Diego, CA 92103-8892, USA

Guy Meyer
Division of Pulmonary and Intensive Care Medicine, Hôpital Européen Georges Pompidou, Assistance Publique Hôpitaux de Paris, Faculté de Médecine, Université Paris Descartes, 75015 Paris, France

Patrick Mismetti
Thrombosis Research Group: EA 3065 – CIE3, University Hospital of Saint-Etienne, Université Jean Monnet, 42055 Saint-Etienne, France

John T. Murchison
Department of Clinical Radiology, Royal Infirmary of Edinburgh, Little France Crescent, Edinburgh EH16 4SA, Scotland, UK

Matthijs Oudkerk
Department of Radiology, Academic Medical Centre Groningen, Hanzeplein 1, P.O. Box 30001, 9700 RB Groningen, The Netherlands

Arnaud Perrier
Division of Angiology and Hemostasis, Department of Internal Medicine, Geneva University Hospital and Faculty of Medicine, Geneva, Switzerland

A. Michael Peters
Department of Nuclear Medicine, Royal Sussex County Hospital, Brighton, UK.

Marjolein Peters
Emma Children's Hospital/Academic Medical Centre, Department of Pediatric Haematology, P.O. Box 22700, 1100 DE Amsterdam, The Netherlands

Paolo Prandoni
Department of Medical and Surgical Sciences, Thromboembolism Unit, University of Padua, Via Ospedale Civile 105, 35128 Padua, Italy

Gary Raskob
College of Public Health, University of Oklahoma Health Sciences Center, 801 NE 13th St, 139/Box 26901, Oklahoma City, OK 73190, USA

Jim A. Reekers
Department of Radiology, Academic Medical Centre, Meibergdreef 9, 1105 AZ Amsterdam, The Netherlands

John H. Reid
Department of Clinical Radiology, Borders General Hospital NHS Trust, Melrose, Roxburghshire TD6 9BS, Scotland, UK

Marc Righini
Division of Angiology and Haemostasis, Department of Internal Medicine, Geneva University Hospital and Faculty of Medicine, 24 rue Micheli-du-Crest, 1211 Geneva 14, Switzerland

Marc A. Rodger
Thrombosis Program, Division of Hematology, Department of Medicine, University of Ottawa, Ottawa and Clinical Epidemiology Program, Ottawa Health Research Institute, The Ottawa Hospital, General Campus, 501 Smyth Road, Box 201, Ottawa, Ontario, Canada K1H 8L6

Frits R. Rosendaal
Departments of Clinical Epidemiology and Haematology, C7-P, Leiden University Medical Centre, P.O. Box 9600, 2300 RC Leiden, The Netherlands

Sebastian M. Schellong
Division of Internal Medicine II, Krankenhaus Dresden-Friedrichstadt, Friedrichstrasse 41, 01067 Dresden, Germany

Maaike Söhne
Department of Vascular Medicine, Academic Medical Center, Meibergdreef 9, 1105 AZ Amsterdam, The Netherlands

Victor Tapson
Division of Pulmonary and Critical Care Medicine, Duke University Medical Center, DUMC 31175, Durham, NC 27710, USA

Edwin J.R. van Beek
Forbes Chair of Medical Imaging, Clinical Research Imaging Centre, University of Edinburgh, Little France Crescent, Edinburgh EH16 4SA, Scotland, UK
Professor of Radiology, Medicine and Biomedical Engineering Carver College of Medicine, University of Iowa, Iowa City, USA

Jan van der Meer
Division of Haemostasis, Thrombosis and Rheology, Department of Haematology University Medical Center Groningen, Hanzeplein 1, 9713 GZ Groningen, The Netherlands

Marjolein van Loveren
Department of Radiology EB 45, University Medical Centre Groningen, University of
Groningen, P.O. Box 30001, 9700 RB Groningen, The Netherlands

C. Heleen van Ommen
Emma Children's Hospital/Academic Medical Center, Department of Pediatric Hematology,
P.O. Box 22700, 1100 DE Amsterdam, The Netherlands

Peter M.A. van Ooijen
Department of Radiology, Academic Medical Centre Groningen, Hanzeplein 1,
P.O. Box 30001, 9700 RB Groningen, The Netherlands
p.m.a.van.ooijen@rad.umcg.nl

Roel Vink
Department of Internal Medicine, Academic Medical Centre, Meibergdreef 9,
1105 AZ Amsterdam, The Netherlands

Philip S. Wells
Division of Hematology, Canada Research Chair, Suite F6-49, 1053 Carling Avenue,
Ottawa Hospital, Civic Campus, Ottawa, Ontario, Canada K1Y 4E9

PART I

Introduction

CHAPTER 1

Causes of Venous Thrombosis

Frits R. Rosendaal

Departments of Clinical Epidemiology and Hematology, Leiden University
Medical Center, Leiden, The Netherlands

THROMBOSIS

Until the mid-1800s, thrombosis was known as 'phlebitis', indicating that for a long time the disease was seen as inflammatory (1). Thrombosis is the process of obstructive clot formation as the end product of an imbalance of procoagulant, anticoagulant and fibrinolytic factors. In contrast to arterial disease, which results from a chronic process of atherosclerosis, the development of a venous clot is a relatively sudden phenomenon which occurs in reaction to acute and transient risk circumstances. In spite of this, symptoms may develop more slowly than in arterial disease and time of onset often remains unclear.

The role of the environment in the occurrence of venous thrombosis, particularly pregnancy and puerperium, was recognized centuries ago. At some stage, it was believed that the thrombosis in puerperium, called 'milk leg', was caused by milk accumulating in the leg. In the late 1700s this led to the first public-health advice to breast-feed as a prevention of milk leg (2,3).

At the basis of our current thinking about the causes of thrombosis stands the pathologist Virchow, who postulated three major causes of thrombosis: changes in the vessel wall, changes in the blood flow and changes in the blood composition (1): '... wir können auch künftig die mehr mechanischen Formen der Thrombose, wie sie bei der Blutstockung vorkommen, von den mehr chemischen oder physikalischen Formen, wie sie durch direkte Sauerstoff-Einwirkung oder veränderte Flächenanziehung zu Stande kommen, unterscheiden', translated as '... we can separately recognize a more mechanical form of thrombosis, such as seen in blood stasis, from the chemical or physical variant, which develops through a direct oxygen effect or by changed vessel wall interaction'.

This postulate is still valid, although not similarly in arterial and venous thrombosis, which is why arterial and venous thrombosis share some, but not all, causes. Vessel wall ('Flächenanziehung') disease dominates arterial disease as atherosclerosis and so do its risk factors, of which hypertension, hyperlipidaemia, smoking and diabetes mellitus are still the most important (4–6). Stasis ('Blutstockung'), however, does not play a role in causing arterial disease, due to the high pressure and flow in the arteries. Hypercoagulability ('chemischen oder physikalischen Formen') mainly plays a role in venous disease, although it is relevant in arterial disease, too. This is shown by the reduced rate of myocardial infarction in patients with

Deep Vein Thrombosis and Pulmonary Embolism Edited by Edwin J.R. van Beek, Harry R. Büller and Matthijs Oudkerk
© 2009 John Wiley & Sons, Ltd

congenital bleeding disorders, and also the increased risk of myocardial infarction in individuals with non-O ABO blood groups, which are associated with increased levels of von Willebrand factor and factor VIII (7–9). Similarly, the use of oral contraceptives increases the risk of all forms of arterial disease (myocardial infarction, ischaemic stroke, peripheral artery disease), and also of venous disease, which is in all likelihood an effect mediated through coagulation, since the effect does not accumulate with prolonged use (10–13).

The contribution of hypercoagulability is much larger in venous than in arterial disease and is about equally important as stasis. Factors causing vessel wall disease are at most weak risk factors for venous disease, probably because vessel wall disease leads to a pro-inflammatory state. Recently, interest has heightened in the link between venous and arterial disease, i.e., the observation that patients with venous thrombosis have an increased risk of subsequent arterial disease and vice versa (14,15).

VENOUS THROMBOSIS

Venous thrombosis most commonly manifests as deep vein thrombosis (DVT) of the leg or pulmonary embolism (PE), although it may also occur in other veins (upper extremities, liver, cerebral sinus, retina, mesenteric), albeit far more infrequently. The incidence of venous thrombosis is one to three individuals per 1000 per year (16–19). DVT may lead to persistent chronic disease, which can be severely disabling due to impaired venous return in the leg, the so-called post-thrombotic syndrome (PTS); this occurs in up to 20% of patients (20). The case-fatality rate of DVT, mainly due to fatal PE, ranges from 1% in young patients to 10% in older patients and is highest in those with underlying malignancies (16–18). A recent population-based study showed that the 30-day case-fatality rate after a first venous thrombosis was 6.4%, with one-year mortality at 21.6% (21) (Figure 1.1). The high mortality in venous thrombosis is largely determined by its relationship with malignancies. However, after patients with cancer were excluded, venous thrombosis still led to a considerable death risk of 3.6% after one month and 12.6% after one year. The one-year

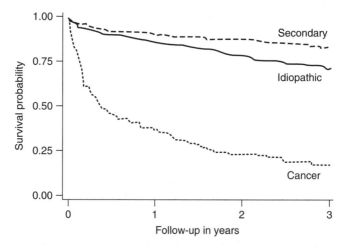

Figure 1.1 Probability of death following a first venous thrombotic event (deep vein thrombosis or pulmonary embolism) for 740 patients diagnosed in a population-based follow-up study including 93 769 individuals in Norway. Reproduced from Figure 2 in (21) Naess *et al.* (21) by permission of Blackwell Publishing.

mortality is equal for DVT and PE, indicating an effect of underlying disease, while the 30-day case-fatality is twice as high in PE as in DVT (10% vs 5%), indicating an effect of the thrombosis itself (21). The natural history of DVT and PE will be discussed in greater detail in Chapter 2.

Men and women are affected about equally by venous thrombosis, with slightly higher rates among women in the younger age groups due to the risk-increasing effects of oral contraceptives, pregnancy and puerperium (18,19,21). The incidence of venous thrombosis is strongly age dependent: it is extremely uncommon (1 in 100 000 per year) in childhood and rises to nearly 1% per year in old age (18,19,21,22).

Venous thrombosis is a multicausal disease, which requires the presence of several risk factors for disease to occur (23,24). The excess risks brought about by each individual factor may, when jointly present, simply add, or exceed additivity (synergy) (24). Therefore, a presentation of individual risk factors is to some extent artificial, since none or very few of them will be able to cause thrombosis on their own and, more importantly, because their effect may differ depending on the presence or absence of other risk factors.

RISK FACTORS FOR VENOUS THROMBOSIS

Venous thrombosis has genetic and acquired causes, of which the former are related to stasis or hypercoagulability and the latter almost invariably to hypercoagulability.

Several causes of venous thrombosis were recognised long ago, such as immobilization, surgery, trauma, plaster casts, pregnancy, puerperium, lupus anticoagulants, cancer and female hormones (25,26). Table 1.1 lists the risk factors for venous thrombosis. The impact of acquired causes of thrombosis has decreased because of the use of prophylactic anticoagulation treatment, but they still lead to a substantial number of thrombotic events (Table 1.2).

The first families with a large number of patients with venous thrombosis were described in the early 20th century. In 1965, Egeberg identified the first defect leading to thrombophilia, when he described a family with hereditary antithrombin deficiency (27). Deficiencies of the other natural anticoagulants protein C and protein S were identified as causes of heritable thrombophilia in the

Table 1.1 Risk factors for venous thrombosis

Acquired	Inherited	Mixed/unknown[a]
Immobilization	Antithrombin deficiency	High levels of factor VIII
Plaster cast	Protein C deficiency	High levels of factor IX
Trauma	Protein S deficiency	High levels of factor XI
Major surgery	Factor V Leiden (FVL)	High levels of fibrinogen
Orthopaedic surgery	Prothrombin 20210A	High levels of TAFI
Malignancy	Dysfibrinogenaemia	Low levels of TFPI
Oral contraceptives	Factor XIII 34val	APC resistance in the absence of FVL
Hormonal replacement therapy	Fibrinogen (G) 10034T	Hyperhomocysteinaemia
Antiphospholipid syndrome		High levels of PCI (PAI-3)
Myeloproliferative disorders		
Polycythemia vera		
Central venous catheters		
Age		
Obesity		

[a]TAFI, thrombin activatable fibrinolysis inhibitor; TFPI, tissue factor pathway inhibitor; PCI, protein C inhibitor; PAI-3, plasminogen activator inhibitor-3.

Table 1.2 Thrombosis risk in acquired risk situations – The Leiden Thrombophilia Study[a]

Risk factor	n(%)		OR	CI95
	Patients (N = 474)	Controls (N = 474)		
Surgery	85 (18)	17 (3.6)	5.9	3.4–10.1
Hospitalization	59 (12)	6 (1.3)	11.1	4.7–25.9
Immobilization	17 (3.6)	2 (0.4)	8.9	2.0–38.2
Pregnancy	8 (5.0)	2 (1.3)	4.2	0.9–19.9
Puerperium	13 (8.2)	1 (0.6)	14.1	1.8–109
Oral contraceptives	109 (70)	65 (38)	3.8	2.4–6.0

[a]The time window for surgery, hospitalization (without surgery) and immobilization (not in the hospital, >13 days) was one year preceding the index date (i.e., date of thrombosis diagnosis in patients, similar date in controls), for puerperium it was delivery 30 days or less prior to the index date and for pregnancy and oral contraceptives it was at the index date. Data on pregnancy, puerperium and oral contraceptive use refer to women of reproductive age.

early 1980s (28,29). More recently, several genetic prothrombotic variants have been identified, that all confer less of a risk increase than deficiencies of antithrombin, protein C and protein S. These variants are also far more frequent than these deficiencies and therefore responsible for a far larger proportion of all venous thrombotic events (16–18,30–32).

Environmental causes of thrombosis

Age

Age is the strongest risk factors for venous thrombosis, with a steep gradient of risk, in which the incidence is 1000-fold higher in the very old than in the very young (18,21,22,33). Why age is such a strong determinant of venous thrombosis is unclear. It seems likely that several factors contribute to the age dependency of the thrombosis incidence, such as decreased mobility, an increased frequency of risk-enhancing diseases, decreased muscular tone, acquisition of other risk factors, and also ageing of the veins themselves and particularly of the valves in the veins. However, research in this area is surprisingly scarce.

Medical causes of thrombosis

Underlying diseases, or conditions such as pregnancy and puerperium, are still the most important causes of thrombosis. They explain, to a large extent, the demographic characteristics of thrombosis, i.e., the higher incidence in young women compared with young men and the increasing incidence with age. These medical causes may exert their risk-increasing effect because of immobilization, as in prolonged bed rest, or because of a hypercoagulable effect, as in the antiphospholipid syndrome, and most often it will be a combination of immobilization and an effect on clotting, as in pregnancy, puerperium and cancer.

Immobilization

All circumstances that lead to stasis in the extremities, i.e., all forms of prolonged immobilization, increase the risk of venous thrombosis. This includes paralysis, bed rest, plaster casts and pregnancy

(34,35). Immobilization leads to reduced action of the calf musculature, which is crucial in pumping the blood upstream through the veins.

Pregnancy and puerperium

Venous thrombosis in young individuals is rare and so is thrombosis following pregnancy and puerperium. Still, given its rarity, about half of all venous thrombotic events in women of reproductive age are related to pregnancy. In a large study of over 72 000 deliveries in Scotland, 62 venous thrombotic events occurred, for an incidence of DVT and PE of 0.86 per 1000 deliveries (36). About two-thirds of these occurred during pregnancy and one-third postpartum. During pregnancy, the risk of thrombosis is highest in the third trimester and most thrombotic events occur in the left leg, probably in relation to the gravid uterus compressing the left common iliac vein (37). The incidence of venous thrombosis during pregnancy and the postpartum period (approximately one per 1000) is at least 10-fold higher than in non-pregnant women (36–38). The risk of thrombosis during pregnancy is affected by the presence of prothrombotic abnormalities and is particularly high in the presence of antithrombin deficiency. Although this rare deficiency is present in only around 1 per 5000 in the general population, it was found in 12% of the patients with thrombosis during pregnancy or puerperium (36). Women with factor V Leiden or prothrombin 20210A, two common prothrombotic genetic variants, have a 30–50-fold increased risk of thrombosis during pregnancy and puerperium, relative to non-pregnant non-carriers (37).

Surgery and trauma

A strikingly high risk of venous thrombosis is brought about by surgery, where for some interventions over 50% of the patients experience thrombosis in the absence of antithrombotic prophylaxis. Orthopaedic surgery and neurosurgery confer the highest risks. Knee and hip surgery lead to thrombosis in 30–50% of patients (39,40). Similarly high event rates follow abdominal surgery (up to 30%), gynaecological surgery and urological surgery (in particular open prostatectomy) (41–43). The risk is increased most in large surgical procedures, which may be related both to the size of the surgical wound and to the duration of the intervention and the related immobilization, but in orthopaedic surgery even minor interventions, such as arthroscopy, have a sizeable effect on the risk of venous thrombosis.

High risks of thrombosis also occur in trauma patients and thrombosis occurs in 50–60% of patients with head trauma, spinal injury, pelvic fractures, femoral fractures and tibial fractures (44–46). Even small injuries, such as muscle ruptures and ankle sprains, affect the risk of thrombosis, increasing (for injuries affecting the leg) the risk of DVT 5-fold (47).

Nowadays, anticoagulant prophylaxis is prescribed in circumstances with high risks of thrombosis, i.e., after surgical interventions, as is advised by the major guidelines for thrombosis prevention (48). Nevertheless, surgery remains a major cause of thrombosis, since even with anticoagulant prophylaxis, high-risk surgery such as total hip or knee replacement leads to symptomatic venous thrombosis in 1–3% of the patients (49). In the Leiden region, where extended anticoagulant prophylaxis is routinely prescribed for most surgical interventions, 18% of patients presenting with a first DVT in the 1990s had had a surgical intervention, which corresponded to a 6-fold risk increase (Table 1.2) (50). In a recent analysis in the same region of over 4000 patients with a first DVT, the risk of symptomatic thrombosis following orthopaedic and major non-orthopaedic surgery was still increased 4-fold (51). Hence surgery remains a major area for thrombosis prevention.

Cancer

Venous thrombosis related to cancer was first identified in 1823 by Bouillaud (52). Subsequently, Trousseau observed that recurrent thrombophlebitis at changing locations (saltans et migrans) was indicative of occult cancer, especially of the pancreas (53). Cancer causes thrombosis by several mechanisms. Many malignant cells produce tissue factor, so the tumour itself may cause a procoagulant state, due to a humoral effect. Apoptosis leads to the formation of microparticles, which may contain tissue factor (54). In cancer patients with thrombosis, microparticles containing tissue factor can be demonstrated (55). In addition to humoral effects, there may be mechanical effects: large tumours may lead directly to venous compression and venous obstruction (56,57). Finally, debilitating disease will lead to immobility and treatment, particularly chemotherapy, may also be thrombogenic (58,59). The mode of treatment may play a role: central venous catheters, often used to administer chemotherapeutics, are the most important cause of symptomatic thrombosis of the arm, occurring in over 10% of patients with a central venous catheter (60).

The presence of a malignancy increases the risk of thrombosis around 5-fold (61). The risk of thrombosis varies by type of cancer. Patients with adenocarcinoma have a several-fold higher risk of thrombosis than patients with squamous cell cancer, with an absolute risk that may be as high as 5–10% per year (62). Therefore, among patients with thrombosis, cancer is often present, either manifest or still undiagnosed. Between 10 and 20% of patients with thrombosis have a known malignancy at the time of the thrombosis and 2–5% will be diagnosed shortly after (61,63). Patients with haematological malignancies have the highest risk of venous thrombosis, followed by lung cancer and gastrointestinal cancer. The risk of venous thrombosis is highest in the first few months after the diagnosis of malignancy and may be up to 60-fold higher than in individuals without cancer, and the presence of distant metastases also greatly increases risk (61). While cancer is a strong risk factor for thrombosis, again it will rarely be a sufficient factor and synergistic effects are seen in the presence of prothrombotic clotting abnormalities, such as factor V Leiden and prothrombin 20210A (61).

Antiphospholipid antibodies

Individuals with antiphospholipid antibodies, both when isolated or in those with systemic lupus erythematodes (SLE), have an increased risk of thrombosis (64–66). A lupus anticoagulant can be found in several percent of patients and increases the risk of thrombosis about 4-fold (67).

Drugs, lifestyle and thrombosis

It appears that immobilization in a sitting position confers a higher risk than other positions, which is likely to be related to additional impediments of the blood stream due to the curvature of the popliteal veins. During World War II and the Battle of Britain, it was observed that a 6-fold increased risk of PE occurred shortly after the air raids, during which people sought shelter in the London Underground, where they were seated in deck-chairs. Replacement of the chairs with bunk beds reduced the risk (68). Massive traffic jams, as occur during public transport strikes, reportedly also lead to cases of DVT (69). An even more contemporary example of thrombosis due to immobilization occurred in a young man who regularly spent 12 hours per day behind a computer screen, which was coined 'eThrombosis' (70).

Long-distance travel

The first cases of venous thrombosis after air travel were reported in the 1950s (71,72). Following the publication of many case reports of thrombosis after air travel, it became known as 'economy class syndrome' or 'travel-associated venous thrombosis' (73,74). Annually, two billion passengers embark on air trips, indicating that even a small excess risk may lead to a considerable burden of thrombotic disease. In 1986, Sarvesvaran performed the first controlled study, comparing causes of death of passengers with sudden death at Heathrow airport, demonstrating an excess of deaths due to PE in the arrival area compared with the departure hall (75). Subsequently, it was shown that patients who developed severe PE shortly after their arrival at Charles de Gaulle airport in Paris had more often flown long than short distances (76). There was a clear graded association of the risk of PE with the duration of the flight, with a 50-fold difference in risk between flights of less than 2500 km and those over 10 000 km (76). Other studies have focused on the magnitude of the risk, the effect of contributing factors and the mechanisms by which air travel leads to thrombosis. In a series of case–control studies, it was shown that long-haul air travel increases the risk of thrombosis about 2-fold (77–82). Individuals with prothrombotic genetic variants, such as factor V Leiden or prothrombin 20210A, oral contraceptive users and those who are obese, very tall of very short have a several-fold higher risk than others when travelling on long-haul trips by air (81). The risk of thrombosis after long trips is not restricted to air travel; prolonged trips by car, bus or train also double the risk of thrombosis relative to non-travellers (81). Nevertheless, particularly in the joint presence of other risk factors, the risk appears highest after air travel (81). This may be related to specific, cabin-related conditions, such as dehydration or hypobaric hypoxia.

Previous observations have suggested that mild hypobaric hypoxia, as can be found in an airplane at high altitude, leads to coagulation activation (83). This was not confirmed, however, in a study in which a large number of volunteers were exposed to a test condition of hypoxic hypobaria and a control condition of normoxic normobaria in climate- and pressure-controlled chambers (84). However, in another study, in which volunteers were exposed to an actual eight-hour flight, clotting activation, as evidenced by increases in thrombin–antithrombin complexes, was observed (85). The differences between studies may be the result of differences in the study population: in the latter study volunteers were selected on the presence of risk factors for thrombosis, particularly factor V Leiden and oral contraceptive use. The clotting activation was most pronounced in those with these risk factors (85). Finally, in a similar study, no clotting activation was observed in male volunteers who were flown from France to La Réunion (86). Dehydration appear to play no role in clotting activation (87). While there can be little doubt that the main factor leading to thrombosis after air travel is prolonged seated immobilization, it seems that the conditions of air travel, e.g., hypoxic hypobaria, may lead to a hypercoagulant response in a minority of individuals, mainly those with prothrombotic risk factors, that further contributes to risk.

For the individual traveller, relative risks are of little relevance: only absolute risks count. In a study of 8755 employees of several large international organizations and companies, it was found that thrombosis affected one in 4500 travellers; this rose to one in 1200 for very long flights, exceeding 16 hours in duration (88).

Lifestyle

Engagement in physical exercise generally reduces the risk of venous thrombosis (89,90). In a large study, including over 3500 patients with venous thrombosis and over 4000 controls, it was shown that regular participation in sports activities reduced the risk of venous thrombosis by 30% (90). This risk reduction was strongest for PE, halving the incidence. This beneficial effect was not related to the frequency of the activity or its intensity. In elderly individuals, regular exercise does not appear to reduce the risk of venous thrombosis and strenuous exercise even increases the risk (91,92). It is plausible that this is related to a higher risk of minor injuries in the elderly and that a beneficial effect of exercise *per se* is offset by a detrimental effect of trauma. It should be noted that this observation only deals with venous thrombosis and that exercise is likely to offer general health benefits, also for the elderly. Participation in exercise and sports also reduces the risk of arm vein thrombosis; however, strenuous sports involving the arms increase the risk of thrombosis in the dominant arm (93). Venous thrombosis of the upper extremity after strenuous exercise of any kind is known as the Paget–Schrötter syndrome and is thought to result from temporary or lasting swelling of the anterior scalenus muscle (94).

Individuals who are overweight or obese have an increased risk of thrombosis (95–98). In recent large case–control study with nearly 4000 patients and over 4500 controls, being overweight [body mass index (BMI) $>25\,kg/m^2$ and BMI $<30\,kg/m^2$] increased the risk of venous thrombosis 1.7-fold and being obese (BMI $>30\,kg/m^2$) led to a 2.4-fold increased risk (99) (Figure 1.2). There was a clear gradient of increasing risk of thrombosis with increasing BMI. Body weight also proved to be a good risk indicator: those weighing over 110 kg had a nearly 3-fold higher risk of thrombosis than those weighing between 50 and 70 kg. Body height had little influence on the risk of thrombosis, except in the very tall, in whom the risk was weakly increased (99). Among women, there was a synergistic effect of excess body weight and use of oral contraceptives on the risk of venous thrombosis, with a 23-fold increased risk for obese women who used oral contraceptives, relative to non-users with normal BMI (99).

As an atherogenic factor, one would not expect smoking to be a risk factor for venous thrombosis, and older studies indeed showed no risk increase, for instance in the Framingham study (100). More recent studies, such as the 'Nurses' Health Study' and the 'Study of Men Born in 1913', however, have demonstrated that the risk of venous thrombosis is increased for smokers, with 2–3-fold increased risks for smokers versus non-smokers (95,101). In the 'Multiple Environmental and Genetic Assessment of Risk Factors for Thrombosis' (MEGA) study, the largest study on venous thrombosis available, the effect of smoking habits was studied in nearly 4000 patients with a first DVT or PE and nearly 5000 controls (102). Smoking appeared to be a mild risk factor for venous thrombosis, increasing the risk by 40%, to a similar extent for DVT and PE. There was also a weak effect in former smokers, with a 20% risk increase. The risk was dependent on the number

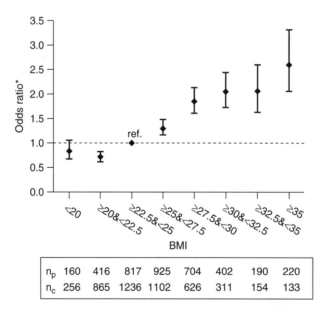

Figure 1.2 Relative risk of venous thrombosis by categories of body mass index (BMI) (kg/m^2). I, 95% confidence interval; n_p, number of patients; n_c, number of control subjects; ref., reference category. *Adjusted for age and sex. Reproduced from Figure 1 in (99) Pomp *et al.* (99) by permission of Blackwell Publishing.

of cigarettes smoked per day, with a relative risk of 1.23 in those who smoked 1–9 cigarettes per day and 1.64 in those who smoked more than 20 cigarettes per day (all relative to never smokers) (102). Smoking modifies the risk brought about by oral contraceptive use, leading to a 9-fold increased risk in smokers who use oral contraceptives, relative to those who do neither. It is unclear how smoking affects risk, but it may be related to a pro-inflammatory effect. Smoking increases fibrinogen levels, which in itself is a risk factor for thrombosis. However, in the MEGA study smoking remained a risk factor even after adjustment for fibrinogen levels.

In contrast to arterial disease, where a protective effect of moderate alcohol intake has been clearly demonstrated, few studies have looked into the association between alcohol intake and venous thrombosis. In the MEGA-study, drinking habits were examined of over 4000 patients with a first venous thrombosis and over 5000 control subjects. Regular alcohol intake proved to be protective against the occurrence of venous thrombosis, with the strongest effect amongst those who drank two to four glasses per day, leading to a 33% risk reduction (103). Figure 1.3 shows the effect of alcohol consumption, for various categories of drinking, on the risk of venous thrombosis. The effect is most pronounced for PE, nearly halving the risk. Alcohol consumption has well-known effects on the coagulation system, affecting factor VII, von Willebrand factor and fibrinogen levels (104). In the MEGA study, it appeared that those drinking categories with the most protection also had the most pronounced reduction of fibrinogen levels, suggestive of a mechanism for the protective effect.

Hormonal drugs

The first oral contraceptive came on the market in 1959 and the first case of thrombotic complications was reported in 1961, when a nurse who used them because of endometriosis developed PE (105), while the first occurrences of arterial thrombosis leading to myocardial infarction and ischaemic stroke in oral contraceptive users were also described (106,107). Subsequent

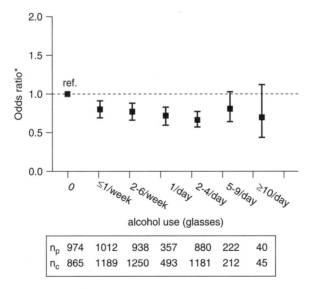

n_p	974	1012	938	357	880	222	40
n_c	865	1189	1250	493	1181	212	45

Figure 1.3 Relative risk of venous thrombosis by level of alcohol consumption. I, 95% confidence interval; n_p, number of patients; n_c, number of control subjects; ref., reference category. *Adjusted for age, sex, body mass index, smoking and pregnancy. Reproduced from Pomp ER, Rosendaal FR, Doggen CJ. Alcohol consumption is associated with a decreased risk of venous thrombosis. Thromb Haemost 2008; 99:59–63, with permission of Schattauer GmbH.

controlled studies have established the association between oral contraceptives and the risk of venous and arterial disease, which still exists for the currently available low-dose oral contraceptives (10–13,108–111).

Most oral contraceptives consist of a combination of an oestrogen and a progestogen. In nearly all brands the oestrogen compound is Fethinylestradiol, while the progestogen compound differs between brands and has changed over time. Currently, the progestogens mainly used are so-called second-generation progestogens (levonorgestrel), third-generation progestogens (desogestrel, gestodene) and the anti-androgen cyproterone acetate and finally drospirenone, which is an anti-mineralocorticoid (112,113). The main change in the oestrogen content over time has been a reduction in dose, which has reduced the risk of thrombosis, although there is still a 2–5-fold increased risk with the current brands (108,114–119). Since the absolute risk of venous thrombosis is low in young women, the annual risk in users of oral contraceptives remains low, at two to three per 10 000 (21,117,120). Oral contraceptives only affect thrombotic risk during actual use and there is no risk increase in former users. The risk is highest during the first year of use, at 12 per 10 000 women per year (for second-generation progestogen-containing oral contraceptives) (121,122).

The type of progestogen affects the risk of venous thrombosis, with a 2-fold higher risk for brands containing a third-generation than a second-generation progestogen (108,123–125). The risk is highest in new users, with an incidence in the first year of 30 per 10 000, but, while becoming less pronounced over time, it remains higher for third- than second-generation users (121). The differential effect of second- and third-generation progestogens may be limited to preparations that also contain an oestrogen (combination oral contraceptives) and not be present in progestogen-only preparations, indicating an interaction between the two compounds (126). Cyproterone acetate-containing oral contraceptives have a substantially higher risk of venous thrombosis than preparations containing a second-generation progestogen (127). Whether drospirenone-containing oral contraceptives are as safe as second-generation oral contraceptives is unclear: the few studies that have been performed have been conflicting and there have been several case reports that have raised concern (128–130).

Oral contraceptives containing oestrogens have multiple effects on the coagulation system, increasing levels of procoagulant factors and reducing levels of natural anticoagulants, notably protein S. The net effect, that of a prothrombotic state, can be quantified with a global test, such as thrombin generation tests (131–135). The variation seen with the thrombin generation-based APC-resistance test associated well with the risk of venous thrombosis, even in women who do not use the contraceptive pill and men, which makes this a laboratory tool to examine the safety of oral contraceptives (136,137). With this test, oral contraceptives containing third-generation progestogens, cyproterone acetate and drospirenone all had a more profound prothrombotic effect on the coagulation system than oral contraceptives containing the second-generation progestogen levonorgestrel (133,138).

Currently used oral contraceptives still increase the risk of venous thrombosis 2–5-fold. However, the risk is again dependent on the presence of other factors. The risk is higher in some women, particularly in those who start using oral contraceptives, older women, obese women, women who smoke and women with prothrombotic abnormalities. In women with deficiencies of natural anticoagulants, i.e., protein C, protein S and antithrombin, the risk is greatly increased with concomitant oral contraceptive use (139,140). Heterozygous factor V Leiden carriers or prothrombin 20210A carriers have a 15–30-fold increased risk of thrombosis when they use oral contraceptives (141,142) and women with high levels of procoagulant factors, notably factor II, factor V and factor XI, also have a several-fold increased risk when they use oral contraceptives (143).

The available literature suggests the preferential use of oral contraceptives with a low dose of oestrogen and a second-generation (levonorgestrel) progestogen and caution in older women,

women with a family history of thrombosis and women with risk factors. Oral contraceptives are contraindicated in women with a personal history of venous thrombosis and with deficiencies of protein C, protein S or antithrombin.

Oestrogens after the menopause have been used for the treatment of symptoms of menopause, to reduce the progression of osteoporosis and to prevent ischaemic heart disease. Only the effect on menopausal symptoms, i.e., reduction of hot flushes, is undisputed. While prolonged treatment reduces osteoporosis progression, there is no consensus that this will reduce fractures (144–150). Recent large trials have refuted the hypothesis that oestrogen therapy would protect against arterial disease and have demonstrated an elevated risk of breast cancer (148,151,152).

Hormonal replacement therapy increases the risk of venous thrombosis 2–4-fold (153–162). In contrast to oral therapy, transdermally administered oestrogen does not have a first-pass effect through the liver and it has been suggested that this might lead to less risk of thrombosis. Although some studies have shown an elevated risk of venous thrombosis with skin patches, a large study and a recent meta-analysis suggest that the risk of venous thrombosis is indeed lower than with oral hormone therapy, if not completely unaffected (157,159,163,164). Most oral preparations contain equine conjugated oestrogens. A recent study suggests that oral preparations containing esterified oestrogens do not increase venous thrombotic risk (165). When compared in a thrombin generation-based APC-resistance test, esterified oestrogens led to less of a prothrombotic state than conjugated oestrogens (166).

Similarly to oral contraceptive use, the risk of thrombosis during postmenopausal hormone replacement is additionally increased in women who begin therapy, in older women, in obese women, in women with prothrombotic abnormalities and in women with a previous venous thrombosis (153,155,159,160,162,167–171).

From a clinical perspective, the use of postmenopausal hormones offers no cardiovascular benefit and a potential positive effect on osteoporosis is offset by an increased risk of venous thrombosis, breast cancer and possibly coronary heart disease. Hence there is no medical indication for prolonged use, while short-term use to counter menopausal symptoms may be indicated in some patients. Oestrogens should be avoided in women with a personal history of thrombosis. It should be borne in mind that postmenopausal hormones will be used by women who are considerably older than women of reproductive age and that therefore in absolute terms this will lead to far more cases of thrombosis and that additional risk factors will have a greater impact.

Genetic causes of thrombosis

Deficiencies of natural coagulation inhibitors

Deficiencies of antithrombin, protein C and its cofactor protein S and are found in less that 1% of the population (antithrombin deficiency in only one per 5000) (172–175). Even among patients with thrombosis, these defects are only found in a few percent (176,177). In families with hereditary thrombophilia they are found more often and these deficiencies can lead to a highly penetrant phenotype, with recurrent thrombosis occurring at a young age, probably due to the co-inheritance of additional defects, that may as yet be unknown (27–29,178–183). Heterozygous individuals with a deficiency of protein C or S have a risk of thrombosis that is at least 10-fold increased, and the risk is probably even higher for antithrombin deficiency (184–187). Homozygous deficiencies are exceedingly rare and lead to a life-threatening thrombotic tendency (purpura fulminans) shortly after birth (188,189).

Factor V Leiden

Factor V Leiden (factor V R506Q, G1691A) was identified in 1994 and is a common genetic prothrombotic defect, with an overall prevalence of carriers among Caucasians of around 5% (190–192). Among patients with venous thrombosis it is found in 20% and in around 50% of patients with familial thrombophilia (192). Factor V Leiden was identified after the discovery of resistance to activated protein C (APC resistance) as a major risk factor for venous thrombosis (193–196). Factor V Leiden is the result of the mutation at the location coding for one of the cleavage sites in factor V, where APC inactivates factor Va (190). Inactivation of the mutant procoagulant factor V occurs less efficiently and the resulting 'factor Va persistence' leads to an increased risk of thrombosis (193–195). The risk of thrombosis is increased 5-fold in heterozygotes and 50–80-fold in homozygotes (192,194,195). Homozygous patients are not extremely rare, at around one per 5000; this may be higher in regions with a high prevalence of the allele, as for instance in southern Sweden (191,192).

Prothrombin 20210A

A mutation in the 3′-untranslated part of the prothrombin gene (G to A, prothrombin 20210A) leads to increased prothrombin (factor II) levels, which are associated with an increased risk of venous thrombosis (197). Similarly to factor V Leiden, the mutation is frequent (several percent carriers) and is almost exclusively found in Caucasians, again with regional differences in its prevalence (198). It increases the risk of venous thrombosis 2–3-fold and is present in around 6% of patients with venous thrombosis (197,199). Because both are common, compound heterozygotes for factor V Leiden and prothrombin 20210A are not exceedingly rare and have a 20-fold increased risk of thrombosis compared with individuals with neither mutation (200).

Blood group

Individuals with non-O ABO blood groups have a 2–4-fold higher risk of thrombosis than those with blood group O, which has been known since the 1960s (201). Non-O blood groups are associated with reduced levels of von Willeband factor and factor VIII, which has been shown to be related to thrombotic risk (202,203). The risk is increased for all non-OO genotypes (A1A1, A1A2, A1O1/A1O2, BB/BO1/BO2, A1B/A2B), except for A2O1/A2O2/A2A2 (202–204).

MTHFR 677T

Methylenetetrahydrofolate reductase (MTHFR) is an enzyme relevant to homocysteine metabolism. The C →T variant at position 677 renders the enzyme thermolabile, resulting in slightly elevated homocysteine levels (205,206). While the variant is common (10% of the general population are homozygous carriers), the elevation of homocysteine levels is minimal. It is therefore not surprising that the studies investigating its relation with thrombotic risk have rendered conflicting results. A meta-analysis pooling the available data suggested a weak effect (relative risk 1.20), but a recent large single study (the MEGA study) showed no association at all (207,208). While this variant is of scientific interest, it has no clinical relevance.

Factor XIII val34leu

The variant FXIII (34leu) is more rapidly activated, which leads to earlier cross-linking of fibrin and thinner fibres (209). Homozygous carriers of the leu-allele, approximately 10% of the population, have a 30% reduced risk of venous thrombosis, and this effect is strongest (50% risk reduction) in those with high fibrinogen levels (210,211).

New genetic variants associated with venous thrombosis

The search for new genetic variants associated with venous thrombosis goes on and follows several paths, first by studying candidate genes and haplotypes in family studies and studies among unrelated subjects, second by genome scans in families and third, just emerging, by whole genome scans in unrelated individuals (32). The next step will be massive deep resequencing of candidate genes. The studies which include a large number of genetic variants have compounded the problem of reports on false-positive findings. Therefore, here only variants that have been confirmed in independent studies will be listed.

A variant in the fibrinogen gamma chain, at position 10 034 (C → T) reduces the fraction of gamma'-fibrinogen (an alternative splice product) in plasma, which is related to the risk of venous thrombosis (212–214). Around 6% of individuals carry the variant, which increases thrombotic risk over 2-fold. Several single nucleotide polymorphisms (SNPs) in all three fibrinogen genes have been associated with the risk of thrombosis, albeit with small risk increases (relative risks 1.2–1.3) (30).

Variants in the promoter region of protein C, that are associated with mildly reduced levels of protein C (positions 2404 and 2418), are associated with a 1.3–1.6-fold increased risk of venous thrombosis (30,215,216).

In a recent study, nearly 20 000 SNPs distributed over 11 000 genes were tested in a serial approach in three independent datasets (from the Leiden Thrombophilia Study and the MEGA study, divided into two datasets), totalling over 3000 patients with a first DVT and over 5000 controls (31). Several SNPs were associated with venous thrombosis in all three datasets, located in CYP4V2 (rs 13146272), SERPINC1 (antithrombin, rs 2227589), GP6 (Glycoprotein VI, rs1613662) and F9 (Factor IX, rs 6048, with a variant protein that is known as Factor IX Malmö). The variant in CYP4V2 is located close to the prekallikrein and factor XI genes and is associated with factor XI levels. The risk-enhancing alleles for these variants are all common, with 18–97% of the population carrying a variant allele, and were associated with mild increases in thrombotic risk, with relative risks varying from 1.2 to 1.5.

Other plasma abnormalities associated with the risk of thrombosis

Hyperhomocysteinaemia

Individuals with a mildly elevated level of plasma homocysteine (over 18 μmol/L), which is found in 5–10% of the population, have a 2-fold increased risk of thrombosis (217–219). It is unclear how hyperhomocysteinaemia increases the risk of thrombosis and there is some debate whether the relation is causal. The high risk of thrombosis seen in classical homocystinuria, caused by homozygous cystathionine beta-synthase (CS) deficiency, renders it plausible that by analogy mildly elevated plasma levels lead to a mildly elevated risk. This is the reason why the association between the MTHFR variant and the risk of thrombosis is of scientific interest, since this association, as it is based on a genetic predisposition, would render it unlikely that some other unknown factor would cause both thrombosis and hyperhomocysteinaemia, leading to a spurious relationship. The effect of MTHFR 677T on homocysteine levels, however, is too weak to give a definite answer. Mild hyperhomocysteinaemia is rarely caused by heterozygous

CS deficiency and commonly by low dietary intake of folate, or vitamin B_6 or B_{12}. Therefore, it is easily treated by supplementation of these vitamins (220). A randomized placebo-controlled trial of homocysteine lowering by vitamins in patients with a first venous thrombosis showed no overall effect in reduction of recurrence (221). A positive finding would have been strong evidence for a causative role of hyperhomocysteinaemia in the aetiology of venous thrombosis.

High levels of clotting factors

Elevated levels of procoagulant factors, notably factor VIII, IX and XI, prothrombin and fibrinogen, are associated with an increased risk of venous thrombosis. Since these are not deficiencies, there is no natural cut-off point and the risk increases gradually with the clotting factor level. Generally, levels in the upper 10th percentile (by definition present in 10% of the population) are associated with a 2–3-fold increased risk of venous thrombosis (197,202,222–225). The same holds true for low levels of Tissue Factor Pathway Inhibitor (TFPI) (226).

It is unclear whether these elevated levels have a genetic or acquired origin, except for high levels of factor VIII, which has been shown to be related to the ABO blood group and for which familial clustering of levels has been shown, even when taking blood group into account (227,228). This also is evidence for a causal role of elevated clotting factor levels in the aetiology of venous thrombosis.

Levels of fibrinolytic factors

High levels of Thrombin Activatable Fibrinolysis Inhibitor (TAFI) increase the risk of thrombosis, again with a doubling of the risk for levels exceeding the 90th percentile of the population distribution (229). The overall fibrinolytic capacity of plasma can be determined with the clot lysis time, a global assay. Individuals with a high clot lysis time, i.e., a low fibrinolytic potential, have a doubling of the risk of thrombosis (those with times in the upper 10% of the distribution) (230,231). It is still unknown which parts of the fibrinolytic system contribute to this effect on thrombotic risk.

Clinical implications

Venous thrombosis is a multicausal disease, where a combination of genetic predisposition and acquired transient risk factors will lead to thrombosis (24). In many instances, the genetic and acquired causes act synergistically, for instance in hormone users by carriers of factor V Leiden. Since genetic risk factors either are rare, or have a weak overall effect, their usefulness for clinical practice is still minimal and there are hardly any indications for screening for such abnormalities: by measuring one or a few factors only part of a more complex profile becomes visible and identification of genetic defects rarely affects treatment. This may change when it becomes possible to create a comprehensive risk profile, i.e., an individual 'thrombosis potential' based on the measurement of all major and common variants. Currently, acquired risk factors still dominate the field, and, since they are usually transient, offer the best opportunity to reduce the burden of thrombosis by improved and individualized anticoagulant prophylaxis.

REFERENCES

1. Virchow R. *Phlogose und Thrombose im Gefäßsystem; Gesammelte Abhandlungen zur Wissenschaftlichen Medizin*. Staatsdruckerei, Frankfurt, 1856.

2. White, C. An inquiry into the nature and cause of that swelling in one or both of the lower extremities which sometimes happen to in-lying women together with the propriety of drawing the breasts of those who do and also who do not give suck. Warrington, London, 1784.

3. Deslandes M. *Traité des Accouchements de M. Puzos*. Desaint & Saillant, Paris, 1759.

4. Khot UN, Khot MB, Bajzer CT, Sapp SK, Ohman EM, Brener SJ, Ellis SG, Lincoff AM, Topol EJ. Prevalence of conventional risk factors in patients with coronary heart disease. *JAMA* 2003; **290**:898–904.

5. Greenland P, Knoll MD, Stamler J, Neaton JD, Dyer AR, Garside DB, Wilson PW. Major risk factors as antecedents of fatal and nonfatal coronary heart disease events. *JAMA* 2003; **290**:891–7.

6. Yusuf S, Hawken S, Ounpuu S, Dans T, Avezum A, Lanas F, McQueen M, Budaj A, Pais P, Varigos J, Lisheng L. Effect of potentially modifiable risk factors associated with myocardial infarction in 52 countries (the INTERHEART study): case–control study. *Lancet* 2004; **364**:937–2.

7. Medalie JH, Levene C, Papier C, Goldbourt U, Dreyfuss F, Oron D, Neufeld H, Riss E. Blood groups, myocardial infarction and angina pectoris among 10,000 adult males. *N Engl J Med* 1971; **285**: 1348–53.

8. Rosendaal FR, Varekamp I, Smit C, Brocker-Vriends AH, van Dijck H, Vandenbroucke JP, Hermans J, Suurmeijer TP, Briet E. Mortality and causes of death in Dutch haemophiliacs, 1973–86. *Br J Haematol* 1989; **71**:71–6.

9. Triemstra M, Rosendaal FR, Smit C, van der Ploeg HM, Briët E. Mortality in patients with hemophilia: changes in a Dutch population from 1986 to 1992 and 1973 to 1986. *Ann Intern Med* 1995; **123**:823–7.

10. World Health Organization. Venous thromboembolic disease and combined oral contraceptives: results of international multicentre case–control study. WHO Collaborative Study of Cardiovascular Disease and Steroid Hormone Contraception. *Lancet* 1995; **346**:1575–82.

11. World Health Organization. Haemorrhagic stroke, overall stroke risk and combined oral contraceptives: results of an international, multicentre, case–control study. WHO Collaborative Study of Cardiovascular Disease and Steroid Hormone Contraception *Lancet* 1996; **348**:505–10.

12. World Health Organization. Ischaemic stroke and combined oral contraceptives: results of an international, multicentre, case–control study. WHO Collaborative Study of Cardiovascular Disease and Steroid Hormone Contraception *Lancet* 1996; **348**:498–5.

13. World Health Organization. Acute myocardial infarction and combined oral contraceptives: results of an international multicentre case–control study. WHO Collaborative Study of Cardiovascular Disease and Steroid Hormone Contraception *Lancet* 1997; **349**:1202–9.

14. van der Hagen PB, Folsom AR, Jenny NS, Heckbert SR, O'Meara ES, Reich LM, Rosendaal FR, Cushman M. Subclinical atherosclerosis and the risk of future venous thrombosis in the Cardiovascular Health Study. *J Thromb Haemost* 2006; **4**:1903–8.

15. Prandoni P. Links between arterial and venous disease. *J Intern Med* 2007; **262**:341–350.

16. Nordström M, Lindblad B, Bergqvist D, Kjellström T. A prospective study of the incidence of deep-vein thrombosis within a defined urban population. *J Intern Med* 1992; **232**:155–160.

17. Anderson FA, Wheeler HB, Goldberg RJ, Hosmer DW, Patwardhan NA, Jovanovic B, Forrier A, Dalen JE. A population based perspective of the hospital incidence and case-fatality rates of deep vein thrombosis and pulmonary embolism. The Worcester DVT study *Arch Intern Med* 1991; **151**: 933–8.

18. Oger E. Incidence of venous thromboembolism: a community-based study in western France. *Thromb Haemost* 2000; **83**:657–60.

19. Cushman M, Tsai AW, White RH, Heckbert SR, Rosamond WD, Enright P, Folsom AR. Deep vein thrombosis and pulmonary embolism in two cohorts: the longitudinal investigation of thromboembolism etiology. *Am J Med* 2004; **117**:19–25.

20. Brandjes DP, Büller HR, Heijboer H, Huisman MV, de Rijk M, Jagt H, Ten Cate JW. Randomised trial of effect of compression stockings in patients with symptomatic proximal-vein thrombosis. *Lancet* 1997; **349**:759–762.

21. Naess IA, Christiansen SC, Romundstad P, Cannegieter SC, Rosendaal FR, Hammerstrøm J. Incidence and mortality of venous thrombosis: a population-based study. *J Thromb Haemost* 2007; **5**:692–9.

22. Rosendaal FR. Thrombosis in the young: epidemiology and risk factors, a focus on venous thrombosis. *Thromb Haemost* 1997; **78**:1–6.

23. Seligsohn U, Zivelin A. Thrombophilia as a multigenic disorder. *Thromb Haemost* 1997; **78**:297–301.

24. Rosendaal FR. Venous thrombosis: a multicausal disease. *Lancet* 1999; **353**:1167–73.

25. Rosendaal FR. Risk factors for venous thrombosis: prevalence, risk and interaction. *Semin Hematol* 1997; **34**:171–187.

26. Heit JA, O'Fallon WM, Petterson TM, Lohse CM, Silverstein MD, Mohr DN, Melton LJ, III. Relative impact of risk factors for deep vein thrombosis and pulmonary embolism: a population-based study. *Arch Intern Med* 2002; **162**:1245–8.

27. Egeberg O. Inherited antithrombin deficiency causing thrombophilia. *Thromb Diath Haemorrh* 1965; **13**:516–30.

28. Griffin JH, Evatt B, Zimmerman TS, Kleiss AJ, Wideman C. Deficiency of protein C in congenital thrombotic disease. *J Clin Invest* 1981; **68**:1370–3.

29. Schwarz HP, Fischer M, Hopmeier P, Batard MA, Griffin JH. Plasma protein S deficiency in familial thrombotic disease. *Blood* 1984; **64**:1297–1300.

30. Smith NL, Hindorff LA, Heckbert SR, Lemaitre RN, Marciante KD, Rice K, Lumley T, Bis JC, Wiggins KL, Rosendaal FR, Psaty BM. Association of genetic variations with nonfatal venous thrombosis in postmenopausal women. *JAMA* 2007; **297**:489–8.

31. Bezemer ID, Bare LA, Doggen CJ, Arellano AR, Tong C, Rowland CM, Catanese J, Young BA, Reitsma PH, Devlin JJ, Rosendaal FR. Gene variants associated with deep vein thrombosis. *JAMA* 2008; **299**:1306–14.

32. Bezemer ID, Rosendaal FR. Predictive genetic variants for venous thrombosis: what's new? *Semin Hematol* 2007; **44**:85–92.

33. Rosendaal FR, van Hylckama Vlieg A, Doggen CJM. Venous thrombosis in the elderly. *J Thromb Haemost* 2007; **5**(Suppl 1):310–7.

34. Gibbs NM. Venous thrombosis of the lower limbs with particular reference to bed-rest. *Br J Surg* 1957; **45**:209–5.

35. Warlow C, Ogston D, Douglas AS. Deep venous thrombosis of the legs after stroke. *Br Med J* 1976; **1**:1178–81.

36. McColl MD, Ramsay JE, Tait RC, Walker ID, McCall F, Conkie JA, Carty MJ, Greer IA. Risk factors for pregnancy associated venous thromboembolism. *Thromb Haemost* 1997; **78**:1183–8.

37. Pomp ER, Lenselink AM, Rosendaal FR, Doggen CJ. Pregnancy, the postpartum period and prothrombotic defects: risk of venous thrombosis in the MEGA study. *J Thromb Haemost* 2008; **6**:632–7.

38. Kierkegaard A. Incidence and diagnosis of deep vein thrombosis associated with pregnancy. *Acta Obstet Gynecol Scand* 1983; **62**:239–3.

39. Cohen SH, Ehrlich GE, Kaufman MS, Cope C. Thrombophlebitis following knee surgery. *J Bone Joint Surg* 1973; **55**:106–111.

40. Hull RD, Raskob GE. Prophylaxis of venous thromboembolic disease following hip and knee surgery. *J Bone Joint Surg* 1986; **68**:146–50.

41. Nicolaides AN, Field ES, Kakkar VV, Yates-Bell AJ, Taylor S, Clarke MB. Prostatectomy and deep-vein thrombosis. *Br J Surg* 1972; **59**:487–8.

42. Mayo M, Halil T, Browse NL. The incidence of deep vein thrombosis after prostatectomy. *Br J Urol* 1971; **43**:738–2.

43. Walsh JJ, Bonnar J, Wright FW. A study of pulmonary embolism and deep vein thrombosis after major gynaecological surgery using labelled fibrinogen, phlebography and lung scanning. *J Obstet Gynaecol Br Commonw* 1974; **81**:311–6.

44. Hjelmstedt A, Bergvall U. Incidence of thrombosis in patients with tibial fractures. *Acta Chir Scand* 1968; **134**:209–8.

45. Myllynen P, Kammonen M, Rokkanen P, Böstman O, Lalla M, Laasonen E. Deep venous thrombosis and pulmonary embolism in patients with acute spinal cord injury: a comparison with nonparalyzed patients immobilized due to spinal fractures. *J Trauma* 1985; **25**:541–3.

46. Geerts WH, Code KI, Jay RM, Chen E, Szalai JP. A prospective study of venous thromboembolism after major trauma. *N Engl J Med* 1994; **331**:1601–6.

47. van Stralen KJ, Rosendaal FR, Doggen CJ. Minor injuries as a risk factor for venous thrombosis. *Arch Intern Med* 2008; **168**:21–6.

48. Geerts WH, Bergqvist D, Pineo GF, Heit JA, Samama CM, Lassen MR, Colwell CW. Prevention of venous thromboembolism: American College of Chest Physicians Evidence-Based Clinical Practice Guidelines (8th Edition) *Chest* 2008; **133**:381S–453S.

49. Eikelboom JW, Quinlan DJ, Douketis JD. Extended-duration prophylaxis against venous thromboembolism after total hip or knee replacement: a meta-analysis of the randomised trials. *Lancet* 2001; **358**:9–15.

50. Koster T. Deep-vein thrombosis. A population-based case–control study: Leiden Thrombophilia Study. Thesis. Rijksuniversiteit Leiden, Leiden, 1995.

51. Bannink L, Doggen CJM, Nelissen RGHH, Rosendaal FR. Increased risk of venous thrombosis after orthopedic and general surgery: results of the MEGA study (abstract). *J Thromb Haemost* 2005; **3**(Suppl 1):P1653

52. Bouillaud, S. De l'oblitération des veines et de son influence sur la formation des hydropisies partielles: considération sur la hydropisies passive et général. *Arch Gen Med* 1823; **1**:188–204.

53. Trousseau A. *Phlegmasia alba dolens; Clinique Médicale de l'Hôtel-Dieu de Paris*. J.B. Ballière et Fils, Paris, 1865, vol **3**, pp. 652–5.

54. Morel O, Toti F, Hugel B, Freyssinet JM. Cellular microparticles: a disseminated storage pool of bioactive vascular effectors. *Curr Opin Hematol* 2004; **11**:156–64.

55. Tesselaar MET, Romijn PHTM, Van der Linden IK, Prins FA, Bertina RM, Osanto S. Microparticle-associated tissue factor activity: a link between cancer and thrombosis? *J Thromb Haemost* 2007; **5**:520–7.

56. Zurborn KH, Duscha H, Gram J, Bruhn HD. Investigations of coagulation system and fibrinolysis in patients with disseminated adenocarcinomas and non-Hodgkin lymphomas. *Oncology* 1990; **47**:376–80.

57. Bick RL. Coagulation abnormalities in malignancy: a review. *Sem Thromb Hemost* 1992; **18**:353–9.

58. Meier CR, Jick H. Tamoxifen and risk of idiopathic venous thromboembolism. *Br J Clin Pharmacol* 1998; **45**:608–2.

59. Weijl NI, Rutten MF, Zwinderman AH, Keizer HJ, Nooy MA, Rosendaal FR, Cleton FJ, Osanto S. Thromboembolic events during chemotherapy for germ cell cancer: a cohort study and review of the literature. *J Clin Oncol* 2000; **18**:2169–78.

60. van Rooden CJ, Rosendaal FR, Barge RM, van Oostayen JA, van der Meer FJ, Meinders AE, Huisman MV. Central venous catheter related thrombosis in haematology patients and prediction of risk by screening with Doppler-ultrasound. *Br J Haematol* 2003; **123**:507–2.

61. Blom JW, Doggen CJ, Osanto S, Rosendaal FR. Malignancies, prothrombotic mutations and the risk of venous thrombosis. *JAMA* 2005; **293**:715–2.

62. Blom JW, Osanto S, Rosendaal FR. The risk of a venous thrombotic event in lung cancer patients: higher risk for adenocarcinoma than squamous cell carcinoma. *J Thromb Haemost* 2004; **2**:1760–5.

63. Nordström M, Lindblad B, Anderson H, Bergqvist D, Kjellström T. Deep venous thrombosis and occult malignancy: an epidemiological study. *BMJ* 1994; **308**:891–4.

64. Ginsberg JS, Wells PS, Brill-Edwards P, Donovan D, Moffatt K, Johnston M, Stevens P, Hirsh J. Antiphospolipid antibodies and venous thromboembolism. *Blood* 1995; **86**:3685–91.

65. Simioni P, Prandoni P, Zanon E, Saracino MA, Scudeller A, Villalta S, Scarano L, Girolami B, Benedetti L, Girolami A. Deep venous thrombosis and lupus anticoaguant. *Thromb Haemost* 1996; **76**:187–9.

66. Mateo J, Oliver A, Borrell M, Sala N, Fontcuberta J and the EMET Group. Laboratory evaluation and clinical characteristics of 2132 consecutive unselected patients with venous thromboembolism – results of the Spanish multicentric study on thrombophilia (EMET-study) *Thromb Haemost* 1997; **77**:444–51.

67. de Groot PG, Lutters B, Derksen RH, Lisman T, Meijers JC, Rosendaal FR. Lupus anticoagulants and the risk of a first episode of deep venous thrombosis. *J Thromb Haemost* 2005; **3**:1993–7.

68. Simpson K. Shelter deaths from pulmonary embolism. *Lancet* 1940; **ii**:744.

69. Eschwège V, Robert A. Strikes in French public transport and resistance to activated protein C. *Lancet* 1996; **347**:206.

70. Beasley R, Raymond N, Hill S, Nowitz M, Hughes R. eThrombosis: the 21st century variant of venous thromboembolism associated with immobility. *Eur Respir J* 2003; **21**:374–6.

71. Louvel J. [Four cases of phlebitis due to air travel]. *Arch.Mal Coeur Vaiss* **44**, 748–9. 1951.

72. Homans J. Thrombosis of the leg veins due to prolonged sitting. *N Engl J Med* 1954; **250**:148–9.

73. Symington IS, Stack BHR. Pulmonary thromboembolism after travel. *Br J Dis Chest* 1977; **71**:138–40.

74. Cruickshank JM, Gorlin R, Jennett B. Air travel and thrombotic episodes: the economy class syndrome. *Lancet* 1988; **ii**:497–8.

75. Sarvesvaran R. Sudden natural deaths associated with commercial air travel. *Med Sci Law* 1986; **26**:35–8.

76. Lapostolle F, Surget V, Borron SW, Desmaizieres M, Sordelet D, Lapandry C, Cupa M, Adnet F. Severe pulmonary embolism associated with air travel. *N Engl J Med* 2001; **345**:779–83.

77. Ferrari E, Chevallier T, Chapelier A, Baudouy M. Travel as a risk factor for venous thromboembolic disease: a case–control study. *Chest* 1999; **115**:440–4.

78. Kraaijenhagen RA, Haverkamp D, Koopman MM, Prandoni P, Piovella F, Büller HR. Travel and risk of venous thrombosis. *Lancet* 2000; **356**:1492–3.

79. Arya R, Barnes JA, Hossain U, Patel RK, Cohen AT. Long-haul flights and deep vein thrombosis: a significant risk only when additional factors are also present. *Br J Haematol* 2002; **116**:653–4.

80. Martinelli I, Taioli E, Battaglioli T, Podda GM, Passamonti SM, Pedotti P, Mannucci PM. Risk of venous thromboembolism after air travel: interaction with thrombophilia and oral contraceptives. *Arch Intern Med* 2003; **163**:2771–4.

81. Cannegieter SC, Doggen CJ, van Houwelingen HC, Rosendaal FR. Travel-related venous thrombosis: results from a large population-based case control study (MEGA study). *PLoS Med* 2006; **3**:e307.

82. Kuipers S, Schreijer AJM, Cannegieter SC, Büller HR, Rosendaal FR, Middeldorp S. Travel and venous thrombosis: a systematic review. *J Intern Med* 2007; **262**:615–4.

83. Bendz B, Rostrup M, Sevre K, Andersen TO, Sandset PM. Association between acute hypobaric hypoxia and activation of coagulation in human beings. *Lancet* 2000; **356**:1657–8.

84. Toff WD, Jones CI, Ford I, Pearse RJ, Watson HG, Watt SJ, Ross JA, Gradwell DP, Batchelor AJ, Abrams KR, Meijers JC, Goodall AH, Greaves M. Effect of hypobaric hypoxia, simulating conditions during long-haul air travel, on coagulation, fibrinolysis, platelet function, and endothelial activation. *JAMA* 2006; **295**:2251–61.

85. Schreijer AJ, Cannegieter SC, Meijers JC, Middeldorp S, Büller HR, Rosendaal FR. Activation of coagulation system during air travel: a crossover study. *Lancet* 2006; **367**:832–8.

86. Boccalon H, Boneu B, Emmerich J, Thalamas C, Ruidavets JB. Long-haul flights do not activate hemostasis in young healthy men. *J Thromb Haemost* 2005; **3**:1539–41.

87. Schreijer AJ, Cannegieter SC, Caramella M, Meijers JC, Krediet RT, Simons RM, Rosendaal FR. Fluid loss does not explain coagulation activation during air travel. *Thromb Haemost* 2008; **99**:1053–9.

88. Kuipers S, Cannegieter SC, Middeldorp S, Robyn L, Büller HR, Rosendaal FR. The absolute risk of venous thrombosis after air travel: a cohort study of 8755 employees of international organizations. *PLoS Med* 2007; **4**:e290.

89. Sidney S, Petitti DB, Soff GA, Cundiff DL, Tolan KK, Quesenberry CP, Jr. Venous thromboembolic disease in users of low-oestrogen combined oestrogen–progestin oral contraceptives. *Contraception* 2004; **70**:3–10.

90. van Stralen KJ, le Cessie S, Rosendaal FR, Doggen CJM. Regular sports activities decrease the risk of venous thrombosis. *J Thromb Haemost* 2007; **5**:517–2.

91. Glynn RJ, Rosner B. Comparison of risk factors for the competing risks of coronary heart disease, stroke and venous thromboembolism. *Am J Epidemiol* 2005; **162**:975–982.

92. van Stralen KJ, Doggen CJM, Lumley T, Cushman M, Folsom AR, Psaty BM, Siscovick DS, Rosendaal FR, Heckbert SR. Exercise in relation to venous thrombosis risk in the elderly. *J Am Geriatr Soc* 2008; **56**:517–22.

93. van Stralen KJ, Blom JW, Doggen CJ, Rosendaal FR. Strenuous sport activities involving the upper extremities increase the risk of venous thrombosis of the arm. *J Thromb Haemost* 2005; **3**:2110–11.

94. Zell L, Kindermann W, Marschall F, Scheffler P, Gross J, Buchter A. Paget–Schroetter syndrome in sports activities – case study and literature review. *Angiology* 2001; **52**:337–42.

95. Goldhaber SZ, Grodstein F, Stampfer MJ, Manson JE, Colditz GA, Speizer FE, Willett WC, Hennekens CH. A prospective study of risk factors for pulmonary embolism in women. *JAMA* 1997; **277**:642–5.

96. Samama MM. An epidemiologic study of risk factors for deep vein thrombosis in medical outpatients: the Sirius study. *Arch Intern Med* 2000; **160**:3415–20.

97. Tsai AW, Cushman M, Rosamond WD, Heckbert SR, Polak JF, Folsom AR. Cardiovascular risk factors and venous thromboembolism incidence: the longitudinal investigation of thromboembolism etiology. *Arch Intern Med* 2002; **162**:1182–9.

98. Abdollahi M, Cushman M, Rosendaal FR. Obesity: risk of venous thrombosis and the interaction with coagulation factor levels and oral contraceptive use. *Thromb Haemost* 2003; **89**:493–8.

99. Pomp ER, le Cessie S, Rosendaal FR, Doggen CJ. Risk of venous thrombosis: obesity and its joint effect with oral contraceptive use and prothrombotic mutations. *Br J Haematol* 2007; **139**:289–96.

100. Goldhaber SZ, Savage DD, Garrison RJ, Castelli WP, Kannel WB, McNamara PM, Gherardi G, Feinleib M. Risk factors for pulmonary embolism. The Framingham Study *Am J Med* 1983; **74**:1023–8.

101. Hansson PO, Eriksson H, Welin L, Svardsudd K, Wilhelmsen L. Smoking and abdominal obesity: risk factors for venous thromboembolism among middle-aged men: 'The Study of Men Born in 1913'. *Arch Intern Med* 1999; **159**:1886–90.

102. Pomp ER, Rosendaal FR, Doggen CJ. Smoking increases the risk of venous thrombosis and acts synergistically with oral contraceptive use. *Am J Hematol* 2008; **83**:97–102.

103. Pomp ER, Rosendaal FR, Doggen CJ. Alcohol consumption is associated with a decreased risk of venous thrombosis. *Thromb Haemost* 2008; **99**:59–63.

104. Lee KW, Lip GY. Effects of lifestyle on hemostasis, fibrinolysis and platelet reactivity: a systematic review. *Arch Intern Med* 2003; **163**:2368–92.

105. Jordan WM. Pulmonary embolism. *Lancet* 1961; **ii**:1146–47.

106. Lorentz I. Parietal lesions and Enavid. *BMJ* 1962; **ii**:1191.

107. Boyce J, Fawcett JW, Noall EWP. Coronary thrombosis and Conovid. *Lancet* 1963; **i**:111.

108. Bloemenkamp KWM, Rosendaal FR, Helmerhorst FM, Büller HR, Vandenbroucke JP. Enhancement by factor V Leiden mutation of risk of deep-vein thrombosis associated with oral contraceptives containing a third-generation progestagen. *Lancet* 1995; **346**:1593–6.

109. Tanis BC, van den Bosch MA, Kemmeren JM, Manger Cats V, Helmerhorst FM, Algra A, van der Graaf, Rosendaal FR. Oral contraceptives and the risk of myocardial infarction. *N Engl J Med* 2001; **345**:1787–93.

110. Kemmeren JM, Tanis BC, van den Bosch MA, Bollen EL, Helmerhorst FM, van der Graaf, Rosendaal FR, Algra A. Risk of Arterial Thrombosis in Relation to Oral Contraceptives (RATIO) study: oral contraceptives and the risk of ischaemic stroke. *Stroke* 2002; **33**:1202–8.

111. van den Bosch MAAJ, Kemmeren JM, Tanis BC, Mali WPTM, Helmerhorst FM, Rosendaal FR, Algra A, van der Graaf Y. The RATIO study: oral contraceptives and the risk of peripheral arterial disease in young women. *J Thromb Haemost* 2003; **1**:439–4.

112. Lachnit-Fixson U. The development and evaluation of an ovulation inhibitor (DIAne) containing an antiandrogen. *Acta Obstet Gynecol Scand Suppl* 1979; **88**:33–42.

113. Muhn P, Fuhrmann U, Fritzemeier KH, Krattenmacher R, Schillinger E. Drospirenone: a novel progestogen with antimineralocorticoid and antiandrogenic activity. *Ann N Y Acad Sci* 1995; **761**:311–35.

114. Gerstman BB, Piper JM, Tomita DK, Ferguson WJ, Stadel BV, Lundin FE. Oral contraceptive oestrogen dose and the risk of deep venous thromboembolic disease. *Am J Epidemiol* 1991; **133**:32–7.

115. Thorogood M, Mann J, Murphy M, Vessey M. Risk factors for fatal venous thromboembolism in young women: a case–control study. *Int J Epidemiol* 1992; **21**:48–52.

116. Farmer RDT, Preston TD. The risk of venous thromboembolism associated with low-oestrogen oral contraceptives. *J Obst Gynecol* 1995; **15**:195–200.

117. Vandenbroucke JP, Rosing J, Bloemenkamp KW, Middeldorp S, Helmerhorst FM, Bouma BN, Rosendaal FR. Oral contraceptives and the risk of venous thrombosis. *N Engl J Med* 2001; **344**:1527–35.

118. Rosendaal FR, Helmerhorst FM, Vandenbroucke JP. Female hormones and thrombosis. *Arterioscler Thromb Vasc Biol* 2002; **22**:201–10.

119. Rosendaal FR, ran Hylckama Vlieg A, Tanis BC, Helmerhorst FM. Oestrogens, progestogens and thrombosis. *J Thromb Haemost* 2003; **1**:1371–80.

120. Jick H, Kaye JA, Vasilakis-Scaramozza C, Jick SS. Risk of venous thromboembolism among users of third generation oral contraceptives compared with users of oral contraceptives with levonorgestrel before and after 1995: cohort and case–control analysis. *BMJ* 2000; **321**:1190–5.

121. Herings RMC, Urquhart J, Leufkens HGM. Venous thromboembolism among new users of different oral contraceptives. *Lancet* 1999; **354**:127–8.

122. Bloemenkamp KWM, Rosendaal FR, Helmerhorst FM, Vandenbroucke JP. Higher risk of venous thrombosis during early use of oral contraceptives in women with inherited clotting defects. *Arch Intern Med* 2000; **160**:49–52.

123. World Health Organization. Effect of different progestagens in low oestrogen oral contraceptives on venous thromboembolic disease. WHO Collaborative Study of Cardiovascular Disease and Steroid Hormone Contraception *Lancet* 1995; **346**:1582–8.

124. Jick H, Jick SS, Gurewich V, Myers MW, Vasilakis C. Risk of idiopathic cardiovascular death and nonfatal venous thromboembolism in women using oral contraceptives with differing progestagen components. *Lancet* 1995; **346**:1589–93.

125. Kemmeren JM, Algra A, Grobbee DE. Third generation oral contraceptives and risk of venous thrombosis: meta-analysis. *BMJ* 2001; **323**:131–4.

126. Kemmeren JM, Algra A, Meijers JC, Bouma BN, Grobbee DE. Effects of second and third generation oral contraceptives and their respective progestagens on the coagulation system in the absence or presence of the factor V Leiden mutation. *Thromb Haemost* 2002; **87**:199–205.

127. Vasilakis-Scaramozza C, Jick H. Risk of venous thromboembolism with cyproterone or levonorgestrel contraceptives. *Lancet* 2001; **358**:1427–9.

128. Sheldon T. Dutch GPs warned against new contraceptive pill. *BMJ* 2002; **324**:869.

129. Dinger JC, Heinemann LA, Kuhl-Habich D. The safety of a drospirenone-containing oral contraceptive: final results from the European Active Surveillance Study on oral contraceptives based on 142,475 women-years of observation. *Contraception* 2007; **75**:344–54.

130. Pearce HM, Layton D, Wilton LV, Shakir SA. Deep vein thrombosis and pulmonary embolism reported in the Prescription Event Monitoring Study of Yasmin. *Br J Clin Pharmacol* 2005; **60**:98–102.

131. Olivieri O, Friso S, Manzato F, Guella A, Bernardi F, Lunghi B, Girelli D, Azzini M, Brocco G, Russo C. Resistance to activated protein C in healthy women taking oral contraceptives. *Br J Haematol* 1995; **91**:465–70.

132. Henkens CM, Bom VJ, Seinen AJ, van der Meer J. Sensitivity to activated protein C; influence of oral contraceptives and sex. *Thromb Haemost* 1995; **73**:402–4.

133. Rosing J, Middeldorp S, Curvers J, Christella M, Thomassen LG, Nicolaes GA, Meijers JC, Bouma BN, Büller HR, Prins MH, Tans G. Low-dose oral contraceptives and acquired resistance to activated protein C: a randomised cross-over study. *Lancet* 1999; **354**:2036–40.

134. Middeldorp S, Meijers JCM, van den Ende AE, van Enk A, Bouma BN, Tans G, Rosing J, Prins MH, Büller HR. Effects on coagulation of levonorgestrel- and desogestrel-containing low dose oral contraceptives: a cross-over study. *Thromb Haemost* 2000; **84**:4–8.

135. Tans G, Curvers J, Middeldorp S, Thomassen MCLGD, Meijers JCM, Prins MH, Bouma BN, Büller HR, Rosing J. A randomized cross-over study on the effects of levonorgestrel- and desogestrel-containing oral contraceptives on the anticoagulant pathways. *Thromb Haemost* 2000; **84**:15–21.

136. Rosing J, Tans G, Nicolaes GA, Thomassen MC, Van Oerle R, Van der Ploeg PM, Heijen P, Hamulyak K, Hemker HC. Oral contraceptives and venous thrombosis: different sensitivities to activated protein C in women using second- and third-generation oral contraceptives. *Br J Haematol* 1997; **97**:233–8.

137. Tans G, van Hylckama Vileg A, Thomassen MC, Curvers J, Bertina RM, Rosing J, Rosendaal FR. Activated protein C resistance determined with a thrombin generation-based test predicts for venous thrombosis in men and women. *Br J Haematol* 2003; **122**:465–70.

138. van Vliet HA, Winkel TA, Noort I, Rosing J, Rosendaal FR. Prothrombotic changes in users of combined oral contraceptives containing drospirenone and cyproterone acetate. *J Thromb Haemost* 2004; **2**:2060–62.

139. Pabinger I, Schneider B and the GTH study group.: Thrombotic risk of women with hereditary antithrombin III-, protein C and protein S-deficiency taking oral contraceptive medication. *Thromb Haemost* 1994; **71**:548–52.

140. Martinelli I, Mannucci PM, De Stefano V, Taioli E, Rossi V, Crosti F, Paciaroni K, Leone G, Faioni EM. Different risks of thrombosis in four coagulation defects associated with inherited thrombophilia: a study of 150 families. *Blood* 1998; **92**:2353–8.

141. Vandenbroucke JP, Koster T, Briët E, Reitsma PH, Bertina RM, Rosendaal FR. Increased risk of venous thrombosis in oral-contraceptive users who are carriers of factor V Leiden mutation. *Lancet* 1994; **344**:1453–7.

142. Martinelli I, Taioli E, Bucciarelli P, Akhavan S, Mannucci PM. Interaction between the G20210A mutation of the prothrombin gene and oral contraceptive use in deep vein thrombosis. *Arterioscler Thromb Vasc Biol* 1999; **19**:700–3.

143. van Hylckama Vlieg A, Rosendaal FR. Interaction between oral contraceptive use and coagulation factor levels in deep venous thrombosis. *J Thromb Haemost* 2003; **1**:2186–90.

144. Hutchinson TA, Polansky SM, Feinstein AR. Post-menopausal oestrogens protect against fractures of hip and distal radius. A case–control study. *Lancet* 1979; **ii**:705–9.

145. Weiss NS, Ure CL, Ballard JH, Williams AR, Daling JR. Decreased risk of fractures of the hip and lower forearm with postmenopausal use of oestrogen. *N Engl J Med* 1980; **303**:1195–8.

146. Doren M, Samsioe G. Prevention of postmenopausal osteoporosis with oestrogen replacement therapy and associated compounds: update on clinical trials since 1995. *Hum Reprod Update* 2000; **6**:419–26.

147. Villareal DT, Binder EF, Williams DB, Schechtman KB, Yarasheski KE, Kohrt WM. Bone mineral density response to oestrogen replacement in frail elderly women: a randomized controlled trial. *JAMA* 2001; **286**:815–20.

148. Rossouw JE, Anderson GL, Prentice RL, Lacroix AZ, Kooperberg C, Stefanick ML, Jackson RD, Beresford SA, Howard BV, Johnson KC, Kotchen JM, Ockene J. Risks and benefits of oestrogen plus progestin in healthy postmenopausal women: principal results from the Women's Health Initiative randomized controlled trial. *JAMA* 2002; **288**:321–33.

149. Hulley S, Furberg C, Barrett-Connor E, Cauley J, Grady D, Haskell W, Knopp R, Lowery M, Satterfield S, Schrott H, Vittinghoff E, Hunninghake D. Noncardiovascular disease outcomes during 6.8 years of hormone therapy: Heart and Oestrogen/progestin Replacement Study follow-up (HERS II) *JAMA* 2002; **288**:58–66.

150. Watts NB. Therapies to improve bone mineral density and reduce the risk of fracture: clinical trial results. *J Reprod Med* 2002; **47**:82–92.

151. Hulley S, Grady D, Bush T, Furberg C, Herrington D, Riggs B, Vittinghoff E, for the Heart and Oestrogen/progestin Replacement Study (HERS) Research Group. Randomized trial of oestrogen plus progestin for secondary prevention of coronary heart disease in postmenopausal women. *JAMA* 1998; **280**:605–13.

152. The ESPRIT team. Oestrogen therapy for prevention of reinfarction in postmenopausal women: a randomised placebo-controlled trial. *Lancet* 2002; **360**:2001–8.

153. Daly E, Vessey MP, Hawkins MM, Carson JL, Gough P, Marsh S. Risk of venous thromboembolism in users of hormone replacement therapy. *Lancet* 1996; **348**:977–980.

154. Daly E, Vessey MP, Painter R, Hawkins MM. Case–control study of venous thromboembolism risk in users of hormone replacement therapy. *Lancet* 1996; **348**:1027.

155. Jick H, Derby LE, Wald Myers M, Vasilakis C, Newton KM. Risk of hospital admission for idiopathic venous thromboembolism among users of postmenopasusal oestrogens. *Lancet* 1996; **348**: 981–3.

156. Grodstein F, Stampfer MJ, Goldhaber SZ, Manson JE, Colditz GA, Speizer FE, Willett WC, Hennekens CH. Prospective study of exogenous hormones and risk of pulmonary embolism in women. *Lancet* 1996; **348**:983–7.

157. Perez Gutthann S, Garcia Rodriguez LA, Castellsague J, Duque Oliart A. Hormone replacement therapy and risk of venous thromboembolism: population based case–control study. *BMJ* 1997; **314**: 796–800.

158. Grady D, Furberg C. Venous thromboembolic events associated with hormone replacement therapy. *JAMA* 1997; **278**:477.

159. Varas Lorenzo C, Garcia Rodriguez LA, Cattaruzzi C, Troncon MG, Agostinis L, Perez Gutthann S. Hormone replacement therapy and the risk of hospitalization for venous thromboembolism: a population-based study in southern Europe. *Am J Epidemiol* 1998; **147**:387–90.

160. Høibraaten E, Abdelnoor M, Sandset PM. Hormone replacement therapy with estradiol and risk of venous thromboembolism – a population-based case–control study. *Thromb Haemost* 1999; **82**:1218–21.

161. Grady D, Wenger NK, Herrington D, Khan S, Furberg C, Hunninghoke D, Vittinghoff E, Hulley S. Postmenopausal hormone therapy increases risk for venous thromboembolic disease. *Ann Intern Med* 2000; **132**:689–96.

162. Cushman M, Kuller LH, Prentice R, Rodabough RJ, Psaty BM, Stafford RS, Sidney S, Rosendaal FR. Oestrogen plus progestin and risk of venous thrombosis. *JAMA* 2004; **292**:1573–80.

163. Scarabin PY, Oger E, Plu-Bureau G. Differential association of oral and transdermal oestrogen-replacement therapy with venous thromboembolism risk. *Lancet* 2003; **362**:428–32.

164. Canonico M, Plu-Bureau G, Lowe GD, Scarabin PY. Hormone replacement therapy and risk of venous thromboembolism in postmenopausal women: systematic review and meta-analysis. *BMJ* 2008; **336**:1227–31.

165. Smith NL, Heckbert SR, Lemaitre RN, Reiner AP, Lumley T, Weiss NS, Larson EB, Rosendaal FR, Psaty BM. Esterified oestrogens and conjugated equine oestrogens and the risk of venous thrombosis. *JAMA* 2004; **292**:1581–7.

166. Smith NL, Heckbert SR, Doggen CJ, Lemaitre RN, Reiner AP, Lumley T, Meijers JC, Psaty BM, Rosendaal FR. The differential association of conjugated equine oestrogen and esterified oestrogen with activated protein C resistance in postmenopausal women. *J Thromb Haemost* 2006; **4**:1701–6.

167. Høibraaten E, Qvigstad E, Arnesen H, Larsen S, Wickstrøm E, Sandset PM. Increased risk of recurrent venous thromboembolism during hormone replacement therapy – results of the randomized, double-blind, placebo-controlled oestrogen in venous thromboembolism trial (EVTET). *Thromb Haemost* 2000; **84**:961–7.

168. Lowe G, Woodward M, Vessey M, Rumley A, Gough P, Daly E. Thrombotic variables and risk of idiopathic venous thromboembolism in women aged 45–64 years: relationships to hormone replacement therapy. *Thromb Haemost* 2000; **83**:530–5.

169. Rosendaal FR, Vessey M, Rumley A, Daly E, Woodward M, Helmerhorst FM, Lowe GDO. Hormonal replacement therapy, prothrombotic mutations and the risk of venous thrombosis. *Br J Haematol* 2002; **116**:851–4.

170. Herrington DM, Vittinghoff E, Howard TD, Major DA, Owen J, Reboussin DM, Bowden D, Bittner V, Simon JA, Grady D, Hulley SB. Factor V Leiden, hormone replacement therapy and risk of venous thromboembolic events in women with coronary disease. *Arterioscler Thromb Vasc Biol* 2002; **22**:1012–7.

171. Curb JD, Prentice RL, Bray PF, Langer RD, Van HL, Barnabei VM, Bloch MJ, Cyr MG, Gass M, Lepine L, Rodabough RJ, Sidney S, Uwaifo GI, Rosendaal FR. Venous thrombosis and conjugated equine oestrogen in women without a uterus. *Arch Intern Med* 2006; **166**:772–80.

172. Tait RC, Walker ID, Perry DJ, Islam SI, Daly ME, McCall F, Conkie JA, Carrell RW. Prevalence of antithrombin deficiency in the healthy population. *Br J Haematol* 1994; **87**:106–12.

173. Tait RC, Walker ID, Reitsma PH, Islam SI, McCall F, Poort SR, Conkie JA, Bertina RM. Prevalence of protein C deficiency in the healthy population. *Thromb Haemost* 1995; **73**:87–93.

174. McColl M, Tait RC, Walker ID, Perry DJ, McCall F, Conkie JA. Low thrombosis rate seen in blood donors and their relatives with inherited deficiencies of antithrombin and protein C: correlation with type of defect, family history and absence of the factor V Leiden mutation. *Blood Coag Fibrinolysis* 1996; **7**:689–94.

175. Rosendaal FR. Risk factors for venous thrombotic disease. *Thromb Haemost* 1999; **82**:610–619.

176. Heijboer H, Brandjes DPM, Büller HR, Sturk A, Ten Cate JW. Deficiencies of coagulation-inhibiting and fibrinolytic proteins in outpatients with deep-vein thrombosis. *N Engl J Med* 1990; **323**:1512–6.

177. Koster T, Rosendaal FR, Briët E, Van der Meer FJM, Colly LP, Trienekens PH, Poort SR, Vandenbroucke JP. Protein C deficiency in a controlled series of unselected outpatients: an infrequent but clear risk factor for venous thrombosis (Leiden Thrombophilia Study). *Blood* 1995; **85**:2756–61.

178. Broekmans AW, Veltkamp JJ, Bertina RM. Congenital protein C deficiency and venous thromboembolism: a study of three Dutch families. *N Engl J Med* 1983; **309**:340–4.

179. Koeleman BPC, Reitsma PH, Allaart CF, Bertina RM. APC-resistance as an additional risk factor for thrombosis in protein C deficient families. *Blood* 1994; **84**:1031–5.

180. Zöller B, Berntsdotter A, Garcia de Frutos P, Dahlbäck B. Resistance to activated protein C as an additional genetic risk factor in hereditary deficiency of protein S. *Blood* 1995; **85**:3518–23.

181. Lensen RPM, Rosendaal FR, Koster T, Allaart CF, De Ronde H, Vandenbroucke JP, Reitsma PH, Bertina RM. Apparent different thrombotic tendency in patients with factor V Leiden and protein C deficiency due to selection of patients. *Blood* 1996; **88**:4205–8.

182. Hasstedt SJ, Bovill EG, Callas PW, Long GL. An unknown genetic defect increases venous thrombosis risk, through interaction with protein C deficiency. *Am J Hum Genet* 1998; **63**:569–76.

183. Van Boven HH, Vandenbroucke JP, Briët E, Rosendaal FR. Gene–gene and gene–environment interactions determine risk of thrombosis in families with inherited antithrombin deficiency. *Blood* 1999; **94**:2590–4.

184. Horellou MH, Conard J, Bertina RM, Samama M. Congenital protein C deficiency and thrombotic disease in nine French families. *Br Med J* 1984; **289**:1285–7.

185. Demers C, Ginsberg JS, Hirsh J, Henderson P, Blajchman MA. Thrombosis in antithrombin III-deficient persons: report of a large kindred and literature review. *Ann Intern Med* 1992; **116**:754–61.

186. Vossen CY, Conard J, Fontcuberta J, Makris M, van der Meer FJ, Pabinger I, Palareti G, Preston FE, Scharrer I, Souto JC, Svensson P, Walker ID, Rosendaal FR. Familial thrombophilia and lifetime risk of venous thrombosis. *J Thromb Haemost* 2004; **2**:1526–32.

187. Vossen CY, Conard J, Fontcuberta J, Makris M, van der Meer FJ, Pabinger I, Palareti G, Preston FE, Scharrer I, Souto JC, Svensson P, Walker ID, Rosendaal FR. Risk of a first venous thrombotic event in carriers of a familial thrombophilic defect. The European Prospective Cohort on Thrombophilia (EPCOT). *J Thromb Haemost* 2005; **3**:459–64.

188. Branson HE, Marble R, Katz J, Griffin JH. Inherited protein C deficiency and coumarin-responsive chronic relapsing purpura fulminans in a newborn. *Lancet* 1983; **ii**:1165–8.

189. Mahasandana C, Suvatte V, Chuansumrit A, Marlar RA, Manco-Johnson MJ, Jacobson LJ, Hathaway WF. Homozygous protein S deficiency in an infant with purpura fulminans. *J Pediatr* 1990; **117**:750–3.

190. Bertina RM, Koeleman RPC, Koster T, Rosendaal FR, Dirven RJ, De Ronde H, Van der Velden PA, Reitsma PH. Mutation in blood coagulation factor V associated with resistance to activated protein C. *Nature* 1994; **369**:64–7.

191. Rees DC, Cox M, Clegg JB. World distribution of factor V Leiden. *Lancet* 1995; **346**:1133–4.

192. Rosendaal FR, Koster T, Vandenbroucke JP, Reitsma PH. High risk of thrombosis in patients homozygous for factor V Leiden (activated protein C resistance). *Blood* 1995; **85**:1504–8.

193. Dahlbäck B, Carlsson M, Svensson PJ. Familial thrombophilia due to a previously unrecognised mechanism characterized by poor anticoagulant response to activated protein C: prediction of a cofactor to activated protein C. *Proc Natl Acad Sci USA* 1993; **90**:1004–8.

194. Koster T, Rosendaal FR, De Ronde H, Briët E, Vandenbroucke JP, Bertina RM. Venous thrombosis due to a poor anticoagulant response to activated protein C. Leiden Thrombophilia Study. *Lancet* 1993; **342**:1503–6.

195. Svensson PJ, Dahlbäck B. Resistance to activated protein C as a basis for venous thrombosis. *N Engl J Med* 1994; **330**:517–522.
196. Dahlbäck B. The discovery of activated protein C resistance. *J Thromb Haemost* 2003; **1**:3–9.
197. Poort SR, Rosendaal FR, Reitsma PH, Bertina RM. A common genetic variation in the 3'-untranslated region of the prothrombin gene is associated with elevated plasma prothrombin levels and an increase in venous thrombosis. *Blood* 1996; **88**:3698–703.
198. Rosendaal FR, Doggen CJM, Zivelin A, Arruda VR, Aiach M, Siscovick DS, Hillarp A, Watzke HH, Bernardi F, Cumming AM, Preston FE, Reitsma PH. Geographic distribution of the 20210 G to A prothrombin variant. *Thromb Haemost* 1998; **79**:706–8.
199. Bank I, Libourel EJ, Middeldorp S, van Pampus EC, Koopman MM, Hamulyak K, Prins MH, van der MJ, Büller HR. Prothrombin 20210A mutation: a mild risk factor for venous thromboembolism but not for arterial thrombotic disease and pregnancy-related complications in a family study. *Arch Intern Med* 2004; **164**:1932–7.
200. Emmerich J, Rosendaal FR, Cattaneo M, Margaglione M, de Stefano V, Cumming T, Arruda V, Hillarp A, Reny JL. Combined effect of factor V Leiden and prothrombin 20210A on the risk of venous thromboembolism – pooled analysis of 8 case–control studies including 2310 cases and 3204 controls. Study Group for Pooled-Analysis in Venous Thromboembolism. *Thromb Haemost* 2001; **86**:809–16.
201. Jick H, Slone D, Westerholm B, Inman WHW, Vessey MP, Shapiro S, Lewis GP, Worcester J. Venous thromboembolic disease and ABO blood type. *Lancet* 1969; **i**:539–42.
202. Koster T, Blann AD, Briët E, Vandenbroucke JP, Rosendaal FR. Role of clotting factor VIII in effect of von Willebrand factor on occurrence of deep-vein thrombosis. *Lancet* 1995; **345**:152–5.
203. Kamphuisen PW, Eikenboom JC, Rosendaal FR, Koster T, Blann AD, Vos HL, Bertina RM. High factor VIII antigen levels increase the risk of venous thrombosis but are not associated with polymorphisms in the von Willebrand factor and factor VIII gene. *Br J Haematol* 2001; **115**:156–8.
204. Morelli VM, De Visser MC, Vos HL, Bertina RM, Rosendaal FR. ABO blood group genotypes and the risk of venous thrombosis: effect of factor V Leiden. *J Thromb Haemost* 2005; **3**:183–5.
205. Kang SS, Zhou J, Wong PWK, Kowlisyn J, Strokosch G. Intermediate homocysteinemia: a thermolabile variant of methyenetetrahydrofolate reductase. *Am J Hum Genet* 1988; **48**:536–45.
206. Frosst P, Blom HJ, Milos R, Goyette P, Sheppard CA, Matthews RG, Boers GHJ, Den Heijer M, Kluijtmans LAJ, Van den Heuvel LPWJ, Rozen R. A candidate genetic risk factor for vascular disease: a common mutation in methylenetetrahydrofolate reductase. *Nat Genet* 1995; **10**:111–3.
207. Den Heijer M, Lewington S, Clarke R. Homocysteine, MTHFR and risk of venous thrombosis: a meta-analysis of published epidemiological studies. *J Thromb Haemost* 2005; **3**:292–9.
208. Bezemer ID, Doggen CJ, Vos HL, Rosendaal FR. No association between the common MTHFR 677C→T polymorphism and venous thrombosis: results from the MEGA study. *Arch Intern Med* 2007; **167**:497–501.
209. Ariëns RA, Philippou H, Nagaswami C, Weisel JW, Lane DA, Grant PJ. The factor XIII V34L polymorphism accelerates thrombin activation of factor XIII and affects cross-linked fibrin structure. *Blood* 2000; **96**:988–95.
210. van Hylckama Vlieg A, Komanasin N, Ariens RA, Poort SR, Grant PJ, Bertina RM, Rosendaal FR. Factor XIII Val34Leu polymorphism, factor XIII antigen levels and activity and the risk of deep venous thrombosis. *Br J Haematol* 2002; **119**:169–75.
211. Vossen CY, Rosendaal FR. The protective effect of the factor XIII Val34Leu mutation on the risk of deep venous thrombosis is dependent on the fibrinogen level. *J Thromb Haemost* 2005; **3**:1102–3.
212. Uitte de Willige S, De Visser MC, Houwing-Duistermaat JJ, Rosendaal FR, Vos HL, Bertina RM. Genetic variation in the fibrinogen gamma gene increases the risk for deep venous thrombosis by reducing plasma fibrinogen gamma' levels. *Blood* 2005; **106**:4176–83.
213. Uitte de Willige S, Rietveld IM, De Visser MC, Vos HL, Bertina RM. Polymorphism 10034C→T is located in a region regulating polyadenylation of FGG transcripts and influences the fibrinogen gamma'/gammaA mRNA ratio. *J Thromb Haemost* 2007; **5**:1243–9.
214. Grunbacher G, Weger W, Marx-Neuhold E, Pilger E, Koppel H, Wascher T, Marz W, Renner W. The fibrinogen gamma (FGG) 10034C→T polymorphism is associated with venous thrombosis. *Thromb Res* 2007; **121**:33–6.
215. Spek CA, Koster T, Rosendaal FR, Bertina RM, Reitsma PH. Genotypic variation in the promoter region of the protein C gene is associated with plasma protein C levels and thrombotic risk. *Arterioscler Thromb Vasc Biol* 1995; **15**:214–8.
216. Aiach M, Nicaud V, Alhenc-Gelas M, Gandrille S, Arnaud E, Amiral J, Guize L, Fiessinger JN, Emmerich J. Complex association of protein C gene promoter polymorphism with circulating protein C levels and thrombotic risk. *Arterioscler Thromb Vasc Biol* 1999; **19**:1573–6.

217. Fermo I, D'Angelo SV, Paroni R, Mazzola G, Calori G, D'Angelo A. Prevalence of moderate hyper-homocysteinemia in patients with early-onset venous and arterial occlusive disease. *Ann Intern Med* 1995; **123**:747–53.
218. Simioni P, Prandoni P, Burlina A, Tormene D, Sardella C, Ferrari V, Benedetti L, Girolami A. Hyper-homocysteinemia and deep-vein thrombosis: a case–control study. *Thromb Haemost* 1996; **76**:883–6.
219. Den Heijer M, Koster T, Blom HJ, Bos GMJ, Briët E, Reitsma PH, Vandenbroucke JP, Rosendaal FR. Hyperhomocysteinemia as a risk factor for deep-vein thrombosis. *N Engl J Med* 1996; **334**:759–62.
220. Den Heijer M, Brouwer IA, Bos GM, Blom HJ, van der Put NM, Spaans AP, Rosendaal FR, Thomas CM, Haak HL, Wijermans PW, Gerrits WB. Vitamin supplementation reduces blood homocysteine levels: a controlled trial in patients with venous thrombosis and healthy volunteers. *Arterioscler Thromb Vasc Biol* 1998; **18**:356–61.
221. Den Heijer M, Willems HP, Blom HJ, Gerrits WB, Cattaneo M, Eichinger S, Rosendaal FR, Bos GM. Homocysteine lowering by B vitamins and the secondary prevention of deep vein thrombosis and pulmonary embolism: a randomized, placebo-controlled, double-blind trial. *Blood* 2007; **109**:139–44.
222. Koster T, Rosendaal FR, Van der Velden PA, Briët E, Vandenbroucke JP. Factor VII and fibrino-gen levels as risk factors for venous thrombosis: a case–control study of plasma levels and DNA polymorphisms: the Leiden Thrombophilia Study (LETS). *Thromb Haemost* 1994; **71**:719–22.
223. van Hylckama Vlieg A, Van der Linden IK, Bertina RM, Rosendaal FR. High levels of factor IX increase the risk of venous thrombosis. *Blood* 2000; **95**:3678–82.
224. Meijers JC, Tekelenburg WL, Bouma BN, Bertina RM, Rosendaal FR. High levels of coagulation factor XI as a risk factor for venous thrombosis. *N Engl J Med* 2000; **342**:696–701.
225. van Hylckama Vlieg A, Rosendaal FR. High levels of fibrinogen are associated with the risk of deep venous thrombosis mainly in the elderly. *J Thromb Haemost* 2003; **1**:2677–8.
226. van Tilburg NH, Rosendaal FR, Bertina RM. Thrombin activatable fibrinolysis inhibitor and the risk for deep vein thrombosis. *Blood* 2000; **95**:2855–9.
227. Kamphuisen PW, Houwing-Duistermaat JJ, van Houwelingen JC, Eikenboom JCJ, Bertina RM, Rosendaal FR. Familial clustering of factor VIII and von Willebrand factor levels. *Thromb Haemost* 1998; **79**:323–7.
228. Kamphuisen PW, Lensen R, Houwing-Duistermaat JJ, Eikenboom JC, Harvey M, Bertina RM, Rosendaal FR. Heritability of elevated factor VIII antigen levels in factor V Leiden families with thrombophilia. *Br J Haematol* 2000; **109**:519–22.
229. Dahm A, van Hylckama Vlieg A, Bendz B, Rosendaal F, Bertina RM, Sandset PM. Low levels of tissue factor pathway inhibitor (TFPI) increase the risk of venous thrombosis. *Blood* 2003; **101**:4387–92.
230. Lisman T, de Groot PG, Meijers JC, Rosendaal FR. Reduced plasma fibrinolytic potential is a risk factor for venous thrombosis. *Blood* 2005; **105**:1102–5.
231. Meltzer ME, Lisman T, Doggen CJ, de Groot PG, Rosendaal FR. Synergistic effects of hypofibrinolysis and genetic and acquired risk factors on the risk of a first venous thrombosis. *PLoS Med* 2008; **5**:e97.

CHAPTER 2

The Natural History of Venous Thromboembolism

Paolo Prandoni

Department of Medical and Surgical Sciences, Thromboembolism Unit,
University of Padua, Padua, Italy

The classic study of the epidemiology of a disease is closely linked to the natural history of the condition. Natural history refers to the evolution of disease in the absence of medical intervention. In the field of venous thromboembolism (VTE), these observational aspects are often compromised by interventions. Thus, the definition 'clinical course' is likely more appropriate for the description of long-term outcomes of venous thromboembolic disorders.

For practical purposes, we will discuss separately the clinical course of isolated calf deep vein thrombosis (DVT), that of DVT involving the proximal-vein system and, finally, the clinical course of pulmonary embolism (PE).

At the end of the chapter, we will include a few considerations on the risk of subsequent cancer in patients with VTE and on the emerging view that VTE is associated with an increased risk of subsequent arterial cardiovascular events.

CLINICAL COURSE OF ISOLATED CALF VEIN THROMBOSIS

Calf vein thrombosis is usually asymptomatic. Calf vein thrombi were a common observation in the past, when the radiofibrinogen uptake test was used to detect DVT arising in patients undergoing general surgery (1). Subsequently, they have been encountered regularly both in the surgical (2,3) and in the medical field (4) in patients who undergo venography before discharge from hospital. The incidence of asymptomatic calf vein thrombi varies widely depending on the patient groups: it ranges from 5 to 30% in general surgery, approximates 15% in hospitalized medical patients and ranges from 40 to 70% in major orthopaedic surgery (5). Most of these thrombi form at or soon after operation, but many disappear because they undergo spontaneous lysis (6) or embolize into the pulmonary circulation where they undergo spontaneous lysis (7). Contrary to popular opinion, calf vein thrombi are associated with PE that is detected postoperatively by pulmonary perfusion scanning in 20–30% of asymptomatic patients who have a positive leg scan of the calf veins (7,8). These emboli are small, almost always asymptomatic and clinically unimportant. The long-term consequences of asymptomatic calf vein thrombosis are unknown but may not be entirely benign (9). Thus, a number of studies have investigated this problem and identified a history of hospital admission over the preceding 6 months as a major risk factor for the occurrence of DVT and PE in ambulatory patients who are seen at the emergency department with confirmed symptomatic VTE (10). It is possible that some of these patients have asymptomatic calf vein thrombosis when discharged from the hospital, which then extends and becomes symptomatic during convalescence at home (10). Whether untreated asymptomatic venous thrombi predispose to the postphlebitic syndrome is also debated (11,12).

Symptomatic calf vein thrombi are usually larger than asymptomatic ones and are important because they occur in 10–45% of symptomatic patients with proven venous thrombosis (13–15). The fate of symptomatic isolated calf DVT is most likely not different from that observed in symptomatic patients with proximal DVT (16). A 29% rate of symptomatic extension or recurrence has been reported for patients with symptomatic calf vein thrombosis if treated with an inadequate course of anticoagulants (17). This recurrence rate was prevented by a 3-month course of anticoagulant therapy (17). Therefore, patients with symptomatic calf vein thrombosis should be managed as usually recommended for those with proximal DVT (18). After discontinuing anticoagulation, patients with symptomatic DVT have a risk of recurrent VTE that is remarkably lower that that observed in patients with proximal DVT (19,20). Accordingly, the rate of late post-thrombotic sequelae is definitely lower (21).

CLINICAL COURSE OF THROMBOSIS INVOLVING THE PROXIMAL VEIN SYSTEM

Thrombosis involving the proximal vein system is usually symptomatic.

Patients with proximal vein thrombosis are usually treated with an initial course of heparin or low molecular weight heparin (LMWH) followed by 3–6 months of oral anticoagulant therapy (18). This treatment regimen reduces the risk for short-term thromboembolic complications to less than 5% (18).

In contrast with the extensive and uniform documentation on the short-term outcome of DVT, sparse and conflicting results are available about the long-term clinical course of this disease. Recurrent VTE and the post-thrombotic syndrome (PTS) are the most important complications of DVT. The cost implications of such complications are relevant (22).

Long-term recurrent VTE

Twelve years ago, we published the results of a prospective cohort study dealing with the long-term follow-up of more than 300 patients after their first episode of proximal DVT of the lower extremities, alone or associated with clinically symptomatic PE (23). All of them had received a short period of anticoagulation therapy, ranging from 3 to 6 months. The cumulative incidence of recurrent VTE was approximately 20% after 2 years, 25% after 5 years and 30% after 8 years. Overall, this risk was found to be considerably higher than previously thought. Among the investigated risk factors of recurrences, those associated with the highest hazard ratio were idiopathic presentation, malignancy and thrombophilia. As a consequence of this and other similar observations (19,24–29), in the last 10 years there has been an increasing tendency to prolong the duration of anticoagulation, adjusting it to individual risk profiles (18).

About 10 years later, we published the results of a new prospective cohort study, dealing with the long-term follow-up of more than 1600 patients with a first episode of DVT and/or PE recruited at several centres in Italy (30). We excluded from the evaluation patients with active cancer, and also all those with indications for indefinite anticoagulation. The analysis started at the time of

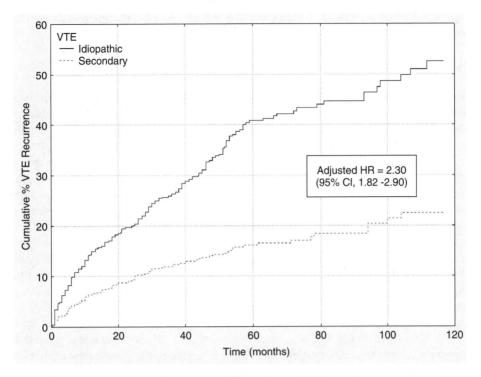

Figure 2.1 Cumulative incidence of recurrent VTE in patients with idiopathic and secondary DVT and/or PE. Reproduced with permission from Prandoni P, Noventa F, Ghirarduzzi A, *et al*. The risk of recurrent venous thromboembolism after discontinuing anticoagulation in patients with acute proximal deep vein thrombosis or pulmonary embolism. A prospective cohort study in 1626 patients. *Haematologica* 2007; **91**:199–205. © Ferrata Storti Foundation, 2007.

coumarin discontinuation. Surprisingly, in spite of the exclusion of patients with active cancer, the cumulative incidence of recurrent VTE was even higher than that reported 10 years earlier, approaching 30% after 5 years, 35% after 8 years and then increasing up to 40% after 10 years. As expected, the recurrence risk was twice higher in patients with idiopathic than in those with secondary thromboembolism (Figure 2.1). Thus, a lot of work still remains to be done in order to improve the long-term prognosis of these patients. Let us start by analysing the risk factors of recurrent VTE.

Persistent acquired risk factors

After stopping anticoagulation, patients with active cancer, especially those with metastatic malignancy and those undergoing chemotherapy, carry a particularly high risk of recurrent VTE (31), and so do patients with chronic medical diseases requiring prolonged immobilization (32). Although there is no conclusive evidence coming from randomized clinical trials, both patient categories should be treated with long-term anticoagulation therapy, consisting of low molecular weight heparins (LMWH) in patients with cancer (33–35) and of conventional oral anticoagulants in medical conditions other than neoplastic diseases (18).

Other conditions associated with a particularly high risk of recurrent VTE and, thus, requiring indefinite anticoagulation are multiple (especially if idiopathic) VTE episodes (36), the insertion of a permanent vena caval filter (whenever anticoagulation is not contraindicated) (37) and antiphospholipid syndrome (18). Whether these subjects require on a routine basis anticoagulation regimens, which are more intense than usual, is controversial (38–40).

Idiopathic presentation

As a result of an impressive series of prospective cohort, population-based and randomized clinical trials performed in recent years (19,20,23–30,41–44), probably the most important advance in the assessment of risk of recurrent VTE after anticoagulant therapy is stopped is recognition that patients whose thrombosis is provoked by a major reversible risk factor, such as surgery or major trauma, have a low risk of recurrence, whereas this risk becomes higher when thrombosis is provoked by a minor reversible risk factor, such as minor leg trauma, oestrogen therapy, pregnancy or puerperium or prolonged air travel, and is particularly high in patients with an idiopathic episode of proximal DVT and/or PE. Accordingly, patients with major transient risk factors, such as major trauma or surgery, should be given 12 weeks of anticoagulation therapy (18). In patients with minor transient risk factors, such as minor trauma, long air travel, pregnancy or puerperium or hormonal therapy, a longer duration may be considered according to each individual case (32). Patients presenting with a first episode of idiopathic proximal DVT should be offered 6–12 months of anticoagulation therapy (18). Whether low-dose warfarin may improve the benefit-to-risk ratio of prolonging anticoagulation is controversial (43,44).

In a recent prospective cohort study, we have shown that the persistence of residual thrombosis after an episode of proximal DVT as detected by repeated ultrasonography is an independent risk factor for recurrent thromboembolism (45). A similar prognostic value of the resolution of the thrombus was observed by others (46,47). Strategies that include such an assessment of thrombotic burden are intuitively attractive, since a patient can potentially be managed based on the individual course of his or her thrombotic disease, rather than by broad guidelines alone (48).

Following the demonstration that a marker of a thrombotic tendency (D-dimer) can be helpful in the risk stratification, and thus ultimately therapeutic guidance, of individual patients with DVT (28,49–51), Palareti *et al.* showed that patients with an abnormal D-dimer level one month after the discontinuation of anticoagulation need indefinite anticoagulation therapy (52). The optimal course of anticoagulation in patients with negative D-dimer level remains to be determined (52).

Inherited thrombophilia

Whether and to what extent carriers of inherited thrombophilia exhibit a higher risk of recurrent VTE is controversial. It is generally accepted, although not conclusively demonstrated, that carriers of antithrombin, protein C and S (53,54), carriers of hyperhomocysteinaemia (55,56), carriers of increased levels of factor VIII or IX (57–59), carriers of multiple abnormalities (29,30), homozygous carriers of factor V Leiden or prothrombin G20210A variant and heterozygous carriers of both mutations (60,61) have a recurrence risk that is higher than that of control subjects. Whether heterozygous carriers factor V Leiden or prothrombin G20210A variant also have a higher risk of recurrence is controversial, as there are data in favour (28,30,62–67) and against this association (27,29,41,43,60,61,68–70). Discrepancies among studies may be related to different selection of inception cohort, length of follow-up, initial treatment of the acute thrombotic disorder, duration of treatment and changes in general management of thrombotic patients (71). As a consequence, whether detection of these abnormalities, which are highly prevalent in western countries, has the potential to identify a subgroup of patients who might benefit from the adoption of individually adjusted prevention strategies following their first thrombotic episode is virtually unknown (18). As in recent years a good number of prospective cohort and randomized clinical trials have appeared, reporting on the long-term outcome of heterozygous carriers of either mutation after discontinuing

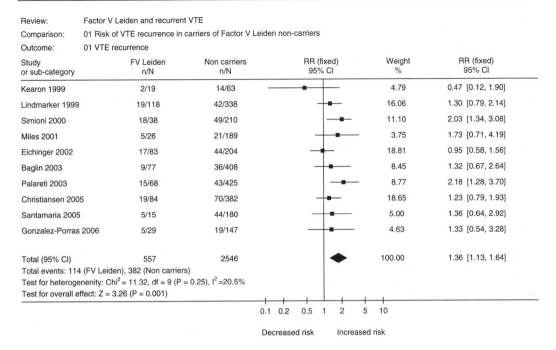

Figure 2.2 Risk of VTE recurrence in heterozygous carriers of FVL. Reproduced with permission from Marchiori A, Mosena L, Prins MH, Prandoni P. The risk of recurrent venous thromboembolism among heterozygous carriers of factor V Leiden or prothrombin G20210A mutation. A systematic review of prospective studies. *Haematologica* 2007; **92**:1107–14. © Ferrata Storti Foundation, 2007.

anticoagulation, we undertook the first systematic review and meta-analysis of available prospective investigations (72). According to the results of our meta-analysis, the heterozygous carriage of FVL confers a definitely increased risk of VTE recurrence (by about 40%), whereas the risk conferred by the heterozygous carriage of prothrombin mutation (PTM) is milder and statistically not significant (72) (Figures 2.2 and 2.3).

Further prospective studies addressing the role of thrombophilia in determining the risk of recurrent VTE are indicated, as are randomized studies addressing the benefit-to-risk ratio of prolonging anticoagulation in carriers of thrombophilic abnormalities.

Other factors

Recently, an unexpected association has been reported between male sex and recurrent VTE, especially in patients with idiopathic VTE (73).

In the recent literature, there are data in favour of (26,27,29,74–78) and against this association (23–25,28,79–81). In a prospective cohort study recently conducted in Italy in a broad cohort of patients, we could only find a slight and non-significant increase in the risk of recurrent VTE in men (30). Even when the analysis was confined to the only patients with idiopathic VTE, we could not show significant differences between men and women in this regard. Therefore, based on current evidence, we think that sex should not be regarded as a qualifying factor in deciding the duration of oral anticoagulant therapy after the first episode of thrombosis.

Old age, which has long been regarded as a risk factor of venous thrombosis (26), has recently been identified as a predictive factor of recurrent VTE (30). Thus, the common practice of

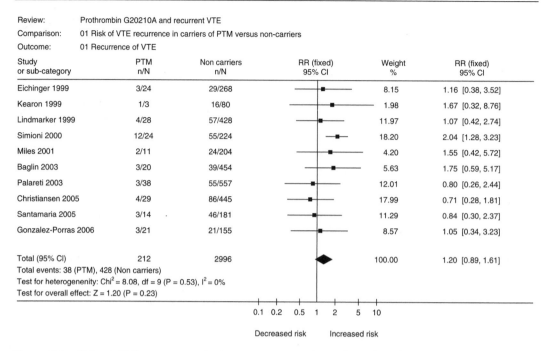

Review: Prothrombin G20210A and recurrent VTE
Comparison: 01 Risk of VTE recurrence in carriers of PTM versus non-carriers
Outcome: 01 Recurrence of VTE

Study or sub-category	PTM n/N	Non carriers n/N	RR (fixed) 95% CI	Weight %	RR (fixed) 95% CI
Eichinger 1999	3/24	29/268		8.15	1.16 [0.38, 3.52]
Kearon 1999	1/3	16/80		1.98	1.67 [0.32, 8.76]
Lindmarker 1999	4/28	57/428		11.97	1.07 [0.42, 2.74]
Simioni 2000	12/24	55/224		18.20	2.04 [1.28, 3.23]
Miles 2001	2/11	24/204		4.20	1.55 [0.42, 5.72]
Baglin 2003	3/20	39/454		5.63	1.75 [0.59, 5.17]
Palareti 2003	3/38	55/557		12.01	0.80 [0.26, 2.44]
Christiansen 2005	4/29	86/445		17.99	0.71 [0.28, 1.81]
Santamaria 2005	3/14	46/181		11.29	0.84 [0.30, 2.37]
Gonzalez-Porras 2006	3/21	21/155		8.57	1.05 [0.34, 3.23]
Total (95% CI)	212	2996		100.00	1.20 [0.89, 1.61]

Total events: 38 (PTM), 428 (Non carriers)
Test for heterogenenity: Chi^2 = 8.08, df = 9 (P = 0.53), I^2 = 0%
Test for overall effect: Z = 1.20 (P = 0.23)

0.1 0.2   0.5   1   2   5   10

Decreased risk   Increased risk

Figure 2.3 Risk of VTE recurrence in heterozygous carriers of prothrombin mutation. Reproduced with permission from Marchiori A, Mosena L, Prins MH, Prandoni P. The risk of recurrent venous thromboembolism among heterozygous carriers of factor V Leiden or prothrombin G20210A mutation. A systematic review of prospective studies. *Haematologica* 2007; **92**:1107–14. © Ferrata Storti Foundation, 2007.

administering old patients lower regimens or shorter periods of anticoagulation because of the fear of haemorrhagic complications should be reconsidered (82).

Women who had their first episode in fertile age are at a higher risk of experiencing recurrent thromboembolism when they are given hormonal treatment or become pregnant. This risk is particularly high in women in whom the first episode had been triggered by hormonal compounds or had developed during pregnancy (83–85).

Whether poor quality of vitamin K antagonists is an additional risk factor of recurrent VTE is controversial (86,87). Interestingly, a family history for VTE does not segregate patients into high- or low-risk categories and is not suitable to identify patients at increased risk for recurrent VTE (88). Obesity, which is a well-known risk factor of venous thrombosis (89,90), does not seem to increase the risk for recurrent VTE (30,91). Finally, it has recently been reported that a number of simple laboratory tests, such as the activated partial thromboplastin time (92) and global coagulation assays measuring thrombin generation (93,94), can help identify patients at a lower or higher risk of recurrent VTE. However, these findings need confirmation.

Post-thrombotic syndrome

At least one of every three patients with DVT of the lower extremities will develop within 5 years (severe) post-thrombotic sequelae. They vary from minor signs (e.g., stasis pigmentation, venous ectasia, slight pain and swelling) to severe manifestations such as chronic pain, intractable oedema and leg ulcer (95). The established PTS remains a significant cause of chronic illness, with considerable socio-economic consequences for both the patient and the healthcare services (96).

Incidence

The precise incidence of the PTS following confirmed DVT is still controversial, as the rate of PTS in the published studies has varied between 20% and 100% (23,24,97–124). In the earlier studies, a surprisingly high rate of severe PTS complications was reported (50–100% of the patients within 4–10 years after the qualifying thrombotic episode) (97–100). This rate decreased sharply in the studies performed in the last 20 years (23,24,101–124), most likely as the result of an improved diagnostic and therapeutic approach to patients with DVT. However, owing to large differences between studies in terms of design, definition of PTS, sample size and length of follow-up, the reported incidence of overall PTS still shows considerable variability, ranging between 20 and 50% of patients (of whom approximately one-fifth have severe manifestations).

According to the results of recent studies, most of the patients who developed post-thrombotic manifestations become symptomatic within 2 years from the acute episode of DVT (23,24,95, 121–124). These findings challenge the general view that the PTS requires a long time to become manifest.

Clinical diagnosis

The syndrome is characterized by aching pain on standing, dependent oedema and the frequent development of brawny, tender induration of the subcutaneous tissues of the medial lower limb, a condition that has been termed 'lipodermatosclerosis'. Pruritus and eczematous skin changes are frequently present and a proportion of patients develop secondary superficial varicose veins as the syndrome evolves. Ulceration, often precipitated by minor trauma, arises in a considerable number of patients and is characteristically chronic and indolent with a high recurrence rate, once healing has been achieved. Uncommonly, patients with persistent obstruction may experience venous claudication, a bursting pain in the leg during exercise, which, in some respects, mimics arterial claudication (125).

The clinical picture of the PTS is aspecific, as conditions other than DVT may result in a comparable set of signs and symptoms to those affecting the lower extremities of patients with a previous DVT, including superficial venous insufficiency, old age, increased body mass index and traumas (126–128).

The diagnosis of PTS is essentially based on the development of the above-mentioned clinical manifestations in patients with a history of DVT, irrespective of the presence of venous abnormalities, as shown by invasive or non-invasive diagnostic procedures. In the absence of signs and symptoms, the demonstration of venous abnormalities (such as venous reflux, persistent venous obstruction or both) does not allow one to define a patient with a history of DVT as having a PTS.

Although the picture of PTS is classical, there are large variations between published studies as to its clinical classification (129). Among the suggested scoring systems, the Villalta scale and the CEAP classification are the most widely adopted (Tables 2.1 and 2.2). The former, based on clinical findings alone, has a high inter-observer agreement (130) and a high sensitivity and specificity for discriminating patients with versus those without PTS and patients with mild versus those with severe PTS (130,131). In addition, this scale correlates well with the patient's perception of the interference of leg complaints with daily life (130,131). The latter, known as the CEAP (Clinical, Etiologic, Anatomic, Pathophysiologic) classification, emanates from the cooperative work of a panel of experts in the field of vascular disease and combines clinical and objective findings into a sophisticated scoring system (132).

Table 2.1 Standardized scale for the assessment of the post thrombotic syndrome: the villalta scale

Subjective symptoms[a]	Objective signs[a]
Heaviness	Pretibial oedema
Pain	Induration of the skin
Cramps	Hyperpigmentation
Pruritus	Venous ectasia
Paresthesia	Redness
	Pain during calf compression
	Ulceration of the skin

Definition of the post-thrombotic syndrome
Severe: score ≥15 at two consecutive visits at least 3 months apart or ulcer in one occasion
Mild to moderate: score between 5 and 14 at two consecutive visits
Absent: score less than 5

[a]Each sign or symptom was graded with a score of 0 (absent), 1 (mild), 2 (moderate) and 3 (severe). The presence or absence of leg ulcer was noted.

Table 2.2 Standardized scale for the assessment of the post-thrombotic syndrome: The CEAP classification

Class	Clinical signs
Class 0	No visible or palpable signs of venous disease
Class 1	Teleangiectases or reticular veins
Class 2	Varicose veins
Class 3	Oedema
Class 4	Skin changes ascribed to venous disease
Class 5	Skin changes as defined above with healed ulceration
Class 6	Skin changes as defined above with leg ulceration

Instrumental diagnosis

If a patient with a history of a previous (documented or highly suspected) DVT develops symptoms and signs compatible with PTS, there is no need for further investigation. As the clinical picture is aspecific (126–128), the need for objective confirmation arises in patients with leg complaints and without likely or proven history of DVT. Ascending phlebography is potentially useful to detect a previous DVT. Suggestive findings include narrowing or occlusion of the deep veins, contrast dye opacification of fewer veins (than normal) or perfusion of superficial or deep collateral veins. Recanalized veins show irregular margins, bizarre-appearing or multi-channelled lumen with webs and usually have reduced calibre due to fibrotic thickening of their walls. Such veins may subsequently become dilated, probably because of loss of their elastic tissue (133). Despite the predictive value of these venographic patterns in patients with possible PTS, the invasive nature and cost of plebography make such an approach inapplicable to most patients with a history of clinically suspected DVT.

We have shown that the combination of standardized clinical evaluation with compression ultrasonography and continuous-wave Doppler analysis can reliably diagnose or exclude a prior proximal vein thrombosis in almost 90% of patients with a suggestive history (134). Compression ultrasonography should be performed first, checking the popliteal and the common femoral veins for compressibility. If either or both veins are incompressible, then a definite diagnosis of previous (proximal) DVT is made. Patients with normal ultrasound test results are interviewed and examined according to a standardized form and subsequently undergo continuous-wave Doppler analysis to test valve function, both in the common femoral vein and in the popliteal vein. The finding of both a popliteal reflux and/or of a clinical score >8 is highly specific for the adjudication of a prior DVT in patients with a normal ultrasound test result. If ultrasound testing is normal, deep venous reflux is absent and the clinical score is <8, then previous proximal DVT is virtually excluded (134). The widespread availability of Duplex scanners renders our approach even more rapid and precise, as they allow for venous flow sampling during direct visualization of the vessels.

In addition to the demonstration of previous episodes of DVT, either invasive or non-invasive methods can be employed to document and quantify the presence of obstruction, reflux or both, that are considered the major determinants of PTS.

Pathophysiology and determinants of PTS development

It is generally believed that PTS develop as a result of the combination of venous hypertension, due to persistent outflow obstruction and/or valvular incompetence, with abnormal microvasculature or lymphatic function (135). Long-standing venous hypertension in the deep vein system ultimately leads to the onset of valve incompetence at the level of a constant series of perforating veins located in the medial ankle area. This allows the direct transmission of the high deep venous pressures (especially during walking) to the venous end of subcutaneous capillaries, resulting in increased endothelial permeability. Escape of large molecules into the interstitial tissue may, in turn, explain the typical pattern of oedema, hyperpigmentation and even ulcer formation (125–127). A few authors speculate that an increased venous pressure on standing or walking causes a reduction in capillary flow rate, resulting in trapping of white blood cells in the leg and the subsequent release of free radicals and proteolytic enzymes ultimately responsible for the venous ulceration (136,137).

The presence of reflux in the proximal veins is considered to be crucial for the development of PTS and so is the persistence of venous obstruction, alone or in combination with venous reflux (109,138–142). However, this is an area of great uncertainty. Recently, we determined the role of residual vein thrombosis and popliteal valve incompetence for the development of PTS, as assessed with the Villalta scale, in 180 consecutive patients who were followed for at least 3 years after an episode of acute proximal DVT (143). Venous abnormalities were searched for in the first 6 months following the thrombotic episode and were detected in 104 patients (60%). PTS developed in 18 of the 76 patients (24%) without vein abnormalities and in 49 of the 104 (47%) with at least one abnormality: in 25 of the 52 (48%) with residual vein thrombosis alone, in 9 of the 24 (37.5%) with popliteal valve incompetence alone and in 15 of the 28 (54%) with both abnormalities. The relative risk of PTS was 1.0 (95% CI, 0.5 to 2.2) in patients with popliteal valve incompetence alone; 1.4 (0.9 to 2.3) in patients with transpopliteal reflux alone or combined with persistent venous obstruction; 1.6 (1.0 to 2.4) in patients with residual vein thrombosis alone; and 1.7 (1.2 to 2.3) in patients with persistent venous obstruction alone or combined with popliteal valve incompetence.

Roumen-Klappe et al. assessed the role of residual thrombosis, reflux and venous outflow resistance in 93 patients with proximal and distal DVT, followed for 6 years; the incidence of PTS was 49% after 1 year and 55% after 2 years, without further increase up to 6 years; reflux had a moderate predictive value; a strong increase in the predictive value was obtained on combining measures of residual thrombus, assessed by a thrombosis score and venous outflow resistance, at 3 months (124). On the basis of these findings, the lack of recanalization within the first 6 months after the thrombotic episode appears to be an important predictor of PTS, whereas the development of transpopliteal venous reflux is not. However, incompetence of the popliteal valve increases the risk of PTS when combined with residual vein thrombosis (124,143).

Whether the initial extent of thrombosis and its degree of occlusiveness are related to the risk of developing PTS is controversial.

A strong relationship between ipsilateral DVT recurrence and the development of PTS has been reported by several authors (23,24,108,110,121). Other parameters that have shown to be associated with an increased risk of developing PTS are old age (121,144), obesity (144,145) and an insufficient quality of oral anticoagulant therapy following the acute thrombotic episode (144). Accordingly, an appropriate conduction of the oral anticoagulant therapy following the initial thrombotic episode in terms of both intensity and duration has the potential to help prevent late post-thrombotic sequelae.

CLINICAL COURSE OF PULMONARY EMBOLISM

The natural course of acute PE depends primarily on whether the embolism has been detected and (appropriately) treated. Among factors affecting the natural course of acute PE, the most important are the extent of embolic obstruction, the degree of haemodynamic severity, the previous state of the cardiopulmonary system, the age of the embolus and the degree of spontaneous thrombolytic activity of the patient's pulmonary vascular endothelium (146).

Mortality and other short-term adverse outcomes

It is generally acknowledged that most patients with PE who are adequately anticoagulated survive the acute episode (147). It should be noted, however, that most information comes from studies that have evaluated patients who survived at least a couple of hours after the onset of symptoms. Hence currently available mortality rates are likely to underestimate the true incidence of PE-related death (146,147). Mean mortality (1 month) rates of treated and untreated PE are 8 and 30%, respectively (148). Acute mortality is correlated with hypotension and right ventricular failure, as shown by echocardiography or other parameters of right ventricular dysfunction (149–152). Patients with pre-existing cardiac disease may not have sufficient right pump reserve to sustain an adequate cardiac output in the face of even a relatively small clot burden (149,153).

Recently, the results of an important prospective cohort study conducted in Spain have become available (154). This study included 1338 consecutive outpatients with objectively confirmed symptomatic PE who were followed up for 3 months after the start of anticoagulant therapy. The authors analysed the time course of death and other adverse events (non-fatal recurrences and non-fatal major bleeding) during the initial 3 months of follow-up. They also assessed and compared risk factors for early death (occurring within the first 7 days after diagnosis of PE) and late death. At 3 months, 142 patients had died, resulting in a cumulative rate of overall mortality of 11%. During the first 7 days, 36 of 1338 (25%) patients with PE died, 61% due to PE. On multivariate analysis, patients with systolic arterial hypotension exhibited a 6.7-fold risk of early death. Risk factors associated with long-term mortality were cancer, immobility and elevated troponin levels (154). These findings are consistent with those of two other cohort studies, one dealing with the clinical course of haemodynamically stable PE (155) and the other with that of PE patients regardless of the severity of their clinical presentation (156). Nijkeuter et al. were able to obtain information for a 3-month period in 673 patients (155). Of these patients, 20 (3.0%) had recurrent VTE. Eleven of 14 patients with recurrent PE had a fatal PE (79%), occurring mostly in the first week after diagnosis of initial PE. In 23 patients (3.4%) a haemorrhagic complication occurred, 10 of which were major bleeds (1.5%) and two were fatal (0.3%). During the 3-month follow-up, 55 patients died (8.2%). Risk factors for recurrent VTE were immobilization for >3 days and being an inpatient; having a chronic obstructive broncopneumopathy or malignancies were risk factors for bleeding. Higher age, immobilization, malignancy and being an inpatient were risk factors for mortality. In a cohort study published 15 years ago, which addressed the 1-year follow-up of a wide series of patients with angiographically proven PE, Carson *et al.* observed a mortality rate of 24%, most deaths being observed in an early phase (22% within a week) (156). The conditions associated with these deaths were cancer, left-sided congestive heart failure and chronic lung disease. The most frequent causes of death were cancer (35%), infection (22%) and cardiac disease (17%). Overall, 2.5% of patients deceased because of PE.

Among factors that have been associated with an unfavourable short-term outcome in patients with PE are echocardiographic findings. The risk of an unfavourable outcome seems definitely higher in patients with right ventricular dysfunction, as shown by echocardiography (150–152157–160). This view has prompted the use of thrombolysis also in patients with submassive PE, provided that they present echocardiographic findings suggestive of right ventricular dysfunction (161). This approach, however, requires caution (162). According to the results of two recent meta-analyses of comparative studies between thrombolysis and heparin in the treatment of acute PE, patients treated with thrombolytic drugs have a more favourable outcome in terms of prevention of short-term recurrent episodes of PE than those treated with heparin alone (163,164). However, mortality is not reduced and the risk of major bleeding is definitely enhanced (163,164). In addition, according to the results of a recent meta-analysis, echocardiographic findings appear to predict an increased mortality rate in patients with haemodynamically unstable PE, but not in those with stable clinical presentation (165).

Other factors that have been associated with increased mortality and/or other adverse short-term clinical outcomes are increased plasmatic levels of troponin I or T (166–175), increased levels of brain natriuretic peptides (176–179), particularly elevated D-dimer levels (180–182), and the severity of pulmonary arteries obstruction as assessed by objective tests performed at patients' referral (183,184). A few clinical scores have been proposed that help predict the outcome of patients with PE (185–190) (Tables 2.3 and 2.4).

Recurrent VTE

For most patients presenting with primary PE, factors that determine the risk for recurrent events do not differ from those described for patients with proximal vein thrombosis.

Table 2.3   Index of wicki for the determination of the severity of PE

Item	Score
Cancer	2
Heart failure	1
Previous venous thromboembolism	1
Blood pressure <100 mmHg	1
PaO$_2$ <60 mmHg	1
Ultrasound proven DVT	1
Categories of risk:	
Probability of favourable outcome	0–2
Probability of unfavourable outcome	3–7

Table 2.4 Index of aujesky for the determination of the severity of PE

Item	Score
Age	Years
Male sex	+10
Cancer	+30
Heart failure	+10
Chronic lung disease	+10
Pulse rate ≥110/min	+20
Systolic blood pressure <100 m Hg	+30
Respiratory rate>30/ min	+20
Body temperature <36°C	+20
Altered mental status	+60
Arterial oxyhaemoglobin saturation <90%	+20
Categories of risk:	
Very low	≤65
Low	66–85
Intermediate	86–105
High	106–125
Very high	>125

In a prospective study conducted in Austria, patients with clinically symptomatic PE were found to be associated with a significantly higher risk of recurrent events than those with symptomatic DVT not associated with PE (191). These findings, however, have not been confirmed by those from a prospective cohort investigation recently carried out at our institution in a much wider series of patients (30). In our study, the rate of recurrent VTE was significantly higher in patients with proximal DVT (alone or associated with clinically symptomatic PE) than in those with PE alone at presentation. Accordingly, there seems to be no reason to adopt systematically a longer duration of anticoagulation therapy in patients with PE than in those with DVT. Our results are consistent with those from a randomized controlled clinical trial, which failed to show an appreciable advantage of prolonging anticoagulation therapy beyond 5 months both in the subgroup of patients with idiopathic and in that of patients with secondary PE (192).

Interestingly, in both the Austrian and Italian cohorts (191,192), and also in a population-based study performed in California (193), patients with clinically symptomatic PE were found to be at a higher risk of recurrent PE than those with DVT alone. As PE is potentially more dangerous than DVT alone, long-term anticoagulation therapy may be considered in selected patients with idiopathic PE, at least in those presenting with life-threatening manifestations (32).

Whether the risk of recurrent VTE is enhanced in patients with persistent right ventricular dysfunction at hospital discharge (160) and in those with persistent residual thrombosis, as shown by repeat lung scanning over time (194), is worth investigating further.

Residual thrombosis and chronic thromboembolic pulmonary hypertension

Data regarding the degree and rate of PE resolution are conflicting. Pulmonary embolism resolves by at least three principal mechanisms: fragmentation, dissolution by endogenous fibrinolytic mechanism and recanalization. The processes of dissolution and recanalization are probably responsible for the late removal of embolic material, occurring within a few weeks following an acute episode.

Several studies using serial perfusion lung scans have documented progressive improvement in non-perfused lung segments with time, although the improvement rate is highly variable (155,194,195). The rate of improvement of perfusion scans is influenced by the severity of the embolic event, the type of the pharmacological treatment and the presence or absence of underlying cardiopulmonary disorders (196). Approximately 50% of patients with submassive PE still have persistent residual thrombosis after 6 months of therapy (197). Patients with large emboli or cardiopulmonary disorders exhibit a slower rate of scintigraphic recovery and, sometimes, the perfusion scan never returns to normal (198).

For reasons that are still unclear, the emboli in a few patients do not resolve completely; rather, they follow an aberrant path of organization and recanalization, leaving endothelialized residua that obstruct or significantly narrow major pulmonary arteries (199). Whether and to what extent residual thrombosis is associated with an increased risk of chronic thromboembolic pulmonary hypertension (CTPH) remain to be established.

The true incidence and prevalence of CTEPH are unknown. Originally, it was believed that 0.1–0.5% of patients who survive an episode of acute PE develop CTPH (199–201). However, in a prospective study of 78 survivors of acute PE, echocardiographic findings suggestive of persistent pulmonary hypertension and/or right ventricular dysfunction were present in 44% of the patients after 1 year (157). Four patients (5.1%) developed definite CTPH and three of these subsequently underwent successful pulmonary embolectomy. The only identifiable risk factors for persistent pulmonary hypertension were an age >70 years and a systolic pulmonary artery pressure >50 mmHg at the initial presentation. An echocardiogram at week 6 after diagnosis of an acute PE was capable of distinguishing between patients with persistent pulmonary hypertension and those with complete recovery (157).

Recently, we performed a prospective long-term follow-up cohort study to assess the incidence of symptomatic CTPH in consecutive patients with the first episode of acute PE (183). In addition, we performed a case–control analysis to assess risk factors for CTPH. For this purpose, we utilized also patients with prior PE. Cases were all PE patients who developed clinically symptomatic CTPH and controls were those PE patients who did not. Patients underwent a follow-up visit every 6 months for the first 2 years and then once yearly. The minimum follow-up was 6 months and the maximum 10 years. The cumulative incidence of symptomatic CTPH was 1.0% at 6 months, 3.1% at 1 year and 3.8% at 2 years. None of the patients with more than 2 years of follow-up developed this complication afterwards. Previous pulmonary embolism, younger age, larger perfusion defects and idiopathic presentation were independently associated with an increased risk of CTPH (183).

It has been appreciated for many years that CTPH may not be explained simply by pulmonary vascular obliteration due to unresolved thromboemboli. Persistent obstruction of pulmonary arteries may result in elevated pulmonary artery pressures and high shear stress in those areas of the pulmonary vasculature that were spared from thromboembolic occlusion. In that scenario, acute PE would be the initiating event, but progression of pulmonary hypertension would result from progressive pulmonary vascular remodelling, i.e., small-vessel disease. Both the extent of proximal occlusion of pulmonary arteries and secondary small-vessel arteriopathy contribute to the elevated pulmonary vascular resistance (202,203).

Several risk factors predisposing to the development of CTPH have been identified, including chronic inflammatory disorders, myeloproliferative syndromes, antiphospholipid syndrome, the presence of a ventriculoatrial shunt and splenectomy. The association with these distinct conditions suggests that chronic infection and/or chronic inflammatory disorders are involved in the pathogenesis of CTPH. This hypothesis is supported by numerous experimental findings showing that inflammation can cause a prothrombotic state and impair resolution of pulmonary thromboemboli (202,203).

Patients with CTEPH typically present in either of two scenarios (202,203):

1. Patients may complain of progressive dyspnea on exertion, haemoptysis and/or signs of right ventricular dysfunction including fatigue, palpitations, syncope or oedema after a single or recurrent episodes of overt PE. A 'honeymoon period' between the acute event and the development of clinical signs of CTEPH is common and may last from a few months to many years.
2. However, up to 63% of patients have no history of acute PE. In these patients, progressive dyspnea on exertion, rapid exhaustion and fatigue are the most common symptoms and the clinical course is often indistinguishable from other forms of severe pulmonary hypertension, especially idiopathic pulmonary arterial hypertension.

Physical signs are often subtle and may include a left parasternal heave, a prominent pulmonary component of S2 and a systolic murmur of trucuspidal regurgitation. A rare clinical finding that is virtually patognomonic for CTEPH is bruits over peripheral lung fields, typically over the lower lobes, which results from turbulent blood flow in partially occluded areas. According to most experts, these bruits can be found in approximately 10% of patients with CTEPH, making this sign one of low sensitivity but probably very high specificity. Signs of right heart failure occur late in the course of the disease and may signal a life-threatening situation (202,203).

The fact that many CTEPH patients have no history of acute PE together with uncertainties about the appropriate diagnostic approach to these patients contributes to a substantial rate of diagnostic misclassification in this patient population.

Echocardiography is widely used as the initial diagnostic tool when pulmonary hypertension is suspected and routine echocardiography 6 weeks after PE has been suggested for identifying patients at risk for developing CTPH (160). Imaging technologies including V/Q scanning, computed tomographic (CT) scanning, magnetic resonance imaging (MRI) and pulmonary angiography are a fundamental part of the diagnostic work-up of patients with suspected CTEPH (202,203).

Prior to current surgical techniques, the prognosis of CTPH was related to the degree of pulmonary hypertension, being extremely serious in all patients with mean pulmonary artery pressure >30 mmHg (198,199). Currently, thromboarteriectomy in selected patients has made this condition a potentially remediable one (199,200,202,203). That is why this condition is probably suspected and recognized more frequently today than in the past.

VTE AND THE RISK OF SUBSEQUENT MALIGNANT DISEASE

Patients with VTE have an increased risk over the general population of developing subsequent manifest cancer. According to the results of the most important studies, this risk has been consistently found to be 4–5 times as high in patients with idiopathic than in patients with secondary thrombosis (204). These data have recently found important confirmation in four very large, retrospective, population-based studies (205–208).

Of interest, although the risk for developing cancer was particularly high in the first 6 months after the diagnosis of VTE, a significant effect persisted for up to 10 years (205,206), suggesting that either a malignant disorder can induce hypercoagulability many years prior to its overt clinical development or that cancer and thrombosis share common risk factors. This view is further supported by the findings from a recent population-based study conducted in England and Scotland, dealing with more than 3000 consecutive men who received the annual determination of a few parameters of hypercoagulability for 4 years (209). Patients with persistent activation of the haemostatic pathway had a statistically significant increase in overall mortality, which was mainly dependent on the development of cancer, especially of the digestive tract. In addition, according to the results of a population-based study conducted in Denmark, in comparison with cancer patients without associated VTE, patients with cancer and associated VTE have a higher risk of development of a second malignancy (particularly in the upper gastrointestinal tract, ovary and prostate) (210). This risk is particularly high in those cancer patients in whom more than 1 year had elapsed between the diagnosis of the first cancer and the associated VTE complication. Finally, antithrombotic drugs have been reported to interfere with the development of cancer or with its evolution. In a prospective randomized study, Schulman and Lindmarker observed a significantly higher rate of cancer development over years in patients with idiopathic VTE who had been administered 6 weeks of anticoagulation therapy than in those who had received 6 months of anticoagulation therapy (211). A meta-analysis of four recent controlled studies (212–215) addressing the survival of cancer patients receiving various doses of LMWH for variable periods of time showed a favourable impact of these compounds on cancer survival regardless of cancer stage (216). Finally, a recent investigation has indeed provided direct genetic evidence for the link between oncogene activation and thrombosis (217).

Despite the conclusive evidence of a strong relationship between idiopathic VTE and the risk for hidden cancer, whether extensive screening for occult malignancy in patients with idiopathic VTE is appropriate is still controversial. Since extensive screening procedures are associated with high costs and themselves carry some morbidity, they are only acceptable if they prove to be cost-effective and have an impact on cancer-related mortality.

A recent publication has raised some concern about the utility of screening for occult malignancy all patients with idiopathic thromboembolism (218). By assessing the survival rate in patients with cancer diagnosed in the first year following the thrombotic episode in comparison with that of matched cancer patients without thrombosis, Sorensen *et al.* found increased mortality in the former group.

The same was true of cancers diagnosed at the time of hospitalization for venous thromboembolism. The results seem discouraging, as it appears that whenever a cancer disease is preceded by a clinical manifestation of thrombosis its prognosis is far worse. However, due to the retrospective nature of the study design, we suppose that the large majority of identified cancers were already symptomatic at the time of detection. The early detection of occult cancers at the time they are totally asymptomatic might still lead to a more favourable clinical outcome. Two adequate studies have recently addressed this issue (219,220).

Monreal and colleagues published the results of a prospective cohort follow-up study in consecutive patients with acute VTE (219). All patients underwent a routine clinical evaluation for malignancy, if negative followed by a limited diagnostic work-up consisting of abdominal and pelvic ultrasound and laboratory markers for malignancy. The routine clinical evaluation was performed in 864 patients and revealed malignancy in 34 (3.9%) of them. Among the remaining 830 patients, the limited diagnostic work-up revealed 13 further malignancies. During follow-up, cancer became symptomatic in 14 patients who were negative for cancer at screening (sensitivity of limited diagnostic work-up, 48%). Malignancies that were identified by the limited diagnostic work-up were early stage in 61% of cases versus 14% in cases occurring during follow-up. Most patients with occult cancer had idiopathic venous thromboembolism and were older than 70 years. According to these study results, a limited diagnostic work-up for occult cancer in patients with VTE has the capacity to identify approximately half of the malignancies, predominantly in an early stage.

We have recently conducted a multicentre randomized clinical trial (the SOMIT study) in apparently cancer-free patients with acute idiopathic venous thrombosis or pulmonary embolism (220). Of 201 patients with a first episode of idiopathic VTE, after initial negative routine battery tests

Table 2.5 Extensive screening procedure according to the SOMIT study

Procedure

- Ultrasound of abdomen/pelvis
- CT scanning of abdomen and pelvis
- Gastroscopy or double contrast barium swallowing
- Flexible sigmoidoscopy or rectoscopy followed by barium enema or colonoscopy
- Haemoccult, sputum cytology, tumour markers (CEA, αFP, CA125)
- Mammography and pap-smear in women
- Transabdominal ultrasound of the prostate and PSA in men

99 were randomized to undergo either extensive screening (Table 2.5) and 102 no further testing for malignancy. All patients were followed until the completion of 2 years of follow-up. Of the 14 malignancies that occurred in the extensive screening group, the screening was able to detect 13 (mostly detected by CT scanning), resulting in sensitivity higher than 90%. The risk for occult cancer was higher among elderly patients and in those without thrombophilic abnormalities. Ten malignancies developed in the follow-up of patients allocated to the control group. Overall, malignancies identified in the extensive screening group were at an earlier stage and the mean delay to diagnosis was reduced from 11 months to 1 month. The earlier discovery and subsequent treatment resulted in a slightly improved cancer-related mortality (2.0% vs 3.9%) and cancer-free survival (5.1% vs 7.9%) of the patients in the extensive screening group. Although these differences were not statistically significant, the reductions observed are in line with the hypothesis and would translate into a number needed to screen of only 50 patients to prevent one cancer-related death at 2 years. The strategy that was associated with the highest cost-effectiveness ratio included abdominal/pelvic CT with or without mammography and/or sputum cytology (221).

Although data from either study do not conclusively demonstrate that early diagnosis ultimately prolongs life, the collective observations make such a beneficial effect likely. The earlier discovery of cancer, which might mean identification of the disease at an attackable state, may be crucial in an unpredictable number of patients, especially nowadays when continuous protocol innovations are providing growing chances of success and eradication of malignancies.

AN ASSOCIATION BETWEEN VTE AND SUBSEQUENT SYMPTOMATIC ATHEROSCLEROSIS

Recently, an unexpected association of VTE with atherosclerosis was found (222).

Whereas subclinical atherosclerosis does not seem to be predictive of VTE (223,224), the opposite is likely true, as seven recent studies consistently showed an increased risk of subsequent symptomatic atherosclerosis and arterial cardiovascular events in patients with previous VTE (76,225–229). This risk seems higher in patients who have an apparently unprovoked VTE episode (225,226) and in those with residual thrombus on follow-up ultrasound scan (229).

These findings have several implications for both research and medical practice. Patients with VTE of unknown origin could be examined for asymptomatic atherosclerosis, in order to modify aggressively the risk profile in those with abnormal test results. Measures could include appropriate counselling about lifestyle changes and control of risk factors for atherosclerosis, and also primary prophylaxis with antiplatelet therapy or statins. Not surprisingly, a diet including more plant food and fish and less red and processed meat has recently been found to be associated with a lower incidence of VTE (230). Interest in statins has increased, given recent data that suggest a potential role both in controlling the development of atherosclerotic lesions and in lowering the risk of venous thromboembolism (231). As far as aspirin is concerned, data on the long-term management of VTE will be provided by two twin studies currently ongoing in Italy (Warfasa) and in Australia and New Zealand (Aspire) (232). Both studies are aimed at assessing the clinical benefit of 100 mg of aspirin given after the completion of anticoagulant treatment in patients with a first episode of unprovoked VTE.

The separate nature of arterial and venous disorders has been challenged. Further studies are needed to clarify the nature of this association, to assess its extent and to evaluate its implications for clinical practice.

REFERENCES

1. Lensing AWA, Hirsh J. ^{125}I-fibrinogen leg scanning: reassessment of its role for the diagnosis of venous thrombosis in post-operative patients. *Thromb Haemost* 1993; **69**:2–7.
2. Quinlan DJ, Eikelboom JW, Dahl OE, Eriksson BI, Sidhu PS, Hirsh J. Association between asymptomatic deep-vein thrombosis detected by venography and symptomatic venous thromboembolism in patients undergoing elective hip or knee surgery. *J Thromb Haemost* 2007; **5**:1438–43.
3. Enoxacan Study group. Efficacy and safety of enoxaparin versus unfractionated heparin for prevention of deep vein thrombosis in elective cancer surgery: a double-blind randomized multicentre trial with venographic assessment. *Br J Surg* 1997; **84**:1099–103.
4. Samama M, Cohen AT, Darmon JY, *et al*. A comparison of enoxaparin with placebo for the prevention of venous thromboembolism in acutely ill medical patients. *N Engl J Med* 1999; **341**:793–800.
5. Geerts WH, Pineo GF, Heit JA, *et al*. Prevention of venous thromboembolism: the seventh ACCP conference on antithrombotic and thrombolytic therapy. *Chest* 2004; **126**: 338–400S.
6. Kakkar VV, Flank C, Howe CT, *et al*. Natural history of postoperative deep vein thrombosis. *Lancet* 1969; **ii**:230–3.
7. Browse NL, Lea Thomas M. Source of non-lethal pulmonary emboli. *Lancet* 1974; **i**:258–9.
8. Doyle DJ, Turpie AGG, Hirsh J, *et al*. Adjusted subcutaneous heparin or continuous intravenous heparin in patients with acute deep vein thrombosis. *Ann Intern Med* 1987; **107**:441–5.
9. Hirsh J, Lensing AWA. Natural history of minimal calf deep vein thrombosis. In Bernstein EF (ed), *Vascular Diagnosis*. CV Mosby, St. Louis, 1993, pp.779–81.
10. Anderson FA, Wheeler HB, Goldberg RJ, *et al*. A population-based perspective of the hospital incidence and case-fatality rates of deep vein thrombosis and pulmonary embolism. The Worcester DVT study. *Arch Intern Med* 1991; **151**:933–8.
11. Lonner JH, Frank J, McGuire K, Lotke PA. Postthrombotic syndrome after asymptomatic deep vein thrombosis following total knee and hip arthroplasty *Am J Orthop* 2006; **35**:469–72.
12. Schindler OS, Dalziel R. Post-thrombotic syndrome after total hip or knee arthroplasty: incidence in patients with asymptomatic deep venous thrombosis. *J Orthop Surg* 2005; **13**:113–9.
13. Cogo A, Lensing AWA, Prandoni P, Hirsh J. Distribution of thrombosis in patients with symptomatic deep vein thrombosis. Implications for simplifying the diagnostic approach with compression ultrasound. *Arch Intern Med* 1993; **153**:2777–80.
14. Markel A, Manzo RA, Bergelin RO, Strandness D. Pattern and distribution of thrombi in acute venous thrombosis. *Arch Surg* 1992; **127**:305–9.
15. Mattos MA, Melendres G, Sumner DS, *et al*. Prevalence and distribution of calf vein thrombosis in patients with symptomatic deep venous thrombosis: a color-flow duplex study. *J Vasc Surg* 1996; **24**:738–44.
16. Philbrick JT, Becker DM. Calf deep venous thrombosis. A wolf in sheep's clothing? *Arch Intern Med* 1988; **148**:2131–8.
17. Lagerstedt CJ, Olsson CG, Fagher BO, Oqvist BW, Albrechtsson U. Need for long-term anticoagulant treatment in symptomatic calf-vein thrombosis. *Lancet* 1985; **ii**:515–8.
18. Büller HR, Agnelli G, Hull RD, Hyers TM, Prins MH, Raskob GE. Antithrombotic therapy for venous thromboembolic disease: The Seventh ACCP Conference on Antithrombotic and Thrombolytic Therapy. *Chest* 2004; **126**: 401–28S.

19. Schulman S, Rhedin AS, Lindmarker P, *et al*. A comparison of six weeks with six months of oral anticoagulant therapy after a first episode of venous thromboembolism. *N Engl J Med* 1995; **332**:1661–5.

20. Pinede L, Ninet J, Duhaut P, *et al*. Comparison of 3 and 6 months of oral anticoagulant therapy after a first episode of proximal deep vein thrombosis or pulmonary embolism and comparison of 6 and 12 weeks of therapy after isolated calf deep vein thrombosis. *Circulation* 2001; **103**:2453–60.

21. Mohr DN, Silverstein MD, Heit JA, Petterson TM, O'Fallon M, Melton LJ. The venous stasis syndrome after deep venous thrombosis or pulmonary embolism: a population-based study. *Mayo Clin Proc* 2000; **75**:1249–56.

22. Bergqvist D, Jendteg S, Johansen L, Persson U, Ödegaard K. Cost of long-term complications of deep venous thrombosis of the lower extremities: an analysis of a defined patient population in Sweden. *Ann Intern Med* 1997; **126**:454–7.

23. Prandoni P, Lensing AWA, Cogo A, *et al*. The long-term clinical course of acute deep venous thrombosis. *Ann Intern Med* 1996; **125**:1–7.

24. Prandoni P, Villalta S, Bagatella P, *et al*. The clinical course of deep-vein thrombosis. Prospective long-term follow-up of 528 symptomatic patients. *Haematologica* 1997; **82**:423–8.

25. Hansson PO, Sorbo J, Eriksson H. Recurrent venous thromboembolism after deep vein thrombosis. Incidence and risk factors. *Arch Intern Med* 2000; **1260**:769–74.

26. Heit JA, Mohr DN, Silverstein MD, Petterson TM, O'Fallon WM, Melton III LJ. Predictors of recurrence after deep vein thrombosis and pulmonary embolism. A population-based cohort study. *Arch Intern Med* 2000; **160**:761–8.

27. Baglin T, Luddington R, Brown K, Baglin C. Incidence of recurrent venous thromboembolism in relation to clinical and thrombophilic risk factors: prospective cohort study. *Lancet* 2003; **362**: 523–6.

28. Palareti G, Legnani C. Cosmi B, *et al*. Predictive value of D-dimer test for recurrent venous thromboembolism after anticoagulation withdrawal in subjects with a previous idiipathic event and in carriers of congenital thrombophilia. *Circulation* 2003; **108**:313–8.

29. Christiansen SC, Cannegieter SC, Koster T, Vandenbroucke JP, Rosendaal FR. Thrombophilia, clinical factors and recurrent venous thrombotic events. *JAMA* 2005; **293**:2352–61.

30. Prandoni P., Noventa F., Ghirarduzzi A., *et al*. The risk of recurrent venous thromboembolism after discontinuing anticoagulation in patients with acute proximal deep vein thrombosis or pulmonary embolism. A prospective cohort study in 1626 patients. *Haematologica* 2007; **91**:199–205.

31. Prandoni P, Falanga A, Piccioli A. Cancer and venous thromboembolism. *Lancet Oncol* 2005; **6**:401–10.

32. Kearon C. Long-term management of patients after venous thromboembolism. *Circulation* 2004; **110**(Suppl. 1):10–8.

33. Lee AY, Levine MN, Baker RI, *et al*. Low-molecular-weight heparin versus a coumarin for the prevention of recurrent venous thromboembolism in patients with cancer. *N Engl J Med* 2003; **349**:146–53.

34. Meyer G, Marjanovic Z, Valcke J, *et al*. Comparison of low-molecular-weight heparin and warfarin for the secondary prevention of venous thromboembolism in patients with cancer. *Arch Intern Med* 2002; **162**:1729–35.

35. Hull RD, Pineo GF, Brant RF, *et al*. Long-term low-molecular-weight heparin versus usual care in proximal-vein thrombosis patients with cancer. *Am J Med* 2006; **119**:1062–72.

36. Schulman S, Granqvist S, Holmstrom M *et al*. The duration of oral anticoagulant therapy after a second episode of venous thromboembolism. *N Engl J Med* 1997; **336**:393–8.

37. Decousus H, Leizorovicz A, Parent F, *et al*. A clinical trial of vena cava filters in the prevention of pulmonary embolism in patients with proximal deep-vein thrombosis. *N Engl J Med* 1998; **338**:409–15.

38. Khamashta MA, Cuadrado MJ, Mujic F, Taub NA, Hunt BJ, Hughes GRV. The management of thrombosis in the antiphospholipid-antibody syndrome. *N Engl J Med* 1995; **332**:993–7.

39. Crowther MA, Ginsberg JS, Julian J, *et al*. A comparison of two intensities of warfarin for the prevention of recurrent thrombosis in patients with the antiphospholipid antibody syndrome. *N Engl J Med* 2003; **349**:1133–8.

40. Finazzi G, Marchioli R, Brancaccio V, *et al*. A randomized clinical trial of high-intensity warfarin vs. conventional antithrombotic therapy for the prevention of recurrent thrombosis in patients with the antiphospholipid syndrome. *J Thromb Haemost* 2005; **3**:848–53.

41. Kearon C, Gent M, Hirsh J *et al*. A comparison of three months of anticoagulation with extended anticoagulation for a first episode of idiopathic venous thromboembolism. *N Engl J Med* 1999; **340**:901–7.

42. Agnelli G, Prandoni P, Santamaria MG, *et al*. Three months versus one year of oral anticoagulant therapy for idiopathic deep venous thrombosis. *N Engl J Med* 2001; **345**:165–9.

43. Ridker PM, Goldhaber SZ, Danielson E, *et al*. Long-term, low-intensity warfarin therapy for the prevention of recurrent venous thromboembolism. *N Engl J Med* 2003; **348**:1425–34.

44. Kearon C, Ginsberg JS, Kovacs MJ, *et al*. Comparison of low-intensity warfarin therapy with conventional-intensity warfarin therapy for long-term prevention of recurrent venous thromboembolism. *N Engl J Med* 2003; **349**:631–9.

45. Prandoni P, Lensing AWA, Prins MH, *et al*. Residual venous thrombosis as a predictive factor of recurrent venous thromboembolism. *Ann Intern Med* 2002; **137**:955–60.

46. Piovella F, Crippa L, Barone M, *et al*. Normalization rates of compression ultrasonography in patients with a first episode of deep vein thrombosis of the lower limbs: association with recurrence and new thrombosis. *Haematologica* 2002; **87**:515–22.

47. Young L, Ockelford P, Milne D, Rolfe-Vyson V, McKelvie S, Harper P. Post treatment residual thrombus increases the risk of recurrent deep vein thrombosis and mortality. *J Thromb Haemost* 2006; **4**:1919–24.

48. Prandoni P, Prins MH, Lensing AWA, *et al*. Ultrasound findings to guide the duration of anticoagulation in patients with deep-vein thrombosis. *Ann Intern Med* in press.

49. Palareti G, Legnani C, Cosmi B, Guazzaloca G, Pancani C, Coccheri S. Risk of venous thromboembolism recurrence: high negative predictive value of D-dimer performed after oral anticoagulation is stopped. *Thromb Haemost* 2002; **87**:7–12.

50. Eichinger S, Minar E, Bialonczyk C, *et al*. D-dimer levels and risk of recurrent venous thromboembolism. *JAMA* 2003; **290**:1071–4.

51. Fattorini A, Crippa L, Viganò D'Angelo S, Pattarini E, D'Angelo A. Risk of deep vein thrombosis recurrence: high negative predictive value of D-dimer performed during oral anticoagulation. *Thromb Haemost* 2002; **88**:162–3.

52. Palareti G, Cosmi B, Legnani C, *et al*. D-dimer testing to determine the duration of anticoagulation therapy. *N Engl J Med* 2006; **355**:1780–9.

53. van den Belt AG, Sanson BJ, Simioni P, *et al*. Recurrence of venous thromboembolism in patients with familial thrombophilia. *Arch Intern Med* 1997; **157**:2227–32.

54. De Stefano V, Simioni P, Rossi E, *et al*. The risk of recurrent venous thromboembolism in patients with inherited deficiency of natural anticoagulants antithrombin, protein C and protein S. *Haematologica* 2006; **91**:695–8.

55. den Heijer M, Blom HJ, Gerrits WB, Rosendaal FR, Wijermans PW, Bos GM. Is hyperhomocysteinaemia a risk factor for recurrent venous thrombosis? *Lancet* 1995; **345**:882–5.

56. Eichinger S, Stümpflen A, Hirschl M, *et al*. Hyperhomocysteinemia is a risk factor of recurrent venous thromboembolism. *Thromb Haemost* 1998; **80**:566–9.

57. Kyrle PA, Minar E, Hirschl M, *et al*. High plasma levels of factor VIII and the risk of recurrent venous thromboembolism. *N Engl J Med* 2000; **343**:457–62.

58. Legnani C, Cosmi B, Cini M, Frascaro M, Guazzaloca G, Palareti G. High plasma levels of factor VIII and risk of recurrence of venous thromboembolism. *Br J Haematol* 2004; **124**:504–10.

59. Weltermann A, Eichinger S, Bialonczyk C, *et al*. The risks of recurrent venous thromboembolism among patients with high factor IX levels. *J Thromb Haemost* 2003; **1**:28–32.

60. De Stefano V, Martinelli I, Mannucci PM, *et al*. The risk of recurrent deep venous thrombosis among heterozygous carriers of both factor V Leiden and the G20210 prothrombin mutation. *N Engl J Med* 1999; **341**:801–6.

61. Margaglione M, D'Andrea G, Colaizzo D, *et al*. Coexistence of factor V Leiden and factor II A20210 mutations and recurrent venous thromboembolism. *Thromb Haemost* 1999; **82**:1583–7.

62. Simioni P, Prandoni P, Lensing AWA, *et al*. The risk of recurrent venous thromboembolism in patients with an Arg506–Gln mutation in the gene for factor V (factor V Leiden). *N Engl J Med* 1997; **336**:399–403.

63. Simioni P, Prandoni P, Lensing AWA, *et al*. Risk for subsequent venous thromboembolic complications in carriers of the prothrombin or the factor V gene mutation with a first episode of deep-vein thrombosis. *Blood* 2000; **96**:3329–33.

64. Ridker PM, Miletich P, Stampfer MJ, *et al*. Factor V Leiden and risks of recurrent idiopathic venous thromboembolism. *Circulation* 1995; **91**:2800–2.

65. Miles JS, Miletich JP, Goldhaber SZ, Hennekens CH, Ridker PM. G20210A mutation in the prothrombin gene and the risk of recurrent venous thromboembolism. *J Am Coll Cardiol* 2001; **37**:215–8.

66. Santamaria MG, Agnelli G, Taliani MR, *et al*. Thrombophilic abnormalities and recurrence of venous thromboembolism in patients treated with standardized anticoagulant treatment. *Thromb Res* 2005; **116**:301–6.

67. Ho WK, Hankey G, Quinlan DJ, Eikelboom J. Risk of recurrent venous thrombembolism in patients with common thrombophilia. *Arch Intern Med* 2006; **166**:729–36.
68. Eichinger S, Pabinger I, Stümpflen A, *et al*. The risk of recurrent venous thromboembolism in patients with and without factor V Leiden. *Thromb Haemost* 1997; **77**:624–8.
69. Eichinger S., Minar E., Hirschl M., *et al*. The risk of early recurrent venous thromboembolism after oral anticoagulant therapy in patients with the G20210A transition in the prothrombin gene. *Thromb Haemost* 1999; **81**:14–7.
70. Lindmarker P, Schulman S, Sten-Linder M, *et al*. The risk of recurrent venous thromboembolism in carriers and non-carriers of the G1691A allele in the coagulation factor V gene and the G20210A allele in the prothrombin gene. *Thromb Haemostas* 1999; **81**:684–9.
71. Simioni P, Tormene D, Spiezia L, *et al*. Inherited thrombophilia and venous thromboembolism. *Semin Thromb Hemost* 2006; **32**:700–8.
72. Marchiori A., Mosena L., Prins M. H., Prandoni P. The risk of recurrent venous thromboembolism among heterozygous carriers of factor V Leiden or prothrombin G20210A mutation. A systematic review of prospective studies. *Haematologica* 2007; **92**:1107–14.
73. Kyrle PA, Minar E, Bialonczyk C, Hirschl M, Weltermann A, Eichinger S. The risk of recurrent venous thromboembolism in men and women. *N Engl J Med* 2004; **350**:2558–63.
74. Nieto JA, Monreal M. Recurrent venous thromboembolism in men and women. *N Engl J Med* 2004; **351**:2015–8.
75. Eriksson H, Lundström T, WÅhlander K, Billing Clason S, Schulman S. Prognostic factors for recurrence of venous thromboembolism (VTE) or bleeding during long-term secondary prevention of VTE with ximelagatran. *Thromb Haemost* 2005; **94**:522–7.
76. Schulman S, Lindmarker P, Holmstrom M, *et al*. Post-thrombotic syndrome, recurrence and death 10 years after the first episode of venous thromboembolism treated with warfarin for 6 weeks or 6 months. *J Thromb Haemost* 2006; **4**:734–42.
77. McRae S, Tran H, Schulman S, Ginsberg J, Kearon C. Effect of patient's sex on risk of recurrent venous thromboembolism: a meta-analysis. *Lancet* 2006; **368**:371–8.
78. Cushman M, Glynn RJ, Goldhaber SZ, *et al*. Hormonal factors and risk of recurrent venous thrombosis: the prevention of recurrent venous thromboembolism trial. *J Thromb Haemost* 2006; **4**:2199–203.
79. Murin S, Romano PS, White RH. Comparison of outcomes after hospitalization for deep venous thrombosis or pulmonary embolism. *Thromb Haemost* 2002; **88**:407–14.
80. Agnelli G, Becattini C, Prandoni P. Recurrent venous thromboembolism in men and women. *N Engl J Med* 2004; **351**:2015–8.
81. Gonzalez-Porras JR, Garcia-Sanz R, Alberca I, *et al*. Risk of recurrent venous thrombosis in patients with G20210A mutation in the prothrombin gene or factor V Leiden mutation. *Blood Coagul Fibrinolysis* 2006; **17**:23–8.
82. Lopez-Jimenez L, Montero M, Gonzalez-Fajardo JA, *et al*. Venous thromboembolism in very elderly patients: findings from a prospective registry. *Haematologica* 2006; **91**:1046–51.
83. Hoibraaten E, Qvigstad E, Arnesen H, Larsen S, Wickstrom E, Sandset PM. Increased risk of recurrent venous thromboembolism during hormone replacement therapy – results of the randomized, double-blind, placebo-controlled oestrogen in venous thromboembolism trial. *Thromb Haemost* 2000; **84**:961–7.
84. Pabinger I, Grafenhofer H, Kaider A, *et al*. Risk of pregnancy-associated recurrent venous thromboembolism in women with a history of venous thrombosis. *J Thromb Haemost* 2005; **3**:949–54.
85. De Stefano V, Martinelli I, Rossi E, *et al*. The risk of recurrent venous thromboembolism in pregnancy and puerperium without antithrombotic prophylaxis. *Br J Haematol* 2006; **135**:386–91.
86. Palareti G, Legnani C, Cosmi B, Guazzaloca G, Cini M, Mattarozzi S. Poor anticoagulation quality in the first 3 months after unprovoked venous thromboembolism is a risk factor for long-term recurrence. *J Thromb Haemost* 2005; **3**:955–61.
87. Prandoni P, Van Dongen CJJ, Hutten BA, Dalla Valle, Pesavento R, Prins MH. Quality of anticoagulant treatment and risk of subsequent recurrent thromboembolism in patients with deep venous thrombosis. *J Thromb Haemost* 2007; **5**: 1555–.
88. Hron G, Eichinger S, Weltermann A, *et al*. Family history for venous thromboembolism and the risk for recurrence. *Am J Med* 2006; **119**:50–3.
89. Stein PD, Beemath A, Olson RE. Obesity as a risk factor in venous thromboembolism. *Am J Med* 2005; **118**:978–80.
90. Glynn RJ, Rosner B. Comparison of risk factors for the competing risks of coronary heart disease, stroke and venous thromboembolism. *Am J Epidemiol* 2005; **162**:975–82.

91. Romualdi E, Squizzato A, Ageno W. Abdominal obesity and the risk of recurrent deep vein thrombosis. *Thromb Res* 2007; **119**:687–90.

92. Grand'maison A, Bates SM, Johnston M, McRae S, Ginsberg JS. 'ProC Global': a functional screening test that predicts recurrent venous thromboembolism. *Thromb Haemost* 2005; **93**:600–4.

93. Hron G, Kollars M, Binder BR, Eichinger S, Kyrle PA. Identification of patients at low risk for recurrent venous thromboembolism by measuring thrombin generation. *JAMA* 2006; **296**:397–402.

94. Hron G, Eichinger S, Weltermann A, Quehenberger P, Halbmayer WM, Kyrle PA. Prediction of recurrent venous thromboembolism by the activated partial thromboplastin time. *J Thromb Haemost* 2006; **4**:752–6.

95. Kahn SR, Ginsberg JS. Relationship between deep venous thrombosis and the postthrombotic syndrome. *Arch Intern Med* 2004; **164**:17–26.

96. Bergqvist D, Jendteg S, Johansen L, Persson U, Ödegaard K. Cost of long term complications of deep venous thrombosis of the lower extremities: an analysis of a defined patient population in Sweden. *Ann Intern Med* 1997; **126**:454–7.

97. Bauer G. Roentgenological and clinical study of the sequelae of thrombosis. *Acta Chir Scand* 1942; **86**(Suppl 74):1–110.

98. Gjores JE. The incidence of venous thrombosis and its sequelae in certain districts of Sweden. *Acta Chir Scand* 1956; **206**(Suppl 1):1–88.

99. O'Donnell TF, Browse NL, Burnand KG, Lea Thomas M. The socioeconomic effects of an ilio-femoral venous thrombosis. *J Surg Res* 1977; **22**:483–8.

100. Shull KC, Nicolaides AN, Fernandes JF, *et al*. Significance of popliteal reflux in relation to ambulatory venous pressure and ulceration. *Arch Surg* 1979; **114**:1304–6.

101. Strandness DE, Langlois Y, Cramer M, Randlett A, Thiele BL. Long-term sequelae of acute venous thrombosis. *JAMA* 1983; **250**:1289–92.

102. Widmer LK, Zemp E, Widmer T, *et al*. Late results in deep vein thrombosis of the lower extremity. *Vasa* 1985; **14**:264–8.

103. Lindner DJ, Edwards JM, Phinney ES, Taylor LM, Porter JM. Long-term hemodynamic and clinical sequelae of lower extremity deep vein thrombosis. *J Vasc Surg* 1986; **4**:436–42.

104. Heldal M, Seem E, Snadset PM, Abildgaard U. Deep vein thrombosis: a 7-year follow-up study. *J Intern Med* 1993; **234**:71–5.

105. Lagerstedt C, Olsson CG, Fagher B, Norgren L, Tengborn L. Recurrence and late sequelae after first-time deep vein thrombosis. Relationship to initial signs. *Phlebology* 1993; **8**:62–7.

106. Monreal M, Martorell A, Callejas JM, *et al*. Venographic assessment of deep vein thrombosis and risk of developing post-thrombotic syndrome: a prospective study. *J Intern Med* 1993; **233**:854–9.

107. Eichlisberger R, Frauchiger B, Widmer MT, Widmer LK, Jager K. Late sequelae of deep venous thrombosis: a 13-year follow-up of 223 patients. *Vasa* 1994; **23**:234–43.

108. Beyth RJ, Cohen AM, Landefeld CS. Long-term outcomes of deep-vein thrombosis. *Arch Intern Med* 1995; **155**:1031–7.

109. Johnson BF, Manzo RA, Bergelin RO, Strandness DE. Relationship between changes in the deep venous system and the development of the postthrombotic syndrome after an acute episode of lower limb deep vein thrombosis: a one- to six-year follow-up. *J Vasc Surg* 1995; **21**:307–13.

110. Saarinen J, Sisto T, Laurikka J, Salenius JP, Tarkka M. Late sequelae of acute deep venous thrombosis: evaluation five and ten years after. *Phlebology* 1995; **10**:106–9.

111. Franzeck UK, Schalch I, Jäger KA, Schneider E, Grimm J, Bollinger A. Prospective 12-year follow-up study of clinical and haemodinamic sequelae after deep vein thrombosis in low-risk patients (Zürich study). *Circulation* 1996; **93**: 74–9.

112. Brandjes DPM, Büller HR, Heijboer H, Huisman MV, de Rijk M, Jagt H. Randomised trial of effect of compression stockings in patients with symptomatic proximal-vein thrombosis. *Lancet* 1997; **349**:759–62.

113. Biguzzi E, Mozzi E, Alatri A, Taioli E, Moia M, Mannucci PM. The post-thrombotic syndrome in young women: retrospective evaluation of prognostic factors. *Thromb Haemost* 1998; **80**:575–7.

114. Masuda EM, Kessler DM, Kistner RL, Eklof B, Sato DT. The natural history of calf vein thrombosis: lysis of thrombi and development of reflux. *J Vasc Surg* 1998; **28**:67–74.

115. McLafferty RB, Moneta GL, Passmann MA, Brant BM, Taylor LM, Porter JM. Late clinical and hemodynamic sequelae of isolated calf vein thrombosis. *J Vasc Surg* 1998; **27**:50–7.

116. Haenen JH, Janssen MCH, van Langen H, *et al*. The postthrombotic syndrome in relation to venous hemodynamics, as measured by means of duplex scanning and strain-gauge plethysmography. *J Vasc Surg* 1999; **29**:1071–6.

117. Holmström M, Åberg W, Lockner C, Paul C. Long term clinical follow-up in 256 patients with deep-vein thrombosis initially treated with either unfractionated heparin or dalteparin: a retrospective analysis. *Thromb Haemost* 1999; **82**:1222–6.

118. Saarinen J, Kallio T, Lehto M, Hiltunen S, Sisto T. The occurrence of the post-thrombotic changes after an acute deep venous thrombosis. A prospective two-year follow-up study. *J Cardiovasc Surg* 2000; **41**:441–6.

119. Mohr DN, Silverstein MD, Heit JA, Petterson TM, O'Fallon M, Melton LJ. The venous stasis syndrome after deep venous thrombosis or pulmonary embolism: a population-based study. *Mayo Clin Proc* 2000; **75**:1249–56.

120. Ziegler S, Schillinger M, Maca TH, Minar E. Post-thrombotic syndrome after primary event of deep venous thrombosis 10 to 20 years ago. *Thromb Res* 2001; **101**:23–33.

121. Prandoni P, Lensing AWA, Prins MH, *et al*. Below-knee elastic compression stockings to prevent the post-thromboric syndrome. A randomized, controlled trial. *Ann Intern Med* 2004; **141**:249–56.

122. Gabriel F, Labios M, Portoles O, *et al*. Incidence of post-thrombotic syndrome and its association with various risk factors in a cohort of Spanish patients after one year of follow-up following acute deep venous thrombosis. *Thromb Haemost* 2004; **92**:328–36.

123. Kahn SR, Kearon C, Julian JA, *et al*. Predictors of the post-thrombotic syndrome during long-term treatment of proximal deep vein thrombosis. *J Thromb Haemost* 2005; **3**:718–23.

124. Roumen-Klappe EM, den Heijer M, Janssen MCH, van der Vleuten C, Thien T, Wollersheim H. The post-thrombotic syndrome: incidence and prognostic value of non-invasive venous examinations in a six-year follow-up study. *Thromb Haemost* 2005; **94**:825–30.

125. Immelman EJ, Jeffrey PC. The postphlebitic syndrome. Pathophysiology, prevention and management. *Clin Chest Med* 1984; **5**:537–50.

126. Raju S. Venous insufficiency of the lower limbs and stasis ulceration. *Ann Surg* 1983; **197**:688–97.

127. Scott TE, LaMorte WW, Gorin DR, Menzoian JO. Risk factors for chronic venous insufficiency: a dual case–control study. *J Vasc Surg* 1995; **22**:622–8.

128. Browse NL, Clemenson G, Lea Thomas M. Is the postphlebitic leg always postphlebitic? Relation between phlebographic appearances of deep-vein thrombosis and late sequelae. *Br Med J* 1980; **281**:1167–70.

129. Kolbach DN, Neumann HA, Prins MH. Definition of the post-thrombotic syndrome, differences between existing classifications. *Eur J Vasc Endovasc Surg* 2005; **30**:404–14.

130. Villalta S, Bagatella P, Piccioli A, Lensing AWA, Prins MH, Prandoni P. Assessment of validity and reproducibility of a clinical scale for the post-thrombotic syndrome. *Haemostasis* 1994; **24**(Suppl. 1): 57a.

131. Kahn SR, Hirsch A, Shrier I. Effect of post-thrombotic syndrome on health-related quality of life after deep venous thrombosis. *Arch Intern Med* 2002; **162**:1144–8.

132. Porter JM, Moneta GL. Reporting standards in venous disease: an update. International Consensus Commitee on Chronic Venous Disease. *J Vasc Surg* 1995; **21**:635–45.

133. Bettmann MA, Paulin S. Leg phlebography: the incidence, nature and modification of undesirable side effects. *Radiology* 1977; **122**:101–4.

134. Villalta S, Prandoni P, Cogo A, *et al*. The utility of non-invasive tests for detection of previous proximal-vein thrombosis. *Thromb Haemost* 1995; **73**:592–6.

135. Carter CJ. Incidence of post-phlebitic syndrome after streptokinase therapy for deep vein thrombosis. *Am J Med* 1990; **89**:697–8.

136. Shami SK, Shields DA, Scurr JH, Coleridge Smith PD: Leg ulceration in venous disease. *Postgrad Med J* 1992; **68**:779–85.

137. Coleridge Smith PD, Thomas P, Scurr JH, Dormandy JA: Causes of venous ulceration: a new hypothesis. *Br Med J* 1988; **296**:1726–7.

138. Lindhagen A, Bergqvist D, Hallböök T, Efsing HO. Venous function five to eight years after clinically suspected deep venous thrombosis. *Acta Med Scand* 1985; **217**:389–95.

139. Markel A, Manzo RA, Bergelin RO, Strandness DE. Valvular reflux after deep vein thrombosis: incidence and time of occurrence. *J Vasc Surg* 1992; **15**:377–84.

140. Franzeck UK, Schalch I, Bollinger A. On the relationship between changes in the deep veins evaluated by Duplex sonography and the postthrombotic syndrome 12 years after deep vein thrombosis. *Thromb Haemost* 1997; **77**:1109–12.

141. Singh H, Masuda EM. Comparing short-term outcomes of femoral-popliteal and iliofemoral deep venous thrombosis: early lysis and development of reflux. *Ann Vasc Surg* 2005; **19**:74–9.

142. Haenen JH, Janssen MC, Wollersheim H, *et al*. The development of postthrombotic syndrome in relationship to venous reflux and calf muscle pump dysfunction at 2 years after the onset of deep venous thrombosis. *J Vasc Surg* 2002; **35**:1184–9.

143. Prandoni P, Frulla M, Sartor D, Concolato A, Girolami A. Vein abnormalities and the post-thrombotic syndrome. *J Thromb Haemost* 2005; **3**:401–2.

144. Van Dongen CJ, Prandoni P, Frulla M, Marchiori A, Prins MH, Hutten BA. Relation between quality of anticoagulant treatment and the development of the postthrombotic syndrome. *J Thromb Haemost* 2005; **3**:939–42.

145. Ageno W, Piantanida E, Dentali F, *et al*. Body mass index is associated with the development of the post-thrombotic syndrome. *Thromb Haemost* 2003; **89**:305–9.

146. Piazza G, Goldhaber SZ. Acute pulmonary embolism: part I: epidemiology and diagnosis. *Circulation* 2006; **114**: e28–32.

147. Piazza G, Goldhaber SZ. Acute pulmonary embolism: part II: treatment and prophylaxis. *Circulation* 2006; **114**: e42–7.

148. Dalen JE, Alpert JS. Natural history of pulmonary embolism. *Prog Cardiovasc Dis* 1975; **17**: 259–70.

149. Goldhaber SZ, Haire WD, Feldstein ML, *et al*. Alteplase versus heparin in acute pulmonary embolism: randomised trial assessing right-ventricular function and pulmonary perfusion. *Lancet* 1993; **341**:507–11.

150. Goldhaber SZ, Visani L, De Rosa M. Acute pulmonary embolism: clinical outcomes in the International Cooperative Pulmonary Embolism Registry. *Lancet* 1999; **353**:1386–9.

151. Konstantinides S, Geibel A, Olschewski M, *et al*. Association between thrombolytic treatment and the prognosis of hemodynamically stable patients with major pulmonary embolism. *Circulation* 1997; **96**:882–8.

152. Grifoni S, Olivotto I, Cecchini P, *et al*. Short-term clinical outcome of patients with acute pulmonary embolism, normal blood pressure and echocardiographic right ventricular dysfunction. *Circulation* 2000; **101**:2817–22.

153. Paraskos JA. Late prognosis of acute pulmonary embolism. *N Engl J Med* 1973; **289**:55–8.

154. Conget F, Otero R, JimÉnez D, Martí D, Escobar C, Rodríguez C, Uresandi F, Cabezudo MA, Nauffal D, Oribe M, Yusen R. Short-term clinical outcome after acute symptomatic pulmonary embolism. *Thromb Haemost* 2008; **100**:937–42.

155. Nijkeuter M, Sohne M, Tick LW, *et al*. The natural course of hemodynamically stable pulmonary embolism: clinical outcome and risk factors in a large prospective cohort study. *Chest* 2007; **131**:517–23.

156. Carson JL, Kelley MA, Duff A, *et al*. The clinical course of pulmonary embolism. *N Engl J Med* 1992; **326**:1240–5.

157. Ribeiro A, Lindmarker P, Johnsson H, Juhlin-Dannfelt P, Jorfeldt L. Pulmonary embolism. One-year follow-up with echocardiography Doppler and five-year survival analysis. *Circulation* 1999; **99**:1325–30.

158. Ribeiro A, Lindmarker P, Johnsson H, Juhlin-Dannfelt A, Jorfeldt L. Pulmonary embolism: a follow-up study of the relation between the degree of right ventricle overload and the extent of perfusion defects. *J Intern Med* 1999; **245**:601–10.

159. Grifoni S, Olivotto I, Cecchini P, *et al*. Short-term clinical outcome of patients with acute pulmonary embolism, normal blood pressure and echocardiographic right ventricular dysfunction. *Circulation* 2000; **101**:2817–22.

160. Grifoni S, Vanni S, Magazzini S, *et al*. Association of persistent right ventricular dysfunction at hospital discharge after acute pulmonary embolism with recurrent thromboembolic events. *Arch Intern Med* 2006; **166**:2151–6.

161. Konstantinides S, Gebel A, Heusel G, *et al*. Heparin plus alteplase compared with heparin alone in patients with submassive pulmonary embolism. *N Engl J Med* 2002; **347**:1143–50.

162. Perlroth DJ, Sanders GD, Gould MK. Effectiveness and cost-effectiveness of thrombolysis in submassive pulmonary embolism. *Arch Intern Med* 2007; **167**:74–80.

163. Agnelli G, Becattini C, Kirschstein T. Thrombolysis vs heparin in the treatment of pulmonary embolism. *Arch Intern Med* 2002; **162**:2537–41.

164. Thabut G, Thabut D, Myers RP, *et al*. Thrombolytic therapy of pulmonary embolism. A meta-analysis. *J Am Coll Cardiol* 2002; **40**:1660–7.

165. ten Wolde M, Sohne M, Quak E, Mac Gillavry MR, Buller HR. Prognostic value of echocardiographically assessed right ventricular dysfunction in patients with pulmonary embolism. *Arch Intern Med* 2004; **164**:1685–9.

166. Douketis JD, Crowther MA, Stanton EB, Ginsberg JS. Elevated troponin levels in patients with sub-massive pulmonary embolism. *Arch Intern Med* 2002; **162**:79–81.

167. Janata K, Holzer M, Laggner AN, Mullner M. Cardiac troponin T in the severity assessment of patients with pulmonary embolism: cohort study. *BMJ* 2003; **326**:312–3.

168. Mehta NJ, Jani K, Khan IA. Clinical usefulness and prognostic value of elevated cardiac troponin I levels in acute pulmonary embolism. *Am Heart J* 2003; **45**:21–5.

169. Pruszczyk P, Bochowicz A, Torbicki A, *et al*. Cardiac troponin T monitoring identifies high-risk group of normotensive patients with acute pulmonary embolism. *Chest* 2003; **123**:1947–52.

170. La Vecchia L, Ottani F, Favero L, *et al*. Increased cardiac troponin I on admission predicts in-hospital mortality in acute pulmonary embolism. *Heart* 2004; **90**:633–7.

171. Aksay E, Yanturali S, Kiyan S. Can elevated troponin I levels predict complicated clinical course and inhospital mortality in patients with acute pulmonary embolism? *Am J Emerg Med* 2007; **25**:138–43.

172. Amorim S, Dias P, Rodrigues RA, *et al*. Goncalves FR. Troponin I as a marker of right ventricular dysfunction and severity of pulmonary embolism. *Rev Port Cardiol* 2006; **25**:181–6.

173. Douketis JD, Leeuwenkamp O, Grobara P, *et al*. The incidence and prognostic significance of elevated cardiac troponins in patients with submassive pulmonary embolism. *J Thromb Haemost* 2005; **3**:508–13.

174. Hsu JT, Chu CM, Chang ST, Cheng HW, Cheng NJ, Chung CM. Prognostic role of right ventricular dilatation and troponin i elevation in acute pulmonary embolism. *Int Heart* 2006; **47**:775–81.

175. Yalamanchili K, Sukhija R, Aronow WS, Sinha N, Fleisher AG, Lehrman SG. Prevalence of increased cardiac troponin I levels in patients with and without acute pulmonary embolism and relation of increased cardiac troponin I levels with in-hospital mortality in patients with acute pulmonary embolism. *Am J Cardiol* 2004; **93**:263–4.

176. Tulevski II, Wolde MT, van Veldhuisen DJ, *et al*. Combined utility of brain natriuretic peptide and cardiac troponine T may improve rapid triage and risk stratification in normotensive patients with pulmonary embolism. *Int J Cardiol* 2007; **116**:161–6.

177. Binder L, Pieske B, Olschewski M, *et al*. N-terminal pro-brain natriuretic peptide or troponin testing followed by echocardiography for risk stratification of acute pulmonary embolism. *Circulation* 2005; **112**:1573–9.

178. Pieralli F, Olivotto I, Vanni S, *et al*. Usefulness of bedside testing for brain natriuretic peptide to identify right ventricular dysfunction and outcome in normotensive patients with acute pulmonary embolism. *Am J Cardiol* 2006; **97**:1386–90.

179. Sohne M, Ten Wolde M, Boomsma F, Reitsma JB, Douketis JD, Buller HR. Brain natriuretic peptide in hemodynamically stable acute pulmonary embolism. *J Thromb Haemost* 2006; **4**:552–6.

180. Aujesky D, Roy PM, Guy M, Cornuz J, Sanchez O, Perrier A. Prognostic value of D-dimer in patients with pulmonary embolism. *Thromb Haemost* 2006; **96**:478–82.

181. Ghanima W, Abdelnoor M, Holmen LO, Nielssen BE, Ross S, Sandset PM. D-dimer level is associated with the extent of pulmonary embolism. *Thromb Res* 2007; **120**:281–8.

182. Grau E, Tenías JM, Soto MJ, *et al*. D-dimer levels correlate with mortality in patients with acute pulmonary embolism: Findings from the RIETE registry. *Crit Care Med* 2007; **35**:1937–41.

183. Pengo V, Lensing AW, Prins MH, *et al*. Incidence of chronic thromboembolic pulmonary hypertension after pulmonary embolism. *N Engl J Med* 2004; **350**:2257–64.

184. Van der Meer RW, Pattynama PM, van Strijen MJ, *et al*. Right ventricular dysfunction and pulmonary obstruction index at helical CT: prediction of clinical outcome during 3-month follow-up in patients with acute pulmonary embolism. *Radiology* 2005; **235**:798–803.

185. Wicki J, Perneger TV, Junod AF, Bounameaux H, Perrier A. Assessing clinical probability of pulmonary embolism in the emergency ward. *Arch Intern Med* 2001; **161**:92–7.

186. Nendaz MR, Bandelier P, Aujesky D, *et al*. Validation of a risk score identifying patients with acute pulmonary embolism, who are at low risk of clinical adverse outcome. *Thromb Haemost* 2004; **91**:1232–6.

187. Aujesky D, Obrosky DS, Stone RA, *et al*. Derivation and validation of a prognostic model for pulmonary embolism. *Am J Respir Crit Care Med* 2005; **172**:1041–6.

188. Aujesky D, Roy PM, Le Manach CP, *et al*. Validation of a model to predict adverse outcomes in patients with pulmonary embolism. *Eur Heart J* 2006; **27**:476–81.

189. Aujesky D, Obrosky DS, Stone RA, *et al*. A prediction rule to identify low-risk patients with pulmonary embolism. *Arch Intern Med* 2006; **166**:169–75.

190. Jiménez D, Yusen RD, Otero R, *et al*. Prognostic models for selecting patients with acute pulmonary embolism for initial outpatient therapy. *Chest* 2007; **132**:7–8.

191. Eichinger S, Weltermann A, Minar E, *et al*. Symptomatic pulmonary embolism and the risk of recurrent venous thromboembolism. *Arch Intern Med* 2004; **164**:92–6.

192. Agnelli G, Prandoni P, Becattini C, *et al*. Extended oral anticoagulant therapy after a first episode of pulmonary embolism. *Ann Intern Med* 2003; **139**:19–25.
193. Murin S, Romano PS, White RH. Comparison of outcomes after hospitalization for deep venous thrombosis or pulmonary embolism. *Thromb Haemost* 2002; **88**:407–14.
194. Riedel M, Stanek V, Widimsky J, Prerovsky I. Longterm follow-up of patients with pulmonary thromboembolism. *Chest* 1982; **81**:151–8.
195. Tow DE, Wagner HN. Recovery of pulmonary arterial blood flow in patients with pulmonary embolism. *N Engl J Med* 1967; **276**:1053–9.
196. Miniati M, Monti S, Bottai M, *et al*. Survival and restoration of pulmonary perfusion in a long-term follow-up of patients after acute pulmonary embolism. *Medicine (Baltimore)* 2006; **85**: 53–62.
197. Nijkeuter M, Hovens MM, Davidson BL, Huisman MV. Resolution of thromboemboli in patients with acute pulmonary embolism: a systematic review. *Chest* 2006; **129**:192–7.
198. Yoo HS, Intenzo CM, Park CH. Unresolved major pulmonary embolism: importance of follow-up lung scan in diagnosis. *Eur J Nucl Med* 1986; **12**:252–3.
199. Moser KM., Auger WR, Fedullo PF. Chronic major-vessel thromboembolic pulmonary hypertension. *Circulation* 1990; **81**:1735–43.
200. Fedullo PF, Auger WR, Kerr KM, Rubin LJ. Chronic thromboembolic pulmonary hypertension. *N Engl J Med* 2001; **345**:1465–72.
201. Becattini C, Agnelli G, Pesavento R, *et al*. Incidence of chronic thromboembolic pulmonary hypertension after a first episode of pulmonary embolism. *Chest* 2006; **130**:172–5.
202. Hoeper MM, Mayer E, Simonneau G, Rubin LJ. Chronic thromboembolic pulmonary hypertension. *Circulation* 2006; **113**:2011–20.
203. Auger WR, Kim NH, Kerr KM, Test VJ, Fedullo PF. Chronic thromboembolic pulmonary hypertension. *Clin Chest Med* 2007; **28**:255–69.
204. Prandoni P, Falanga A, Piccioli A. Cancer and venous thromboembolism. *Lancet Oncol* 2005; **6**:401–10.
205. Sorensen HT, Mellemkjaer L, Steffensen H, Olsen JH, Nielsen GL. The risk of a diagnosis of cancer after primary deep-venous thrombosis or pulmonary embolism. *N Engl J Med* 1998; **338**:1169–73.
206. Baron JA, Gridley G, Weiderpass E, Nyren G, Linet M. Venous thromboembolism and cancer. *Lancet* 1998; **351**:1077–80.
207. Murchison JT, Wylie L, Stockton DL. Excess risk of cancer in patients with primary venous thromboembolism: a national, population-based cohort study. *Br J Cancer* 2004; **91**:92–5.
208. White RH, Chew HK, Zhou H, *et al*. Incidence of venous thromboembolism in the year before the diagnosis of cancer in 528,693 adults. *Arch Intern Med* 2005; **165**:1782–7.
209. Miller GJ, Bauer KA, Howarth DJ, Cooper JA, Humphries SE, Rosenberg RD. Increased incidence of neoplasia of the digestive tract in men with persistent activation of the coagulant pathway. *J Thromb Haemost* 2004; **2**:2107–14.
210. Sorensen HT, Pedersen L, Mellemkjaer L, *et al*. The risk of a second cancer after hospitalization for venous thromboembolism. *Br J Cancer* 2005; **93**:838–41.
211. Schulman S, Lindmarker P. Incidence of cancer after prophylaxis with warfarin against recurrent venous thromboembolism. *N Engl J Med* 2000; **342**:1953–8.
212. Kakkar AK, Levine MN, Kadziola Z, *et al*. Low molecular weight heparin, therapy with dalteparin and survival in advanced cancer: the Fragmin Advanced Malignancy Outcome Study. *J Clin Oncol* 2004; **22**:1944–8.
213. Klerk CPW, Smorenburg SM, Otten HYM, *et al*. The effect of low-molecular-weight heparin on survival in patients with advanced malignancy. *J Clin Oncol* 2005; **23**:2130–5.
214. Altinbas M, Coskun HS, Er O, *et al*. A randomized clinical trial of combination chemotherapy with and without low-molecular-weight heparin in small cell lung cancer. *J Thromb Haemost* 2004; **2**:1266–71.
215. Sideras K, Schaefer PL, Okuno SH, *et al*. Low-molecular-weight heparin in patients with advanced cancer: a phase 3 clinical trial. *Mayo Clin Proc* 2006; **81**:758–67.
216. Lazo-Langner A, Goss GD, Spaans JN, Rodger MA. The effect of low-molecular-weight heparin on cancer survival. A systematic review and meta-analysis of randomized trials. *J Thromb Haemost* 2007; **5**:729–37.
217. Boccaccio C, Sabatino G, Medico E, *et al*. The MET oncogene drives a genetic programme linking cancer to haemostasis. *Nature* 2005; **434**:396–400.
218. Sorensen HT, Mellemkjaer L, Olsen JH, Baron JA. Prognosis of cancers associated with venous thromboembolism. *N Engl J Med* 2000; **343**:1846–50.
219. Monreal M, Lensing AWA, Prins MH, *et al*. Screening for occult cancer in patients with acute deep vein thrombosis or pulmonary embolism. *J Thromb Haemost* 2004; **2**:876–81.

220. Piccioli A, Lensing AWA, Prins MH, *et al*. Estensive screening for occult malignant disease in idiopathic venous thromboembolism. *J Thromb Haemost* 2004; **2**:884–9.

221. Di Nisio M, Otten HM, Piccioli A, *et al*. Decision analysis for cancer screening in idiopathic venous thromboembolism. *J Thromb Haemost* 2005; **3**:2391–6.

222. Prandoni P, Bilora F, Marchiori A, *et al*. An association between atherosclerosis and venous thrombosis. *N Engl J Med* 2003; **348**:1435–41.

223. Reich LM, Folsom AR, Key NS, *et al*. Prospective study of subclinical atherosclerosis as a risk factor for venous thromboembolism. *J Thromb Haemost* 2006; **4**:1909–13.

224. van der Hagen PB, Folsom AR, Jenny NS, *et al*. Subclinical atherosclerosis and the risk of future venous thrombosis in the Cardiovascular Health Study. *J Thromb Haemost* 2006; **4**:1903–8.

225. Becattini C, Agnelli G, Prandoni P, *et al*. A prospective study on cardiovascular events after acute pulmonary embolism. *Eur Heart J* 2005; **26**:77–83.

226. Prandoni P, Ghirarduzzi A, Prins MH, *et al*. Venous thromboembolism and the risk of subsequent symptomatic atherosclerosis. *J Thromb Haemost* 2006; **4**:1891–6.

227. Bova C, Marchiori A, Noto A, *et al*. Incidence of arterial cardiovascular events in patients with idiopathic venous thromboembolism. A retrospective cohort study. *Thromb Haemost* 2006; **96**:132–6.

228. Sørensen HT, Horvath-Puho E, Pedersen L, Baron JA, Prandoni P. Venous thromboembolism and subsequent hospitalization due to acute cardiovascular events – a 20 year cohort study. *Lancet* 2007; **370**:1773–9.

229. Young L, Ockelford P, Milne D, Rolfe-Vyson V, McKelvie S, Harper P. Post treatment residual thrombus increases the risk of recurrent deep vein thrombosis and mortality. *J Thromb Haemost* 2006; **4**:1919–24.

230. Steffen LM, Folsom AR, Cushman M, *et al*. Greater fish, fruit and vegetable intakes are related to lower incidence of venous thromboembolism. *Circulation* 2006; **115**:188–95.

231. Squizzato A, Romualdi E, Ageno W. Why should statins prevent venous thromboembolism? A systematic literature search and a call for action. *J Thromb Haemost* 2006; **4**:1925–7.

232. Agnelli G, Becattini C. Venous thromboembolism and atherosclerosis: common denominators or different diseases? *J Thromb Haemost* 2006; **4**:1886–90.

PART II

Clinical Presentation

CHAPTER 3

Clinical Presentation of Deep Vein Thrombosis

Maaike Söhne[1], Roel Vink[2] and Harry R. Büller[1]

[1]Department of Vascular Medicine, Academic Medical Center,
Amsterdam, The Netherlands.
[2]Department of Internal Medicine, Academic Medical Center,
Amsterdam, The Netherlands.

GENERAL INTRODUCTION TO THE CLINICAL PRESENTATION OF DEEP VEIN THROMBOSIS AND PULMONARY EMBOLISM

The clinical spectrum of signs and symptoms suggestive of deep vein thrombosis (DVT) or pulmonary embolism (PE) are common in the general population, fit in a long list of differential diagnoses and are frequently a motive to seek medical expertise. With the introduction of contrast venography in 1940 (1) and pulmonary angiography in 1963 (2,3), it became obvious that the clinical diagnosis of venous thromboembolism (VTE) is inaccurate and signs and symptoms are non-specific. The first study that highlighted the limited value of the clinical diagnosis in suspected DVT was the study by Haeger in 1969, which showed that only 46% of clinically diagnosed DVT patients had phlebographic proof of thrombus (4). Overestimation of DVT remains prevalent, as in contemporary studies the disease is confirmed by objective testing in only 20–30% of patients with suspected disease referred for diagnostic testing. This percentage has not markedly changed over the past 25 years. The introduction of computed tomography (CT) for PE diagnosis has decreased the prevalence in tested patients to less than 10% (see Chapter 7). On the other hand, it is important to realise that the diagnosis is also frequently missed in clinical practice, as revealed by the high incidence of VTE in autopsy studies (5,6). This could partly be explained by the asymptomatic nature of VTE. Several studies have demonstrated that 50–80% of the patients diagnosed with PE have DVT confirmed with objective tests, although these patients do not experience any symptoms of the lower extremity (7,8). Also, in at least half of the patients with confirmed DVT, asymptomatic PE is present (9).

Thus, the clinical spectrum of VTE varies from asymptomatic to circulatory collapse or phlegmasia cerulea dolens, the most extreme clinical presentations of PE and DVT, respectively. Therefore, objective diagnostic strategies are mandatory to confirm or exclude the disease safely. Many diagnostic management studies have been performed in the past decades in order to achieve this (see

Part IV). However, a diagnostic management strategy can only be initiated when the clinical suspicion for DVT or PE has arisen. Early recognition of the clinical signs and symptoms that are associated with VTE is therefore of critical importance. A recent large Italian registry showed that in daily clinical practice a significant proportion of patients with either DVT or PE receive a delayed objective diagnosis. In this registry, which contained more than 2000 cases with VTE, 20% of the patients with DVT and 16% of those with PE had their diagnosis confirmed more than 10 days after the initial onset of symptoms (10). The study did not distinguish between the time from onset of symptoms to seeking medical attention and from referral to objective testing. Although the first period seems to play the most important role (11), the delay in confirmation of the diagnosis partly explains the high incidence of VTE in autopsy studies and underline the necessity for early recognition.

Although early recognition and initiation of a full diagnostic evaluation for DVT or PE are extremely important, it is equally essential to prevent access to diagnostic tests without any threshold. Unrestrained use of a diagnostic investigation might lead to a reduced prevalence of the disease among those patients tested, as has been shown for CT pulmonary angiography. This causes a decrease in the predictive values of the diagnostic methods used, leading to either overtreatment with resultant unnecessary bleeding with initiation of anticoagulation or a missed diagnosis which may result in death. Therefore, the challenge for physicians is to prevent a decrease in the prevalence of confirmed cases among suspected patients. This raises the questions of what can be assumed to be a clinical suspicion of DVT or PE and when a diagnostic work-up should be initiated.

This chapter and Chapter 4 describe the prevalence and value of the spectrum of clinical signs and symptoms of venous thrombosis and the abnormalities that might be present with early investigations that could or should raise clinical suspicion of DVT and PE.

CLINICAL PRESENTATION OF DEEP VEIN THROMBOSIS

The signs and symptoms of DVT reflect the clinical situation of a clot that causes obstruction in one or more veins within the lower extremity. This obstruction causes a range of pathophysiological changes, depending on the anatomical location of the thrombus and its extent. Since a remarkable proportion of the patients with PE have asymptomatic DVT, chest symptoms may be the initial symptom of DVT. This broad clinical spectrum leads to the issue of when a DVT should be considered within the differential diagnosis and hence when to initiate a diagnostic management strategy.

Before discussing the signs and symptoms that can occur with an episode of acute DVT, some comments should be made about the general clinical situation of the patient, which might cause the initial clinical suspicion of DVT. This refers to the risk factors associated with VTE (see Part I), which are almost all explained by the Virchow triad, the founder of the pathophysiological mechanism of the basis for venous thrombosis. This triad, described in 1860, consists of vessel wall damage, stasis of blood and hypercoagulability (12,13). In immobilised, post-surgical or admitted patients, patients with malignancy, a lower extremity fracture with plaster cast or in patients with previous venous thromboembolism, even minor symptoms of one of the lower extremities could easily draw the physician's attention to a suspicion of DVT. Several thrombophilic factors, such as the factor V Leiden mutation, protein C or S deficiency, antithrombin deficiency or lupus anticoagulans, may also have this effect.

Clinical signs and symptoms that can be present with DVT are calf tenderness or tenderness along the course of the veins involved, pain on dorsiflexion of the foot (Homans' sign), unilateral leg swelling, warmth and erythema. Other signs include distension of superficial veins and appearance of prominent venous collaterals. Rarely, DVT of the leg initially presents itself as a condition named *phlegmasia cerulea dolens*, when deoxygenated haemoglobin in stagnant veins can give a cyanotic appearance of the limb. This situation, at the severe end of the clinical spectrum of DVT of the leg, needs therapy instantly in order to preserve it.

Signs and symptoms of deep vein thrombosis

Pain and tenderness of the calf or thigh are the most frequently occurring symptom in patients with and also in patients without confirmed DVT. The pain is not characteristic and varies from an ache to cramping, from dull to sharp and from mild to severe. It may be intermittent or constantly present, but it is usually aggravated by movement and standing up and relieved with elevation of the leg. The location of the pain is not associated with the site of thrombosis and severity bears no relationship to the size or extent of thrombosis. Many other diseases are associated with pain or tenderness of the lower extremity, some of which can be easily differentiated with a thorough history and physical examination. Arterial insufficiency usually presents more suddenly in onset, shows a cold and pale leg, without detectable pulses and without oedema. The pain in neurogenic compression of the sciatic nerve or the lateral cutaneous nerve of the thigh is sharp and intensified by movements that stretch the nerve. Nevertheless, an alternative diagnosis in patients with suspected DVT is normally not considered to be definite unless thrombosis is excluded by objective testing.

A positive *Homans' sign*, pain in the calf with forced dorsiflexion of the foot, is assumed to be predictive for the presence of DVT (14). John Homans (1877–1954) was a surgeon in Boston who had an important influence on the development of vascular surgery (15). He named it the 'dorsiflexion sign' and did not attribute much value of this sign for the diagnosis of DVT (16). Nevertheless, it is still universally used in the physical examination of patients with calf pain, although its predictive value for the presence or absence of DVT is very low. Of all patients with symptomatic DVT, approximately 30–40% have a positive Homans' sign, and at least half of the clinically suspected patients without DVT also experience calf pain with dorsiflexion of the foot.

In addition to Homans' sign, a series of other signs, named after the physicians who first described them, can be found in literature. Lowenberg's sign (pain in the calf when inflating a cuff up to 180 mmHg on the thigh), Moses' sign (an increased severity of pain when the calf is compressed in a frontal backward direction compared with lateral compression), Pratt's sign (distension of pretibial veins) and Peabody's sign (spasm of the calf muscles on elevating the leg with a stretched foot) (17–20). All of these signs are insensitive and non-specific and have no value in the clinical examination. Homans' sign is the only one broadly known or used these days.

Oedema is defined as a clinically apparent increase in the interstitial fluid volume. Oedema may be localized or have a generalized distribution. Oedema of the unilateral leg in patients with confirmed DVT is assumed to be caused either by obstruction of proximal veins or by inflammation of perivascular tissues. Due to local obstruction in venous drainage, the hydrostatic pressure in the capillary bed downstream to the obstruction increases so that more fluid than normal is transferred from the vascular to the interstitial space. Oedema usually occurs distal to the site of obstruction and may be painless. When inflammation exists, the site is associated with pain, tenderness or erythema. Oedema of one leg can be present in many other clinical entities. Muscle strain or trauma, a ruptured Baker's cyst, lymphedema, external compression of the iliac vein by tumour, haematoma, abscess, cellulites and erysipelas should all be considered in the differential diagnosis. Accompanying symptoms could give direction to a specific diagnosis, but diagnostic evaluation with either laboratory investigation, for example C-reactive protein, a white blood cell count, haemoglobin or D-dimer, or radiological imaging, i.e., ultrasonography, is often necessary.

Venous distension or a palpable cord are two signs of thrombosis that are relatively uncommon to observe with physical examination. Distension of superficial vessels might occur with obstruction, but is equally present after a long walk in high temperatures. A thrombosed vessel may be palpable as a solid cord (Figure 3.1). The cord is usually tender and may be felt in the popliteal fossa or the groin. It is difficult to distinguish a venous cord from oedema or haematoma. Residual thrombosis of a previous DVT can still be present and thus also be palpable. With superficial thrombophlebitis the vessel is usually palpable. However, this is easily differentiated from DVT, because of its immediate subcutaneous location and its specific anatomical sites.

Phlegmasia alba dolens is the clinical situation of an iliofemoral vein thrombosis associated with arterial spasm, which is relatively rare. This causes a clinical picture of a very pale and cold leg with weak or absent arterial pulses. In the early stage swelling may be minimal, but as the spasm continues, the leg may become swollen and the skin might show a mottled blue appearance. However, an arterial occlusion with a different origin can result in an identical clinical presentation.

Phlegmasia cerulea dolens is another rare complication of DVT with total or near total venous occlusion of the lower extremity. It is associated with a high degree of morbidity and may result in venous gangrene, the compartment syndrome, arterial compromise, systemic hypovolemic shock and even death. The clinical presentation of the syndrome usually consists of pain, swelling, rubor and cyanosis. The cyanosis is caused by extensive venous obstruction that involves not only the deep veins of the lower extremity, but also the superficial and the collateral veins. Severe oedema

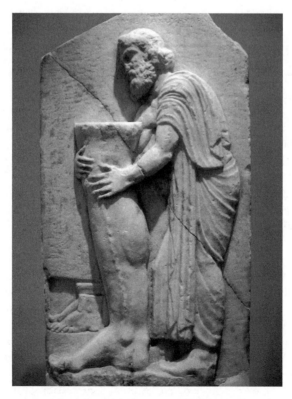

Figure 3.1 Hippocrates treating thrombophlebitis on a relief located at the National Archaeological Museum, Athens, Greece. Image courtesy of Professor Edwin J.R. van Beek.

develops rapidly, which may impair arterial inflow and thus produce marked tissue ischaemia. Hypotension occurs while there is marked pooling of the blood in the affected leg. Phlegmasia cerulea dolens has been associated with malignancy (21).

Treatment of phlegmasia cerulea and alba dolens is primarily aimed at the prevention of ischaemia by decreasing oedema and prevention of the compartment syndrome by fasciotomy. Immediate anticoagulation should be initiated, but, due to the very low prevalence of phlegmasia cerulea dolens, treatment has not yet been clearly established. Recently, intravenous thrombolysis has been suggested as a treatment modality, which might prevent progression to gangrene or amputation (22,23). Most importantly, it is essential to recognise this rapidly as venous thrombosis rather than arterial insufficiency.

Post-thrombotic syndrome

The post-thrombotic syndrome (PTS) is a complicating factor in the clinical presentation of patients with a history of DVT. PTS is thought to be caused by venous hypertension, which occurs as a consequence of either recanalization of major vein thrombi that lead to valve destruction or as a result of persistent outflow obstruction produced by residual thrombotic burden. Valve destruction and recanalization might result in malfunction of the muscular pump of the leg, causing an increased pressure in the deep calf veins. This high pressure ultimately renders the perforating veins of the calf incompetent. Due to these non-functioning perforating veins, the blood flow is directed from the deep into the superficial vein system during muscular contraction and the clinical signs of PTS become apparent (24,25). The syndrome consists of complaints of pain and swelling of the affected leg as well as itching or tingling. In the severe form, even venous ulceration can occur. Typically the symptoms become worse at the end of the day or after a period of standing, while they are relieved by rest and leg elevation. PTS is a chronic clinical entity; however, some of the patients present themselves with repeated episodes of increasing oedema and calf pain. This resemblance with the clinical picture of an acute DVT frequently encourages the physician to initiate diagnostic evaluation, often with ultrasonography. Post-thrombotic sequelae develop in almost half of the patients with a proximal DVT, usually within 2 years of the acute thrombotic episode.

REFERENCES

1. Bauer G. A venographic study of thromboembolic problems. *Acta Chir Scand* 1940; **84**:Suppl. 61.
2. Williams JR, Wilcox, C, *et al*. Angiography in pulmonary embolism. *JAMA* 1963; **184**:473–6.
3. Sasahara AA, Stein M, Simon M, Littmann D. Pulmonary angiography in the diagnosis of thromboembolic disease. *N Engl J Med* 1964; **270**:1075–81.
4. Haeger K. Problems of acute deep vein thrombosis. The interpretations of signs and symptoms. *Angiology* 1969; **20**:219–23.
5. Stein PD, Henry JW. Prevalence of acute pulmonary embolism among in a general hospital and at autopsy. *Chest* 1995; **108**:978–81.
6. Ryu JH, Olson EJ, Pellikka PA. Clinical recognition of pulmonary embolism: problem of unrecognized an asymptomatic cases. *Mayo Clin Proc* 1998; **73**:873–9.
7. Hull RD, Hirsh J, Carter CJ, *et al*. Pulmonary angiography, ventilation lung scanning and venography for clinically suspected pulmonary embolism with abnormal perfusion lung scan. *Ann Intern Med* 1983; **98**:891–9.
8. Kruit WH, de Boer AC, Sing AK, *et al*. The significance of venography in the management of patients with clinically suspected pulmonary embolism. *J Intern Med* 1991; **230**:333–9.
9. Huisman MV, Büller HR, ten Cate JW, *et al*. Unexpected high prevalence of silent pulmonary embolism in patients with deep vein thrombosis. *Chest* 1989; **95**:498–502.

10. Ageno W, Agnelli G, Imberti D, *et al*. Factors associated with the timing of diagnosis of venous thromboembolism: Results from the MASTER registry. *Thromb Res* 2008; **121**(6):751–6.
11. Elliott CG, Goldhaber SZ, Jensen RL. Delays in diagnosis of deep vein thrombosis and pulmonary embolism. *Chest* 2005; **128**:3372–6.
12. Virchow R. *Cellular Pathology as Based upon Physiological and Pathologic Histology: Local Formation of Fibrin*. Churchill, London, 1860.
13. Kahn SR. The clinical diagnosis of deep vein thrombosis. *Arch Intern Med* 1998; **158**:2315–23.
14. Levi M, Hart W, Büller H. R. Fysische diagnostiek – het teken van Homans. *Ned Tijdschr Geneesk* 1999; **143**:1861–3.
15. Barker WF. To the memory of John Homans, MD, 1877–1954. *Major Probl Clin Surg* 1966; **4**: v–vii.
16. Crawford ES. The seventh John Homans lecture: heroes in vascular surgery. *J Vasc Surg* 1992; **15**:417–23.
17. Moses WR. The early diagnosis of phlebothrombosis. *N Engl J Med* 1946; **234**:288–91.
18. Lowenberg R. Early diagnosis of phlebothrombosis with aid of a new clinical test. *JAMA* 1946; **155**, 1566–70.
19. Pratt GH. An early sign of femoral thrombosis. *JAMA* 1949; **140**:476–7.
20. Peabody CN. An objective sign of thrombophlebitis. *Angiology* 1964; **15**:434–5.
21. Perkins JM, Magee JR, Galland RB. Phlegmasia caerulea dolens and venous gangrene. *Br J Surg* 1996; **83**:19–23.
22. Tardy B, Moulin N, Mismetti P, Decousus H, Laporte S. Intravenous thrombolytic therapy in patients with phlegmasia cerulea dolens. *Haematologica* 2006; **91**:281–2.
23. Bhatt S, Wehbe C, Dogra VS. Phlegmasia cerulea dolens. *J Clin Ultrasound* 2007; **35**:401–4.
24. Hirsh J, Hull RD. Natural history and clinical features of venous thrombosis. In Colman RW, Hirsh J, Marder VJ, Salzman EW (eds), *Hemostasis and Thrombosis*. Lippincott, Philadelphia, PA, 1987, pp. 1208–19.
25. Kahn SR, Ginsberg JS. Relationship between deep vein thrombosis and the post thrombotic syndrome. *Arch Intern Med* 2004; **164**:17–26.

CHAPTER 4

Clinical Presentation of Pulmonary Embolism

Maaike Söhne[1], Roel Vink[2] and Harry R. Büller[1]

[1]Department of Vascular Medicine, Academic Medical Center, Amsterdam, The Netherlands
[2]Department of Internal Medicine, Academic Medical Center, Amsterdam, The Netherlands

INTRODUCTION

Pulmonary embolism (PE) is diagnosed by demonstrating intravascular filling defects on compute tomography (CT) or angiography or by mismatched perfusion defects with normal ventilation on lung scintigraphy. Venous thrombi are intravascular deposits predominantly composed of fibrin, red blood cells and a variable platelet and leukocyte component. In addition to the fibrin clots, there are different other emboli that can obstruct the pulmonary vasculature. These other syndromes generally have a clear aetiology and a different clinical presentation. Fat embolisms are usually caused by fracture of the long bones, particularly the femur, and also occur during orthopaedic procedures requiring bone marrow manipulation (intramedullary nails or total hip replacement). Infected clots originating from systemic veins or a bacterial endocarditis of the right side of the heart are the basis for septic emboli and amniotic fluid might cause pulmonary problems during or shortly after labour.

The fibrin clots in the pulmonary arteries generally originate in the veins of the lower extremities. When (part of) the thrombus is dislodged by the bloodstream, it migrates via the inferior caval vein, the right atrium and right ventricle to the lungs and causes obstruction of one or more pulmonary arteries, which defines PE.

SYMPTOMS OF PULMONARY EMBOLISM

PE symptoms can vary greatly, depending on the size of the clot, the extent of obstruction of the pulmonary vascular bed and the overall physical condition of the patient, especially the presence or absence of underlying lung or heart disease.

Deep Vein Thrombosis and Pulmonary Embolism   Edited by Edwin J.R. van Beek, Harry R. Büller and Matthijs Oudkerk
© 2009 John Wiley & Sons, Ltd

Chest pain or discomfort is one of the most frequent complaints for which patients seek medical attention (1) and approximately 70% of patients with confirmed PE have this symptom at presentation (2). It is of importance to distinguish potentially life-threatening conditions such as PE, coronary artery disease or aortic dissection from other causes of chest pain. However, to decide whether the chest discomfort is a manifestation of one of the above-mentioned conditions or of an innocent condition such as musculoskeletal problems is not straightforward. A focused medical history, physical examination and often additional diagnostic tests are necessary to arrive at the correct diagnosis. The chest pain in patients with PE is most often of pleuritic origin. Pleural pain usually has a restricted distribution, rather than a diffuse pattern. The most important characteristic is its clear relationship to respiratory movements and pleural pain typically increases on taking a deep breath. Acute pleurisy is due to irritation of the pleura, which may also be seen in, for instance, a peripheral pneumonia, an acute pneumothorax and PE. Intercostal neuritis may resemble pleural pain, but does not involve the pleura and tends to be along the affected nerve's distribution. In PE, the pain is thought to be associated with infarction of a segment of the lung that is adjacent to the pleura. Pleural pain is even more prevalent than pulmonary infarction, which is detected by chest X-ray or spiral CT in patients with confirmed PE. Approximately 10% of patients with PE will progress to pulmonary infarction. This is mainly caused by the fact that the lung depends on two circulatory sources of oxygen, i.e., the bronchial circulation and the pulmonary circulation. Since pulmonary infarction develops only when both sources are compromised simultaneously, it is not surprising that its prevalence is not high. A less common type of pain in patients with PE is chest pain located substernally and resembling that of acute myocardial infarction or angina pectoris. This pain is usually described as aching or compressing and occasionally occurs in patients with massive (sometimes saddle) embolism, often accompanied by other signs of circulatory compromise.

Dyspnea could be defined as the subjective experience of a hampered respiration, whereas *tachypnea* is the objective observation of an increased number of breaths per time period. Dyspnea is the most frequent symptom in patients suspected of acute PE. The presence of dyspnea, however, is equally prevalent in those suspected of PE in whom the diagnosis is confirmed as in those in whom it is refuted, occurring in approximately 75%. Dyspnea has a long list of differential diagnoses, ranging from neurogenic to cardiogenic and metabolic. Most importantly, as with chest pain, one needs to differentiate between an acute onset of the pain, a short duration and on the other hand long-term chronic dyspnea. PE usually gives a relatively acute dyspnea, which increases with time. The mechanism of dyspnea in PE is likely to be related to the ventilation/perfusion imbalance, shunting, decreased lung compliance produced by congestive atelectasis, pulmonary infarction and regional pulmonary oedema.

Coughing is an essential defence mechanism to protect the airways from the potential harmful effects of inhaled noxious substances and it clears the airways from retained secretions. Normal, healthy, non-smoking individuals seldom cough since the amount of daily bronchial secretions produced is sufficiently small to be removed by mucociliary action alone. Coughing can be divided into a productive cough, which usually implies an underlying inflammatory process such as infection, or in a non-productive 'dry' cough, indicating a mechanical or other irritating stimulus. It is not the most frequently present symptom in patients with PE and usually points to another pulmonary disease, especially when it is productive. When a productive cough comprises streaks of blood, it is called haemoptysis and PE should be included in the differential diagnosis.

Haemoptysis, the expectoration of blood or blood-stained sputum, is a symptom of pulmonary pathology of which a considerable proportion of patients appear to have serious disease, most importantly malignancy. To be sure that it is blood from the bronchi and not from the gastrointestinal tract, the pH can be measured, which will be low if originated from the stomach or oesophagus. In general, haemoptysis is clearly reddish, whereas haematemesis shows a darker to brownish colour. Accompanying symptoms might point to the different clinical diagnoses. In patients with malignancy of the lung, weight loss and tiredness (and also a smoking history) are likely to be present also, whereas fever is usually seen in pneumonia. In confirmed PE, haemoptysis is present only in a minority of patients (Table 4.1). Its presence indicates alveolar haemorrhage caused by pulmonary infarction or congestive atelectasis. It may get worse with the initiation of anticoagulant therapy, but it is rarely massive and usually does not create a significant clinical problem.

Table 4.1 Clinical spectrum, prevalence and differential diagnosis of pulmonary embolism(21,22)

Clinical presentation	Prevalence of sign or symptom in patients with PE with no prior cardiopulmonary disease (%)	Differential diagnosis of sign or symptom
Circulatory collapse	8–10	Cardiogenic shock (myocardial infarction, cardiac arrythmia), hypovolaemic shock (bleeding, ruptured aortic aneurysm, fluid loss), obstructive shock (pericardial tamponade, tension pneumothorax, aortic dissection), distributive shock (sepsis, anaphylaxis), intoxication (benzodiazepines, opiates)
Acute dyspnea as only symptom	36	Asthma, COPD, asthma cardiale, pleural fluid, pneumonia, bronchitis, pneumothorax, corpus alienum, hyperventilation syndrome, neuromuscular disease
Dyspnea in combination with other symptoms	73–80	
Pleuritic chest pain Chest pain/discomfort	27–44	Coronary artery disease, pericarditis, aortic dissection, pleuritis, pneumonia, bronchitis, pneumothorax, tumour, intercostal muscle cramps or neuritis, costochondritis, herpes zoster
Haemoptysis	5–13	Nasopharyngeal bleeding, neoplasm, bronchitis, bronchiectasis, foreign body, lung abscess, pneumonia, tuberculosis, congestive heart failure, Wegener's granulomatosis, lung contusion, mycetoma, Goodpasture's syndrome
Cough	34–40	Infectious disease, corpus alienum, bronchitis, COPD, smoking
Symptoms of DVT	30–40	Trauma, cellulites, erysipelas, ruptured Baker's cyst, haematoma, lymphangitis, chronic venous insufficiency, post-thrombotic syndrome, inguinal tumour

Symptoms of the leg, suggesting DVT, should alert the physician managing a patient with chest symptoms. These symptoms were described in Chapter 3.

CLINICAL SIGNS OF PULMONARY EMBOLISM

Circulatory collapse suggests massive PE, but this is not necessarily the case in all patients. Especially in patients with underlying cardiopulmonary disease, small emboli can cause circulatory problems. In clinical studies where PE was confirmed in enrolled patients, circulatory collapse was present in less than 10%. However, a proportion of patients with haemodynamic instability will probably have died before the diagnosis was confirmed. Therefore, exact numbers cannot be calculated. The origin of the circulatory problems in patients with PE appears to be the right ventricle. The pathophysiology of right ventricular dysfunction might be initiated through the hypoxaemia and the release of vasoconstrictors such as serotonin. This causes a concomitant reflex pulmonary vasoconstriction which results in pulmonary arterial hypertension and secondary right ventricular dysfunction. Right ventricular dilatation also leads to interventricular septum shift and relative compromise of the left ventricle. Additional factors such as acute inflammation and increased platelet activation, as implicated in animal studies of PE, may contribute to ongoing subclinical right ventricular dysfunction (3,4).

The prevalence of right ventricular dysfunction varies from 40–50% in patients with haemo-dynamically stable PE to 70% in those with circulatory instability. Its presence is associated with an increased mortality. Absolute differences in short-term PE-related mortality in normotensive patients between patients with and without right ventricular dysfunction are approximately 5% (5). These differences are somewhat higher in studies that included haemodynamic stable and haemo-dynamic unstable patients. Echocardiography may be helpful in these patients to assess severity of disease and response to treatment (see Chapter 11).

The prevalences of the above-mentioned signs and symptoms in patients with PE are summa-rized in Table 4.1. It should be kept in mind that the percentages in this table are from studies investigating diagnostic strategies for acute PE. The clinical characteristics of these patients were sufficient to alert physicians to the diagnosis of PE and to enrol them in clinical studies.

DIAGNOSTIC TESTS

Several baseline diagnostic tests are often carried out in patients presenting with one or more chest symptoms before a specific diagnostic management strategy for PE is initiated. These include laboratory measurement of parameters for infection such as C-reactive protein (CRP) and white blood cell count and also an arterial blood gas analysis. An electrocardiogram (ECG) and chest X-ray are generally also performed and the results could give rise to a suspicion of PE.

Arterial blood gas analysis

An arterial blood gas analysis is regularly performed in those patients presenting with tachypneu or dyspnea. In the diagnostic work-up of patients with suspected PE, arterial blood gases have been extensively evaluated. The ultimate goal of these studies was to find some combination of normal arterial blood gases combined with a normal $P(A-a)O_2$ gradient that may be used to exclude acute PE safely. This was based on some observations that in patients with confirmed PE and no prior cardiac or pulmonary disease, 93% have hypoxaemia or hypocapnia and 98% have an increased P(A-a)O$_2$ gradient or hypocapnia (6). However, several studies have documented that no combination of blood gas results could be identified that reliably excluded PE (7–11).

Hypoxaemia is a consistent and important clinical feature of PE, although this feature is classical for different other pulmonary diseases also, and can be absent even in patients with major vascular obstruction. The actual mechanism of hypoxaemia in PE is incompletely understood. Intrapulmonary shunting, right to left intracardiac shunting, ventilation/perfusion mismatching and also impaired diffusion have all been suggested as plausible contributory causes. Hypoxaemia has been related to the degree of pulmonary vascular obstruction as measured with pulmonary angiography or helical CT (12).

Electrocardiogram

The electrocardiogram (ECG) is often one of the initial diagnostic tests performed in patients presenting with dyspnea and is essential in the assessment of patients with acute chest pain. Abnormalities might be diagnostic for conditions present in the differential diagnosis of patients with suspected PE, but might also alert the physician to PE which he or she had not considered before. It is important to recognize the frequently seen abnormalities in this group of patients. Any cause of acute cor pulmonale can give ECG abnormalities. This includes acute PE, pneumothorax or acute bronchospasm. A sinus tachycardia is most frequently seen, whereas other rhythm abnormalities are relatively rare (13).

The findings on an ECG may vary from normal to completely pathological. The ECG can be abnormal in up to 70% of the patients with confirmed PE who had no prior cardiac or pulmonary disease (2). Many abnormalities on the ECG have been described in patients with PE. The classical finding on the ECG in a patient with PE is the S1Q3T3 pattern (Figure 4.1). It was first described by McGinn and White in 1935 (14). S1Q3T3 is a triad consisting of a prominent S wave in lead I, a prominent Q wave in lead III and an inverted T wave in lead III. Although classical, this pattern occurs in only 2–15% of patients with PE (13,15). Other abnormalities found may vary from alterations in rhythm (sinustachycardia, atrial flutter and atrial fibrillation) to non-specific abnormalities of the ST segment or the T wave, T wave inversion in the right pre-cordial leads, low amplitude deflexions, rightward QRS complex axis shift and a right bundle branch block (2).

The genesis of some ECG abnormalities is not completely understood, but the majority of changes result from the right-sided heart strain pattern. Thrombus formation and obstruction in the pulmonary arteries result in acute dilatation of the right atrium and ventricle and increased myocardial wall tension. This can cause pulmonary hypertension and a decreased blood return to the left ventricle, resulting in decreased cardiac output and coronary perfusion. A right bundle branch block is probably due to the increased pressure within the right ventricle, resulting in compression of the bundle branch.

In massive PE, ECG changes are more likely to be present. This seems to be common sense considering that patients with massive PE have a fall in blood pressure indicating diminished left ventricular function and also right ventricle function. Some of the ECG changes may be very transient and disappear with only a relatively small improvement in the haemodynamic state.

Although the value of an ECG for diagnostic purposes is modest, it could be used as a tool in risk stratification in major PE, as suggested in recent studies. Massive PE and right ventricular failure are associated with an increased risk of death (16). Some ECG abnormalities (right bundle branch block, ST segment changes, T wave inversion) have a good specificity to identify right ventricular dysfunction, which indicates that the presence of any of these features is suggestive of right ventricular dysfunction, but their absence does not rule it out. T wave inversion in leads V1–V3 was the most accurate criterion for right ventricular dysfunction (17). In a large study

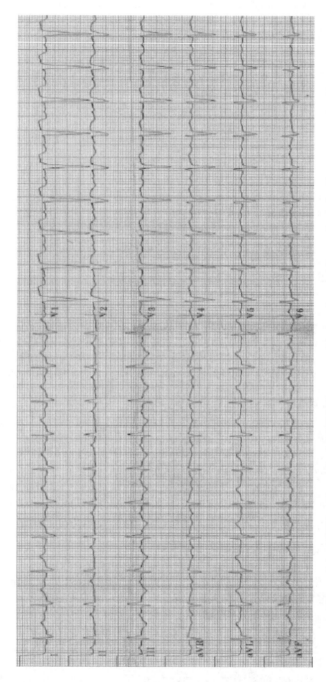

Figure 4.1   ECG with typical S1Q3T3 pattern in a patient with confirmed pulmonary embolism.

with approximately 500 patients with acute major PE, the presence of the above-mentioned ECG abnormalities was a predictor of poor outcome (18). Thorough research should be performed in order to decide whether therapeutic consequences can be based on ECG changes, possibly in combination with other prognostic instruments such as brain natriuretic peptide or troponin measurement.

In conclusion, the ECG makes a limited contribution to the diagnostic evaluation of patients with suspected PE. A completely normal ECG is not at all sensitive to rule out PE. Nevertheless, an ECG has the great power to exclude other life-threatening diseases with comparable symptoms to PE, such as myocardial infarction. Therefore, the ECG should always be obtained in patients with acute chest pain and dyspnea.

Chest radiograph

It was not long after the discovery of the Roentgen rays in 1895 that chest radiography became available. And although it could therefore be regarded as an antique diagnostic tool, it is still the most frequently requested radiological investigation as it tends to be the first-line examination in patients presenting with cardiac or pulmonary signs or symptoms and it is commonly used in the assessment of the general condition of a patient.

In patients with suspected PE, spiral CT angiography has recently become the diagnostic procedure to detect pulmonary vascular filling defects. A chest radiograph, however, is frequently performed in the diagnostic work-up and can be considered a useful tool in the clinical evaluation. There are several reasons to perform a chest radiograph in patients with suspected PE. The main advantage of chest radiography is its ability easily to exclude or confirm alternative diseases that may be considered in the differential diagnosis, such as pneumonia or pleural effusion. In patients with chronic pulmonary diseases, a comparison with previous radiographs can detect differences and could therefore be helpful to decide whether the clinical symptoms are due to a previously existing illness. With respect to diagnosing PE, the main purpose of chest radiography is to search for different radiographic findings that are associated with the presence of PE.

In two large series of patients with proven PE, the results of a chest X-ray were abnormal in approximately 75–90% of the patients (19,20). The radiographic findings varied according to the size and number of emboli and the haemodynamic features of the pulmonary circulation. In the case of a smaller embolism (without overt cor pulmonale), radiographic changes have time to develop. After 24–72 hours, loss of pulmonary surfactant often causes atelectasis and alveolar infiltrates that are indistinguishable from pneumonia. Many other features have been described in the literature. Cardiomegaly and an elevated hemidiaphragm are common abnormalities. Pulmonary artery enlargement (Fleischner's sign) can be caused by increased pulmonary pressure, by the clot itself or even by pulmonary artery aneurysm (Figure 4.2).

Pleural effusion is seen in 20–50% of patients presenting with PE (2,19). Pulmonary oedema occurred only in a minority of the patients. On rare occasions, the chest X-ray may show focal oligaemia (Westermark's sign), which is thought to be caused by dilatation of the pulmonary vessels proximal to an embolism in combination with collapse of the distal vessels. This reduction in local blood volume combined with changes in the lung volume can cause oligaemia in the involved lung. If the presence of PE causes infarction of the lung parenchyma, the chest radiograph shows a wedge-shaped consolidation that is located in the lung periphery. This is called the Hampton hump (Figure 4.3). The prevalence of infarction in patients presenting with acute PE ranges between 5 and 10% (19). Plate-like atelectasis, if present, appears early in patients with PE and disappears completely after a few days, possibly as perfusion recovers.

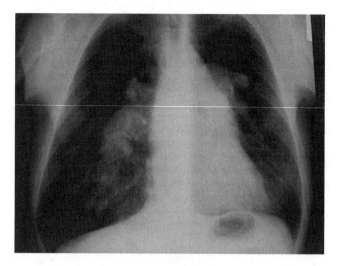

Figure 4.2   Pulmonary artery enlargement (Fleischner's sign) on chest X-ray.

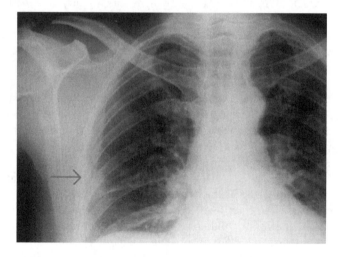

Figure 4.3   Hampton hump on chest X-ray in patient with pulmonary embolism.

Once a thrombus has formed in the deep veins of the lower extremities or the embolus has migrated to the pulmonary arteries, different pathophysiological mechanisms assist the physician to come to the diagnosis.

Due to partly or completely occluded vessels and initiation of local inflammation, signs and symptoms occur that raise the suspicion of DVT or PE. This information from medical history and physical examination can be used in quantitative clinical scores that help the physician in increasing or decreasing its probability. However, the value of the individual signs and symptoms remains low due to their non-specific nature. As a result, once a suspicion arises, the clinician should try to stratify patients into those where PE is more or less likely and order diagnostic tests to gain an objective diagnosis.

REFERENCES

1. Goldman L. Chest discomfort and palpitation. In Fauci AS, Braunwald E, Isselbacher KJ, Wilson JD, Martin JB, Kasper DL, Hauser SL, Longo DL (eds), *Harrison's Principles of Internal Medicine*. McGraw-Hill, New York, 1998, pp. 58–65.

2. Stein PD, Terrin ML, Hales CA, *et al*. Clinical, laboratory, roentgenographic and electrocardiogrpahic findings in patients with acute pulmonary embolism and no pre-existing cardiac or pulmonary disease. *Chest* 1991; **100**:598–603.

3. Elliot CG. Pulmonary physiology during pulmonary embolism. *Chest* 1992; **101**: 163–71S.

4. Stratmann G, Gregory GA. Neurogenic and humoral vasoconstriction in acute pulmonary thromboembolism. *Anesth Analg* 2003; **97**:341–54.

5. ten Wolde M, Söhne M, Quak E, MacGillavry MR, Büller HR. Prognostic value of echocardiographic assessed right ventricular dysfunction in patients with pulmonary embolism. *Arch Intern Med* 2004; **164**:1686–9.

6. Cvitanic O, Marino PL. Improved use of arterial blood gas analysis in suspected pulmonary embolism. *Chest* 1989; **95**:48–51.

7. Stein PD, Goldhaber SZ, Henry JW. Arterial blood gas analysis in the assessment of suspected acute pulmonary embolism. *Chest* 1996; **109**:78–81.

8. Jones JS. Use of the alveolar–arterial oxygen gradient in the assessment of acute pulmonary embolism. *Am J Emerg Med* 1998; **16**:333–7.

9. Prediletto R, Miniati M, Tonelli L *et al*. Diagnositc value of gas exchange tests in patients with clinical suspicion of pulmonary embolism. *Crit Care* 1999; **3**:111–6.

10. Masotti L, Ceccarelli E, Cappelli R, *et al*. Arterial blood gas analysis and alveolar–arterial oxygen gradient in diagnosis and prognosis of elderly patients with suspected pulmonary embolism. *J Gerontol A Biol Sci Med Sci* 2000; **55A**:M761–M764.

11. Rodger MA, Carrier M, Jones GN, *et al*. Diagnostic value of arterial blood gas measurement in suspected pulmonary embolism. *Am J Resp Crit Care Med* 2000; **162**:2105–8.

12. Metafratzi ZM, Vassiliou MP, Maglaras GC, *et al*. Acute pulmonary embolism: correlation of CT pulmonary artery obstruction index with blood gas values. *AJR* 2005; **186**:213–9.

13. Petruzzelli S, Palla A, Peraccini F, *et al*. Routine electrocardiography in screening for pulmonary embolism. *Respiration* 1986; **50**:233–43.

14. McGinn S, White PD. Acute cor pulmonale resulting from pulmonary embolism. *JAMA* 1935; **104**:1473–80.

15. Richman PB, Loutf, H, Lester SJ, *et al*. Electrocardiographic findings in emergency department patients with pulmonary embolism. *J Emerg Med*. 2004; **27**:121–6.

16. Laporte S, Mismetti P, Decousus H, *et al*. Clinical predictors for fatal pulmonary embolism in 15 520 patients with venous thromboembolism. Findings from the Registro Informatizado de la Enfermedad TromboEmbolica Venosa (RIETE) Registry. *Circulation* 2008; **117**:1711–6.

17. Punukollu G, Gowda RM, Vasavada BC, Khan IA. Role of electrocardiography in identifying right ventricular dysfunction in acute pulmonary embolism. *Am J Cardiol* 2005; **96**:450–2.

18. Geibel A, Zehender M, Kasper W, *et al*. Prognostic value of the ECG on admission in patients with acute major pulmonary embolism. *Eur Respir J* 2005; **25**:843–8.

19. Elliot CG, Goldhaber SZ, Visani L, DeRosa M. Chest radiographs in acute pulmonary embolism: results from the international cooperative pulmonary embolism registry. *Chest* 2000; **118**:33–8.

20. Worsley DF, Alavi A, Aronchick JM, *et al*. Chest radiographic findings in patients with acute pulmonary embolism: observations from the PIOPED study. *Radiology* 1993; **189**:133–6.

21. Manganelli D, Palla A, Donnamaria V, Giuntini C. Clinical features of pulmonary embolism: doubts and certainties. *Chest* 1995; **107**(1 Suppl):22S–32S.

22. Stein PD, Beemath A, Matta F, *et al*. Clinical characteristics of patients with acute pulmonary embolism: data from PIOPED II. *Am J Med*. 2007; **120**:871–9.

PART III

Diagnostic Procedures

CHAPTER 5

Clinical prediction rules for diagnosis of venous Thromboembolism

Grégoire Le Gal[1,2] **and Marc A. Rodger**[3,4]

[1]Department of Internal Medicine and Chest Diseases, Brest University Hospital, Brest, France;
[2]Thrombosis Program, Division of Hematology, Department of Medicine, University of Ottawa, Ontario, Canada;
[3]Division of Hematology, The Ottawa Hospital, General Campus Ontario, Canada;
[4]Clinical Epidemiology Program, Ottawa Health Research Institute, The Ottawa Hospital, Ontario, Canada

INTRODUCTION

Clinical probability assessment has become a mandatory step in the investigation of patients with clinically suspected venous thromboembolism (VTE). The objective of this chapter is to understand why we need clinical prediction rules and specifically why they are desirable in the field of VTE. The questions to be addressed are: What is clinical probability? What are clinical prediction rules? How do they work? How they are developed? How should we use them? What are their limitations? What are the existing clinical prediction rules for venous thromboembolism? What are their strengths and weaknesses?

DIAGNOSTIC TESTS AND CLINICAL PROBABILITY: HOW DO THEY WORK?

The objective of a diagnostic test is to define the presence or absence of a disease or condition. Diagnosis is then usually used to inform a therapeutic decision. The ideal diagnostic test is simple to apply, widely available, inexpensive, has no complications and provides a 'yes or no' answer. Diagnostic tests, however, rarely are perfectly accurate. They are often evaluated in comparison to a 'gold standard', which is usually as close to 'perfect' as possible.

Deep Vein Thrombosis and Pulmonary Embolism Edited by Edwin J.R. van Beek, Harry R. Büller and Matthijs Oudkerk
© 2009 John Wiley & Sons, Ltd

In diagnostic accuracy studies, a group of patients being investigated for the study's disease of interest undergoes both the gold standard test(s) and the test under evaluation (experimental test). One of the quality criteria for this type of study is that the interpretation and conduct of the new test should be blind from the final diagnosis obtained with the gold standard test(s). A 2 × 2 table is then generated, in which patients are divided according to the results of both the experimental test and the gold standard test(s) (Table 5.1). Ideally, all patients with the disease will test positive (i.e., they are all true positive with no false positives) and all patients without the disease will test negative (i.e., they are all true negative with no false negatives). However, in reality this rarely occurs, and we often observe patients without the disease who test positive (false positive) and patients with disease who test negative (false negative). Accuracy indices can be computed to describe the degree of experimental test imperfection. The sensitivity of a test is the percentage of patients who test positive within the pool of patients with the disease [as per the gold standard test(s)] (i.e., A/(A + C) in Table 5.1). The specificity of a test is the percentage of patients who test negative when the disease is absent (i.e., D/(B + D) in Table 5.1). These two characteristics of diagnostic tests are said intrinsic to the test and will not be influenced by the population in which the test is 'tested'. From a clinical perspective, two other measures of diagnostic accuracy are even more relevant: the probability of disease in patients who test positive [positive predictive value (PPV)] and the probability of disease in those who test negative [negative predictive value (NPV)]. The PPV is the percentage of patients with disease in the pool of patients who test positive [i.e., A/(A + B) in Table 5.1]. The NPV is the percentage of patients without disease in the pool of patients with a negative test [i.e., D/(C + D) in Table 5.1]. It is very important to realize that, unlike sensitivity and specificity, the PPV and NPV are highly dependent on the prevalence (that is, the proportion of subjects who have the disease) in the test population. Indeed, in each row of the 2 × 2 table, not only will the absolute numbers of patients in each box vary according to sensitivity and specificity, but these numbers also depend on the prevalence of disease.

The evaluation of a diagnostic test should also include an assessment of its reproducibility. Indeed, the same test in the same patient may not always give the same result, which may be due to a whole variety of reasons, including test variability and observer interpretation. Hence reproducibility, and the reasons for any variability and its extent, should be investigated. One of the simplest ways to assess reproducibility is to compute the Cohen's kappa statistic, which provides a measure of agreement between two observers. It corresponds to the percentage of patients in whom both observers agreed (on the presence of a clinical sign, for example), adjusted on the amount of agreement that could be expected due to chance alone. A kappa score above 0.8 is considered excellent inter-observer reliability, 0.6–0.8 is good inter-observer reliability, 0.4–0.6 is moderate inter-observer reliability, 0.2–0.4 is fair inter-observer reliability and below 0.2 is poor inter-observer reliability.

Bayes' theorem allows us to compute the post-test probability of a disease in groups who test positive and groups who test negative based on knowledge of a test's sensitivity and specificity and pre-test probability of disease in a population. The pre-test probability is simply the prevalence

Table 5.1 Evaluation of diagnostic test, comparison with gold standard

	Gold standard positive (disease present)	Gold standard negative (disease absent)
Test positive	True positive A	False positive B
Test negative	False negative C	True negative D

of the disease in a population in which the test is to be applied. In order to increase the utility of diagnostic tests, we exploit this characteristic of diagnostic tests by determining the probability of disease before applying the test, in other words, the clinical pre-test probability. Applying Bayes' theorem is particularly useful when simple and accurate tests are not available in clinical practice. The latter is probably why this approach has been widely adopted in the management of suspected VTE.

Deep vein thrombosis (DVT) and pulmonary embolism (PE) are serious conditions that are potentially fatal if left untreated (1). However, treatment with anticoagulants is very effective, albeit complex (due to the narrow therapeutic window, it requires a close monitoring of its efficacy by blood test and frequent dose adjustments), of long duration (months), accompanied by dietary and lifestyle modifications and has serious adverse effects, mainly a 1–3% annual risk of major bleeding (2–5), of which approximately 15% are fatal (6). Hence enough diagnostic certainty must be reached before such anticoagulant treatment is introduced. In other words, we neither want to miss a patient with VTE, nor expose a patient without VTE to anticoagulants. However, the gold standard tests, which are pulmonary angiography for PE and venography for DVT (see Chapters 10 and 13), are invasive, expensive and not without risk, leading to the efforts of the two last decades to avoid their use by employing less invasive diagnostic tests [plasma D-dimer measurement, lower limb vein ultrasonography, ventilation–perfusion lung scan and, most recently, chest computed tomography (CT); these tests are discussed more fully in the following chapters].

The use of clinical probability assessment became mainstream after the PIOPED study (7). This diagnostic accuracy study compared ventilation–perfusion lung scintigraphy (V/Q) (the experimental test) with pulmonary angiography (the gold standard) in patients with suspected PE. V/Q scan as a stand-alone test was disappointing: 12% of patients with a low probability V/Q had PE on angiography, which is too high a proportion to rely on this result alone to rule out PE. Conversely, 88% of patients with a high probability V/Q had PE on angiography. Therefore, considering all patients with a high V/Q as having PE, one out of nine would receive unnecessary anticoagulant therapy. The only clinically useful result of V/Q as a stand-alone test was limited to the 14% of patients who had a normal V/Q in whom the proportion of PE on angiography was low enough to rule out the diagnosis [which was later confirmed by a management outcome study (8)]. In the PIOPED study, expert physicians were asked to assign a clinical pre-test probability to each patient based on their expert intuitive evaluation of the probability of PE and to classify patients into three probability groups: 0–19%, 20–79% and 80–100%. Combining this clinical pre-test probability assessment and the results of the V/Q scan allowed the investigators to increase significantly the diagnostic yield of the V/Q scan. Patients with both low clinical pre-test probability and low-probability V/Q had a low enough proportion of PE on pulmonary angiography to rule out the diagnosis, whereas almost all patients with both high clinical pre-test probability and high-probability V/Q had PE on angiography. Conversely, the proportion of PE was unacceptably high (about 40%) in patients with a low-probability V/Q but a high clinical pre-test probability and unacceptably low (about 60%) in patients with high-probability V/Q but a low clinical pre-test probability.

Clinical pre-test probability assessment has since been increasingly used in diagnostic strategies for VTE. It allows not only a clinically useful interpretation of the results of the V/Q scan, but also, as outlined in other chapters, identifies a subgroup of patients with a low clinical probability of VTE in whom a simpler work-up can be performed using plasma D-dimer measurement and VTE be ruled out with no diagnostic imaging. As discussed in the next chapter, D-dimers are cross-linked fibrin derivatives that are produced by fibrin degradation by plasmin. D-dimer has a very high sensitivity for VTE, which in turn results in a high negative predictive value. Thus, in a low pre-test probability population, a negative D-dimer test makes the post-test probability of VTE low enough to rule out the diagnosis of VTE without any other testing (9). However, if the pre-test probability of VTE is above a certain threshold the negative predictive value of D-dimer is not sufficiently high to exclude VTE comfortably. For these reasons, D-dimers are used in combination with clinical pre-test probability. Most D-dimer tests can safely rule out the diagnosis in patients with a low pre-test probability of disease, whereas a highly sensitive D-dimer test can even exclude the diagnosis in patients with a low or intermediate clinical pre-test probability. The safety of such an approach has been confirmed in multiple management outcome studies (10–12).

CLINICAL PREDICTION RULES: WHY DO WE NEED THEM?

Determining clinical pre-test probability of VTE can be performed empirically by a physician, taking into account a patient's medical history and physical examination, based on the physician's experience and clinical judgement (i.e., intuitive or 'gestalt' approach to pre-test probability assessment). This intuitive approach to pre-test probability assessment was indeed conducted in the PIOPED study and was demonstrated to be relatively accurate. However, this intuitive approach to clinical pre-test probability assessment is probably highly dependent on the physician's experience, cannot be standardized and is not reproducible. In an inter-observer reliability study of 110 consecutive patients seen for suspected PE and assessed by two independent physicians, the reproducibility of the physician's intuitive evaluation of clinical probability (or 'gestalt') was inadequate (kappa coefficient 0.33) (13). The importance of the poor reproducibility of intuitive clinical pre-test probability assessment cannot be understated. Patients with suspected VTE are referred to the emergency room, where they are often seen by different physicians at different steps of their management, younger physicians or physicians in training or after-hours physicians who are not experts in the field of VTE. Moreover, given the direct consequences on patient management in suspected VTE, physicians often feel uncomfortable when assessing the clinical probability. Indeed, clinical probability assessment may affect the extensiveness of the diagnostic work-up, the therapeutic management while awaiting the results of the tests and the decision to admit or discharge a patient. This underlines the need for a reliable and reproducible clinical probability assessment tools.

Clinical prediction rules are decision-making tools using combinations of simple available clinical predictors to define a probability of disease which then leads to a diagnostic or therapeutic course of action. Clinical prediction rules allow us to standardize clinical probability assessment and to select and combine the best independent predictors, risk factors, symptoms, clinical signs and results of simple diagnostic tests for VTE. Not unlike a diagnostic test, the most useful clinical prediction rules are accurate, reproducible, simple and easy to apply to facilitate introduction and use in clinical practice. Given the importance of accuracy and reproducibility in clinical pre-test probability assessment for VTE diagnosis, investigators have focused on developing clinical prediction rules for the VTE diagnosis. The importance of the use of clinical prediction rules for pre-test probability assessment for VTE is highlighted by a cohort study of 1529 consecutive outpatients seen in 117 emergency departments, which showed that the inappropriate diagnostic management of patients with suspected PE was associated with a significantly poorer outcome: the 3-month thromboembolic risk was 7.7% in patients with inappropriate management versus 1.2% in those in whom the diagnosis was ruled out according to internationally validated criteria. In this study, the lack of a written guideline including a clinical prediction rule was associated with a two-fold increased risk of inappropriate management (14).

HOW ARE CLINICAL PREDICTION RULES BUILT?

Clinical prediction rules should be sensible, i.e., have a clear purpose, be relevant, demonstrate content validity, be concise and be easy to use in the intended clinical application. The use of the rule should provide a probability of disease and should imply a course of action. The construction of valid, accurate and reproducible clinical prediction rules follows a strict methodology. Standards for their development and validation were first published more than 20 years ago (15) and were recently updated (16).

   The first step is the derivation of the clinical prediction rule. If the goal of the rule is to predict the probability of PE, the derivation should be performed in a group of patients with suspected PE as similar as possible to the clinical setting in which the rule is planned to be used (e.g., emergency room patients, inpatient, all comers). A description of inclusion and exclusion criteria in the derivation study, and also of clinical and demographic characteristics of participants, is important to ensure generalizability and applicability of the results. Participants should represent a wide spectrum of disease (not only patients who clearly have and clearly do not have the condition). The outcome or diagnosis to be predicted must be clearly defined and clinically important and the assessment of the outcome must be blinded (i.e., the final arbiter of outcome must have no prior knowledge of potential predictive variables under study). The final diagnosis should be obtained using a standardized and valid gold standard. Prior to the start of the study, a list of all candidate predictors should be established through a thorough literature search. The potential predictors must be clearly defined *a priori*. To avoid observation bias, their assessment must be done without knowledge of the outcome (i.e., blinded). To ensure valid predictor data collection, data collection should be prospective and recorded on a standardised data collection form. The reproducibility of each individual predictor should also be assessed and only those predictors with a good reproducibility (e.g., kappa > 0.6) should be considered for inclusion in the clinical prediction rule. The statistical techniques used to derive the rule must be identified and valid. The sample size should be determined to ensure that all relevant predictor variables could be included in the rule. A commonly accepted criterion is that $5-10$ outcome events in the smallest outcome category (e.g., PE) per predictor in the final rule are required. A univariate analysis is first performed, comparing the frequency (or mean in case of continuous variables) of all candidate predictors in patients with and without confirmed disease (e.g., PE). Those found to be statistically significantly associated with the final diagnosis are included in a multivariate logistic regression model. The threshold for the *p*-value for variable selection is often increased (e.g., $p > 0.20$), to be able to include all candidate predictors (including those whose univariate association with the diagnosis may be confounded by another predictor) in the multivariate model. Continuous variables can be dichotomized at their best discriminate cut-off value to facilitate use, memorability and implementation of the final clinical prediction rule. The final multivariate model is an equation that gives the probability of disease (e.g., PE) according to the presence or absence of those predictors that are independently associated with the disease, each of them with a multiplication coefficient reflecting the strength of its association with the diagnosis. To simplify the computation of the score, these coefficients are often replaced by simple integer numbers. The score is then computed for all patients in the study. The proportion of patients with each possible value of the score and the proportion of confirmed disease in each of these groups are then determined. Thresholds for dividing clinical probability groups are then chosen, according to the desired repartition of patients across groups and to the desired proportion of with disease in each group. For example, a common objective is to separate out the largest possible group of patients that have a low enough prevalence to exclude the disease. The definition of the 'low enough prevalence' is dependent on the clinical condition, subsequent diagnostic testing planned and the characteristics of the subsequent diagnostic tests (accuracy, invasiveness, expense). For example, in PE, the accuracy of the D-dimer test used in each institution helps to determine the threshold at which a negative result makes the post-test probability of disease low enough to rule out the diagnosis safely. Conversely, the prevalence of PE in the highest probability group should be high enough to justify an extensive and more invasive work-up. The accuracy of the clinical prediction rule in classifying patients with the outcome (i.e., sensitivity) and without the outcome (i.e., specificity) should be demonstrated.

A second step after derivation of the clinical prediction rule is the validation of the rule in an independent cohort of patients. In fact, the rule is built as a 'tailored suit' for the derivation cohort. It is therefore important to check the proportion of patients classified by the rule in the different clinical probability groups, and also its accuracy (e.g., overall ability to identify patients with and without PE) and calibration (ability to predict a number of PE that corresponds to observed numbers of PE across the entire spread of the data) in a different cohort of patients. In other words, it is important to ensure that the 'suit' will fit all the populations in which it is intended to be applied. This cohort should again represent an unselected group of patients with a wide spectrum of disease severity and the predictors for the rule should again be collected blinded from the final diagnosis.

Finally, the impact of use of the rule, its clinical utility and safety of managing patients on the basis of the rule 'in the real world' should be demonstrated in a prospective management outcome study. In these studies, use of the rule in usual practice is measured along with the performance of the rule in usual practice.

HOW DO WE KNOW THAT A RULE IS READY TO BE USED?

Levels of evidence can be attributed to clinical prediction rules depending on whether or not they went through all the methodological steps described above. Level 4 corresponds to a rule that is derived but not prospectively validated: it needs to be further evaluated before clinical application. Level 3 rules have been prospectively validated but only in one narrow sample: physicians may consider their use with caution and only if patients in their clinical setting are similar to those included in validation study. Level 2 rules have demonstrated their accuracy in either a large prospective study including a broad spectrum of the disease or in several different smaller settings. They can be used in various settings with confidence in their accuracy. Level 1 rules have been prospectively validated in a different population and the impact of use of the rule has been measured and demonstrates a change in clinician behaviour with beneficial consequences. Level 1 rules can be used with the confidence that they can change clinician behaviour and improve patients' outcomes (16).

WHICH PREDICTION RULES ARE AVAILABLE FOR PE DIAGNOSIS?

A first attempt to build a clinical prediction tool for pre-test probability assessment for PE was derived by expert consensus (17). This tool allowed the classification of patients into three risk categories, based on the presence of a list of 'typical signs and symptoms of PE', the existence of 'an alternative diagnosis as or more likely than that of PE' and on a list of risk factors for VTE (17). This complex model was then validated in an independent cohort of patients and proved to be able to classify patients with suspected PE into three groups with increasing proportions of confirmed PE. Although explicit, the main limitations of this model were that the 'typical signs and symptoms of PE' and 'likelihood of an alternative diagnosis' required expert clinical evaluation, which, like the intuitive approach to pre-test probability assessment, would be difficult to standardize. Moreover, even if based on literature review and experts' consensus, important predictors might have been omitted during the development of the rule.

Subsequently, various clinical prediction rules to assess the clinical pre-test probability for PE in patients with suspected PE have been published (18–23). Two of them have been more widely used and validated in diagnostic strategies based on their estimates and reached level 1 evidence: the Wells' score and the Geneva score. They are presented in Table 5.2. A characteristic of the Wells' score is the use of a predictor requiring an estimation of the likelihood of PE, as compared with that of alternative diagnoses, 'PE as or more likely than any alternative diagnosis'. This criterion has been shown to be a strong predictor of PE and thus carries a major weight in the score. Although this is a strength of this clinical prediction tool, it also constitutes its main limitation. In fact, it is difficult to conceive that this estimation of 'PE as or more likely than any alternative diagnosis' can be standardized and indeed the reproducibility of this predictor has been demonstrated to be low (13). The Wells' score has been widely validated, in different countries and clinical settings. Presence of PE ranged from 38 to 91% in the high clinical probability group, as compared with 28–40% and 1–28% in the intermediate and the low clinical probability groups, respectively (24). The original Geneva rule used the results of chest X-ray and arterial blood gas (ABG) analysis while breathing room air, both of which appeared to be strong predictors of PE. This also turned out to be a limitation of this clinical prediction rule. In fact, in the validation study (25), ABG results were not available for about 20% of patients, either because the physician felt that a patient's condition was not serious enough to warrant this invasive test or at the other end of the spectrum because patients with severe respiratory distress were treated with oxygen since their admission and before the ABG could be performed. The revised Geneva score attempts to answer the limitations of existing scores, providing a model that is independent of clinical judgement and/or the results of diagnostic tests (18). Interestingly, but not surprisingly, some clinical variables, which are the strongest predictors, are common to most clinical prediction rules: a history of VTE, the presence of an active malignancy, tachycardia and haemoptysis.

Table 5.2 Clinical prediction rules for PE

Wells' score (19)		Revised Geneva score (45)	
Active cancer	+1	Age >65 years	+1
Haemoptysis	+1	Active cancer	+2
History of previous DVT or PE	+1.5	Haemoptysis	+2
Heart rate >100/ min	+1.5	History of previous DVT or PE	+3
Surgery or bedrest ≥3 days within 1 month	+1.5	Surgery or lower limb fracture within one month	+2
Clinical signs or symptoms of DVT	+3	Unilateral oedema and pain at palpation	+4
No alternative diagnosis as or more likely than PE	+3	Spontaneously reported calf pain	+3
		Heart rate 75–94/ min	+3
		Heart rate ≥95/min	+5

Clinical probability	Points	PE (%)	Clinical probability	Points	PE (%)
Low	<2	2–6	Low	0–3	7–12
Intermediate	2–6	17–24	Intermediate	4–10	22–31
High	>6	54–78	High	≥11	58–82
Unlikely	≤ 4	8–13			
Likely	>4	37–56			

Which one should be the preferred clinical prediction rule? The diagnostic accuracy of these rules has been shown to be comparable when retrospectively applied in one study (26). The safety and accuracy of each rule has been demonstrated in large management outcome studies or randomized control trials in which the diagnostic work-up was based on the results of these scores (27–29). The decision to implement a clinical prediction rule in diagnostic strategies for PE at an institutional level is certainly much more important than the choice among available rules.

More recently, another type of clinical prediction rule has been developed in order to assess the clinical probability of PE, not in patients with suspected PE but to identify which patients should be suspected of having PE and conversely, in which patients PE should not be suspected and where no work-up is required. In fact, in recent years, an important decrease in the proportion of confirmed PE cases among patients with suspected PE has been documented in studies examining the diagnosis of PE, suggesting that the threshold for clinical suspicion has been significantly lowered. In the PIOPED study, one out of three patients with suspected PE were confirmed to have PE (7). This proportion has decreased during the last two decades and recent studies in North America report the prevalence of PE among the tested population to be as low as 5% (31,32). This, even with the use of D-dimer testing, has resulted in an important increase in the number of patients needed to be investigated by imaging tests to find one case of PE (30). Therefore, an emerging new challenge is to define more precisely who should be suspected of having PE. Indeed, searching for PE in all patients with dyspnea or chest pain will probably lead to increases in cost and test complications without improvements in health. Kline *et al.* (33) have built a clinical prediction rule in emergency department patients to identify those at such low risk of PE on clinical grounds that they would not need either D-dimer testing or any other investigation. The overall prevalence of PE was 11% in this derivation set. The final model comprised eight negative variables significantly associated with *absence* of PE: age <50 years, pulse <100 bpm, SaO_2>94%, no unilateral leg swelling, no haemoptysis, no recent trauma or surgery, no history of VTE and no estrogen use. If all criteria were absent then PE should not be suspected. In a validation set of 1427 patients with a prevalence of PE of 8%, the rule was negative (all criteria met) in 25%. Among them, the proportion of PE was only 1.4% (5/362, 95% CI 0.4 to 3.2), and the authors contend that such patients would not need to be tested for PE. The same figure was obtained in a prospective validation study of 8138 emergency room patients who were included if the physician in charge ordered any objective diagnostic test for PE; 24% of those patients were classified in the low-risk group and 1.3% of them had PE at the initial work-up or during the 45 days of follow-up (34).

WHICH PREDICTION RULES ARE AVAILABLE FOR DVT DIAGNOSIS?

For DVT, the Wells' score is by far the most validated and used clinical prediction rule (see Table 5.3). It was derived (35) and externally validated (36) 10 years ago in outpatients with suspected DVT. It first included nine items, among them three risk factors for VTE (active cancer; paralysis, paresis or recent plaster immobilization of the lower extremities; bed rest for more than 3 days or major surgery), five clinical signs of DVT (localised tenderness along the distribution of the deep venous system, entire leg swollen, calf swelling by more than 3 cm when compared with the asymptomatic leg, pitting oedema, collateral superficial veins) and the presence of an alternative diagnosis as likely or greater than that of DVT. All items scored one point, while the presence of an alternative diagnosis scored −2 points. It classified patients into three groups of low (<1 point), intermediate (1 or 2 points) and high (>2 points) clinical probability.

In 2004, a systematic review reported 15 studies in which the Wells' score was used to assess the clinical probability of DVT in a total of 7122 patients. In these studies, prevalence of DVT ranged

Table 5.3 The dichotomized Wells' score for DVT (11)

Clinical characteristics	Points
Active cancer (patient receiving treatment for cancer within the previous 6 months or currently receiving palliative treatment)	+1
Paralysis, paresis or recent plaster immobilization of the lower extremities	+1
Recently bedridden for 3 days or more or major surgery within the previous 12 weeks requiring general or regional anaesthesia	+1
Localized tenderness along the distribution of the deep venous system	+1
Entire leg swollen	+1
Calf swelling at least 3 cm larger than that on the asymptomatic side (measured 10 cm below tibial tuberosity)	+1
Pitting oedema confined to the symptomatic leg	+1
Collateral superficial veins (non-varicose)	+1
Previously documented DVT	+1
Alternative diagnosis at least as likely as DVT	−2

Total score	Clinical probability	Prevalence of DVT
<2 points	DVT unlikely	5.5% (95% CI: 3.8 to 7.6%)
≥ 2 points	DVT likely	27.9% (95% CI: 23.9 to 31.8%)

from 0 to 13% in the low, from 0 to 38% in the intermediate and from 17 to 85% in the high clinical probability groups. The summary area under the receiver operating characteristic (ROC) curve was 0.78 (95% CI: 0.73 to 0.82) (24). The rule may be used in various clinical settings. In fact, in this systematic review, about 800 patients were inpatients. Other studies suggested that the rule could be applied to orthopaedic (37) or cancer patients (38).

More recently, this score has been modified to include a new item (a history of previously documented DVT) and to allow its use in a dichotomized approach in a diagnostic strategy that only uses two clinical probability groups (Table 5.3). Patients are classified as having either DVT 'unlikely' or 'likely'. Prevalence of confirmed DVT in these two groups was 5.5% (95% CI 3.8 to 7.6%) and 27.9% (95% CI 23.9 to 31.8) (11).

Other prediction rules have been proposed for DVT (39–42), some of them focusing on specific settings such as ambulatory practice (41) or inpatients (39).

WHAT ARE THE LIMITATIONS OF EXISTING CLINICAL PREDICTION RULES?

A first limitation is that it is difficult to build rules that meet all criteria, i.e., are simple, explicit, standardized, including easily and reproducibly collected clinical predictors, which in turn are accurate, reproducible, accepted in clinical practice and change clinical practice. In a study of a diagnostic strategy for PE based on the original Geneva score, physicians were allowed to override the results of the score in case of disagreement with their own clinical judgement: this occurred in almost 20% of patients (25). The main reason advocated for override was the absence among the rule's criteria of a risk factor or clinical sign that the patient presented with and that was deemed important by the physician (e.g., recent long travel, ongoing pregnancy).

Another limitation is the difficulty in memorizing the items of the score and the points given to each item and the points threshold to classify patients into risk groups. Attempts to simplify the use of clinical prediction rules for VTE diagnosis have been made. For example, strategies have validated using a dichotomized version of the Wells' PE and DVT scores, classifying patients into two instead of three clinical probability groups (28,29). Another approach is to simplify further the computation of these scores, attributing one point to all criteria whatever the weight they carried in the original model. This has been shown not to alter the diagnostic accuracy of both the Wells' and the revised Geneva score (43,44). The use of reminder tools may help with implementation of clinical prediction rules, for example by including the rule in local written guidelines for the diagnosis of PE, in diagnostic tests requisitions or in medical calculator software downloaded on personal digital assistants.

CONCLUSION

Current diagnostic strategies for VTE diagnosis almost all include an assessment of the pre-test clinical probability, in order to enable the interpretation of diagnostic tests and to select low-risk patients in whom a less intensive work-up can safely rule out the diagnosis without any imaging test. Clinical prediction rules are decision-making tools that provide a reliable and reproducible estimate of the clinical probability. They are built and validated following methodological standards. They use combinations of simple available clinical predictors to define a probability of disease which leads to a diagnostic or therapeutic course of action. Several clinical prediction rules are available for VTE diagnosis; all have completed required validation steps. The safety and usefulness of their use in diagnostic strategies have been demonstrated. Their implementation in local guidelines for VTE diagnosis has been shown to be associated with better patients' outcomes. Their use should be encouraged; further research efforts are required to ease their use in daily clinical practice.

REFERENCES

1. Barritt DW, Jordan SC. Anticoagulant drugs in the treatment of pulmonary embolism. A controlled trial. *Lancet* 1960; **1**(7138):1309–12.
2. Agnelli G, Prandoni P, Santamaria MG, Bagatella P, Iorio A, Bazzan M, *et al*. Three months versus one year of oral anticoagulant therapy for idiopathic deep venous thrombosis. *N Engl J Med* 2001; **345**(3):165–69.
3. Kearon C, Gent M, Hirsh J, Weitz J, Kovacs MJ, Anderson DR, *et al*. Extended anticoagulation compared to placebo after three months of therapy for a first episode of idiopathic venous thromboembolism. *N Engl J Med* 1999; **340**(12):901–7.
4. Kearon C, Ginsberg JS, Kovacs MJ, Anderson DR, Wells P, Julian JA, *et al*. Comparison of low-intensity warfarin therapy with conventional-intensity warfarin therapy for long-term prevention of recurrent venous thromboembolism. *N Engl J Med* 2003; **349**(7):631–39.
5. Ridker PM, Goldhaber SZ, Danielson E, Rosenberg Y, Eby CS, Deitcher SR, *et al*. Long-term, low-intensity warfarin therapy for the prevention of recurrent venous thromboembolism. *N Engl J Med* 2003; **348**(15):1425–34.
6. Linkins LA, Choi PT, Douketis JD. Clinical impact of bleeding in patients taking oral anticoagulant therapy for venous thromboembolism: a meta-analysis. *Ann Intern Med* 2003; **139**(11):893–900.
7. The PIOPED Investigators. Value of the ventilation/perfusion scan in acute pulmonary embolism. Results of the prospective investigation of pulmonary embolism diagnosis (PIOPED). *JAMA* 1990; **263**(20):2753–59.
8. Hull RD, Raskob GE, Coates G, Panju AA. Clinical validity of a normal perfusion lung scan in patients with suspected pulmonary embolism. *Chest* 1990; **97**(1):23–26.

9. Roy PM, Colombet I, Durieux P, Chatellier G, Sors H, Meyer G. Systematic review and meta-analysis of strategies for the diagnosis of suspected pulmonary embolism. *BMJ* 2005; **331**(7511):259.

10. Perrier A, Roy PM, Sanchez O, Le Gal G, Meyer G, Gourdier AL, *et al*. Multi-detector row computed tomography in outpatients with suspected pulmonary embolism. *N Engl J Med* 2005; **352**:1760–68.

11. Wells PS, Anderson DR, Rodger M, Forgie M, Kearon C, Dreyer J, *et al*. Evaluation of D-dimer in the diagnosis of suspected deep-vein thrombosis. *N Engl J Med* 2003; **349**(13):1227–35.

12. Wells PS, Anderson DR, Rodger M, Stiell I, Dreyer JF, Barnes D, *et al*. Excluding pulmonary embolism at the bedside without diagnostic imaging: management of patients with suspected pulmonary embolism presenting to the emergency department by using a simple clinical model and D-dimer. *Ann Intern Med* 2001; **135**(2):98–107.

13. Rodger MA, Maser E, Stiell I, Howley HE, Wells PS. The inter-observer reliability of pretest probability assessment in patients with suspected pulmonary embolism. *Thromb Res* 2005; **116**(2):101–107.

14. Roy P-M, Meyer G, Vielle B, Le Gall C, Verschuren F, Carpentier F, *et al*. Appropriateness of diagnostic management and outcomes of suspected pulmonary embolism. *Ann Intern Med* 2006; **144**(3):157–164.

15. Wasson JH, Sox HC, Neff RK, Goldman L. Clinical prediction rules. Applications and methodological standards. *N Engl J Med* 1985; **313**(13):793–799.

16. Stiell IG, Wells GA. Methodologic standards for the development of clinical decision rules in emergency medicine. *Ann Emerg Med* 1999; **33**(4):437–447.

17. Wells PS, Ginsberg JS, Anderson DR, Kearon C, Gent M, Turpie AG, *et al*. Use of a clinical model for safe management of patients with suspected pulmonary embolism. *Ann Intern Med* 1998; **129**(12):997–1005.

18. Le Gal G, Righini M, Roy PM, Sanchez O, Aujesky D, Bounameaux H, *et al*. Prediction of pulmonary embolism in the emergency department: the revised Geneva score. *Ann Intern Med* 2006; **144**(3):165–171.

19. Wells PS, Anderson DR, Rodger M, Ginsberg JS, Kearon C, Gent M, *et al*. Derivation of a simple clinical model to categorize patients probability of pulmonary embolism: increasing the models utility with the SimpliRED D-dimer. *Thromb Haemost* 2000; **83**(3):416–420.

20. Wicki J, Perneger TV, Junod AF, Bounameaux H, Perrier A. Assessing clinical probability of pulmonary embolism in the emergency ward: a simple score. *Arch Intern Med* 2001; **161**(1):92–97.

21. Miniati M, Monti S, Bottai M. A structured clinical model for predicting the probability of pulmonary embolism. *Am J Med* 2003; **114**(3):173–179.

22. Stollberger C, Finsterer J, Lutz W, Stoberl C, Kroiss A, Valentin A, *et al*. Multivariate analysis-based prediction rule for pulmonary embolism. *Thromb Res* 2000; **97**(5):267–273.

23. Hoellerich VL, Wigton RS. Diagnosing pulmonary embolism using clinical findings. *Arch Intern Med* 1986; **146**(9):1699–1704.

24. Tamariz LJ, Eng J, Segal JB, Krishnan JA, Bolger DT, Streiff MB, *et al*. Usefulness of clinical prediction rules for the diagnosis of venous thromboembolism: a systematic review. *Am J Med* 2004; **117**(9):676–684.

25. Chagnon I, Bounameaux H, Aujesky D, Roy PM, Gourdier AL, Cornuz J, *et al*. Comparison of two clinical prediction rules and implicit assessment among patients with suspected pulmonary embolism. *Am J Med* 2002; **113**(4):269–275.

26. Klok FA, Kruisman E, Spaan J, Nijkeuter M, Righini M, Aujesky D, *et al*. Comparison of the revised Geneva score with the Wells rule for assessing clinical probability of pulmonary embolism. *J Thromb Haemost* 2008; **6**(1):40–44.

27. Righini M, Le Gal G, Aujesky D, Roy PM, Sanchez O, Verschuren F, *et al*. Diagnosing pulmonary embolism by multi-detector computed tomography alone or combined with lower limb venous ultrasonography: a randomized non-inferiority trial. *Lancet* 2008; **371**:1343–52.

28. Anderson DR, Kahn SR, Rodger MA, Kovacs MJ, Morris T, Hirsch A, *et al*. Computed tomographic pulmonary angiography vs ventilation-perfusion lung scanning in patients with suspected pulmonary embolism: a randomized controlled trial. *JAMA* 2007; **298**(23):2743–53.

29. Writing Group for the Christopher Study Investigators. Effectiveness of managing suspected pulmonary embolism using an algorithm combining clinical probability, D-dimer testing and computed tomography. *JAMA* 2006; **295**(2):172–179.

30. Le Gal G, Bounameaux H. Diagnosing pulmonary embolism: running after the decreasing prevalence of cases among suspected patients. *J Thromb Haemost* 2004; **2**(8): 1244–46.

31. Dunn KL, Wolf JP, Dorfman DM, Fitzpatrick P, Baker JL, Goldhaber SZ. Normal D-dimer levels in emergency department patients suspected of acute pulmonary embolism. *J Am Coll Cardiol* 2002; **40**(8): 1475–78.

32. Runyon MS, Webb WB, Jones AE, Kline JA. Comparison of the unstructured clinician estimate of pretest probability for pulmonary embolism to the Canadian score and the Charlotte rule: a prospective observational study. *Acad Emerg Med* 2005; **12**(7): 587–593.

33. Kline JA, Mitchell AM, Kabrhel C, Richman PB, Courtney DM. Clinical criteria to prevent unnecessary diagnostic testing in emergency department patients with suspected pulmonary embolism. *J Thromb Haemost* 2004; **2**: 1247–55.

34. Kline JA, Courtney DM, Kabrhel C, Moore CL, Smithline HA, Plewa MC, *et al*. Prospective multicenter evaluation of the pulmonary embolism rule-out criteria. *J Thromb Haemost* 2008; **6**(5): 772–780.

35. Wells PS, Hirsh J, Anderson DR, Lensing AW, Foster G, Kearon C, *et al*. A simple clinical model for the diagnosis of deep-vein thrombosis combined with impedance plethysmography: potential for an improvement in the diagnostic process. *J Intern Med* 1998; **243**(1): 15–23.

36. Wells PS, Anderson DR, Bormanis J, Guy F, Mitchell M, Gray L, *et al*. Value of assessment of pretest probability of deep-vein thrombosis in clinical management. *Lancet* 1997; **350**(9094): 1795–98.

37. Riddle DL, Hoppener MR, Kraaijenhagen RA, Anderson J, Wells PS. Preliminary validation of clinical assessment for deep vein thrombosis in orthopaedic outpatients. *Clin Orthop Relat Res* 2005(432): 252–257.

38. Di Nisio M, Rutjes AW, Buller HR. Combined use of clinical pretest probability and D-dimer test in cancer patients with clinically suspected deep venous thrombosis. *J Thromb Haemost* 2006; **4**(1): 52–57.

39. Constans J, Nelzy ML, Salmi LR, Skopinski S, Saby JC, Le Metayer P, *et al*. Clinical prediction of lower limb deep vein thrombosis in symptomatic hospitalized patients. *Thromb Haemost* 2001; **86**(4): 985–990.

40. Kahn SR, Joseph L, Abenhaim L, Leclerc JR. Clinical prediction of deep vein thrombosis in patients with leg symptoms. *Thromb Haemost* 1999; **81**(3): 353–357.

41. Oudega R, Moons KG, Hoes AW. Ruling out deep venous thrombosis in primary care. A simple diagnostic algorithm including D-dimer testing. *Thromb Haemost* 2005; **94**(1): 200–205.

42. Subramaniam RM, Chou T, Heath R, Allen R. Importance of pretest probability score and D-dimer assay before sonography for lower limb deep venous thrombosis. *AJR Am J Roentgenol* 2006; **186**(1): 206–212.

43. Gibson NS, Sohne M, Kruip MJ, TICK L, Gerdes VE, Bossuyt PM, *et al*. Further validation and simplification of the Wells clinical decision rule in pulmonary embolism. *Thromb Haemost* 2008; **99**: 229–234.

44. Klok FA, Mos ICM, Nijkeuter M, Righini M, Perrier A, Le Gal G, *et al*. Simplification of the Revised Geneva Score for assessing clinical probability of pulmonary embolism *Arch Intern Med* 2008; **168**: 2131–36.

45. Le Gal G, Righini M, Roy P-M, Sanchez O, Aujesky D, Bounameaux H, *et al*. Prediction of pulmonary embolism in the emergency department: the Revised Geneva Score. *Ann Intern Med* 2006; **144**(3): 165–171.

CHAPTER 6

Plasma D-Dimer and Venous Thromboembolic Disease

Marc Righini, Henri Bounameaux and Arnaud Perrier

Division of Angiology and Hemostasis, Department of Internal Medicine,
Geneva University Hospital and Faculty of Medicine,
Geneva, Switzerland

INTRODUCTION

Clinical suspicion of venous thromboembolism (VTE) mandates objective testing, such as compression ultrasonography (CUS) or computed tomography (CT), to confirm or exclude the diagnosis (1–3). As VTE is a frequent, often suspected disease, the realization of an easily performed plasma test allowing physicians to rule out the disease without further testing in an important proportion of patients is of utmost interest. Plasma D-dimer, specific cross-linked fibrin derivatives, partially fulfil these criteria.

D-DIMER FORMATION

D-dimer (DD) units are generated by the action of factor XIIIa on fibrin monomers and polymers and when the endogenous fibrinolytic system degrades cross-linked fibrin present in the organism (Figure 6.1). These units consist of two identical subunits derived from two fibrin molecules. DD is the final fragment of the plasmin-mediated degradation of cross-linked fibrin and its molecular weight is around 180 000 Da. Unlike fibrin/fibrinogen degradation products, which are derived from both fibrinogen and fibrin, DD fragments are end products of the action of plasmin on cross-linked fibrin; however, monoclonal antibodies used in the so-called DD assays also recognize many fragments from cross-linked fibrin without prior proteolysis by plasmin (4). Because 2–3% of plasma fibrinogen is physiologically converted to fibrin and then degraded, small amounts of D-dimer-containing species are detectable in the plasma of healthy individuals. However, the D-dimer concentration in blood is increased under all conditions associated with enhanced fibrin formation and subsequent degradation by plasmin. D-dimer represents the most frequently used laboratory marker of coagulation and fibrinolysis activation (5). Plasma levels demonstrate an

Deep Vein Thrombosis and Pulmonary Embolism   Edited by Edwin J.R. van Beek, Harry R. Büller and Matthijs Oudkerk
© 2009 John Wiley & Sons, Ltd

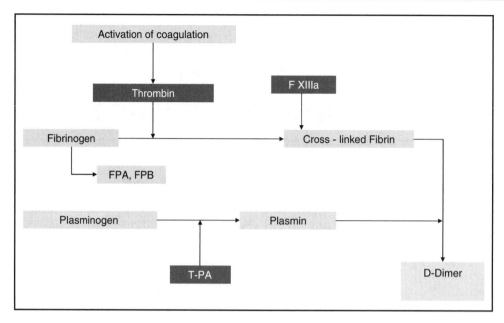

Figure 6.1   Schematic representation of D-dimer formation. Activated coagulation results in thrombin formation. Thrombin cleaves fibrinopeptides A and B (FPA and PPB) from the fibrinogen molecule, turning it into a fibrin monomer that polymerizes into soluble fibrin. Simultaneously, thrombin activates coagulation factor XIII (F XIII a), which then stabilizes the soluble fibrin. The activation of plasmin by the tissue-type plasminogen activator begins fibrin degradation and leads to the generation of D-dimer. A full colour version of this image appears in the plate section of this book.

average 8-fold increase in patients with proven VTE compared with controls, with a level falling to approximately one-quarter of the initial value between week 1 and 2 following the acute event, especially on anticoagulant treatment (6). The plasma half-life of DD fragments is approximately 8 hours and clearance occurs via the kidney and the reticuloendothelial system (7).

ASSAYS FOR MEASURING D-DIMER LEVEL

Description of the different assays

Measurement of DD level has been made possible by the development of monoclonal antibodies, which bind to epitopes on DD fragments that are absent on fibrinogen and non-cross-linked fragments of fibrin (8). Table 6.1 summarizes the main characteristics of the most commonly used DD tests. The detection of the resulting complexes occurs by enzyme-linked immunosorbent assay (ELISA), immunofiltration, sandwich-type or agglutination techniques. The classic microplate ELISA technique was considered the gold standard and this technique was used in early clinical studies to assess the value of DD for VTE diagnosis. The sensitivity and negative predictive value (NPV) were high enough to use the assay as exclusion test in diagnostic strategies for deep vein thrombosis (DVT) or pulmonary embolism (PE). Unfortunately, this kind of test

Table 6.1 Characteristics of various commercial DD assays (non-exhaustive list)

Technique	Examples	Sensitivity	Specificity	Comments
Microplate ELISA	Asserachrom Ddi (Stago) Enzygnost (Behring)[a] Dimertest Gold (Agen)[a]	High	Low	Considered as the gold standard; suitable for batch analysis and not useful for real-time single testing; observer independent
ELISA and fluorescence (ELFA)	Vidas DD (bioMérieux) AxSym D-dimer (Abbott) Stratus D-dimer (Behring)	High	Low	Similar sensitivity as classic microplate ELISA; quantitative; suitable for real-time use; observer independent
ELISA and chemi-luminescence	Immulite (Siemens) Pathfast (Mitsubishi)	High	Low	Similar sensitivity as classic microplate ELISA; quantitative; suitable for real-time use; observer-independent
ELISA and time-resolved fluorescence	Innotrac Aio!	–	–	No clinical study available; observer independent
Immunofiltration and sandwich-type	NycoCard (Nycomed)	High–intermediate	Low–intermediate	Reduced sensitivity compared with classic microplate ELISAs; quantitative; suitable for real-time use; observer independent
	Cardiac D-dimer (Roche)	High	High	Few clinical studies available, promising results
Semi-quantitative latex agglutination	Dimertest latex, (IL); Fibrinosticon (bioMérieux) Ddi latex (Stago)	Inter-mediate	Inter-mediate	Rapid, but insufficiently sensitive to be clinically useful; observer dependent
Manual whole-blood agglutination	SimpliRED (Agen) Clearview Simplify D-dimer (Agen)	High–inter-mediate	Inter-mediate	Rapid, can be performed on whole blood. Exclusion of VTE only in association with low clinical probability; observer dependent
Second-generation latex agglutination (immunoturbidi-metric)	TinaQuant (Roche) Liatest (Stago) Automated Dimertest (Agen) MDA D-dimer (bioMérieux) Turbiquant (Dade-Behring) Miniquant D-dimer (Trinity) HemosIL Dimertest HS (IL) Innovance D-dimer (Dade-Behring)	High	Inter-mediate	Rapid and quantitative; comparable sensitivity to microplate ELISA; observer independent

[a]No longer available.

is cumbersome, labour intensive and appropriate only for batch analysis, rendering it ill-suited for routine emergency use (9,10). However, using these assays established the concept and the usefulness of DD measurement for VTE exclusion (11–13). Subsequently, a single, fast (about 30 minutes) and fully automated ELISA was developed in which capture antibodies are coated on tips and reagents are located in a strip. Further modified ELISA assays that are more rapid and suited for single samples were developed later. After the sample has been transferred into the dedicated hole, the analysis proceeds automatically (14). A batch calibration curve assay is performed by the manufacturer and is stored in a database by bar-code reading. The usual cut-off for VTE exclusion, as determined in clinical studies by receiver operating characteristic (ROC) curve analysis, is the optimal point within the measuring range, which confers a good analytical sensitivity to that particular assay. VTE exclusion by a DD level below the cut-off has been validated in outcome studies, i.e., studies in which patients with clinically suspected VTE are left untreated on the basis of a normal DD test and are systematically followed up for a 3-month period to detect possible thromboembolic events (15,16). These ELISA tests (e.g., Vidas D-dimer, bioMérieux, Marcy l'Etoile, France; Stratus CS D-dimer, Dade Behring, Newark, DE, USA; AxSYM D-dimer, Axis-Shield Diagnostics, Dundee, UK) combine the ELISA technique with a final detection by fluorescence [D-dimer enzyme-linked immunofluorescence assay (ELFA)], chemiluminescence (PATHFAST, Mitsubishi Kagabu Iatron, Chiba, Japan and Immulite, Siemens, Eschborn, Germany, in particular) or time-resolved fluorescence (Innotrac Aio!, Turku, Finland) are fully automated, provide a result within 15–35 min and can be used for single sample testing (17–19). The main limitation for these assays is the requirement of a dedicated immunoanalyser.

Another rapid format is immunofiltration, in which capture antibodies are coated on to a permeable membrane. Sample, washing solution and second antibody undergo passive filtration. Signal is generated by a colloid gold-labelled tag antibody and quantified with a reflectometer (Nyco-Card D-dimer, Axis-Shield, Oslo, Norway). A fully automated sandwich-type assay on a dedicated device, using colloid gold-labelled tag antibody, is also available (Cardiac Reader D-dimer, Roche Diagnostics, Mannheim, Germany).

In some assay systems, DD is measured in anticoagulated whole blood (Cardiac Reader, Pathfast and Innotrac Aio!). In the Stratus assay, an anticoagulated whole blood sample is introduced into the device and centrifugation proceeds automatically.

Latex-based systems rely on the ability of the analyte to agglutinate latex beads coated with the antibody. This implies that fragments possessing either only one epitope or epitopes made unavailable by masking complexes escape determination. Usually, latex assays are performed with native or slightly diluted plasma, whereas microplate or membrane ELISA techniques require high dilutions. Two types of latex tests are available: semi-quantitative slide assays and quantitative assays. The simplest and least expensive systems are semi-quantitative agglutination methods (Dimertest latex, Instrumentation Laboratory, Lexington, MA, USA; Fibrinosticon, bioMérieux, Marcy l'Etoile, France; Ddi latex, Diagnostica Stago, Paris, France), because they are fast and do not require complicated instrumentation. However, as reading is most often visual, some inter-observer variability in estimating the presence of agglutination is unavoidable. Various clinical evaluations have shown a low sensitivity (between 51 and 96%, with an average around 80%) for acute DVT or PE (20,21), clearly insufficient for excluding these conditions.

More recently, quantitative, automated agglutination methods have been developed. These are photometric or turbidimetric methods, designed to be performed on routine coagulation or clinical chemistry analysers. They do not need dedicated instruments (e.g., Tinaquant, Roche Mannheim, Germany; STA Liatest, Diagnostica Stago, Paris, France; IL test, Instrumentation Laboratory, Lexington, MA, USA; BC D-dimer Plus, Dade-Behring, Marburg, Germany; MDA, Organon Teknika, Oss, The Netherlands) (Table 6.1). Results are usually available in 5–10 minutes, are dependent and full automation reduces other sources of variability. However, the analytical sensitivity and the low limit of detection may be a cause of concern The calibration curve usually covers a wide range of concentrations, but the upper reference range of normal values and the detection limit for VTE exclusion often lies on the lower part of the calibration curve where the signal is weak (22), In spite of these laboratory limitations, the clinical performances of turbidimetric DD have been shown to be excellent and close to those of ELISA DD tests. In recent meta-analyses, the diagnostic performances of DD ELISA tests and DD tests using latex turbidimetric methods appear to have operating characteristics similar to those of ELISA methods (23).

Other available manual and semiquantitative DD tests that use whole blood can be performed at the patient's bedside. For example, the SimpliRED test (AGEN Biomedical, Brisbane, Australia) is a red blood cell agglutination assay designed for use with fresh capillary or venous whole blood. It provides a result in less than 5 minutes and is therefore suitable for point-of-care testing. This assay is based on the use of a hybrid monoclonal antibody, which reacts with DD and human erythrocytes, leading to haemagglutination in the presence of fibrin compounds containing the DD epitope. Study results with this assay have been variable, with an average sensitivity of 69% for DVT and 75% for PE according to the meta-analysis of Di Nisio *et al.* (24). Published studies indicate that the sensitivity and NPV of this test are high enough to rule out VTE but only in the presence of a *low* clinical probability. As readings are visual, some inter-observer variability has been reported (25,26), and it may be that the sensitivity is highest when the test is performed by experienced personnel.

Recently, a novel qualitative immunochromatographic method (Clearview Simplify D-dimer, Agen Biomedical, Brisbane, Australia) was described. This technique does not require instrumentation because reading is visual, which, however, raises concern regarding inter-observer variability (27). The diagnostic performance of this test was compared with venography in a sample of 187 outpatients with suspected DVT in an emergency department (28). The sensitivity and NPV were 94% and 95%, respectively, but confidence intervals remained large in relation to the relatively small sample size (28). Moreover, more recent studies reported significantly worse performance of this test (29,30).

An unresolved and complex issue: standardization of D-dimer tests

One of the main problems with DD measurement is the confusion raised by the multiplicity of commercial assays, with various techniques, cut-offs, systems of units [DD units or FEU (fibrinogen equivalent units): thus, the calibrators for DD units are purified DD fragments whereas the calibration material for FEU is obtained from controlled plasmin digestion of purified fibrinogen clotted in the presence of factor XIII], operational characteristics and clinical validity. This demonstrated heterogeneity (31) led to sustained attempts to standardize or at least harmonize the expression of test results. Standardization is a process based on the application of a comprehensive reference system including a reference method, primary standard and the use of SI units. Standardization can only be obtained when the entity measured in the assay can be clearly defined. As D-dimer is not a single entity but a complex mixture of degradation products of different sizes, standardization is probably not an option to make the test results of different assays comparable. Therefore, despite all of the attempts that have been made, standardization is still an unresolved problem (32,33). As a consequence, comparison of results obtained with different methods is impossible and every result is method specific. The second option could be harmonization of test results. Harmonization is based on the application of a mathematical model to make test results comparable (34). Some models of harmonization of D-dimer tests have been proposed (33,35,36), without reaching a consensus, but such a discussion is beyond the scope of this chapter.

D-DIMER AS A DIAGNOSTIC TEST

Choosing a D-dimer assay

The cut-off level used in diagnostic strategies for acute venous thromboembolism is not a true reference or a normality range. Rather, each diagnostic system has its own decisional levels that help to identify patients without the disease, explaining why different cut-offs are reported. This point highlights the fact that clinicians have to know which test is used, its performance and, obviously, its cut-off. Also, it underlines the fact that only D-dimer assays which have been correctly validated in prospective management studies or directly compared with assays validated in outcome studies should be used. When choosing the type of D dimer assay to use in diagnostic strategies for acute DVT or PE, the main attention should obviously be paid to sensitivity, as false-negative results can lead to potentially fatal consequences. Therefore, preference should be given to highly sensitive D-dimer assay.

Although specificity is also an issue, because it determines the proportion of true-negative results, i.e., the diagnostic yield of the test, it is not a determinant factor for choosing a D-dimer assay. Indeed, more specific assays have a lower sensitivity and their use should be restricted to patients with a low clinical probability of VTE, thereby offsetting the theoretical advantage of a higher true-negative rate. Also, specificity is affected by the patient population and clinical context in addition to a particular assay's characteristics. For instance, the diagnostic yield of D-dimer is very low in hospitalized patients (37) due to the variety of conditions potentially elevating D-dimer in those patients or in the elderly because of the rise of the D-dimer concentrations in a normal ageing population (38). A useful index allowing one to compare the diagnostic yield of various D-dimer assays or of a specific assay in various clinical settings is the 'number-needed-to-test', i.e., the number of patients in whom D-dimer must be measured to rule out one DVT or one PE (39). For instance, if the prevalence of PE in theoretical population of 100 patients is 20%, 80 patients will not have PE. If the specificity of the D-dimer assay is 40%, it will rule out PE in 32 of those 80 patients, i.e., 32% of the overall population. Therefore, 3.1 patients will require testing to rule out one PE.

Other important characteristics include sample turnaround time, which should be achieved in under 30 minutes (to allow its use in the emergency room), and observer dependence of results. Generally, observer-independent methods are to be preferred, particularly as results obtained in clinical studies with well-trained readers can probably not be extrapolated to real clinical practice with an emergency staff functioning 24 hours per day (40).

Another important point when choosing a D-dimer test is its role in the local diagnostic strategy. If the D-dimer is used as a first-step test and other tests are not performed in the presence of a negative test, the method of choice should be the most sensitive one, for example an ELISA test with a sensitivity as close to 100% as possible, in order to minimize the proportion of false-negative results. In contrast, if the D-dimer test is used in association with other tests such as compression ultrasonography, a less sensitive test may be appropriately chosen.

Nowadays, D-dimer tests are used mainly to assess outpatients in whom the presence of other conditions that are associated with increased D-dimer levels is lower. In contrast, the clinical usefulness of the test in hospitalized patients is reduced owing to the many causes for false-positive results due to comorbid conditions (41).

D-dimer to make a positive diagnosis of DVT or PE

The positive predictive value for VTE rises as D-dimer levels increase progressively above the chosen threshold. In a study evaluating 671 outpatients with suspected PE, the specificity of a D-dimer test (Asserachrom Ddi ELISA) was 93% when levels exceeded 4000 ng/mL, in the presence of a non-low clinical probability. However, this resulted in a limited positive predictive value because of the low prevalence of PE, particularly in patients with a low clinical probability. Moreover, it is well recognized that PE and DVT should always be diagnosed by an imaging method and, therefore, clinicians would be reluctant to rule in the diagnosis on the sole basis of a positive D-dimer test (1,42). Finally, although potentially elegant, the concept of using two different cut-offs for the same test to refute or prove the presence of VTE may be confusing in busy real-life settings and has not been shown to be safe in clinical practice. Therefore, at this stage, D-dimer levels should only be used as an exclusion test for VTE.

D-dimer assays in the diagnostic work-up of DVT

The SimpliRED test

As previously discussed, the SimpliRED test (Agen Biomedical, Brisbane, Australia) is a manual semi-quantitative latex test using whole blood that can be performed at the patient's bedside.

In the first study assessing the performances of this test in the presence of suspected DVT, the test had a sensitivity of 89%, a specificity of 77% and an NPV of 96% for the exclusion of DVT compared with the reference standard, contrast venography (43). However, some authors reported values of sensitivity as low as 66% compared with contrast venography (20).

In a subsequent management study, patients with a low clinical probability of DVT and a normal SimpliRED D-dimer test had a 3-month thromboembolic rate of 1.8% (95% CI: 0.9 to 3.3%). (44) A negative SimpliRED test reduced the prevalence of DVT in the low clinical probability classification (Wells' rule) in two independent Canadian studies from 2.5 and 5.6%, respectively, to less than 1% during a 3-month follow-up period (3,45) (Table 6.2). Therefore, although its diagnostic performances suggest that the test is not sensitive enough as a stand-alone test for the exclusion of DVT, there are convincing data which demonstrate that the association of a low clinical probability and a negative test may safely rule out DVT.

The Vidas D-dimer test

A normal quantitative ELISA Vidas D-dimer test (cut-off <500 ng/mL) was reported to have a 100% sensitivity when compared with contrast venography in two studies (13,46). In three large management studies of outpatients with suspected DVT, the sensitivity of this test varied between 98 and 99% in 2239 patients irrespective of clinical probability assessment (15,47–49).

Table 6.2 Role of a negative SimpliRED test in combination with a low clinical probability to rule out DVT

| Study | Low Clinical Probability (Wells' Score) | | Negative Simplired: |
	No. Of Patients	Prevalence Of Dvt (%)	3-Month Te Risk (%)
Kearon et al. (45)	206	2.5	0.6
Wells et al. (3)	317	5.6	0.9
Anderson et al. (102)	313	4.5	0.9
Kraaijenhagen et al. (44)	561	8.0	1.8
Tick et al. (103)	250	11.0	2.0
Blattler W. et al. (104)	94	5.3	2.4

The rapid automated turbidimetric tests

In two large management studies, the sensitivity of a normal (cut-off <500 ng/mL) turbidimetric assay (Tinaquant, Roche Diagnostics, Mannheim, Germany) for the exclusion of DVT varied from 91 to 98% and the specificity from 44 to 51% (48–50). In one prospective outcome study, the combination of a normal Tinaquant test result with a low clinical probability had a negative predictive value of more than 99% without the need for CUS testing (50).

D-dimer assays in the diagnostic work-up of PE

The SimpliRED test

In a large prospective study of 1117 patients with suspected PE (prevalence of PE: 17%), the SimpliRED test had a sensitivity of 85%, a specificity of 68% and an NPV of 96% for exclusion of PE (51). Using the Wells' scoring system (Table 6.3), the prevalence of PE in the patients with a low clinical probability (Wells score <2 points) was very low (1.3–3.4%) in two prospective clinical outcome studies. Combining a negative SimpliRED test result in those patients excluded PE with a negative predictive value of 99–99.5% (51,52). The safety of this strategy has recently

Table 6.3   Most commonly used prediction rules for suspected PE

Wells' score (105)		Geneva score (106)		Revised Geneva score (107)	
Items	**Score**	**Items**	**Score**	**Items**	**Score**
Previous PE or DVT	1.5	Previous PE or DVT	2	Age >65 years	1
Heart rate >100	1.5	Heart rate >100	1	Previous DVT or PE	3
Recent surgery or immobilization	1.5	Recent surgery	3	Surgery or fracture within 1 month	2
		Age:			
		60–79 years	1		
Clinical signs of DVT	3	>80 years	2	Active malignancy	2
Alternative diagnosis less likely than PE	3	Arterial blood gases: CO_2 (kPa):		Unilateral lower limb pain	3
		<4.8	2		
Haemoptysis	1	4.8–5.19	1	Haemoptysis	2
Cancer	1	O_2 (kPa):		Heart rate:	
		<6.5	4	75–94	3
		6.5–7.99	3	>95	5
		8–9.49	2	Pain on lower limb deep vein palpation and unilateral oedema	4
		9.5–10.99	1		
		Chest X-ray			
		Atelectasia	1		
		Elevated hemidiaphragm	1		
Clinical probability		**Clinical probability**		**Clinical probability**	
Low	<2	Low	0–4	Low	0–3
Intermediate	2–6	Intermediate	5–8	Intermediate	4–10
High	>6	High	>9	High	>11
'Dichotomized' (58)					
PE unlikely	<4				
PE likely	>4				

been confirmed in 373 patients with a low clinical probability and a negative SimpliRED test in patients randomly assigned into a non-imaging arm versus an arm with additional testing using lung scintigraphy (53). None of 182 patients assigned to D-dimer testing and no additional diagnostic procedures in case of a negative result had a VTE event during follow-up, compared with one patient in the additional perfusion lung scan group (53).

Rapid ELISA D-dimer assays

When compared with the reference standard, pulmonary angiography, in a validation study or in large cross-sectional studies with prospective data collection, the rapid ELISA Vidas D-dimer assay had a sensitivity and an NPV of 95–100% for the exclusion of DVT and PE during the subsequent 3 months of follow-up (13,15,46,48). These data suggest that in the presence of a negative ELISA Vidas D-dimer (cut-off <500 ng/mL), the post-test probability of VTE is close to zero, irrespective of the clinical score. Whether a negative ELISA Vidas D-dimer test predicts an uneventful 3 months of follow-up was confirmed in prospective management studies. The test was first validated in 195 outpatients with suspected PE (54). All 56 (29%) patients with a negative ELISA Vidas D-dimer test had PE excluded and had an uneventful 3 months of follow-up. In an other prospective study of 444 outpatients with suspected PE, the sensitivity and the NPV of this test were 100% and the specificity was 46% (15).

In a third study, of 965 patients with suspected PE, a normal rapid ELISA Vidas D-dimer level (<500 ng/mL) ruled out PE with an NPV of 98.8% and a specificity of 38% (55). The test allowed PE to be ruled out in 29% of patients. Two recent prospective management studies confirmed that it is safe to rule out PE by a normal rapid ELISA Vidas D-dimer test with a sensitivity and NPV of 100%, irrespective of clinical assessment (56,57). Therefore, there are good data suggesting that ELISA Vidas D-dimer tests are mostly independent of clinical assessment. However, due to the theoretically limited NPV of a D-dimer test in patients with a high prevalence of the disease, the latest British Thoracic Society guidelines (42) suggested that the test should not be performed in patients with a high clinical probability. Moreover, it would be difficult for physicians to accept that a normal D-dimer test result overrules their clinical judgement of a high clinical suspicion of PE in a particular patient. In a recent multicentre study including 1819 patients, the D-dimer test allowed the exclusion of PE in 561 patients with a non-high clinical probability as no thromboembolic events occurred in the 3-month follow-up of patients with D-dimer <500 ng/mL. (CT-PE4 study). Table 6.4 displays the diagnostic performances of the Vidas D-dimer test for suspected PE in prospective outcome studies.

ELISA Vidas and Tinaquant D-dimer test

The Christopher study (58) was a prospective outcome study which enrolled 3306 patients with suspected PE. The diagnostic strategy was based on assessment of clinical probability by a modified Wells' rule, which separated patients as PE 'unlikely' and PE 'likely', D-dimer test and CT pulmonary angiography. The combination of PE unlikely (Wells score ⩽4 points) and a normal D-dimer (either Vidas ELISA or Tinaquant) occurred in 1057 patients (32% of the total group), of whom 1028 did not receive anticoagulant treatment. Subsequent non-fatal VTE occurred in five patients (0.5%) and two were lost to follow-up. At the usual threshold (500 ng/mL), the Vidas ELISA test had a sensitivity of 100% for PE exclusion. The five false-negative D-dimer tests in the Christopher study were all in the group tested with Tinaquant. Therefore, the incidence of VTE was five of 624 (0.8%) in the Tinaquant group (58).

Table 6.4 Exclusion of pulmonary embolism by a normal rapid ELISA Vidas D-dimer test in prospective studies

Study	Clinical Probability	Cut-Off (Ng/Ml)	No. Of Patients	Prevalence of PE (%)	Sensitivity (%)	Npv (%)
de Moer-loose et al. (54)	Low/intermediate/high	<500	196	24	100	100
Perrier et al. (15)	Low/intermediate/high	<500	444	23	100	100
Kruip et al. (55)	Low/intermediate/high	<500	234	22	98	99
Perrier et al. (75)	Low/intermediate/high	<500	965	21	100	100
Perrier et al. (56)	Non-High (Geneva Score <9)	<500	756	26	100	100
Kucher et al. (57)	Non-High (Wells' rule <6 Points)	<780	191	45	100	100
Christopher Study (58)	Unlikely (Revised Wells' Score ≤4)	<500	428	20	100	100
Righini et al. (Ct-Pe 4 Study) (110)	Non-High (Revised Geneva Score <11 Points)	<500	1819	21	100	100

Summary of diagnostic performances of D-dimer in suspected DVT and PE

In a recent extensive meta-analysis (24), Di Nisio et al. calculated the diagnostic performances of several D-dimer tests, based on 113 individual studies. They separated D-dimer tests into the following categories: D-dimer enzyme-linked immunofluorescence assay (ELFA), microplate enzyme-linked immunosorbent assay (ELISA); membrane ELISA; latex quantitative assay; latex semi-quantitative assay, latex qualitative assay; and whole blood assay. The comprehensive results on diagnostic performances are shown in Table 6.5. Overall, compared with other D-dimer assays, the ELFA, microplate ELISA and latex quantitative assays have a higher sensitivity but lower specificity, resulting in a more confident exclusion of the disease at the expense of potentially more additional imaging testing (24). The whole blood agglutination assays display a lower sensitivity (about 85% compared with 95% or more for the ELISAs, the ELFA and the quantitative automated latex tests) but are more specific (about 70% compared with approximately 50% for the high-sensitivity assays), which allows VTE to be safely ruled out in populations with a low prevalence of the disease. One year earlier, Stein et al. published similar results in a careful meta-analysis of 78 studies of D-dimer assays used for either DVT or PE diagnosis (59). They included all types of D-dimer assays, grouped into seven categories, and included studies using a mixture of reference tests. The authors pooled the sensitivities and specificities by assay type and evaluated how these test characteristics varied by several explanatory variables using a regression model. For DVT diagnosis, the pooled sensitivities of the assays were highest for the ELISA and quantitative rapid ELISA assays, with sensitivities of 95% (95% CI, 91 to 99%) and 96% (95%

Table 6.5 Summary estimates of sensitivity and specificity of D-dimer methods. Adapted from (24)

	DVT		PE	
	Sensitivity (95% CI)	Specificity (95% CI)	Sensitivity (95% CI)	Specificity (95% CI)
ELISA microplate	94 (86 to 97)	53 (38 to 68)	95 (84 to 99)	50 (29 to 71)
ELFA	96 (89 to 98)	46 (31 to 61)	97 (88 to 99)	43 (23 to 65)
Membrane immunofiltration	89 (76 to 95)	53 (37 to 68)	91 (73 to 98)	50 (29 to 72)
Latex:				
Qualitative	69 (27 to 93)	99 (94 to 100)	75 (25 to 96)	99 (92 to 100)
Semiquantitative	85 (68 to 93)	68 (53 to 81)	88 (66 to 97)	66 (43 to 83)
Quantitative	93 (89 to 95)	53 (46 to 61)	95 (88 to 98)	50 (36 to 64)
Manual whole-blood assays	83 (67 to 93)	71 (57 to 82)	87 (64 to 96)	69 (48 to 84)

CI, 90 to 100%), respectively. For PE diagnosis, the pooled sensitivities of the assays were again highest for the ELISA and quantitative rapid ELISA assays, with sensitivities of 96% (95% CI, 88 to 100%) and 97% (95% CI, 87% to 100%), respectively. Pooled specificities were in the 40–50% range for these assays. The authors concluded that the NPVs for ELISA assays, particularly the quantitative rapid ELISA assays, are sufficiently high to consider that these assays should be able to stand alone in excluding a diagnosis of DVT or PE (59).

Limits of D-dimer tests

A reduced diagnostic yield of D-dimer testing has been observed in many clinical settings, such as in inpatients (60), post-surgical patients (41), during pregnancy or postpartum (61,62), in patients with a high clinical probability (63) or with previous venous thromboembolic disease (64) and in elderly patients (65). Indeed, in these settings, although the sensitivity and NPV of the test remain high enough to rule out VTE safely, its clinical usefulness, i.e., the proportion of patients in whom VTE can be ruled out on the basis of a negative D-dimer, is greatly diminished. Some of these situations are described hereafter and Table 6.6 displays the number of patients needed to test to rule out one PE in various medical conditions.

Hospitalized patients

Most patients with comorbid conditions and/or inpatients have D-dimer levels higher than the diagnostic cut-off value, thereby questioning its usefulness in ruling out VTE. In a study applied to a population of hospitalized, surgical and medical patients with suspected PE and using an ELISA D-dimer assay, this test turned out to be negative in only 5 of 73 (7%) patients. Therefore, the test is of very limited utility, if any, in hospitalized patients with suspected PE (41).

Elderly patients

Several investigators have reported a significant decrease in specificity and hence in clinical usefulness of the D-dimer test with age (38,66). In a study by our group (65), a cohort of 1029

Table 6.6 Number-needed-to-test (NNT) to rule out one PE in various medical situations

Study	Clinical conditions	Number-needed-to-test to rule out one PE[a]
Righini *et al.* (63)	Patients with a high clinical probability	9.1
	Patients with a non-high clinical probability	2.2
Righini *et al.* (74)	Cancer patients	9.1
	Non-cancer patients	3.1
Le Gal *et al.* (64)	Patients with previous VTE	6.3
	Patients without previous VTE	3.1
Chabloz *et al.* (61)	Pregnancy before the 30th week	2.6
	Pregnancy between 30th week and 42nd week	4
Perrier *et al.* (15)	Outpatients with suspected PE	3.3
Righini *et al.* (65)	Elderly outpatients of more than 80 years	20
Miron *et al.* (41)	Inpatients (non-surgical patients)	30
	Inpatients (surgical patients)	Infinite (no patient with negative D-dimers in this cohort)

[a]The number-needed-to-test (NNT) reflects the number of patients in whom D-dimer measurement has to be performed to rule out one PE.

Table 6.7 Influence of age on the diagnostic characteristics of ELISA D-dimer and clinical usefulness of ELISA D-dimer. Adapted from (65)

Age (years)	Sensitivity (%) (95% CI)	Specificity (%) (95% CI)	Patients with a DD <500 µg/L (%)
<40	100 (86 to 100)	67 (60 to 74)	58
40–49	100 (86 to 100)	67 (59 to 75)	56
50–59	100 (83 to 100)	56 (47 to 65)	49
60–69	100 (94 to 100)	40 (3 to 49)	26
70–79	99 (93 to 100)	26 (19 to 34)	17
80+	100 (95 to 100)	9 (4 to 18)	5
Total	99 (98–100)	47(44–51)	18

patients was divided into six classes of increasing age (by decade) and diagnostic performances were calculated for each class of age. The specificity of D-dimer according to age is shown in Table 6.7. D-dimer allowed PE to be ruled out in almost two-thirds of patients aged less than 40 years, but in only 5% of patients above 80 years. This highlights the clinical usefulness of the test in young patients but questions its application to very elderly patients.

The limited usefulness of D-dimer measurement in elderly patients may explain why clinicians are reluctant to perform the test in that population and explains why adapted diagnostic strategies without D-dimer have been proposed for elderly patients (67). However, a frequently asked question is the extent to which – and in particular until which age – the D-dimer assay should

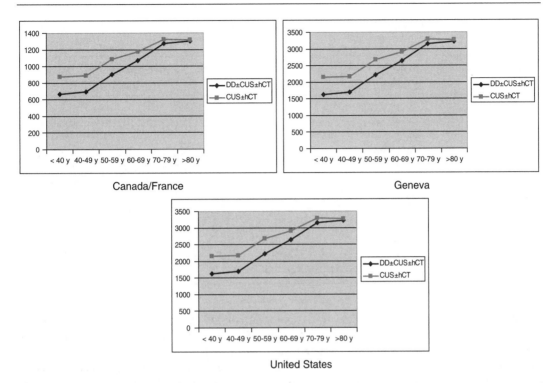

Figure 6.2 Costs in dollars of diagnostic strategies with and without ELISA D-dimer according to age and to the costs in different countries. Adapted from reference 68. A full colour version of this image appears in the plate section of this book.

be performed. To answer this question, a cost-effectiveness analysis as a function of age was published recently (68). Figure 6.2 shows that whatever the diagnostic strategy, using D-dimer was cost-saving until the age of 79 years. After 80 years, there was no clear cost benefit of the D-dimer measurement, as costs of strategies with or without D-dimer testing in this age group are very similar. However, even at this age, D-dimer-using strategies were never more expensive than competing strategies without D-dimer measurement. Therefore, measuring D-dimer in outpatients older than 80 years may be performed at the discretion of the physician. On the one hand, it could be argued that the clinical usefulness is so limited that D-dimer measurement is not indicated. On the other hand, D-dimer measurement does not increase the costs of diagnostic strategies. To avoid complicated recommendations or age-adapted diagnostic strategies (for example, not doing D-dimer in elderly patients), systematic measurement may be proposed, at least in outpatients. Moreover, D-dimer might still be justified in patients over 80 years old when the availability of other diagnostic tests is limited or when the risk of imaging using CT pulmonary angiography is higher because of (for instance) impaired renal function.

Clinical usefulness of D-dimer in elderly patients: can it be increased?

Some authors have attempted to increase the specificity and hence the clinical usefulness of D-dimer in elderly people by increasing the diagnostic threshold, for example from 500 to 600 or 700 μg/L (69). A retrospective analysis was performed on the data in a database of patients with suspected PE included in a prospective management study (70). The effect of raising the threshold of D-dimer in patients above 70 years of age is shown in Table 6.8. Increasing the

Table 6.8 Effect of varying D-dimer cut-off on D-dimer diagnostic performances in patients aged above 70 years ($n = 359$). Adapted from (70)

D-dimer cut-off (μg/L)	Sensitivity (%) (95% CI)	Specificity (%) (95% CI)	Positive LR (95% CI)	Negative LR (95% CI)
500	99.3 (96 to 100)	18.5 (13 to 23)	1.2 (1.1 to 1.3)	0.0 (0.0 to 0.3)
600	96.6 (92 to 98)	23.2 (17 to 28)	1.3 (1.2 to 1.4)	0.1 (0.1 to 0.4)
700	95.9 (91 to 98)	28.9 (22 to 35)	1.4 (1.2 to 1.5)	0.1 (0.1 to 0.3)
800	95.3 (90 to 98)	40.7 (34 to 47)	1.6 (1.4 to 1.8)	0.1 (0.1 to 0.2)
900	95.3 (90 to 98)	47.9 (41 to 54)	1.8 (1.6 to 2.0)	0.1 (0.0 to 0.2)
1000	94.6 (89 to 97)	56.9 (50 to 63)	2.2 (1.9 to 2.6)	0.1 (0.0 to 0.2)

cut-off from 500 to 600 μg/L resulted in a more than 3% fall in sensitivity. Thus, four patients (out of 359) with a D-dimer concentration between 500 and 600 μg/L had a PE confirmed by the subsequent diagnostic work-up. Moreover, at a cut-off value of 600 μg/L, the corresponding increase in specificity and, hence, the test's clinical usefulness were marginal. Indeed, in order for the specificity of D-dimer in older patients to reach that observed in the entire cohort, i.e., 47% (65), the cut-off should be set at 900 μg/L. At that cut-off value, however, the sensitivity of D-dimer is only 95%, yielding an NPV as low as 91% when taking into account the higher prevalence of PE (40%) in these patients. Therefore, increasing the D-dimer cut-off seems unsafe as the number of false negatives increases rapidly. Such a policy would be particularly risky in a diagnostic strategy in which D-dimer measurement would be used as the initial step, PE being ruled out in patients with a concentration below the cut-off.

It is important to note that all these results are based on data analysis obtained in outpatients. As D-dimer concentration is known to increase in the presence of cancer and inflammatory, infectious and cardiopulmonary diseases, the rate of normal D-dimer levels in elderly and hospitalized patients may be assumed to be even lower and the clinical utility of the test in this particular population is certainly further diminished.

Cancer patients

In cancer patients with clinically suspected DVT, two recently published studies have drawn opposite conclusions about the clinical usefulness of the same whole blood agglutination D-dimer assay (71,72). ten Wolde *et al.* published the results of a management study, in which a moderately sensitive D-dimer assay (SimpliRED, Agen Biomedical, Brisbane, Australia) was used to rule out DVT in cancer and non-cancer patients (71). Of 217 cancer patients, 63 (29%) had a normal D-dimer test and a normal ultrasound at the day of referral and were, therefore, not treated with anticoagulants. Only one thromboembolic event occurred during follow-up (1.6%; 95% CI: 0 to 8.5%). In contrast, in another study, by Lee *et al.*, the NPV of D-dimer was only 79% in cancer patients compared with 97% in patients without cancer (72). However, in a retrospective analysis of three prospective series (72), the sensitivity of D-dimer was similar in patients with (86%) and without cancer (83%) and the lower NPV was entirely due to a three-fold higher prevalence of DVT in cancer patients (49% versus 15%).

In cancer patients with suspected PE, limited data are available about the clinical usefulness of D-dimer tests (73). To the best of our knowledge, only two recently published studies have analysed this particular issue. The first study suggested a high sensitivity (100%; 95% CI: 82 to 100%) and NPV (100%; 95% CI: 72 to 100%) in a sample of 72 cancer patients (73). These data were confirmed in a second, larger study (74). In this study, the clinical usefulness and safety of an ELISA D-dimer test for ruling out PE were analysed in a large cohort of 1721 outpatients with ($n = 164$) and without cancer previously included in two outcome studies on the diagnosis of PE (75,76). The D-dimer test result was below the cut-off value of 500 ng/mL in 494 (32%; 95% CI: 30 to 34%) of the 1554 patients suspected of PE and without a history of cancer, compared with 18 (11%; 95% CI: 6 to 16%) out of the 164 with a known malignancy ($p < 0.0001$). Accordingly, the number of patients needed to test by D-dimer to rule out one PE rose from 3.1 in patients without cancer to 9.1 in those with an active malignancy. In patients in whom PE was considered ruled out by a negative D-dimer test and who did not receive oral anticoagulant treatment, there were no thromboembolic events during the 3-month follow-up, either in patients with (0/18; 0%; 95% CI: 0 to 18%) or without cancer (0/469; 0%; 95% CI: 0 to 0.8%). Therefore, the sensitivity and NPV of D-dimer were 100% in both cancer and non-cancer patients. However, the 95% CIs in cancer patients were much wider, owing to the small number of patients. The specificity of the D-dimer test was definitely lower in patients with cancer: 16% (95% CI: 11 to 24%) versus 41% (95% CI: 39 to 44%) in patients without cancer. Table 6.9 displays the diagnostic performances of various D-dimer tests patients with and without the presence of cancer.

In summary, these data suggest that ELISA D-dimer assays are probably safe to rule out PE in patients with cancer in the emergency department. However, the test's clinical usefulness is reduced because around only one of ten patients with cancer and suspected PE will have a normal D-dimer test result (74).

Table 6.9 Diagnostic performances of various D-dimer tests in cancer and non-cancer patients

Study	Patient type	Sample size	Kind of D-dimer	Prevalence of DVT/PE (%)	Sensitivity (%)	Specificity (%)	NPV (%) (95% CI, when available)
Suspected DVT							
Wells *et al.* (43)	No cancer	184	SimpliRED	25.0	78.3	81.9	91.9
	Cancer	29		51.7	86.7	35.7	71.4
Ginsberg *et al.* (108)	No cancer	350	SimpliRED	13.4	87.2	85.2	97.7
	Cancer	48		45.8	86.4	46.2	80.0
Kearon (109)	No cancer	413	SimpliRED	10.9	82.2	79.9	97.4
	Cancer	44		50.0	86.4	59.1	81.3
ten Wolde *et al.* (71)	No cancer	217	SimpliRED	20.0	93	64	97 (96 to 98)
	Cancer	1522		37	98	48	97 (89 to 100)
Lee *et al.* (72)	No cancer	947	SimpliRED	14.6	82.6	82.2	96 (95 to 98)
	Cancer	121		48.8	86.4	48.4	79 (63 to 90)
Suspected PE							
Di Nisio *et al.* (73)	No cancer	447	Tinaquant	19	93	53	97 (95 to 99)
	Cancer	72	D-dimer	26	100	21	100 (72 to 100)
Righini *et al.* (74)	No cancer	1554	Vidas	33.0	100	41	100 (99 to 100)
	Cancer	164	D-dimer	23.0	100	16	100 (82 to 100)

Patients with previous DVT/PE

Diagnosing recurrent VTE is a difficult challenge (77,78). Plasma D-dimer measurement is widely used as a first-line test in patients with suspected DVT or PE (56,59). However, recent research has shown that patients at risk for recurrence are also at higher risk of having persistently elevated D-dimer levels, which might limit the clinical usefulness of the D-dimer test in the case of a suspected recurrence. Recently, some authors reported on the value of D-dimer testing to predict the recurrence of VTE. Among patients who were given a 6-month anticoagulant course for a first episode of VTE, 40% still had an elevated D-dimer level 1 month after withdrawal of oral anticoagulant treatment, probably reflecting the persistence of a hypercoagulable state. This was compounded by a higher recurrence rate in such patients (79), Obviously, a high proportion of patients with persistent D-dimer elevation may limit the clinical usefulness of D-dimer in the case of a suspected recurrent event in patients with previous VTE.

In the setting of DVT, Rathbun *et al.* (80) reported the results of a management study in which a highly sensitive D-dimer test was used to exclude DVT in 300 patients with a previous episode of DVT who were suspected of a recurrent event. The final prevalence of DVT was 54/300 (18%) and 134 (45%) patients had a negative D-dimer test. During the 3-month follow-up, only one of the latter patients experienced proven recurrent VTE (1/134; 0.8%; 95% CI: 0 to 4%)

A recent study assessed the safety and usefulness of D-dimer in patients suspected of PE who had experienced previous VTE (Table 6.10). In this study, PE was ruled out by a negative D-dimer test in 33% (462/1411) of patients without previous VTE but in only 16% (49/308) of patients with previous VTE, $p < 0.0001$. The 3-month thromboembolic risk was 0% (95% CI: 0.0 to 7.9%) in patients with previous VTE and a negative D-dimer test. The two-fold lower chance of obtaining a negative D-dimer result in patients with previous VTE was independent of older age, active malignancy, fever and recent surgery. These data suggest that in patients suspected of PE with a history of previous VTE, a negative ELISA D-dimer test allows the diagnosis to be safely ruled out. However, the usefulness of the test is reduced because the proportion of patients with a history of VTE and a negative D-dimer test is lower than observed in patients without previous VTE.

Table 6.10   Performance of D-dimer test in patients with and without a history of VTE. Adapted from (64)

Characteristics	History of VTE ($n = 308$)	No history of VTE ($n = 1411$)	P
Negative D-dimer test	49 (15.9)	462 (32.7)	<0.0001
Three-month follow-up:			
OAT for other indication than VTE	4	18	
Lost of follow-up	0	3	
No. of events in patients with negative D-dimer test and not receiving OAT[a]	0/45	0/441	
3-month risk (95% CI)	0.0% (0.0 to 7.9)	0.0% (0.0 to 0.9)	
Number-needed-to-test to rule out one PE	6.3	3.1	
Sensitivity (%) (95% CI)	100 (97 to 100)	100 (99 to 100)	
Specificity (%) (95% CI)	27 (21 to 33)	41 (38 to 44)	

[a]OAT, oral anticoagulant therapy.

Pregnant women

It is well known that D-dimer levels increase as pregnancy progresses and, obviously, this will diminish the specificity of the test and will limit its clinical usefulness. Nevertheless, in a previous prospective study on the evolution of fibrinolytic markers throughout pregnancy, the proportion of pregnant women with a normal D-dimer value was still 39% before the 30th week of gestation and 25% before the 42nd week (62,81). Therefore, a substantial proportion of D-dimer measurements may be negative during pregnancy and this would be particularly important as a means to avoid ionizing radiation required as part of the radiological work-up.

A recent prospective study suggested a high sensitivity (100; 95% CI: 77 to 100%) and a high negative predictive value (100%; 95% CI: 95 to 100%) in pregnant women with suspected DVT using another D-dimer test (SimpliRED D-dimer, Agen Biomedical, Brisbane, Australia). However, it was not a management study and the limited number of patients explains the wide CIs (82). However, there is no evidence from any of the situations in which D-dimer has a lower specificity [patients with cancer or with previous VTE or in the elderly (64,65,74)] that sensitivity might also be affected. Therefore, although there is at present no prospective study confirming the safety of not treating a pregnant woman with suspected VTE on the basis of a normal D-dimer test, it is probably safe to do so.

Other situations which limit the diagnostic performances of the test

At least three situations may be associated with a decreased sensitivity of D-dimer tests. These situations, limited size of thrombus, time lag between the onset of symptoms and laboratory test and anticoagulation already started at the time of measurement, may lead to a decrease in sensitivity with a subsequent increase in the probability of false-negative results.

Patients with a small thrombus burden

It has been shown that D-dimer levels are correlated with thrombus extension. Obviously, a large thrombus will be associated with large deposits and subsequent lysis of the fibrin and will result in higher D-dimer levels than a small peripheral thrombus. This may explain why reduced sensitivities for D-dimer have been reported in the presence of calf and infra-popliteal vein thromboses or subsegmental PE (83). In a prospective study of 314 consecutive inpatients and outpatients with suspected PE, De Monyé *et al.* (83) investigated the relation between the diagnostic accuracy of D-dimer plasma concentration and pulmonary embolus location. Plasma D-dimer levels were measured using a quantitative immunoturbidimetric method. A strict protocol of ventilation–perfusion scintigraphy, CT pulmonary angiography and catheter pulmonary angiography was used to reach a final diagnosis and to assess the largest pulmonary artery in which embolus was visible. There was a strong correlation between plasma D-dimer concentration and embolus location (Kruskal-Wallis, $p < 0.001$). Thus, the assay showed greater accuracy in excluding segmental or larger emboli (sensitivity = 93%) than subsegmental emboli (sensitivity = 50%) (83), In another study, Galle *et al.* suggested that D-dimer levels above 4000 ng/mL were associated with perfusion defects of more than 50% on ventilation–perfusion lung scan (84). The situation is identical in the presence of suspected DVT. In a study where the diagnostic performances of a standard plasma D-dimer and of a quantitative microlatex test measurement were compared with contrast venography, both tests has a diminished sensitivity for calf DVT. In this study, the sensitivity and NPV were 98.5% and 96%, respectively, for diagnosing proximal DVT, but only 84% and 85%, respectively, in the diagnosis of distal DVT (85). However, despite this limited sensitivity for calf DVT, many management studies using ELISA D-dimer tests confirmed the safety of not treating patients with suspected DVT and normal D-dimer levels (15,54).

Patients with a prolonged duration of symptoms

There is also an inverse relation between D-dimer levels and duration of symptoms. D-dimer concentrations tend to decrease when the patient presents symptoms several days before testing. In a study published more than 10 years ago, dealing with suspected DVT, the time elapsed from the onset of symptoms was negatively associated with D-dimer levels both in patients with and in those without DVT. In these patients, the D-dimer values already decreased to 25% of the initial value after 1–2 weeks (6).

Patients already on anticoagulant treatment

Anticoagulant therapy, both with heparin and with oral anticoagulants, reduces the formation and deposition of fibrin and thus reduces D-dimer levels. Based on the literature, some authors calculated that the mean D-dimer levels decrease by 25% within 24 hours after starting heparin therapy in patients with acute VTE (86). This 25% decrease in D-dimer levels resulted in a decrease in sensitivity from 95.5% (95% CI: 90 to 99%) to 89% (95% CI: 84 to 95%). Therefore, D-dimer measurement performed after starting anticoagulation therapy should be interpreted with caution as a higher frequency of false-negative results is expected under these circumstances (86,87).

D-DIMER AS A PROGNOSTIC MARKER IN PATIENTS WITH PE

As previously discussed, D-dimer levels are associated with the extent and burden of thromboembolic disease. Risk assessment is important for selecting the appropriate management strategy in patients with PE. In particular, selected patients with a low risk of recurrence or of an unfavourable outcome could be treated as outpatients. Risk stratification may be based on clinical prediction rules (88,89), biomarkers or right ventricular imaging by echocardiography or CT (90–93). In addition, a recently published study suggested that D-dimer could be a good predictor of mortality after symptomatic PE. Patients who died had higher median D-dimer levels than patients who survived (4578 versus 2946 ng/mL; $p = 0.005$) (94). When D-dimer levels were separated in quartiles, mortality increased with increasing D-dimer level, rising from 1.1% in the first quartile (<1500 ng/mL) to 9.1% in the fourth quartile (>5500 ng/mL). The sensitivity and NPV for mortality associated with a D-dimer level less than 1500 ng/mL were 95% (95% CI: 74 to 100%) and 99% (95% CI: 94 to 100%), respectively. Therefore, these data suggest that patients with confirmed PE and D-dimer levels below 1500 ng/mL have a very low mortality risk. Hence D-dimer combined with other prognostic tools might be useful to identify low-risk patients who could be treated more readily on an outpatient basis (94).

D-DIMER TESTING TO DECIDE THE DURATION OF ANTICOAGULATION

The optimal duration of oral anticoagulant therapy for VTE is uncertain as the disease tends to recur after vitamin K antagonist (VKA) withdrawal, irrespective of the duration of treatment. The WODIT-DVT (95) and WODIT-PE (96) studies, and also the DOTAVK (97) study, have shown that the benefit associated with VKA prolongation is not maintained after therapy is discontinued. A potential strategy would consist of an individual assessment of risk of recurrence with the stratification of patients at low or high risk. Currently, the duration of anticoagulation therapy is mainly based on the clinical context of the index event (provoked versus unprovoked VTE and existence of a persistent risk factor such as high-risk thrombophilia or active cancer). In the case of a VTE triggered by a transient risk factor, anticoagulation treatment is recommended for at least 3 months, whereas in the case of a first episode of unprovoked or idiopathic VTE the Seventh American College of Chest Physicians (AACP) Conference on Antithrombic and Thrombolytic Therapy (98) recommends treatment with a VKA for at least 6–12 months (Grade 1) with the suggestion of considering such patients for indefinite anticoagulant therapy (Grade 2).

D-dimer measurement might play a role in assessing the individual need for prolonged anticoagulation. D-dimer during antithrombotic treatment and after its withdrawal has been studied in many prospective cohort studies in relation to late recurrence. These studies show that around 15% of patients with VTE have persistently high D-dimer levels, in spite of adequate anticoagulation. Moreover, D-dimer remained elevated (more than 500 ng/mL with the Vidas ELISA test) in a significantly higher proportion of patients with an idiopathic DVT (24%) than patients with a permanent risk factor (15%) and subjects with a transient risk factor (8%). Finally, elevated D-dimer levels during anticoagulation have been shown to be associated with a higher risk of recurrences after treatment discontinuation. Therefore, measuring D-dimer during VKA treatment would be clinically relevant. However, this approach would miss patients in whom D-dimer increases after anticoagulation withdrawal.

D-dimer after anticoagulation has been stopped

The value of D-dimer as a risk factor for recurrence after VKA withdrawal was studied first by Palareti et al. in a cohort study of 396 patients after a first episode of VTE (DVT and/or PE either idiopathic or secondary to a permanent or transient risk factor) with a follow-up of 21 months (79). D-dimer (Vidas ELISA D-dimer, bioMérieux, Marcy l'Etoile, France, cut-off 500 ng/mL) was measured on the day of VKA withdrawal and 3–4 weeks (T2) and 3 months (T3) thereafter. D-dimer was found to be increased in 15.5% of cases on the day of VKA withdrawal, in 40.3% at 3 weeks and in 46.2% at 3 months. During follow-up, VTE recurred in 10.1% of all patients, in 10.8% of subjects with idiopathic VTE, in 34% of subjects with permanent risk factors, such as cancer or chronic inflammatory disease, and in 4.3% of subjects with transient risk factors. The hazard ratio for recurrence associated with abnormal D-dimer was 2.45 (95% CI: 1.28 to 4.53). The NPV of a normal D-dimer level was 95.5% (95% CI: 92 to 98%) when measured at 3 months. Only five idiopathic recurrences occurred in the 186 patients with consistently normal D-dimer. The results of this study suggest that D-dimer has a high NPV for VTE recurrence even when performed after anticoagulation withdrawal.

The predictive value of D-dimer for recurrent VTE was confirmed by another study including 610 patients with a first idiopathic VTE event (99). D-dimer was measured with Asserachrom D-d (Boehringer Mannheim, Mannheim, Germany) 3 weeks after VKA withdrawal with a mean follow-up of 38 months. D-dimer levels less than 250 ng/mL were associated with a cumulative recurrence rate at 2 years of only 3.7% and a 60% risk reduction of recurrence when compared with higher levels. Patients with plasma D-dimer levels higher than 250 ng/mL had a recurrence rate of 11.5%.

In another prospective study (100), 599 patients with a previous VTE episode were repeatedly examined for D-dimer after VKA withdrawal and screened for inherited thrombophilic alterations, which were detected in 130 (22%), the most prevalent being factor V Leiden ($n = 70$, two of whom homozygotes) and prothrombin mutation ($n = 38$). Recurrent events were recorded in 58 subjects during a follow-up of 871 patient-years. Elevated D-dimer at month 1 after VKA withdrawal was associated with a higher rate of subsequent recurrences in all subjects investigated and especially in those with an idiopathic qualifying VTE event (hazard ratio 2.43; 95% CI: 1.18 to 4.61) and in those with thrombophilia (hazard ratio 8.34; 95% CI: 2.72 to 17.43). The NPV of D-dimer was 93 and 96% in subjects with either an unprovoked qualifying event or with thrombophilia, respectively. These data indicate that D-dimer levels measured 1 month after VKA withdrawal have a high NPV for recurrence in subjects with idiopathic VTE, whether or not carriers of congenital thrombophilia.

The PROLONG study

A randomized study evaluated the safety of withholding VKA in patients with normal D-dimer 30 days after VKA withdrawal has recently been published (101). Patients with a first idiopathic event received oral anticoagulants for a 3–6-month period and underwent a D-dimer measurement 1 month after VKA withdrawal with a qualitative whole blood test (Clearview Simplify D-dimer assay, Instrumentation Laboratory). Patients with normal D-dimer did not resume anticoagulation. Patients with abnormal D-dimer were randomized either to resume or to discontinue anticoagulation. The aims of the study were the following: to evaluate the safety of withholding VKA in patients with normal D-dimer 1 month after VKA withdrawal; to establish the risk of recurrence in patients with altered D-dimer 1 month after VKA interruption; and to evaluate the protective effect of VKA in the latter group. Patients with normal D-dimer in whom anticoagulants were discontinued had a thromboembolic rate of 6.3% (24/385). Patients with abnormal D-dimer test results, who were randomized to resume VKA anticoagulation, had a thromboembolic rate of 2.9% (3/103), while the recurrence rate was 15% (18/20) in the patients with elevated D-dimer randomized to discontinue anticoagulation. The relative risk of recurrence was 2.3 times greater in patients with elevated D-dimer concentrations who discontinued anticoagulation than in patients in whom anticoagulants were discontinued on the basis of a normal D-dimer (relative risk 2.27; 95% CI: 1.15 to 4.46). Resuming anticoagulation in patients with positive D-dimer induced a four-fold reduction in the recurrence risk (relative risk 4.26; 95% CI: 1.23 to 14.6). The authors concluded that patients with an abnormal D-dimer test who resumed anticoagulation had a significantly lower combined incidence of recurrent venous thromboembolism than those in whom anticoagulants were discontinued. However, the use of a positive D-dimer test to select patients at high risk of recurrence may be viewed as puzzling as the positive predictive value appears very low. As shown in Table 6.11, the positive predictive value varies between 10 and 16%. These data and the characteristics of the test suggest that D-dimer cannot be used to identify high-risk patients who would require prolonged anticoagulation, as the D-dimer level is probably offset by clinical characteristics such as idiopathic or unprovoked type of the event and the male gender, both being highly predictive of recurrence.

Unresolved issues

Different D-dimer methods may yield different results when their predictive value for recurrence is assessed. Moreover, the cut-off values for recurrence may differ from the cut-off values employed for diagnosis. As persisting high D-dimer levels under anticoagulation are associated with an increased risk of recurrence, a better understanding of the relationship between D-dimer and therapeutic international normalized ratio (INR) in patients who present with elevated D-dimer levels while on anticoagulant treatment would help to establish whether a stricter monitoring of INR value in these patients or higher INR therapeutic values are warranted in these patients.

Table 6.11 Performance of D-dimer measurement to predict recurrent thromboembolic disease

Study	DD cut-off (ng/mL)	Kind of test	Δ T	Recurrence rate (%) in patients with normal D-dimer levels	Recurrence rate (%) in patients with abnormal D-dimer levels	Hazard ratio for recurrence rate for abnormal D-dimer (95% CI)	PPV (%) (95% CI)	NPV (%) (95% CI)
Palareti et al., 2002 (79)	500	Quantitative, Vidas ELISA	Day 0–3 months	4.1	10.1	2.45 (1.28 to 3.53)	10 (5 to 19)	96 (87 to 100)
Palareti et al., 2003 (100)	500	Quantitative, Vidas ELISA	1 month	7.0	16.5	2.43 (1.18 to 4.61)	16 (12 to 22)	94 (91 to 96)
Eichinger et al., 2003 (99)	250	Quantitative, Asserachrom ELISA	3 weeks	7.6	15.7	2.24 (1.26 to 4.0)	16 (13 to 20)	92 (88 to 95)
Palareti et al., 2006 (101)	–	Qualitative, Simplify D-dimer test	1 month	6.2	15	2.27 (1.15 to 4.46)	15 (10 to 22)	94 (91 to 96)

CONCLUSIONS

There is an impressive literature dealing with D-dimer, clearly highlighting the perceived importance of the test. Many accuracy and management studies have been performed, in particular in outpatients. These studies demonstrate that ELISA D-dimer tests and latex turbidimetric tests are associated with the highest sensitivity and with virtually no inter-observer differences. Latex test and whole blood tests are less sensitive but have other advantages, including fast patient bedside realization and lack of labour intensity. Some ELISA D-dimer assays have been shown to rule out PE and/or DVT reliably, irrespective of clinical assessment. However, the theoretical concern of a lower NPV in patients with a high clinical probability, and hence a high prevalence of the disease, explain why recent guidelines suggest that these tests should be used to rule out VTE only in non-high clinical probability patients. Less sensitive tests can be used, but they should be restricted to ruling out VTE in patients with a low clinical probability and even so only provided that the true prevalence of VTE in that clinical probability category does not exceed 5%. The main limitation of D-dimer tests for diagnostic purposes is their reduced usefulness in specific patient categories or clinical settings which are correlated with increased plasma D-dimer levels themselves. Indeed, an important diminution of specificity and hence clinical usefulness has been reported in elderly patients, in cancer patients, in patients with previous VTE and in pregnant and postpartum women, although the test retains its high sensitivity in those situations.

Recently, many studies have evaluated various D-dimer tests for predicting the risk of recurrence after a first VTE event and showed that D-dimer measurement has a high NPV (>92%) for VTE recurrence. One intervention randomized study confirmed that in patients who stopped anticoagulation therapy, the adjusted hazard ratio for a recurrent event among those with an abnormal D-dimer test compared with those with a normal test was doubled, a finding that requires careful analysis before being used in clinical practice. Nevertheless, these recent and highly interesting data suggest that clinical indications for D-dimer have not been completely investigated yet and suggest other clinical uses for D-dimer in the near future.

REFERENCES

1. Task Force on Pulmonary Embolism, European Society of Cardiology. Guidelines on diagnosis and management of acute pulmonary embolism. *Eur Heart J* 2000; **21**:1301–36.
2. Elias A, Mallard L, Elias M, *et al.* A single complete ultrasound investigation of the venous network for the diagnostic management of patients with a clinically suspected first episode of deep venous thrombosis of the lower limbs. *Thromb Haemost* 2003; **89**:221–7.
3. Wells PS, Anderson DR, Rodger M, *et al.* Evaluation of D-dimer in the diagnosis of suspected deep-vein thrombosis. *N Engl J Med* 2003; **349**:1227–35.
4. Chapman CS, Akhtar N, Campbell S, *et al.* The use of D-dimer assay by enzyme immunoassay and latex agglutination techniques in the diagnosis of deep vein thrombosis. *Clin Lab Haematol* 1990; **12**:37–42.
5. Sie P. The value of laboratory tests in the diagnosis of venous thromboembolism. *Haematologica* 1995; **80**:57–60.
6. D'Angelo A, D'Alessandro G, Tomassini L, *et al.* Evaluation of a new rapid quantitative D-dimer assay in patients with clinically suspected deep vein thrombosis. *Thromb Haemost* 1996; **75**:412–6.
7. Hager K, Platt D. Fibrin degeneration product concentrations (D-dimers) in the course of ageing. *Gerontology* 1995; **41**:159–65.
8. Reber G, de Moerloose P. D-dimer assays for the exclusion of venous thromboembolism. *Semin Thromb Hemost* 2000; **26**:619–24.
9. Elms MJ, Bunce IH, Bundesen PG, *et al.* Measurement of crosslinked fibrin degradation products – an immunoassay using monoclonal antibodies. *Thromb Haemost* 1983; **50**:591–4.

10. Hart R, Bate I, Dinh D, *et al*. The detection of D-dimer in plasma by enzyme immunoassay: improved discrimination is obtained with a more specific signal antibody. *Blood Coagul Fibrinolysis* 1994; **5**:227–32.
11. Bounameaux H, Schneider PA, Reber G, *et al*. Measurement of plasma D-dimer for diagnosis of deep venous thrombosis. *Am J Clin Pathol* 1989; **91**:82–5.
12. Elias A, Aptel I, Huc B, *et al*. D-dimer test and diagnosis of deep vein thrombosis: a comparative study of 7 assays. *Thromb Haemost* 1996; **76**:518–22.
13. Freyburger G, Trillaud H, Labrouche S, *et al*. D-dimer strategy in thrombosis exclusion – a gold standard study in 100 patients suspected of deep venous thrombosis or pulmonary embolism: 8 DD methods compared. *Thromb Haemost* 1998; **79**:32–7.
14. Pittet JL, de Moerloose P, Reber G, *et al*. VIDAS D-dimer: fast quantitative ELISA for measuring D-dimer in plasma. *Clin Chem* 1996; **42**:410–5.
15. Perrier A, Desmarais S, Miron MJ, *et al*. Non-invasive diagnosis of venous thromboembolism in outpatients. *Lancet* 1999; **353**:190–5.
16. Perrier A, Bounameaux H, Morabia A, *et al*. Diagnosis of pulmonary embolism by a decision analysis-based strategy including clinical probability, D-dimer levels and ultrasonography: a management study. *Arch Intern Med* 1996; **156**:531–6.
17. Reber G, Bounameaux H, Perrier A, *et al*. A new rapid point-of-care D-dimer enzyme-linked immunosorbent assay (Stratus CS D-dimer) for the exclusion of venous thromboembolism. *Blood Coagul Fibrinolysis* 2004; **15**:435–8.
18. Dempfle CE, Suvajac N, Elmas E, *et al*. Performance evaluation of a new rapid quantitative assay system for measurement of D-dimer in plasma and whole blood: PATHFAST D-dimer. *Thromb Res* 2007; **120**:591–6.
19. Lippi G, Salvagno GL, Rossi L, *et al*. Analytical performances of the D-dimer assay for the Immulite 2000 automated immunoassay analyser. *Int J Lab Hematol* 2007; **29**:415–20.
20. Janssen MC, Verbruggen H, Wollersheim H, *et al*. D-dimer determination to assess regression of deep venous thrombosis. *Thromb Haemost* 1997; **78**:799–802.
21. Legnani C, Pancani C, Palareti G, *et al*. Comparison of new rapid methods for D-dimer measurement to exclude deep vein thrombosis in symptomatic outpatients. *Blood Coagul Fibrinolysis* 1997; **8**: 296–302.
22. Freyburger G, Labrouche S. Comparability of D-dimer assays in clinical samples. *Semin Vasc Med* 2005; **5**:328–39.
23. Brown MD, Lau J, Nelson RD, *et al*. Turbidimetric D-dimer test in the diagnosis of pulmonary embolism: a metaanalysis. *Clin Chem* 2003; **49**:1846–53.
24. Di Nisio M, Squizzato A, Rutjes AW, *et al*. Diagnostic accuracy of D-dimer test for exclusion of venous thromboembolism: a systematic review. *J Thromb Haemost* 2007; **5**:296–304.
25. Mauron T, Baumgartner I, Z'Brun A, *et al*. SimpliRED D-dimer assay: comparability of capillary and citrated venous whole blood, between-assay variability and performance of the test for exclusion of deep vein thrombosis in symptomatic outpatients. *Thromb Haemost* 1998; **79**:1217–9.
26. de Monye W, Huisman MV, Pattynama PM. Observer dependency of the SimpliRED D-dimer assay in 81 consecutive patients with suspected pulmonary embolism. *Thromb Res* 1999; **96**:293–8.
27. Cini M, Legnani C, Cavallaroni K, *et al*. A new rapid bedside assay for D-dimer measurement (Simplify D-dimer) in the diagnostic work-up for deep vein thrombosis. *J Thromb Haemost* 2003; **1**:2681–3.
28. Neale D, Tovey C, Vali A, *et al*. Evaluation of the Simplify D-dimer assay as a screening test for the diagnosis of deep vein thrombosis in an emergency department. *Emerg Med J* 2004; **21**:663–6.
29. Hogg K, Dawson D, Mackway-Jones K. The emergency department utility of Simplify D-dimer to exclude pulmonary embolism in patients with pleuritic chest pain. *Ann Emerg Med* 2005; **46**: 305–10.
30. Kline JA, Runyon MS, Webb WB, *et al*. Prospective study of the diagnostic accuracy of the simplify D-dimer assay for pulmonary embolism in emergency department patients. *Chest* 2006; **129**:1417–23.
31. Jennings I, Woods TA, Kitchen DP, *et al*. Laboratory D-dimer measurement: improved agreement between methods through calibration. *Thromb Haemost* 2007; **98**:1127–35.
32. Gaffney PJ, Edgell TA. The International and 'NIH' units for thrombin – how do they compare? *Thromb Haemost* 1995; **74**:900–3.
33. Nieuwenhuizen W. A reference material for harmonisation of D-dimer assays. Fibrinogen Subcommittee of the Scientific and Standardization Committee of the International Society of Thrombosis and Haemostasis. *Thromb Haemost* 1997; **77**:1031–3.
34. Favaloro EJ. Standardization, regulation, quality assurance and emerging technologies in hemostasis: issues, controversies, benefits and limitations. *Semin Thromb Hemost* 2007; **33**:290–7.

35. Dempfle CE, Zips S, Ergul H, *et al*. The Fibrin Assay Comparison Trial (FACT): evaluation of 23 quantitative D-dimer assays as basis for the development of D-dimer calibrators. FACT Study Group. *Thromb Haemost* 2001; **85**:671–8.

36. Meijer P, Haverkate F, Kluft C, *et al*. A model for the harmonisation of test results of different quantitative D-dimer methods. *Thromb Haemost* 2006; **95**:567–72.

37. van Beek EJ, Schenk BE, Michel BC, *et al*. The role of plasma D-dimers concentration in the exclusion of pulmonary embolism. *Br J Haematol* 1996; **92**:725–32.

38. Masotti L, Ceccarelli E, Cappelli R, *et al*. Plasma D-dimer levels in elderly patients with suspected pulmonary embolism. *Thromb Res* 2000; **98**:577–9.

39. Perrier A. D-dimer for suspected pulmonary embolism: whom should we test? *Chest* 2004; **125**:807–9.

40. Dempfle CE. Use of D-dimer assays in the diagnosis of venous thrombosis. *Semin Thromb Hemost* 2000; **26**:631–41.

41. Miron MJ, Perrier A, Bounameaux H, *et al*. Contribution of noninvasive evaluation to the diagnosis of pulmonary embolism in hospitalized patients. *Eur Respir J* 1999; **13**:1365–70.

42. British Thoracic Society guidelines for the management of suspected acute pulmonary embolism. *Thorax* 2003; **58**:470–83.

43. Wells PS, Brill-Edwards P, Stevens P, *et al*. A novel and rapid whole-blood assay for D-dimer in patients with clinically suspected deep vein thrombosis. *Circulation* 1995; **91**:2184–7.

44. Kraaijenhagen RA, Piovella F, Bernardi E, *et al*. Simplification of the diagnostic management of suspected deep vein thrombosis. *Arch Intern Med* 2002; **162**:907–11.

45. Kearon C, Ginsberg JS, Douketis J, *et al*. Management of suspected deep venous thrombosis in outpatients by using clinical assessment and D-dimer testing. *Ann Intern Med* 2001; **135**:108–11.

46. van der Graaf F, van den Borne H, van der Kolk M, *et al*. Exclusion of deep venous thrombosis with D-dimer testing – comparison of 13 D-dimer methods in 99 outpatients suspected of deep venous thrombosis using venography as reference standard. *Thromb Haemost* 2000; **83**:191–8.

47. Michiels JJ, Gadisseur A, van der Planken M, *et al*. Different accuracies of rapid enzyme-linked immunosorbent, turbidimetric and agglutination D-dimer assays for thrombosis exclusion: impact on diagnostic work-ups of outpatients with suspected deep vein thrombosis and pulmonary embolism. *Semin Thromb Hemost* 2006; **32**:678–93.

48. Oudega R, Moons KG, Hoes AW. Ruling out deep venous thrombosis in primary care. A simple diagnostic algorithm including D-dimer testing. *Thromb Haemost* 2005; **94**:200–5.

49. Oudega R, Hoes AW, Moons KG. The Wells rule does not adequately rule out deep venous thrombosis in primary care patients. *Ann Intern Med* 2005; **143**:100–7.

50. Schutgens RE, Ackermark P, Haas FJ, *et al*. Combination of a normal D-dimer concentration and a non-high pretest clinical probability score is a safe strategy to exclude deep venous thrombosis. *Circulation* 2003; **107**:593–7.

51. Wells PS, Ginsberg JS, Anderson DR, *et al*. Use of a clinical model for safe management of patients with suspected pulmonary embolism. *Ann Intern Med* 1998; **129**:997–1005.

52. Wells PS, Anderson DR, Rodger M, *et al*. Excluding pulmonary embolism at the bedside without diagnostic imaging: management of patients with suspected pulmonary embolism presenting to the emergency department by using a simple clinical model and d-dimer. *Ann Intern Med* 2001; **135**:98–107.

53. Kearon C, Ginsberg JS, Douketis J, *et al*. An evaluation of D-dimer in the diagnosis of pulmonary embolism: a randomized trial. *Ann Intern Med* 2006; **144**:812–21.

54. de Moerloose P, Desmarais S, Bounameaux H, *et al*. Contribution of a new, rapid, individual and quantitative automated D-dimer ELISA to exclude pulmonary embolism. *Thromb Haemost* 1996; **75**:11–3.

55. Kruip MJ, Slob MJ, Schijen JH, *et al*. Use of a clinical decision rule in combination with D-dimer concentration in diagnostic workup of patients with suspected pulmonary embolism: a prospective management study. *Arch Intern Med* 2002; **162**:1631–5.

56. Perrier A, Roy PM, Sanchez O, *et al*. Multi-detector row computed tomography in outpatients with suspected pulmonary embolism. *N Engl J Med* 2005; **352**:1760–8.

57. Kucher N, Kohler HP, Dornhofer T, *et al*. Accuracy of D-dimer/fibrinogen ratio to predict pulmonary embolism: a prospective diagnostic study. *J Thromb Haemost* 2003; **1**:708–13.

58. van Belle A, Buller HR, Huisman MV, *et al*. Effectiveness of managing suspected pulmonary embolism using an algorithm combining clinical probability, D-dimer testing and computed tomography. *JAMA* 2006; **295**:172–9.

59. Stein PD, Hull RD, Patel KC, *et al*. D-dimer for the exclusion of acute venous thrombosis and pulmonary embolism: a systematic review. *Ann Intern Med* 2004; **140**:589–602.

60. Raimondi P, Bongard O, de Moerloose P, *et al*. D-dimer plasma concentration in various clinical conditions: implication for the use of this test in the diagnostic approach of venous thromboembolism. *Thromb Res* 1993; **69**:125–30.

61. Chabloz P, Reber G, Boehlen F, *et al*. TAFI antigen and D-dimer levels during normal pregnancy and at delivery. *Br J Haematol* 2001; **115**:150–2.

62. Epiney M, Boehlen F, Boulvain M, *et al*. D-dimer levels during delivery and the postpartum. *J Thromb Haemost* 2005; **3**:268–71.

63. Righini M, Aujesky D, Roy PM, *et al*. Clinical usefulness of D-dimer depending on clinical probability and cutoff value in outpatients with suspected pulmonary embolism. *Arch Intern Med* 2004; **164**:2483–7.

64. Le Gal G, Righini M, Roy PM, *et al*. Value of D-dimer testing for the exclusion of pulmonary embolism in patients with previous venous thromboembolism. *Arch Intern Med* 2006; **166**:176–80.

65. Righini M, Goehring C, Bounameaux H, *et al*. Effects of age on the performance of common diagnostic tests for pulmonary embolism. *Am J Med* 2000; **109**:357–61.

66. Tardy B, Tardy-Poncet B, Viallon A, *et al*. Evaluation of D-dimer ELISA test in elderly patients with suspected pulmonary embolism. *Thromb Haemost* 1998; **79**:38–41.

67. Righini M, Le Gal G, Perrier A, *et al*. The challenge of diagnosing pulmonary embolism in elderly patients: influence of age on commonly used diagnostic tests and strategies. *J Am Geriatr Soc* 2005; **53**:1039–45.

68. Righini M, Nendaz M, G LEG, *et al*. Influence of age on the cost-effectiveness of diagnostic strategies for suspected pulmonary embolism. *J Thromb Haemost* 2007; **5**:1869–77.

69. Linkins LA, Bates SM, Ginsberg JS, *et al*. Use of different D-dimer levels to exclude venous thromboembolism depending on clinical pretest probability. *J Thromb Haemost* 2004; **2**:1256–60.

70. Righini M, de Moerloose P, Reber G, *et al*. Should the D-dimer cut-off value be increased in elderly patients suspected of pulmonary embolism? *Thromb Haemost* 2001; **85**:744.

71. ten Wolde M, Kraaijenhagen RA, Prins MH, *et al*. The clinical usefulness of D-dimer testing in cancer patients with suspected deep venous thrombosis. *Arch Intern Med* 2002; **162**:1880–4.

72. Lee AY, Julian JA, Levine MN, *et al*. Clinical utility of a rapid whole-blood D-dimer assay in patients with cancer who present with suspected acute deep venous thrombosis. *Ann Intern Med* 1999; **131**:417–23.

73. Di Nisio M, Sohne M, Kamphuisen PW, *et al*. D-dimer test in cancer patients with suspected acute pulmonary embolism. *J Thromb Haemost* 2005; **3**:1239–42.

74. Righini M, Le Gal G, De Lucia S, *et al*. Clinical usefulness of D-dimer testing in cancer patients with suspected pulmonary embolism. *Thromb Haemost* 2006; **95**:715–9.

75. Perrier A, Roy PM, Aujesky D, *et al*. Diagnosing pulmonary embolism in outpatients with clinical assessment, D-dimer measurement, venous ultrasound and helical computed tomography: a multicentre management study. *Am J Med* 2004; **116**:291–9.

76. Perrier A, Roy PM, Sanchez O, *et al*. Multidetector-row computed tomography in suspected pulmonary embolism. *N Engl J Med* 2005; **352**:1760–8.

77. Koopman MM, Buller HR, ten Cate JW. Diagnosis of recurrent deep vein thrombosis. *Haematologica* 1995; **25**:49–57.

78. Prandoni P, Cogo A, Bernardi E, *et al*. A simple ultrasound approach for detection of recurrent proximal-vein thrombosis. *Circulation* 1993; **88**:1730–5.

79. Palareti G, Legnani C, Cosmi B, *et al*. Risk of venous thromboembolism recurrence: high negative predictive value of D-dimer performed after oral anticoagulation is stopped. *Thromb Haemost* 2002; **87**:7–12.

80. Rathbun SW, Whitsett TL, Raskob GE. Negative D-dimer result to exclude recurrent deep venous thrombosis: a management trial. *Ann Intern Med* 2004; **141**:839–45.

81. Boehlen F, Epiney M, Boulvain M, *et al*. [Changes in D-dimer levels during pregnancy and the postpartum period: results of two studies]. *Rev Med Suisse* 2005; **1**:296–8.

82. Chan WS, Chunilal S, Lee A, *et al*. A red blood cell agglutination D-dimer test to exclude deep venous thrombosis in pregnancy. *Ann Intern Med* 2007; **147**:165–70.

83. De Monyé W, Sanson BJ, MacGillavry MR, *et al*. Embolus location affects the sensitivity of a rapid quantitative D-dimer assay in the diagnosis of pulmonary embolism. *Am J Respir Crit Care Med* 2002; **165**:345–8.

84. Galle C, Papazyan JP, Miron MJ, *et al*. Prediction of pulmonary embolism extent by clinical findings, D-dimer level and deep vein thrombosis shown by ultrasound. *Thromb Haemost* 2001; **86**:1156–60.

85. Escoffre-Barbe M, Oger E, Leroyer C, *et al*. Evaluation of a new rapid D-dimer assay for clinically suspected deep venous thrombosis (Liatest D-dimer). *Am J Clin Pathol* 1998; **109**:748–53.

86. Estivals M, Pelzer H, Sie P, *et al*. Prothrombin fragment 1 + 2, thrombin–antithrombin III complexes and D-dimers in acute deep vein thrombosis: effects of heparin treatment. *Br J Haematol* 1991; **78**:421–4.

87. Couturaud F, Kearon C, Bates SM, *et al*. Decrease in sensitivity of D-dimer for acute venous thromboembolism after starting anticoagulant therapy. *Blood Coagul Fibrinolysis* 2002; **13**:241–6.

88. Wicki J, Perrier A, Perneger TV, *et al*. Predicting adverse outcome in patients with acute pulmonary embolism: a risk score. *Thromb Haemost* 2000; **84**:548–52.

89. Aujesky D, Obrosky DS, Stone RA, *et al*. A prediction rule to identify low-risk patients with pulmonary embolism. *Arch Intern Med* 2006; **166**:169–75.

90. Becattini C, Agnelli G. Acute pulmonary embolism: risk stratification in the emergency department. *Intern Emerg Med* 2007; **2**:119–29.

91. Giannitsis E, Katus HA. Risk stratification in patients with confirmed pulmonary embolism: what to do when echocardiography is not available. *Crit Care Med* 2006; **34**:2857–8.

92. Logeart D, Lecuyer L, Thabut G, *et al*. Biomarker-based strategy for screening right ventricular dysfunction in patients with non-massive pulmonary embolism. *Intensive Care Med* 2007; **33**:286–92.

93. Scridon T, Scridon C, Skali H, *et al*. Prognostic significance of troponin elevation and right ventricular enlargement in acute pulmonary embolism. *Am J Cardiol* 2005; **96**:303–5.

94. Aujesky D, Roy PM, Guy M, *et al*. Prognostic value of D-dimer in patients with pulmonary embolism. *Thromb Haemost* 2006; **96**:478–82.

95. Agnelli G, Prandoni P, Santamaria MG, *et al*. Three months versus one year of oral anticoagulant therapy for idiopathic deep venous thrombosis. Warfarin Optimal Duration Italian Trial Investigators. *N Engl J Med* 2001; **345**:165–9.

96. Agnelli G, Prandoni P, Becattini C, *et al*. Extended oral anticoagulant therapy after a first episode of pulmonary embolism. *Ann Intern Med* 2003; **139**:19–25.

97. Pinede L, Ninet J, Duhaut P, *et al*. Comparison of 3 and 6 months of oral anticoagulant therapy after a first episode of proximal deep vein thrombosis or pulmonary embolism and comparison of 6 and 12 weeks of therapy after isolated calf deep vein thrombosis. *Circulation* 2001; **103**:2453–60.

98. Buller HR, Agnelli G, Hull RD, *et al*. Antithrombotic therapy for venous thromboembolic disease: the Seventh ACCP Conference on Antithrombotic and Thrombolytic Therapy. *Chest* 2004; **126**:401S–428S.

99. Eichinger S, Minar E, Bialonczyk C, *et al*. D-dimer levels and risk of recurrent venous thromboembolism. *JAMA* 2003; **290**:1071–4.

100. Palareti G, Legnani C, Cosmi B, *et al*. Predictive value of D-dimer test for recurrent venous thromboembolism after anticoagulation withdrawal in subjects with a previous idiopathic event and in carriers of congenital thrombophilia. *Circulation* 2003; **108**:313–8.

101. Palareti G, Cosmi B, Legnani C, *et al*. D-dimer testing to determine the duration of anticoagulation therapy. *N Engl J Med* 2006; **355**:1780–9.

102. Anderson DR, Kovacs MJ, Kovacs G, *et al*. Combined use of clinical assessment and D-dimer to improve the management of patients presenting to the emergency department with suspected deep vein thrombosis (the EDITED Study). *J Thromb Haemost* 2003; **1**:645–51.

103. Tick LW, Ton E, van Voorthuizen T, *et al*. Practical diagnostic management of patients with clinically suspected deep vein thrombosis by clinical probability test, compression ultrasonography and D-dimer test. *Am J Med* 2002; **113**:630–5.

104. Blattler W, Martinez I, Blattler IK. Diagnosis of deep venous thrombosis and alternative diseases in symptomatic outpatients. *Eur J Intern Med* 2004; **15**:305–311.

105. Wells PS, Anderson DR, Rodger M, *et al*. Derivation of a simple clinical model to categorize patients' probability of pulmonary embolism: increasing the models utility with the SimpliRED D-dimer. *Thromb Haemost* 2000; **83**:416–20.

106. Wicki J, Perneger TV, Junod AF, *et al*. Assessing clinical probability of pulmonary embolism in the emergency ward: a simple score. *Arch Intern Med* 2001; **161**:92–7.

107. Le Gal G, Righini M, Roy PM, *et al*. Prediction of pulmonary embolism in the emergency department: the revised Geneva score. *Ann Intern Med* 2006; **144**:165–71.

108. Ginsberg JS, Kearon C, Douketis J, *et al*. The use of D-dimer testing and impedance plethysmographic examination in patients with clinical indications of deep vein thrombosis. *Arch Intern Med* 1997; **157**:1077–81.

109. Kearon C. Diagnosis of a first deep vein thrombosis in outpatients:interim analysis of a management based on clinical evaluation and D-dimer result [abstract]. *Thromb Haemost* 1997; **78**:588.

110. Righini M, Le Gal G, Aujesky D, *et al*. Diagnosis of pulmonary embolism by multidetector CT alone or combined with venous ultrasonography of the leg: a randomised non-inferiority trial. *Lancet* 2008; **371**(9621):1343–52.

CHAPTER 7

Computed Tomography for Thromboembolic Disease

Lawrence R. Goodman[1] and Edwin J.R. van Beek[2]

[1]Diagnostic Radiology & Pulmonary Medicine & Critical Care, Thoracic Imaging, Medical College of Wisconsin, Wisconsin, USA

[2]Department of Radiology, Carver College of Medicine, Iowa City, USA

INTRODUCTION

Two events merged in the 1990 s that propelled computed tomography (CT) to the forefront of pulmonary embolism (PE) diagnosis. The PIOPED I Study showed that ventilation/perfusion (V/Q) scanning, first introduced in the 1960s, gave excellent definitive diagnosis when read as *high probability* or *normal* (1). Unfortunately, approximately three-quarters of patients fell into *other* categories and only a probability statement could be offered. This often left the clinician in a quandary or required the addition of pulmonary angiography and/or studies of the deep venous system of the legs. Pulmonary angiography – although relatively safe – was invasive, involved a high radiation dose, was perceived as having significant complications and required a skilled operator. Many times, clinicians chose to forego angiography and treat on the basis of the 'best clinical estimate'. Since the lower extremities are the source of the majority of emboli, venography could be used as an adjunct for the global diagnosis of venous thromboembolic (VTE) disease. Contrast-enhanced leg venography had many of the disadvantages of pulmonary angiography and was also underutilized. Lower-extremity ultrasound, which is probably less sensitive and specific, however, gave clinically useful information and was rapidly accepted as a patient- and physician-friendly alternative, even though only approximately 30% of patients with proven PE had DVT demonstrated by ultrasonography (2). Second, the introduction of helical CT scanning and electron beam CT, in the early 1990s, permitted scans of the chest to be performed within a single breath hold (20–30 seconds) using 5 mm axial images. This provided direct visualization of the PE. Initial studies showed that computed tomographic pulmonary angiography (CTPA) had good sensitivity and specificity in the main lobar and segmental vessels, but was less accurate in detecting clot in the segmental and subsegmental vessels (3–6). It was clear to many that CTPA had great potential for PE diagnosis and it often demonstrated the cause for the patient's symptoms when PE was excluded (7–9). As the number of CT detectors increased and gantry speed increased, thinner sections and the possibility of high-quality multiplanar reconstructions

Deep Vein Thrombosis and Pulmonary Embolism Edited by Edwin J.R. van Beek, Harry R. Büller and Matthijs Oudkerk
© 2009 John Wiley & Sons, Ltd

propelled CT to the forefront. Numerous studies in the last 15 years have documented sensitivity and specificity and clinical outcomes satisfactory for clinical use.

With the introduction of CT venography (CTV), radiologists could now offer simplified testing for VTE (10–13). CTV provided extra assurance that if CTPA was falsely negative, a large clot was not lurking in the veins of the leg. When both PE and DVT were detected, the additional information sometimes aided management decisions. This combination became rapidly popular in some institutions, but the widespread introduction of combined CTPA and CTV has not been forthcoming due to the difficulty in weighing the advantages and the pelvic radiation delivered. Given the recent renewed discussion regarding the influence of CT imaging on the population's radiation dose, this will likely remain a point of contention in the foreseeable future (14,15).

This chapter (1) discusses the major clinical studies of sensitivity, specificity and outcome, (2) looks at some of the technical and radiation considerations in the use of helical CT for the diagnosis of VTE and (3) outlines some remaining controversies.

SENSITIVITY, SPECIFICITY AND CLINICAL OUTCOMES

Most investigators agree that a single-slice helical scan is adequate for the diagnosis of central PE but cannot always provide reliable diagnosis for the exclusion of more peripheral segmental and smaller PE. At the four-slice level, CT becomes of more definitive clinical value. The large, multicentre PIOPED II Study ($N = 824$), which utilized predominantly four-slice scanners, found a sensitivity for CTPA of 83% and a specificity of 96%. When CTV or an objective pre-imaging clinical assessment score was added, the sensitivity rose to approximately 90% without lowering specificity (16). PIOPED II also found that when CTPA and the Wells score were discrepant (e.g., high clinical probability/negative CTPA or vice versa), CTPA was not always reliable. Fortunately, less than 4% of patients fell into this category. Kappa values for CTPA, V/Q and pulmonary angiography were 0.73, 0.54 and 0.66, respectively, demonstrating the increased robustness of CTPA as a routine diagnostic modality (16). PIOPED II used composite clinical and imaging results as its 'gold standard'. Those composite standards had some inherent limitations themselves and perhaps explain the lower sensitivity of PIOPED II compared with other smaller clinical trials.

There have been numerous other studies of CTPA with sensitivities varying from 83 to 100% and specificities generally in the mid-90s. Below are some representative additional studies, all completed within the last few years. Qanadli *et al.*, comparing dual-slice CTA with pulmonary angiography ($N = 158$), showed a sensitivity of 90% and specificity of 94% (17). When the six (2%) technically inadequate CTPA studies were omitted, sensitivity and specificity rose to 95% and 97%, respectively. The kappa statistic for CTPA was 0.86 and for angiography 0.78. Using four-slice scanning and pulmonary angiography ($N = 93$), Winer-Muram *et al.* showed a sensitivity and specificity of 100% and 89%, respectively, and kappa values of 0.71 for CTPA and 0.83 for angiography (18). Revel *et al.* reported similar results and a CTPA kappa statistic of 0.88 (19). In a study of 179 patients comparing CTPA with V/Q scanning, the sensitivity and specificity for CTPA were 94% and 94% and for V/Q 81% and 81%, respectively. The kappa statistic for CTPA was 0.72 and for V/Q 0.22 (20). A less optimistic report of 299 cases of D-dimer-positive patients showed a CTPA sensitivity of 70%, a specificity of 91% and a kappa statistic of 0.85 (21). Most workers in the field believe that with 16- and 64-slice scanning, sensitivity in the low- to mid-90s and specificity in the mid-90s is achievable. Inter-observer agreement also improves with newer scanners. Residents and staff ($N = 122$) have 80% concordant reading with four-slice scanners and 94% with 16-slice scanners (22).

If the sensitivity of CTA is less than perfect, what is the outcome of patients who have a negative CTA and who are not anticoagulated? Quiroz *et al.* recently reviewed 15 clinical outcome studies involving 3500 patients (23). The likelihood of a subsequent PE in the next 3 months was 0.9% and the likelihood of death from PE was 0.6%. Moores *et al.* reviewed 4657 patients in studies from 1997 to 2004 and found a subsequent PE rate of 1.4% and a fatal PE rate of 0.5% (24). Another study followed 198 CTPA-negative patients for 3 months and found a 1% clinical recurrence rate. At the same time, 188 of 350 patients who under went V/Q scintigraphy had a normal result and none developed PE. Of 162 patients with a very low-probability reading, five (3.1%) returned with a PE (25). Thus, the negative clinical predictive value of CTPA appears to be approximately 99%, about the same as a negative perfusion scan or angiogram. A recent study compared two groups of patients using a combination of CTPA, clinical assessment and D-dimer testing with or without the additional use of ultrasound of the leg veins (26). In two groups, of 855 and 838 patients, the 3-month thromboembolic risk was 0.3% in each group, albeit that 53 patients (9%) in the ultrasound group did not undergo CTPA.

How does one explain the imperfect sensitivity of CTPA versus the near-perfect negative predictive value of CTPA? Outcome studies are a measure of clinical management results, whereas sensitivity measures the ability of a radiologist to detect a PE on CTPA compared with a 'gold standard'. Stein, from PIOPED II data, calculated that 11% of patients had intermediate pre-test clinical probability and many of these patients probably also had a false-negative CT. Since the CTPA studies were of good quality, one can assume that small emboli were missed (27). PIOPED I showed that two of 20 patients (10%) with untreated missed emboli at pulmonary angiography had clinical evidence of recurrence in the next 3 months. Thus, the 10% of 11% equals 1.1%, approximately the rate shown in clinical outcome studies. Stein calculated that a similar treatment of the data from two large European studies would also yield a 1% recurrence rate (28,29). Finally, these results are replicated in a critical review of catheter pulmonary angiography, which demonstrated improving outcomes after 1990, but still showed a recurrence rate of 1.1% in patients with normal angiogram findings during 3 months of clinical follow-up (30). In conclusion, it appears that the most sensitive tests will still lead to an approximately 1% thromboembolism recurrence rate during 3 months of follow-up and that this is the basis against which any diagnostic strategy should be tested.

Another aspect of clinical outcome has to do with clinician confidence. Rightly or wrongly, physicians feel more comfortable with a negative CTPA than with a negative V/Q. Anderson *et al.* found that when the V/Q with ultrasound was negative, additional studies were ordered in 31 of 640 (5%) of patients (31). Nine of these 31 patients (29%) showed the presence of PE. In comparison, when CTPA and ultrasonography were performed, only three of 694 (0.4%) had additional studies performed, none of which were positive. Perhaps experience has taught clinicians that when there is a discrepancy between their clinical judgments and imaging results, a combination of V/Q and ultrasound is less reliable than the combination of CT and ultrasound (31). CTPA may also uncover an equally plausible alternative diagnosis: a great aid in an emergency room setting (Figure 7.1) (32,33).

TECHNICAL ASPECTS

Equipment

Both the gantry rotation time and the slice thickness decreased as helical CT scanners progressed from single-detector, via four-detector, to 16-detector and 64-detector technology (Table 7.1). Better temporal and spatial resolution improved our ability to visualize smaller vessels and increase the confidence with which these can be evaluated (34). Ghaye *et al.* showed that 3 mm helical images demonstrated 82% of subsegmental vessels, whereas 1.25 mm slices demonstrated 94%

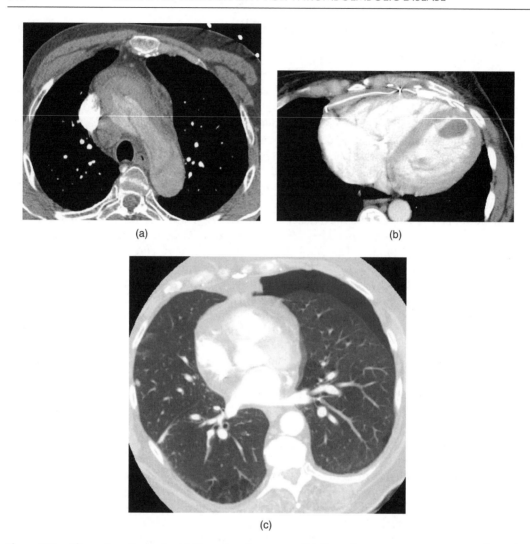

(a)

(b)

(c)

Figure 7.1 Alternative diagnosis. (a) There is a large type 'A' dissecting aneurysm, unsuspected, on this patient studied for a possible pulmonary embolus. The pulmonary artery opacification is suboptimal. (b) Left ventricular clot and apical left ventricular aneurysm in a patient with a negative study for pulmonary embolism. (c) Moderate left pneumothorax. This was not seen on the portable chest X-ray done the day before. CT showed no evidence of pulmonary embolus.

(35). Schoepf *et al.* subsequently showed that subsegmental pulmonary emboli were visible twice as often when viewing 1 mm rather than 3 mm images (36). The number of 'indeterminate' readings was cut by two-thirds and agreement between readers (kappa statistic) more than doubled. Thin-section multidetector CTPA is now the standard and a minimum of 16-detector CT has become routine. One can assume that the new dual-headed scanners, 256-detector scanners and dual-energy capability will improve diagnosis further, because scan time will decrease, diminishing respiratory and cardiac motion further. It is not clear whether thinner sections will provide additional advantages, as noise may increase, and the increased number of images in turn increases the opportunity to miss small emboli by the radiologist.

Table 7.1 CT scanning parameters commonly employed for CT pulmonary. Modified from Reference 89

Scan range:	Lung base to lung apex
Tube voltage:	120 kVp (may go down to 80 kVp in selected patients)
Section thickness:	4-slice scanners: $4 \times 1–1.25$ mm
	8-slice scanners: $8 \times 1–1.25$ mm
	16-slice scanners: $16 \times 0.75–1.5$ mm
	64-slice scanners: 64×0.625 mm
Pitch:	1.25–2 depending on scanner properties
Slice reconstruction:	1.0–1.5 mm; 2.0 mm in obese patients;
Slice reconstruction:	2.5–3.0 mm in dyspneic patients
Increment:	0.7–1.5 mm
Gantry rotation time:	1 s (4-slice CT) to 0.33 s (64-slice CT)
Scan duration:	3–4 s (64-slice CT) up to 25 s (4-slice CT)

Optimizing vessel contrast

Improved intravenous contrast management has also led to better quality CTA. A timing bolus or CT bolus tracking systems ensures that the pulmonary arteries are imaged at maximum opacification. Likewise, shorter scanning times mean that correct timing of the contrast bolus is easier to achieve. Faster injection rates of 4–5 mL/s provide better pulmonary artery opacification. A saline chase of 50 mL after contrast injection clears the venous system of contrast and provides for better contrast enhancement (37). Nonionic contrast is less likely to cause nausea, which may interfere with the study. Hyperextension of the arm being injected should be avoided. This will decrease the likelihood of impeded blood flow, as the subclavian vein passes between the clavicle and first rib. A moderate inspiration – avoiding a Valsalva manoeuvre – produces more uniform contrast flow.

A recent study suggested that adjusting the contrast volume, based on patient weight, could maximize quality and minimize contrast volume (38). It was found that approximately 1.2 mL/kg of a contrast medium containing 350 mg/mL of iodine, injected at a 4 mL/s flow rate, achieved satisfactory opacification (250 HU; HU = Hounsfield units). A 64-MDCT system allowed a 17% reduction in contrast requirements compared with a 16-MDCT scanner, mainly due to decreased scan time (5.7 vs 9.5 s). This decrease in contrast could be applied if one is only performing CTPA, as the addition of CTV would require a full contrast injection in order to achieve adequate peripheral venous opacification.

Another recent approach to improving vessel contrast, while decreasing radiation dose, is the use of a lower kilovoltage technique, which allows for greater absorption of photons by the high-density contrast agent. Schueller-Weidekamm *et al.* compared CTA using 140 kVp with 100 kVp and demonstrated that the average pulmonary artery density (HU) increased by 40–50% (39). At the same time, the calculated CT dose index (an estimate of radiation) decreased by 70%. Subjective grading of images showed no difference in quality. Heyer *et al.* compared 30 patients at 120 or 100 kVp and showed that the vessel density increased by 70 HU (22%) with a decrease in mean effective dose from 2.44 to 1.37 mSv, but without a change in signal-to-noise ratio (40). Neither study utilized real-time mA dose modulation, which is now available on most routinely used CT scanner systems. As a lower kV can take advantage of the K-edge of iodine, this may be an important improvement as dual-energy CT scanners come on the market.

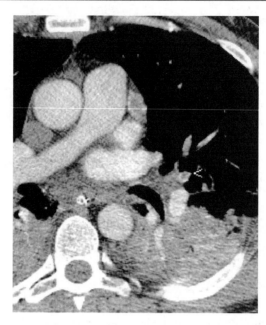

Figure 7.2 Suboptimal CT, but diagnostic. CT shows suboptimal opacification, with a pulmonary artery measuring 138 HU. The image is also somewhat noisy. Nonetheless, there is a definite pulmonary embolus in the anterior segment of the left upper lobe (arrowhead).

How much contrast enhancement is required for an adequate study? This has not been studied methodically. As a rule of thumb, clots in large vessels can generally be detected at 150–200 HU, whereas 250 HU or more is minimal to exclude PE in small vessels confidently (Figure 7.2). The overall evaluation of the adequacy of a CTA is a somewhat subjective combination of vessel density, vessel noise and motion (41).

CT quality is often suboptimal in markedly obese patients. The combination of increased scatter and increased X-ray absorption, and perhaps a larger blood volume diluting contrast, make for a noisier image. PIOPED II found that 5% of CTAs on very obese patients (BMI>35) were uninterpretable, whereas 2.3% were uninterpretable in the remaining population (16). Some improvement can be obtained by increasing the kVp and mA and by increasing the amount of iodinated contrast delivered. Reconstructing images at 2.5 mm, rather than at 1.25 mm, decreases noise, albeit at some minor expense in terms of visualization of the most distal arteries.

Minimizing motion artefact

Most studies show that somewhere between 3 and 7% of CT scans are technically inadequate. Motion artefact is 2–3 times more likely than poor vessel contrast enhancement to cause an inadequate study (16,41,42). Therefore, every attempt should be made to:

1. Work with the patient on breath holding. Quiet (shallow) breathing is preferable to uncertain breath holding. Ventilators should be held in apnea or turned to very low frequency. A caudo-cranial scanning direction is preferable as this will lead to least motion artefact at diaphragm level.

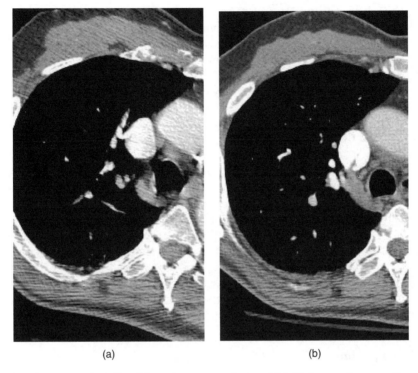

(a)   (b)

Figure 7.3 Respiratory motion. Possible pulmonary embolus. (a) Initial scan shows motion in the right upper lobe vessels. An embolus cannot be excluded. (b) A repeat study of just the upper lobes, following patient coaching, demonstrates no embolus.

2. Use the shortest scan times possible, which may be achieved by decreasing the gantry rotation time (sub-second rotation times are routinely available on all 16-MDCT and 64-MDCT systems now) and by increasing the table feeding speed.
3. If a portion of the scan is uninterpretable due to motion and it is felt that the patient can cooperate with additional coaching, repeated imaging of that portion of the examination using a 50–75 cm^3 contrast bolus may be contemplated. (Figure 7.3).

EKG gated helical CT has been explored as a method of decreasing the motion artefacts adjacent to the heart (43). Gating appears to improve lower lobe vessel depiction by decreasing cardiac motion, but there are several drawbacks to this technique, such as the increased complexity of the study, the doubling or tripling of the acquisition time and the frequent need for premedication to diminish the cardiac rate. The advantages of prospective or retrospective gating have yet to be proven for CTPA.

Multiplanar reconstruction

The value of multiplanar reconstructions in the diagnosis of pulmonary embolism is controversial – some use it routinely, others seldom use it (44). As temporal and spatial resolution has improved, the quality of both the axial and multiplanar reconstructions has improved dramatically. The use of raw data images (often 0.625 mm), rather than the final images (often 1.25 or 2.5 mm), provide optimal multiplanar images. Multiplanar images can now be rapidly reconstructed at the technologist's console or many PACS systems are capable of rapid reconstruction at the reading station. If the reconstructions are performed routinely by the technologist and sent with the axial images, they will be used considerably more frequently, than if one has to stop interpretation and reconstruct the images. They help in a minority of cases when the axial images are equivocal, when distinguishing between clot and adjacent soft tissue, when vessel bifurcations are problematic, assessing artefacts and when chronic pulmonary emboli are being sought.

Computer-assisted diagnosis

As the number of CTPA investigations being performed increases and the number of images per case increases (the term 'information overload' has been suggested), computer-assisted diagnosis (CAD) of PE becomes attractive to the (busy) radiologist. There are several small feasibility studies in the literature suggesting the software may in fact be helpful. Buhmann *et al.* showed the sensitivity of CAD for central vessels to be 74% vs 97% for the reader. Sensitivity for peripheral vessels was 82% vs 70% for the reader (45). There were approximately four false positives per patient. They did find that when CAD was used as a 'second reader', there was a 26% increase in diagnosis, predominantly in the peripheral vessels. There was no outside measure of 'truth'. Two recent studies, using similar software but different research protocols, reached conflicting conclusions (46,47). This will undoubtedly be an area of fruitful research.

CT perfusion scanning

CT perfusion scanning (although this term is somewhat misleading – it is actually a demonstration of moving blood volume – and should not be confused with true assessment of lung perfusion) has been under investigation for several years as a research tool and an adjunct to the CTPA. Most previous work has been limited by the need to scan the patient twice, either with a preliminary non-contrast CT or the use of delayed images (46,48). The latest generation of scanners, whether dual- or single-headed, have the possibility to provide dual energy acquisition and subtraction. As the K-edge of iodine is closer to the lower kVp, it may be possible to detect true lung perfusion in the same pass as the CTPA. This should improve the sensitivity of CTPA and perhaps will improve reading speed, and can help quantify the obstruction of the pulmonary vasculature to determine more or less aggressive treatment strategies.

DIAGNOSTIC CRITERIA

The diagnostic criteria for acute and chronic pulmonary embolism have been well worked out and standardized over the last decade (49).

Acute PE

1. Arterial occlusion – failure to opacify the entire lumen due to central filling defect. The artery may enlarge or develop indistinct margins (Figure 7.4a).

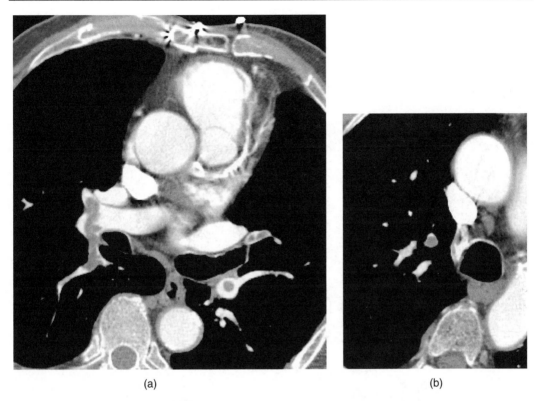

(a)   (b)

Figure 7.4   Acute pulmonary emboli. (a) There is a central clot in the left lower lobe pulmonary artery with a rim of contrast around it. The vessel is imaged perpendicular to the lung axis. The truncus inferior, on the right, has a clot filling the lumen and is visualized parallel to the lung axis. (b) Clot completely fills and expands the vessel in an image perpendicular to the vessel.

2. Partial filling defects surrounded by contrast in the cross-sectional imaging or 'railroad tracking' in the longitudinal image (Figure 7.4b).
3. Peripheral intraluminal defect making an acute angle with the arterial wall.

Chronic PE

1. Complete occlusion but the vessel is smaller than its peers or adjacent bronchus.
2. Eccentric or crescentic thickening of the vessel wall, forming an obtuse angle or thick-walled vessel with central contrast flow (recanalization) (Figure 7.5a). Multiplanar reconstructions often help visualize extent (Figure 7.5b).
3. Web or flap within the contrast-filled artery.
4. Calcification within the pulmonary artery lumen.
5. Secondary signs: extensive bronchial collateral circulation or mosaic lung perfusion seen on lung windows (Figure 7.5c).

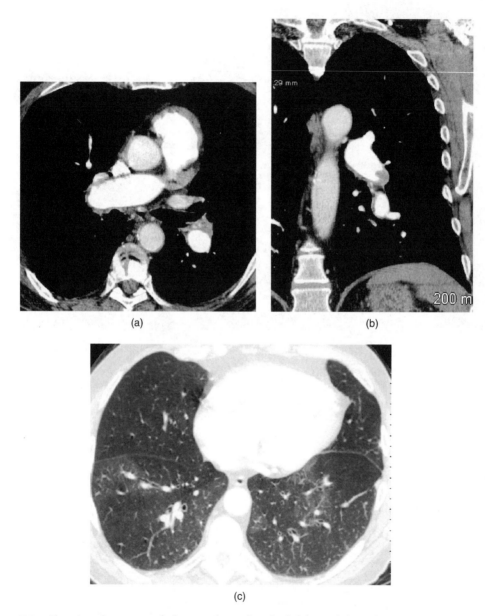

(a)

(b)

(c)

Figure 7.5 Chronic pulmonary embolus. (a) The wall to the left lower lobe pulmonary artery is questionably thickened. There is also some density laterally that may be a node or a thick wall. The posterior wall of the right pulmonary artery is also questionably thickened. (b) Coronal reconstruction shows thickening along the medial wall of the left main and left lower pulmonary artery. There is also a larger intramural clot that also appeared chronic. The right main pulmonary artery is also slightly thickened (not shown). (c) Lung windows show a severe mosaic perfusion pattern. Vessels in the lower attenuation areas are small, whereas the vessels in the higher attenuation areas are large.

Avoiding pitfalls

With faster scans, thinner sections, multiplanar reconstructions and interactive digital viewing, images are now easier to read. Nonetheless, there are still pitfalls to be avoided (49).

1. Clots are usually several centimetres long – a PE is not likely to be 1.25 mm long. We do not tend to diagnose PE based on a single filling defect in one image.
2. Respiratory motion can often simulate a filling defect. These defects are often bilateral or in multiple vessels on the same slice and lung windows reveal marked respiratory motion (Figure 7.3). A 50–75 mL re-injection focused on the area of motion is often helpful, or repeating the study later, after the patient has been stabilized and is better able to cooperate, may be necessary.
3. Vessel bifurcations occasionally simulate a filling defect. Sagittal and coronal reconstructions are extremely helpful in such situations and should clarify the matter. Unenhanced veins can be identified on serial images or lung windows.
4. Very dense arterial opacification may obscure a small intraluminal clot. A wide window of 700–1000 HU will uncover the thrombus.
5. In patients with emphysema, fibrosis or distortion of the lung parenchyma due to other lung diseases, the peripheral vessels often just fade out and cannot be properly evaluated. This should not be confused with peripheral pulmonary emboli.
6. If the contrast in the main pulmonary arteries is less than 250 HU, one may not be able to confidently rule out peripheral pulmonary emboli. A reinjection and local scanning may resolve the issue.
7. Mucous-filled bronchi can be distinguished on lung windows and should not be misinterpreted as pulmonary embolism.
8. Lymph nodes or mediastinal tissue may simulate vessel wall thickening (chronic PE). Coronal and sagittal reconstructions usually make differentiation possible (Figure 7.5a,b).

CT VENOGRAPHY

PIOPED II and other studies have shown that CT venography increases the likelihood of diagnosis of VTE by 7–26% when done in conjunction with CTPA (Figure 7.6) (13,16,50,51). A dissenting study by Perrier *et al.* showed little additional value of lower-extremity imaging with ultrasound after a CTPA (28). Furthermore, a recent study showed little benefit in evaluating the leg veins inmost patients being evaluated in an emergency room setting (26). The use and need for CTV remain, therefore, controversial, especially as the quality of CTPA improves and multiple outcome studies show a very low rate of subsequent PE after a negative CTPA alone. (CTV will be covered in greater depth in other sections.)

CT venography begins 3 minutes after CTPA and it provides a complete evaluation for venous thromboembolic disease in one test (11,13). At least 120 mL of iodinated contrast are required to ensure adequate contrast enhancement of the deep veins. A density of over 90 HU is ideal, 70–90 HU is passable and <70 HU is inadequate. The technique varies from institution to institution, but generally a low-dose technique to minimize gonadal radiation is preferred. (See the following section.)

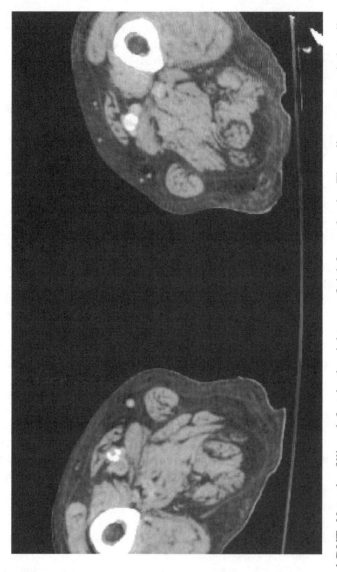

Figure 7.6 Isolated DVT. Note the filling defect in the right superficial femoral vein. The adjacent artery is heavily calcified. The vein is larger than the left superficial femoral vein. The pulmonary embolus study was negative.

RADIATION ISSUES

CT angiography

CTPA is now the most frequently used imaging examination for PE (52). Several recent articles have expressed concern about possible radiation-induced malignancies caused by CT (14,44,53–55). Although the science is imprecise, with much of the data extrapolated downwards from Hiroshima data, all agree that reducing exposure, especially in younger patients, is an important goal.

Dosage varies with the CT manufacturer, the age of the scanner, the number of detectors and the protocol used. PIOPED II estimated radiation dose using a four-slice scanner of 4 mSv for CTA, 6 mSv for the pelvis and 3 mSv for the thigh (unpublished data) (CTV utilized continuous helical scanning from the iliac crest to the knees). Of special concern is the dose to the breast in younger women. Hurwitz *et al.* (55), using a 64-slice scanner, and Parker *et al.* (56), using a four-slice scanner, estimated a breast dose of approximately 20 mSv or the equivalent of 15–20 mammogram studies. Hurwitz *et al.* estimated a breast dose of 18–32 mSv for EKG-gated coronary angiography. They estimated that the relative risk of breast cancer induction in girls and women varies from 1.042 to 1.004 for a single examination (55). For patients over the age of 55 years, the additional risk is negligible. However, in 15- and 25-year-old women, the additional risk estimate ranges from approximately 1.7 to 5.5%. Similar relative risks are given for the induction of lung cancer in both sexes. Multiple examinations cause cumulative risk. CTV delivers a high ovarian and testicular dose, of particular concern in patients of childbearing age. Below are some important strategies to reduce radiation from CT angiography and venography:

1. With the increasing popularity of CTPA, the percentage of PE-positive cases has diminished to <10% in many institutions (58). Better screening methods are required to determine who does not require imaging and to develop imaging strategies that produce lower radiation. Recent guidelines stress that pre-imaging screening using D-dimer and an objective clinical prediction tool (such as the Wells score, the Geneva score or the Pisa score) can safely eliminate the need for scanning in approximately 20–30% of outpatients and ER patients (31,44,57,59). Unfortunately, most physicians utilize an unstructured estimate (60). A patient with low or intermediate clinical probability and a negative D-dimer test does not require imaging. There is an approximately 0.5% likelihood of these patients developing a VTE in the following 3 months (28,29,57).
2. When imaging is required, a V/Q is usually definitive in patients with a normal chest X-ray and delivers approximately 90% less radiation (61). This is especially valuable in younger patients without lung disease. Lung scintigraphy may not be as readily available, especially on nights and weekends.
3. The most potent tool for reducing patient radiation from CTPA is real-time mA modulation, which alters mA based on the density of the part of the body being scanned. This is available on all modern scanners. Calculated dose length product for a single 170-pound patient scanned using a standard CTPA protocol on a 64-slice MDCT scanner was:
   (a) 717 mGy at fixed mA
   (b) 626 mGy with Z axis modulation
   (c) 587 mGy with XYZ modulation (Table 7.2). This corresponds to a 25% dose reduction.
4. As discussed earlier, a lower kVp decreases dosage while increasing vessel density (39,40).
5. When using Z-axis modulation, careful restriction of imaging to the required volume of inter-est (**chest only!**), excluding the lower neck and infradiaphragmatic areas, can result in an approximately 50% decrease in dosage (62).

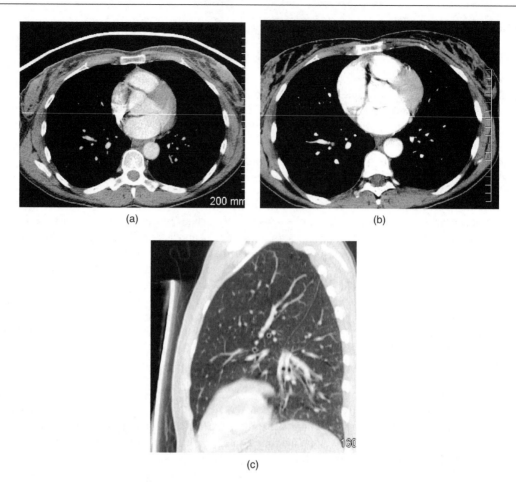

(a)   (b)

(c)

Figure 7.7   Breast shield. (a) CTA with breast shield in place. Note good-quality demonstration of lower lobe pulmonary arteries. There is minimal increased noise in the soft tissue of the breast. (b) CT done on the same patient, a year earlier, without breast shield, for comparison. (c) Sagittal reconstruction of the lung showing no perceptible difference in the image above and below the level of the breast shield.

6. Proper centring of the patient in the gantry isocentre results in an average dose saving of 15% (63).
7. Bismuth breast shields decrease breast dose by about 20% with no perceptible change in image quality (Figure 7.7) (64,65). Many centres now use these routinely in all women under 50 years of age.

CT venography

Radiation is, of course, a concern in the pelvis. PIOPED II data has suggested several strategies to diminish radiation from CTV.

1. In PIOPED II, isolated IVC and iliac clot were found in only 3% of patients, all of whom had visible PE (16). Kalva *et al.* found only two isolated DVTs in the pelvis in 2,074 (0.1%) of

Table 7.2 Differing radiation doses to a patient undergoing CT venography resulting from different scanning parameters[a]

Scanning parameter	Dose–length product (mSv)
Scan from iliac crest to knees[b]	
5 mm helical	
Fixed mA[c]	9.1
Automated mA	8.3
5 mm axial, 15 mm skip	
Fixed mA[d]	4.5
Automated mA	3.0
Scan from acetabulum to knees[e]	
5 mm helical	
Fixed mA[c]	7.4
Automated mA	6.3
5 mm axial, 15 mm skip	
Fixed mA[d]	3.3
Automated mA	2.0
Total reduction in radiation from 9.10 to 2.0 mSv	78%

[a]Calculations were made using a 64-MDCT scanner (LS-VCT, General Electric Healthcare) and 120 kVp was used for all examinations. The patient was a 5 ft 10 in (177.8 cm), 185 lb (83 kg) male.
[b]From low inferior vena cava to popliteal veins.
[c]180 mA, 0.984:1 pitch.
[d]180 mA.
[e]Femoral and popliteal veins.
Reproduced with permission from Goodman LR, Stein PD, Beemath A, Sostman HD, Wakefield TW, Woodard PK, Yankelevitz DF. CT venography: continuous helical images versus reformatted discontinuous images using PIOPED II data. AJR 2007; 189:409–412 (Table 7.5).

patients and in 2/121 (2%) of patients with DVT (66). Starting at the acetabulum, rather than at the iliac crest, reduces anatomic coverage by 40% with little loss of diagnostic information (16).
2. Likewise, 5 mm axial scans every 2 cm yield approximately equal diagnostic quality to continuous helical scanning and also diminishes radiation considerably (67). These two strategies combined reduce radiation by approximately 75%. CT venography and compression ultrasonography are diagnostically equivalent and the latter is preferable in patients of reproductive age or less (68). Thus, CTV should not be routinely performed in patients under the age of 40 years. (Lower-extremity ultrasonography and CT and MR venography are discussed in other sections.)

REMAINING CONTROVERSIES

Small pulmonary emboli/incidental pulmonary emboli

Concerning small pulmonary emboli, traditional teaching, based on several small studies in the 1960s, before there was adequate imaging for pulmonary emboli, suggested that the mortality rate of untreated PE was 30% or more (69). These were, of course, large emboli in order to be clinically detectable. With such a high perceived mortality rate, when heparin and warfarin became available they were rapidly embraced with essentially no controlled studies to show their benefits and risk/benefit ratio (70,71). Few studies have subsequently assessed the need for anticoagulant therapy due to the perceived high *a priori* risk to the patient. One randomized trial in patients with deep vein thrombosis suggested that inadequate early anticoagulation with heparin resulted in propagation of thrombus and also an increased recurrence rate over 6 months of follow-up (72). Hence it appears that a prothrombotic state persists in (at least some) patients.

Imaging studies such as V/Q, pulmonary angiography and CT have reduced estimated mortality rates to the 5–10% range, because they also diagnose small PE – which are less likely to be fatal (70,73–75). Also, large studies have shown that approximately 3–5% of patients who have routine contrast-enhanced chest CT have unsuspected pulmonary emboli that would have otherwise been missed (76,77). These patients would not have been anticoagulated if the CT had not been performed. PIOPD I, retrospectively, uncovered 20 patients with small, unreported PE, missed on initial reading. Only two (10%) returned with PE – one fatal (78). In a study of 90 moderate-to-severe trauma patients without symptoms of PE, scanned 3–7 days after admission, a CT showed 24% had PE, five at the segmental level or higher. None of the 17 subsegmental PE patients were treated and limited follow-up showed no evidence of subsequent PE (79).

Studies such as these have led to the questions, 'Do otherwise healthy patients who have an isolated small embolus need anticoagulation?' (Figure 7.8) (70,78,80,81) and 'What is the cost/benefit ratio of treating small PEs versus the mortality, morbidity and cost of anticoagulation?' (82,83).

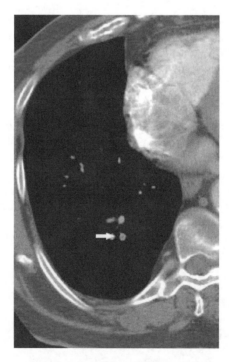

Figure 7.8 Incidental pulmonary embolus. Small but definite subsegmental embolus in the right lower lobe. This study was an unexpected finding in a healthy middle-aged patient.

Suboptimal CT

Most large studies report an incidence of 3–7% suboptimal studies (16,84). This has probably fallen with the use of higher-end equipment. Nonetheless, they do occur and one has to be prepared to deal with them. Some institutions will ensure that every CT is evaluated for the adequacy of the pulmonary embolus study before the patient leaves the CT table. If there is suboptimal opacification or motion in part of the study, this part may be re-imaged, using 50–75 mL of additional contrast and using adjusted bolus timing if necessary. If the suboptimal study is due to respiratory motion or perhaps due to some communication problem with the patient, a study may need to be repeated using new breathing instructions to ensure that the patient can follow them. If the patient cannot hold his/her breath, the study may be repeated the next day after the patient has been stabilized or after the patient has been intubated. If the initial CT shows the lung parenchyma is normal or near normal, a perfusion scan may be preferable to a second CTPA to reduce the radiation dose.

Eyer *et al.* found that in 9% of 1435 patients studied with an 8- or 16-slice scanner, the reader expressed some uncertainty about the peripheral pulmonary vessels, concluding that a 'small PE could not be excluded' (84). They identified 132 patients with inconclusive studies; three were treated presumptively for PE and 16 were already anticoagulated for other reasons. A total of 113 received no anticoagulation. Thirty-two of 132 (24.2%) had at least one other negative imaging study within 72 hours. Five patients returned within 3 months with signs or symptoms of PE. All had a negative work-up for recurrent PE. It is probable that small PEs were missed in a small percentage of these patients, but no PE symptoms recurred over the next 3 months to suggest a pulmonary embolus (84). More often than not, a suboptimal scan is not adequate to rule out small peripheral emboli, but does rule out lobar and segmental emboli. If the patient is of low or moderate clinical probability and has relatively good cardiopulmonary reserve, then a negative imaging study of the legs (CTV or ultrasound) may be all that is necessary to withhold coagulation confidently. Serial leg vein imaging may be a good alternative in such cases, using compression ultrasonography as a preferred method (41,80,81,85).

What is the gold standard for PE diagnosis?

Pulmonary angiography has long been the 'gold standard'. However, a closer look at pulmonary angiography shows some glaring deficiencies. Two angiographers will agree on the presence or absence of a pulmonary embolus in *only* 80 and 90% of patients (1,86). Quinn *et al.* showed that three angiographers will agree on the presence of subsegmental emboli in only 13% of cases (87). Thus, angiography has problems at the small vessel level, just as CT (or any other diagnostic test) has trouble at this level. Wittram *et al.* examined the 20 PIOPED II cases where CTPA and pulmonary angiography disagreed (88). A panel of experienced CT and angiogram readers determined that one patient had a false-positive finding at angiography, 13 had false-negative findings at angiography and two had false-negative findings at CTPA. In four cases, CTPA was thought to be true negative with a PE occurring in the time between the CT study and catheter angiography. Clinical outcome studies of CTPA show a 99% negative predictive value. Many experts now consider CTPA to be the new diagnostic reference standard for PE (23–25,44).

CONCLUSION

Over the last two decades, CTPA has evolved from a promising procedure to the procedure of choice for VTE diagnosis. With current technology, it has replaced invasive pulmonary angiography as the 'gold standard'. It provides reliable evidence of PE and the diagnoses of other pulmonary diseases in a significant minority of patients. Its popularity has led to overuse and strategies are being developed to triage patients better and diminish radiation dose.

REFERENCES

1. PIOPED Investigators. Value of the ventilation/perfusion scan in acute pulmonary embolism: results of the Prospective Investigation of Pulmonary Embolism Diagnosis (PIOPED). *JAMA* 1990; **263**:2753–59.
2. Turkstra F, Kuijer PMM, van Beek EJR, *et al*. Value of compression ultrasonography for the detection of deep venous thrombosis in patients suspected of having pulmonary embolism. *Ann Intern Med* 1997; **126**:775–81.
3. Teigen CL, Maus TP, Sheedy PF, *et al*. Pulmonary embolism: diagnosis with contrast-enhanced electron-beam CT and comparison with pulmonary angiography. *Radiology* 1995; **194**:313–9.
4. Remy-Jardin M, Remy J, Wattinne L, Giraud F. Central pulmonary thromboembolism: diagnosis with spiral volumetric CT with the single-breath-hold technique – comparison with pulmonary angiography. *Radiology* 1992; **185**:381–7.
5. Goodman LR, Curtin JJ, Mewissen MW, *et al*. Detection of pulmonary embolism in patients with unresolved clinical and scintigraphic diagnosis: helical CT versus angiography. *Am J Roentgenol* 1995; **164**:1369–74.
6. van Beek EJR, Brouwers EMJ, Bongaerts AH, Oudkerk M. Lung scintigraphy and helical computed tomography in the diagnosis of pulmonary embolism: a meta-analysis. *Clin Appl Thromb Hemost* 2001; **7**:87–92.
7. Goodman LR, Lipchik RJ. Diagnosis of acute pulmonary embolism: time for a new approach. *Radiology* 1996; **199**:25–7.
8. Gurney JW. No fooling around: direct visualization of pulmonary embolism. *Radiology*, 1993; **188**:618–9.
9. Van Rossum AB, Pattynama PM, Ton ER, *et al*. Pulmonary embolism: valudation of spiral CT angiography in 149 patients. *Radiology* 1996; **201**:467–70.
10. Loud PA, Grossman ZD, Klippenstein D, Ray CE. Combined CT venography and pulmonary angiography: a new diagnostic technique for suspected thromboembolic disease. *Am J Roentgenol*, 1998; **170**:951–4.
11. Loud PA, Klippenstein DL. Lower extremity deep venous thrombosis in cancer patients: correlation of presenting symptoms with venous sonographic findings. *J Ultrasound Med* 1998; **17**:693–696; quiz 697–8.
12. Ghaye B, Szapior D, Willems V, Dondelinger RF. Combined CT venography of the lower limbs and spiral CT angiography of pulmonary arteries in acute pulmonary embolism: preliminary results of a prospective study. *JBR-BTR* 2000; **83**:271–8.
13. Garg K, Mao J. Deep venous thrombosis: spectrum of findings and pitfalls in interpretation on CT venography. *Am J Roentgenol* 2001; **177**:319–23.
14. Brenner DJ, Hall EJ. Computed tomography – an increasing source of radiation exposure. *N Engl J Med* 2007; **357**:2277–84.
15. Wrixon AD. New recommendations from the International Commission on Radiological Protection – a review. *Phys Med Bull* 2008; **53**:R41–R60.
16. Stein PD, Fowler SE, Goodman LR, Gottschalk A, Hales CA, Hull RD. Multidetector computed tomography for acute pulmonary embolism. [PIOPED II]. *N Engl J Med* 2006; **354**:2317–27.
17. Qanadli SD, Hajjam ME, Mesurolle BB, *et al*. Pulmonary embolism detection: prospective evaluation of dual-section helical CT versus selective pulmonary arteriography in 157 patients. *Radiology* 2000; **217**:447–55.
18. Winer-Muram HT, Rydberg J, Johnson MS, *et al*. Suspected acute pulmonary embolism: evaluation with multi-detector row CT versus digital subtraction pulmonary arteriography. *Radiology* 2004; **233**:806–15.
19. Revel MP, Petrover D Hernigou A, Lefort C, Meyer G, Frija G. Diagnosing Pulmonary embolism with four-detector row helical CT: prospective evaluation of 216 outpatients and inpatients. *Radiology* 2005; **234**:265–73.
20. Blachere H, Latrabe V, Montaudon M, *et al*. Pulmonary embolism revealed on helical CT angiography: comparison with ventilation–perfusion radionuclide lung scanning. *Am J Roentgenol* 2000; **174**:1041–7.

21. Perrier A, Jowarth N, Didier D, *et al*. Performance of helical computed tomography in unselected outpatients with suspected pulmonary embolism. *Ann Intern Med* 2001; **135**:88–97.
22. Rufener SL, Patel S, Kazerooni EA, Schipper M, Kelly AM. Comparison of on-call radiology resident and faculty interpretation of 4- and 16-row multidetector CT pulmonary angiography with indirect CT venography. *Acad Radiol* 2008; **15**:71–6.
23. Quiroz R, Kucher N, Zou KH, *et al*. Clinical validity of a negative computed tomography scan in patients with suspected pulmonary embolism: a systematic review. *JAMA* 2005; **293**:2012–7.
24. Moores LK, Jackson WL, Shorr AF, Jackson JL. Meta-analysis: outcomes in patients with suspected pulmonary embolism managed with computed tomographic pulmonary angiography. *Ann Intern Med* 2004; **141**:866–74.
25. Goodman LR, Lipchik RJ, Kuzo RS, Liu Y, Mcauliffe TL, O'Brien DJ. Subsequent pulmonary embolism: risk after a negative helical CT pulmonary angiogram – prospective comparison with scintigraphy. *Radiology* 2000; **215**:535–42.
26. Righini M, Le Gal G, Aujesky D, *et al*. Diagnosis of pulmonary embolism by multidetector CT alone or combined with venous ultrasonography of the leg: a randomized non-inferiority trial. *Lancet* 2008; **371**:1343–52.
27. Stein PD. Outcome studies of pulmonary embolism versus accuracy. In *Pulmonary Embolism*, 2nd edn. Blackwell Futura, Malden, MA, 2007, Chapter 78.
28. Perrier A, Roy PM, Sanchez O, *et al*. Multidetector-row computed tomography in suspected pulmonary embolism. *N Engl J Med* 2005; **352**:1760–8.
29. Writing Group for the Christopher Study. Effectiveness of managing suspected pulmonary embolism using an algorithm combining clinical probability, D-dimer testing and computed tomography. *JAMA* 2006; **295**:172–9.
30. Van Beek EJR, Brouwers E, Song B, Stein PD, Oudkerk M. Clinical validity of a normal pulmonary angiogram in patients with suspected pulmonary embolism – a critical review. *Clin Radiol* 2001; **56**:838–42.
31. Anderson DR, Kahn SR, Rodger MA, *et al*. Computed tomographic pulmonary angiography vs ventilation–perfusion lung scanning in patients with suspected pulmonary embolism. A randomized controlled trial. *JAMA* 2007; **298**:2743–53.
32. Van Rossum AB, Treurniet FE, Kieft GH, Smith SJ, Schepers-Bok R. Role of spiral volumetric computed tomographic scanning in the assessment of patients with clinical suspicion of pulmonary embolism and an abnormal ventilation/perfusion lung scan. *Thorax* 1996; **51**:23–8.
33. Richman PB, Courtney M, Friese JJ, Field A, Petri R, Kline JA. Prevalence and significance of nonthromboembolic findings on chest computed tomography angiography performed to rule out pulmonary embolism: a multicenter study of 1,025 emergency department patients. *Acad Emerg Med* 2004; **11**:642–7.
34. Patel S, Kazerooni EA, Cascade PN. Pulmonary embolism: optimization of small pulmonary artery visualization at multi-detector row CT. *Radiology* 2003; **227**:455–60.
35. Ghaye B, Szapiro D, Mastora I, *et al*. Peripheral pulmonary arteries: how far in the lung does multi-detector row spiral CT allow analysis? *Radiology* 2001; **219**:629–36.
36. Schoepf UJ, Holzknecht N, Helmberger TK, *et al*. Subsegmental pulmonary emboli: improved detection with thin-collimation multi-detector row spiral CT. *Radiology* 2002; **222**:483–90.
37. Hopper KD, Mosher TJ, Kasales CJ, *et al*. Thoracic spiral CT: delivery of contrast material pushed with injectable saline solution in a power injector. *Radiology* 1997; **205**:269–71.
38. Bae KT, Tao C, Gürel S, *et al*. Effect of patient weight and scanning duration on contrast enhancement during pulmonary multidetector CT angiography. *Radiology* 2007; **242**:582–9.
39. Schueller-Weidekamm C, Schaefer-Prokop CM, Weber M, *et al*. CT Angiography of pulmonary arteries to detect pulmonary embolism: improvement of vascular enhancement with low kilovoltage settings. *Radiology* 2006; **241**:899–907.
40. Heyer CM, Mohr PS, Lemburg SP, *et al*. Image quality and radiation exposure at pulmonary CT angiography with 100- or 120-kVp protocol: prospective randomized study. *Radiology* 2007; **245**:577–83.
41. Jones SE, Wittram C. The indeterminate CT pulmonary angiogram: imaging characteristics and patient clinical outcome. *Radiology* 2005; **237**:329–37.
42. Bruzzi JF, Remy-Jardin M, Kirsch J, *et al*. Sixteen-slice multidetector computed tomography pulmonary angiography: evaluation of cardiogenic motion artifacts and influence of rotation time on image quality. *J Comput Assist Tomogr* 2005; **29**:805–14.
43. D'Agostino AG, Remy-Jardin M, Khalil C, *et al*. Low-dose ECG-gated 64-slices helical CT angiography of the chest: evaluation of image quality in 105 patients. *Eur Radiol* 2006; **16**:2137–46.

44. Remy-Jardin M, Pistolesi M, Goodman LR, *et al*. Management of suspected acute pulmonary embolism in the era of CT angiography: a statement from the Fleischner Society. *Radiology* 2007; **245**:315–29.

45. Buhmann S, Herzog P, Liang J, *et al*. Clinical evaluation of a computer-aided diagnosis (CAD) prototype for the detection of pulmonary embolism. *Acad Radiol* 2007; **14**:651–8.

46. Schoepf UJ, Schneider A, Das M, Wood S, Cheema JI, Costello P. Pulmonary embolism: computer-aided detection at multidetector row spiral computed tomography. *J Thorac Imag* 2007; **22**:319–23.

47. Maizlin ZV, Vos PM, Godoy MB, Cooperberg PL. Computer-aided detection of pulmonary embolism on CT angiography: initial experience. *J Thorac Imag* 2007; **22**:324–9.

48. Suga K, Kawakami Y, Iwanaga H, *et al*. Automated breath-hold perfusion SPECT/CT fusion images of the lungs. *Am J Roentgenol* 2007; **189**:455–63.

49. Washington L, Goodman LR, Gonyo MB. CT for thromboembolic disease. *Radiol Clin North Am* 2002; **40**:751–71.

50. Ghaye B, Mchimi A, Noukoua CT, Dondelinger RF. Does multi-detector row CT pulmonary angiography reduce the incremental value of indirect CT venography compared with single-detector row CT pulmonary angiography? *Radiology* 2006; **240**:256–62.

51. Katz DS, Loud PA, Bruce D, *et al*. Combined CT venography and pulmonary angiography: a comprehensive review. *Radiographics* 2002; **22**:S3–19; discussion S20–24.

52. Stein PD, Kayali F, Olson RE. Trends in the use of diagnostic imaging in patients hospitalized with acute pulmonary embolism. *Am J Cardiol* 2004; **93**:1316–7.

53. Einstein AJ, Henzlova MJ, Rajagopalan S. Estimating risk of cancer associated with radiation exposure from 64-slice computed tomography coronary angiography. *JAMA* 2007; **298**:317–23.

54. Mayo JR, Aldrich J, Muller NL. Radiation exposure at chest CT: a statement of the Fleischner Society. *Radiology* 2003; **228**:15–21.

55. Hurwitz LM, Reiman RE, Yoshizumi TT, *et al*. Radiation dose from contemporary cardiothoracic multidetector CT protocols with an anthropomorphic female phantom: implications for cancer induction. *Radiology* 2007; **245**:742–50.

56. Parker MS, Hui FK, Camacho MA, *et al*. Female breast radiation exposure during CT pulmonary angiography. *Am J Roentgenol* 2005; **185**:1228–33.

57. Stein PD, Woodard PK, Weg JG, *et al*. Diagnostic pathways in acute pulmonary embolism: recommendations of the PIOPED II investigators. *Radiology* 2007; **242**:15–21.

58. Prologo JD, Gilkeson RC, Diaz M, Asaad J. CT pulmonary angiography: a comparative analysis of utilization patterns in emergency department and hospitalized patients between 1998 and 2003. *Am J Roentgenol* 2004; **183**:1093–6.

59. Wells PS, Anderson DR, Rodger M, *et al*. Excluding pulmonary embolism at the bedside without diagnostic imaging: management of patients with suspected pulmonary embolism presenting to the emergency department by using a simple clinical model and d-dimer. *Ann Intern Med* 2001; **135**:98–107.

60. Weiss CR, Haponik EF, Diette GB, *et al*. Pretest risk assessment in suspected acute pulmonary embolism. *Acad Radiol* 2008; **15**:3–14.

61. Forbes KP, Reid JH, Murchison JT. Do preliminary chest X-ray findings define the optimum role of pulmonary scintigraphy in suspected pulmonary embolism? *Clin Radiol* 2001; **56**:397–400.

62. Campbell J, Kalra MK, Rizzo S, Maher MM, Shepard JA. Scanning beyond anatomic limits of the thorax in chest CT: findings, radiation dose and automatic tube current modulation. *Am J Roentgenol* 2005; **185**:1525–30.

63. Li J, Udayasankar UK, Toth TL, Seamans J, Small WC, Kalra MK. Automatic patient centering for MDCT: effect on radiation dose. *Am J Roentgenol* 2007; **188**:547–52.

64. Hopper KD, King SH, Lobell ME, TenHave TR, Weaver JS. The breast: in-plane X-ray protection during diagnostic thoracic CT – shielding with bismuth radioprotective garments. *Radiology* 1997; **205**:853–8.

65. Yilmaz MH, Albayram S, Yasar D, *et al*. Female breast radiation exposure during thorax multidetector computed tomography and the effectiveness of bismuth breast shield to reduce breast radiation dose. *J Comput Assist Tomogr* 2007; **31**:138–42.

66. Kalva SP, Jagannathan JP, Hahn PF, Wicky ST. Venous thromboembolism: indirect CT venography during CT pulmonary angiography – should the pelvis be imaged? *Radiology* 2008; **246**:605–11.

67. Goodman LR, Stein PD, Beemath A, *et al*. CT venography: continuous helical images versus reformatted discontinuous images using PIOPED II data. *Am J Roentgenol* 2007; **189**:1–7.

68. Goodman LR, Stein PD, Matta F, *et al*. CT venography and compression sonography are diagnostically equivalent: data from PIOPED II. *Am J Roentgenol* 2007; **189**:1071–6.

69. Barrit DW, Jordan SC. Anticoagulant drugs in the treatment of pulmonary embolism. A controlled study. *Lancet* 1960; **i**:1309–12.

70. Goodman LR. *Small pulmonary emboli: what do we know? Radiology* 2005; **234**:654–658.

71. Padove SJ, Dalen JE. Does anticoagulant therapy reduce mortality of acute pulmonary embolism? *Arch Intern Med* 2002; **162**:720.
72. Brandjes DP, Heijboer H, Buller HR, de Rijk M, Jagt H, ten Cate JW. Acenocoumarol and heparin compared with acenocoumarol alone in the initial treatment of proximal-vein thrombosis. *N Engl J Med* 1992; **327**:1485–9.
73. Dalen JE, Alpert JS. Natural history of pulmonary embolism. *Progr Cardiovasc Dis* 1975; **17**:259–70.
74. Le Gal G, Righini M, Roy PM, *et al.* Prediction of pulmonary embolism in the emergency department: the revised Geneva Score. *Ann Intern Med* 2006; **144**:165–71.
75. Glassroth J. Imaging of pulmonary embolism: too much of a good thing? *JAMA* 2007; **298**:2788–9.
76. Verschakelen JA, Vanwijck E, Bogaert J, Baert AL. Detection of unsuspected central pulmonary embolism with conventional contrast-enhanced CT. *Radiology* 1993; **188**:847–50.
77. Storto ML, Di Credico A, Guido F, Larici AR, Bonomo L. Incidental detection of pulmonary emboli on routine MDCT of the chest. *Am J Roentgenol* 2005; **184**:264–7.
78. Stein PD, Henry JW, Relya B. Untreated patients with pulmonary embolism. *Chest* 1995; **107**:931–5.
79. Schultz DJ, Brasel KJ, Washington L, *et al.* Incidence of asymptomatic pulmonary embolism in moderately to severely injured trauma patients. *J Trauma* 2004; **56**:727–31.
80. Hull RD, Raskob GE, Ginsberg JS, *et al.* A noninvasive strategy for the treatment of patients with suspected pulmonary embolism. *Arch Intern Med* 1994; **154**:289–97.
81. Stein PD, Hull RD, Raskob GE. Withholding treatment in patients with acute pulmonary embolism who have a high risk of bleeding and negative serial noninvasive leg tests. *Am J Med* 2000; **109**:301–06.
82. Van der Meer FJM, Rosendaal FR, Vandenbroucke JP, Briët E. Bleeding complications in oral anticoagulant therapy. An analysis of risk factors. *Arch Intern Med* 1993; **153**:1557–62.
83. Levine MN, Raskob G, Landefeld S, Hirsh J. Hemorrhagic complications of anticoagulant treatment. *Chest* 1995; **108**(Suppl 4): 276S–290S.
84. Eyer BA, Goodman LR, Washington L. Clinicians' response to radiologists' reports of isolated subsegmental pulmonary embolism or inconclusive interpretation of pulmonary embolism using MDCT. *Am J Roentgenol* 2005; **184**:623–8.
85. Hull RD, Pineo GF, Raskob GE. A noninvasive approach for the treatment of patients with suspected pulmonary embolism. *J Thromb Thrombolysis* 1996; **3**:5–8.
86. Van Beek EJ, Bakker AJ, Reekers JA. Pulmonary embolism: interobserver agreement in the interpretation of conventional angiographic and DSA images in patients with non-diagnostic lung scan results. *Radiology* 1996; **198**:721–4.
87. Quinn MF, Lundell CJ, Klotz TA, *et al.* Reliability of selective pulmonary arteriography in the diagnosis of pulmonary embolism. *Am J Roentgenol* 1987; **149**:469–71.
88. Wittram C, Waltman AC, Shepard JA, *et al.* Discordance between CT and angiography in the PIOPED II study. *Radiology* 2007; **244**:883–9.
89. Schaefer-Prokop C, Prokop M. MDCT for the diagnosis of acute pulmonary embolism. *Eur Radiol* 2005; **15**(Suppl 4): D37–D41.

CHAPTER 8

Lung Scintigraphy

Jane A.E. Dutton[1]**, Heok K. Cheow**[2] **and A. Michael Peters**[2]

[1]Department of Nuclear Medicine, Addenbrooke's Hospital,
Cambridge, UK
[2]Department of Nuclear Medicine, Royal Sussex County Hospital,
Brighton, UK

INTRODUCTION

In comparison with other imaging modalities for pulmonary embolism (PE), lung scintigraphy has been around for a very long time. Ventilation imaging arrived first in 1955 (1) with the inhalation of radioactive Xe-133 gas, but it was a further 10 years before regional pulmonary blood flow was assessed with radioactive agents (2). Except for a few small refinements, including the choice of radioactive agents employed, the techniques for assessment of lung ventilation (V) and perfusion (Q) remain essentially unchanged to this day. Lung scintigraphy, however, continues to hold a pivotal role in the diagnosis of pulmonary embolism in many hospitals.

Scintigraphy for suspected PE involves simultaneous imaging of the distributions of pulmonary blood flow and alveolar ventilation, so-called ventilation/perfusion (V/Q) scintigraphy. The principle underlying the diagnosis of pulmonary vascular disease, which is most commonly due to PE, is that, whereas pulmonary perfusion is abnormal, the pulmonary parenchyma usually remains intact as a result of its bronchial blood supply and ventilation remains normal. This gives rise to the so-called mismatched perfusion defect, the hallmark of pulmonary embolic disease (Figure 8.1). V/Q scintigraphy is not only used in the diagnosis of PE, but is also employed to diagnose and quantify derangement of cardiopulmonary haemodynamics in other entities, such as congenital disorders of the lung, lung volume reduction surgery in patients with chronic obstructive lung disease (Figure 8.2) (where quantification of lung function may predict postoperative lung reserve) and to stratify the degree of alveolar damage in pneumonitis (3).

A different approach to imaging thromboembolism is to target it with radiolabelled components of the clotting system, such as platelets (4), fibrinogen (5), monoclonal antibodies to platelets or fibrinogen (6,7), fragments of fibrin which re-combine with pre-formed fibrin but not fibrinogen and peptides which bind to activated fibrinogen receptors on platelets (8,9). These agents, however, have not found a place in routine imaging and will not be discussed further.

Deep Vein Thrombosis and Pulmonary Embolism   Edited by Edwin J.R. van Beek, Harry R. Büller and Matthijs Oudkerk
© 2009 John Wiley & Sons, Ltd

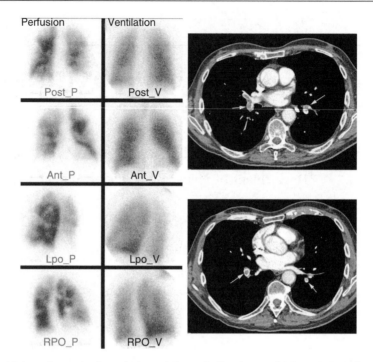

Figure 8.1 Multiple mismatched perfusion defects indicating a high scintigraphic probability of pulmonary embolism. The ventilation images were obtained with Kr-81m. CT PA confirmed multiple emboli, visible in the pulmonary arteries (arrows).

Despite developments in other imaging techniques, V/Q imaging underpins the routine assessment of patients with suspected PE, and its position in the diagnostic pathway for patients with suspected PE is discussed in a later chapter. It is worthwhile at this stage, however, to point out that as a result of the evolution of multidetector computed tomography (MDCT) and the improvements in intravenous contrast medium enhancement by bolus tracking software, CT pulmonary angiography (CT PA) has largely replaced not only conventional pulmonary angiography but also, to a certain extent, V/Q scintigraphy. Despite the inconclusive results that may arise from a CT PA study, owing for instance to suboptimal contrast bolus, respiratory motion or other artefact, a recent survey in the USA found that 87% of clinicians believed that CT PA is the most useful modality for patients with suspected PE (10). The absorbed radiation dose attributable to CT pulmonary angiography (CTPA) is 8 mSv. This is equivalent to 400 chest radiographs (11), which is substantially more than a V/Q scan which gives a dose of approximately 1.5 mSv. When choosing which of these tests to use, the benefit of a higher diagnostic yield from CT must be balanced against the increased radiation burden. This is particularly true in young (female) patients, who are likely to live long enough to be fully exposed to the radiation risk.

IMAGING REGIONAL PULMONARY BLOOD FLOW – THE Q SCAN

Perfusion lung imaging is based on the trapping of a radiotracer in the lungs after intravenous injection and passage through the right side of the heart. There are two available classes of tracer: particles and inert gases. The latter rely on their ability to diffuse rapidly into alveolar gas after intravenous injection in aqueous solution. The inert gases are essentially obsolete for clinical

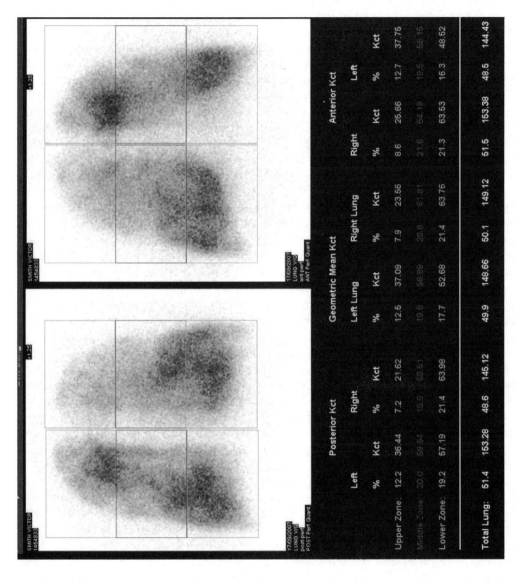

	Posterior Kct				Geometric Mean Kct				Anterior Kct			
	Left		Right		Left Lung		Right Lung		Right		Left	
	%	Kct	%	Kct	%	Kct	%	Kct	%	Kct	%	Kct
Upper Zone:	12.2	36.44	7.2	21.62	12.5	37.09	7.9	23.56	8.6	25.66	12.7	37.75
Middle Zone:	20.0	69.64	19.9	59.51	19.8	58.89	20.8	61.81	21.6	64.19	19.5	58.15
Lower Zone:	19.2	57.19	21.4	63.98	17.7	52.68	21.4	63.76	21.3	63.53	16.3	48.52
Total Lung:	51.4	153.28	48.6	145.12	49.9	148.66	50.1	149.12	51.5	153.38	48.5	144.43

Figure 8.2 Quantification of lung perfusion in a patient with severe emphysema, performed with Tc-99m MAA prior to lung volume reduction surgery.

work but still have a role in clinical research. The workhorse of clinical lung perfusion imaging is microparticulate human protein labelled with technetium-99 m (Tc-99 m). After intravenous injection, the particles microembolize in the lung vascular bed in a distribution representative of regional pulmonary blood flow.

Particles of macroaggregated human serum albumin (MAA), with a size range of 10–100 nm, are routinely used for the clinical diagnosis of PE. For patients with a right-to-left shunt, there is a theoretical (negligible) risk of systemic tissue ischaemia as a result of vessel occlusion from shunted particles at the upper end of the size range (12). Similarly, in patients with pulmonary hypertension, there is a risk of further occlusion of an already compromised vascular bed. However, the safety margin is huge since the pulmonary vascular bed is effectively an open meshwork of intercommunicating capillaries, the number of which is of the order of 10^{12} in normal subjects and far exceeds the number of particles administered (200 000–500 000), even in pulmonary vascular disease. The occlusion is temporary as the particles are biodegradable and have a biological half-time in the lung of 6–8 hours. Pertechnetate elutes from the particles faster and by 24 hours most of the remaining activity is visible in the gut and kidneys. Provided that the particles mix completely in the blood prior to microembolization, the distribution of radioactivity is proportional to the distribution of pulmonary blood flow. Not only is photon emission itself a random event, but so is particle distribution. A distribution of radioactivity which is proportional to the distribution of pulmonary blood flow is, therefore, also dependent on the injection of a sufficiently large number of particles (>60 000) in addition to the amount of injected radioactivity (13). In some situations, principally the pregnant patient with suspected PE, practitioners may choose to perform a perfusion scan only, using a reduced dose of radioactivity, as opposed to a routine full V/Q scan. The benefit of this choice is the reduced radiation dose to the uterus/foetus. One of the potential pitfalls of this approach, however, is that the reduced number of particles may result in inhomogeneous images owing to poor count statistics, potentially rendering the study uninterpretable. The Tc-99 m MAA given should preferably be freshly dispensed, since this will increase the proportion of radioactivity successfully bound to MAA. This 'cut-corner' imaging should be reserved for young patients (pregnant women are likely to be in a young age group) and in those without a past history of lung disease. A normal Q scan excludes PE (as discussed later in this chapter), but an abnormal study requires further investigation. This may take the form of repeating the low-dose MAA study on the following day and additionally performing a ventilation scan. The total dose associated with this imaging strategy is then equal to having performed a complete V/Q scan initially and there will have been a slight delay in diagnosis. In some institutions a low-dose MAA scan is performed initially and then followed only with a ventilation study on the next day. This imaging protocol assumes that perfusion in the lungs remains the same from the initial day to the next. This concept will be discussed later.

A Tc-99 m lung perfusion study gives an effective dose of 1 mSv for the standard 100 MBq of activity injected in adults (14). The quantity of injected radioactivity is proportionally reduced in children (15). The MAA particles should be injected while the patient performs a series of deep inspirations in order to promote a more homogeneous distribution of pulmonary blood flow. Since the material readily adheres to foreign surfaces, injection through central venous lines should be avoided (Figure 8.3) as a considerable fraction is likely to be retained. Injection through a butterfly is acceptable, especially in children, although up to one-third of the activity may be retained, even if the line is flushed with saline following the injection. Withdrawal of blood into the syringe prior to injection promotes clumping of the particles and should be avoided. If this happens, then the resulting images may show inhomogeneous radioactivity in the lungs. Because the pressure in the pulmonary circulation is low, the distribution of pulmonary blood flow is influenced by gravity (16). In the erect position, mean apical alveolar pressure exceeds both pulmonary arterial and venous pressures and there is very little apical flow (16). In the mid-zones, blood flow is

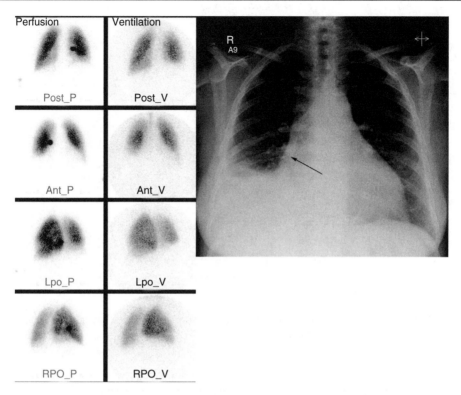

Figure 8.3   Tc-99m MAA was administrated via a left peripherally inserted central catheter (PICC) (arrow). A 'hot spot' from clumped MAA is seen at the tip of the catheter. It is not seen on the ventilation images because they are acquired using the higher energy window required for Kr-81m.

determined by the arterio-alveolar pressure gradient and in the lower zones by the arterio-venous gradient. This explains why the patient should be injected in the supine position, promoting blood flow to the apices, which would be poorly visualized if the patient was injected in the erect position. Normally, more than 95% of the administered Tc-99 m is trapped in the lungs (17), the majority of non-trapped radioactivity being probably unbound Tc-99 m, which may give rise to faint thyroid and gastric activity (Figure 8.4). Free Tc-99 m is excreted in the urine and taken up by the renal parenchyma, and, if present in significant amounts (usually as a result of poor labelling of the protein), also gives images of the kidneys (Figure 8.5). This, however, can be distinguished from anatomical right-to-left shunting of the particles (Figure 8.6) by the absence of splenic and cerebral activity (17).

VENTILATION IMAGING

There is a choice of agents for lung ventilation scintigraphy: either they are radioactive aerosols or radioactive inert gases.

The most commonly used aerosol tracer is Tc-99 m-DTPA (diethylenetriaminepentaacetic acid). This is a low-cost, easily manufactured and readily available substance. In healthy cigarette smokers, the alveolar-to-blood transfer rate (or clearance rate) is 3–4 times faster than in non-smokers (18–20). This may result in a significant loss of counts in the lungs before completion of ventilation imaging, giving rise to poor count statistics. Interestingly, this increased clearance seen in smokers

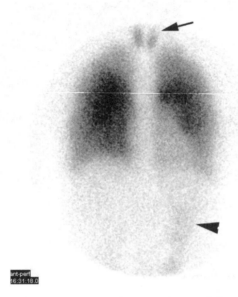

Figure 8.4   Poor labelling of Tc-99m MAA, with accumulation of dissociated pertechnetate visible in the thyroid gland (arrow) and stomach (arrowhead).

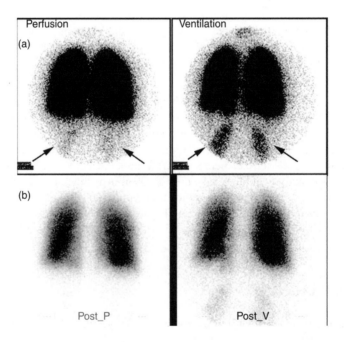

Figure 8.5   Renal parenchymal tracer accumulation (arrows) is noted on the Tc-99m DTPA aerosol ventilation images as a result of unstable labelling. On the perfusion image, renal activity is only visible when the intensity of the grey scale is increased to near maximum (A) but not on the routine viewing scale (B).

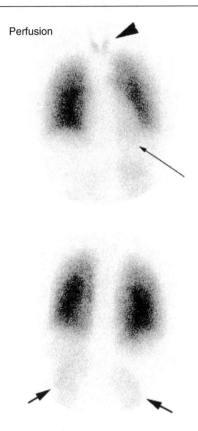

Figure 8.6 Images obtained after intravenous injection of Tc-99m-MAA in a patient with a pulmonary arterio-venous malformation showing first-pass renal (arrow), spleen (long arrow) and thyroid (arrowhead) tracer retention.

is not related to the length of time smoked but to their blood carboxyhaemoglobin concentration (18), which depends on the number of cigarettes smoked in the previous few days. Technegas is another commonly used agent. This is a technetium-labelled carbon particle of extremely small size, suitable for inhalation. Like Tc-99 m-DTPA aerosol, it is cheap and readily available but has a much lower gas-to-blood transfer rate, even in smokers. Another agent with a slow gas-blood transfer rate is Tc-99 m-MIBI (methoxyisobutylisonitrile), which has recently been shown to have a transfer rate even slower in smokers than non-smokers (21). This latter agent has not yet been adopted in clinical practice.

The other group of ventilation agents includes the radioactive inert gases Kr-81m, Xe-133 and Xe-127. Kr-81m has an ultra-short half-life of 13 seconds and is the optimum ventilation imaging agent. Continuous inhalation of Kr-81m produces a constant regional count rate, reflecting the distribution of ventilation, when dynamic equilibrium is achieved, very rapidly, between inhalation and physical decay (with a small contribution from exhalation). Dynamic equilibrium is also achieved with Xe-133, but this is much slower because there is no contribution from physical decay (half-life 5.2 days) and therefore equilibration is between inhalation and exhalation and reflects regional lung volume.

A digression into the physical/mathematical relationship between lung ventilation (V), regional lung volume (ϖ), radioactive physical decay constant (δ) and alveolar (C_a) and inspired (C_i) concentrations of gas helps explain the different imaging properties of Xe-133 (long half-life, low δ) and Kr-81m (ultra-short half-life, high δ):

$$C_i V = C_a V (V/\varpi + \delta) \qquad (8.1)$$

The recorded count rate is proportional to ϖC_a, the quantity of gas in the lung region. Rearranging:

$$\varpi C_a = V C_i / (V/\varpi + \delta) \qquad (8.2)$$

Xe-133 has a long half-life of 5.3 days, so δ is negligible and equation (8.2) reduces to

$$C_a / C_i = 1 \qquad (8.3)$$

i.e., at equilibrium the alveolar concentration is equal to the inspired concentration, giving rise to a constant count rate proportional to regional lung volume. In contrast, the decay constant for Kr-81m is high so that, during quiet breathing, V/ϖ is negligible in comparison and equation (8.2) reduces to

$$\varpi C_a = V C_i / \delta \qquad (8.4)$$

i.e., the count rate is constant and proportional to regional ventilation. During hyperventilation or in small children, V/ϖ increases and is not negligible compared with δ, so the count rate underestimates V and their relationship becomes non-linear.

Although cheap and readily available, Xe-133 gives images of poor resolution because of its low photon energy of 80 keV. Following a period of inhalation, the so-called wash-in phase, an image of the regional distribution of ventilation is acquired. With continuing inhalation and approaching equilibrium, the distribution of radioactivity increasingly reflects regional lung volume. Following termination of inhalation, this equilibrium phase is followed by the wash-out phase. Regions of air trapping within the lung may become evident as areas of relatively increased count rate. Although this dynamic approach may give useful information, particularly regarding air trapping, it can only be conveniently performed in one projection, usually the posterior. This is a disadvantage because, owing to its low energy, Xe-133 (80 keV) has to be administered before Tc-99 m (140 keV) at a time when the location of any perfusion abnormalities, if present, is not known. Nevertheless, wash-in images acquired during limited periods of inhalation can be obtained in multiple projections, such as posterior and both posterior oblique views (22). Alternatively, the lungs can be imaged in these three projections during the wash-out phase, since regional hypoventilation is often associated with air trapping. Xe-127, another long-lived radioactive inert gas, has a higher energy (203 keV) than Tc-99 m and so can be administered following perfusion imaging in a selected projection, namely the one which best shows any perfusion defects, a significant advantage over Xe-133 (23).

Because of its very short half-life, Kr-81m (190 keV) effectively gives information only from wash-in studies since it has almost completely decayed by the time it is exhaled. Kr-81m is the metastable radioactive decay daughter of rubidium-81(Rb-81), which is delivered in a canister from a cyclotron unit. The canister is connected to an air cylinder and has an outlet port through which cylinder air is delivered to the patient for continuous inhalation (Figure 8.7).

The principal advantage of Kr-81m is that it can be continuously inhaled and images acquired in any projection with minimal patient cooperation. It can also be freely used in patients with chronic obstructive pulmonary disease. Perfusion and ventilation images are obtained, without moving the patient, either in sequence by alternating the photo peak settings on the gamma camera between Kr-81m and Tc-99 m or simultaneously by setting two different photo peak windows on the gamma

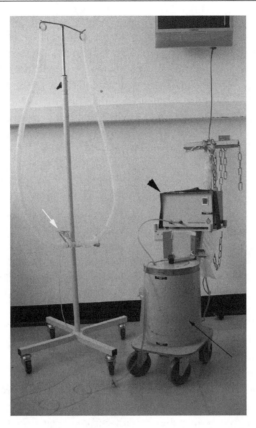

Figure 8.7 A typical Kr-81m generator (black arrow) with heavy lead shielding and an air generator (black arrowhead) mounted on a trolley. Ventilation tubing and mouthpiece (white arrow) are also shown.

camera (dual photon acquisition). For the sequential approach, 'down-scatter' of the higher energy photons of Kr-81m into the Tc-99 m window is not an issue since the Kr-81m supply can be switched off. Residual gas clears rapidly, mainly by radioactive decay, and therefore does not interfere with the Tc-99 m images. Rb-81 has a half-life of 4.7 hours, giving a Kr-81m generator a useful life span of one working day. Currently, an Rb-81:Kr-81m generator costs approximately £300 ($430; €340) in the UK. Offering an alternate day V/Q imaging service based on Kr-81m is an acceptable strategy to reduce costs, reserving aerosol studies on the intervening days for patients in whom deferment for 24 hours would be clinically unacceptable. Alternatively, for hospitals in close proximity to each other, a daily Rb-81:Kr-81m generator can be shared. One hospital can have the facility in the morning, the other in the afternoon. This would give a maximum wait of <24 hours for a V/Q scan at any one hospital. This should be clinically acceptable and financially reduces the burden for both hospitals. The value of Kr-81m imaging is illustrated in patients who have an 'unstable' distribution of ventilation (i.e., changing with time and therefore potentially different from one projection to another). This may give rise to diagnostic confusion but is difficult to detect with any other ventilation agent. Unstable ventilation has been noted, particularly in children (24) and may be posture dependent. It calls into question the reliability of injecting MAA in the supine position and administering the ventilation agent in the erect position. It also questions the wisdom of performing perfusion and ventilation images on separate days, for example in pregnant women when the perfusion study is done first in the hope of avoiding the ventilation study.

Because of the financial limitations of Kr-81m, Tc-99 m aerosols are a widely used alternative because they are cheap, practical and readily manufactured. Aerosol ventilation imaging is therefore widely used. Because of technical improvements in the delivery systems and reduction in aerosol particle size, chronic lung disease is not an immediate contraindication for a V/Q study based on aerosol ventilation imaging. Aerosols are usually generated from Tc-99 m-DTPA but other materials may be used such as Tc-99 m-colloids. Aerosol administration requires patient cooperation because of the need to breathe through a mouthpiece, with a nose-clip in place, for several minutes. It is therefore impractical to achieve ventilation imaging by this method in children, acutely ill patients and in those who are unable to cooperate. As with Xe-133, ventilation imaging with Tc-99 m-aerosols should precede the administration of the perfusion agent since the count rates achieved with aerosols are generally much lower than those with Tc-99 m-MAA. If given after Tc-99 m-MAA, computerized image subtraction will be necessary. This is not ideal since identical patient positioning for the two sets of images cannot be guaranteed. As with Kr-81m, images can be acquired in multiple projections, facilitating comparison with the subsequent perfusion images and SPECT (single photon emission computed tomography) can be performed (25). In so far as the regional distribution of radioactivity depicts regional ventilation at the time of inhalation, aerosol imaging is similar to Tc-99 m MAA perfusion imaging in that the distribution of agent is captured at the time of administration, but is unlike Kr-81m, which continuously and dynamically depicts the distribution of ventilation as the patient breathes the gas.

Another type of aerosol is Technegas (26), which is an ultra-fine dispersion of Tc-99 m-labelled carbon particles generated by combustion of pertechnetate at 2500 °C in a graphite crucible in an atmosphere of 100% argon. The Technegas 'generator' is portable, producing an agent that gives ventilation images with a quality approaching that of Kr-81m (27). Once the generator has been purchased, ventilation imaging can be performed immediately on request, so the technique is convenient. Deposition of particles in the central airways, which may be a problem with conventional DTPA aerosols, particularly in patients with chronic lung disease, appears to be less with Technegas because of the smaller particle size. As with Tc-99 m DTPA aerosol, subtraction of the Technegas signal from the subsequent perfusion signal (or vice versa) may be necessary.

Movement of gas in the peripheral airways, beyond the sixteenth generation of airway, is by molecular diffusion at a rate which is inversely proportional to molecular size (28). Aerosol particles are therefore presumably deposited mainly in distal airways rather than alveoli, although their kinetic energy may carry them into the alveolar sac. Following inhalation, Tc-99 m DTPA dissolves in airspace fluid and, as a hydrophilic solute, diffuses across the distal airway epithelium and pulmonary vascular endothelium (or bronchial if deposited more proximally) via inter-epithelial and inter-endothelial junction gaps, respectively. Epithelial permeability is 10 times less than endothelial permeability and is therefore the rate-limiting membrane as far as rate of clearance into pulmonary blood is concerned. In normal, non-smoking subjects, Tc-99 m DTPA clears from the lung via the blood–gas barrier with a half-disappearance time of about 80 minutes (29). It is much faster in smokers (18,19) and by the time scintigraphy is performed, activity is often already visible in the renal collecting systems. It is also often visible as swallowed activity in the upper gastrointestinal tract as a result of particle deposition in the mouth and in the proximal airways of patients with chronic lung disease as a result of particle deposition from turbulent air flow. Larger particles tend to be deposited in the proximal airways (Figure 8.8) and it is towards the elimination of this problem that the technical improvements in aerosol production and delivery have largely been aimed.

A minimum of four views is recommended for V/Q lung scanning: anterior, posterior and both posterior oblique views. Occasionally, lateral and anterior oblique views may also be useful. SPECT may have a role in V/Q lung scanning, particularly when ventilation imaging is performed with Kr-81m (25), Technegas (30) or Tc-99 m-MIBI. If clinically relevant, V/Q lung imaging

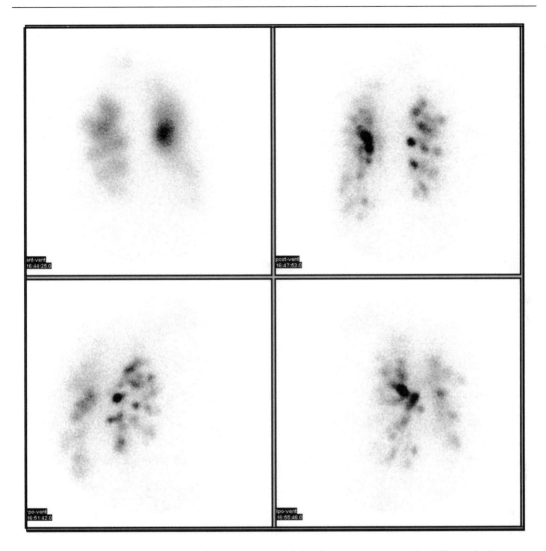

Figure 8.8 'Hot spots' from clumped DTPA aerosol droplets in a patient with airflow turbulence.

should be performed with little hesitation in pregnant women because of the obvious undesirability of anticoagulation in such circumstances. Dosimetry of ventilation agents is somewhat imprecise, depending on efficiency of delivery, and therefore difficult to estimate. In the case of Kr-81m, however, the radiation dose is negligible and so it can be freely used in special groups such as children, pregnant women and lactating women. Perfusion-only lung imaging may be adequate for a pregnant patient (Figure 8.9), provided that she is a non-smoker, has a normal chest radiograph and has no history of chronic lung disease. Reducing the injected dose to less than about 50 MBq provides an opportunity for a follow-up scan, although, for statistical reasons, the number of particles injected should not be reduced (13). Tc-99 m is excreted in breast milk (31,32), so nursing mothers should express their milk and discard it for 14 hours from the time of injection to allow for radionuclide physical decay (14). If early warning is given before the test is performed, then the nursing mother may have an opportunity to express sufficient milk to sustain the infant in the period following the test, when breastfeeding is withheld.

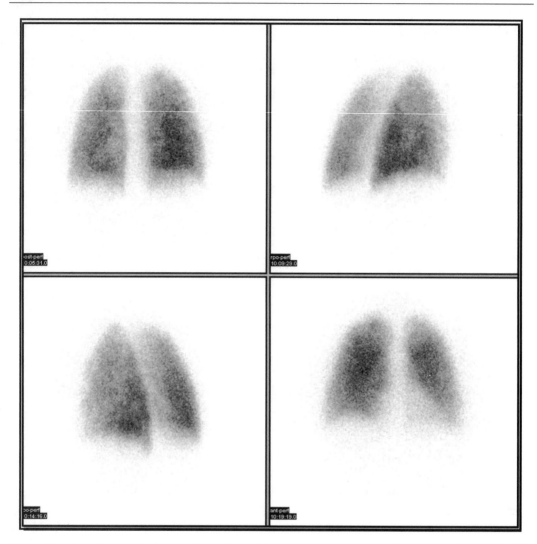

Figure 8.9 Low-dose perfusion study performed in a pregnant woman. The images show a slightly inhomogeneous distribution of radioactivity but no clear perfusion defects.

INTERPRETATION OF V/Q SCINTIGRAPHY FOR SUSPECTED PULMONARY EMBOLISM

The diagnostic feature of PE on a V/Q lung scan is a perfusion defect in a region of normally ventilated lung. This is the so-called mismatched perfusion defect (Figure 8.10). However, it is important to appreciate that mismatched or unmatched perfusion defects point to pulmonary vascular disease and not specifically to embolic disease. In the appropriate clinical setting, the great majority of unmatched perfusion defects arise from embolic disease.

The size of a perfusion defect in pulmonary thromboembolism is important and may range from appreciably smaller than a segment (subsegmental), to about the size of a segment (segmental) or even a lobe or whole lung. A non-segmental defect is one that does not correspond to segmental anatomy and, although less likely to be due to an embolus, it is not always clear whether a defect

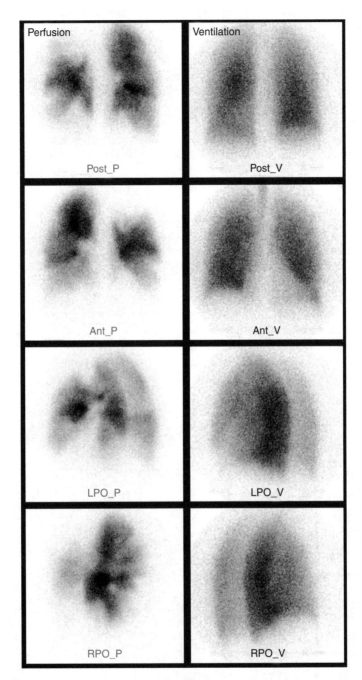

Figure 8.10 Multiple mismatched perfusion defects indicating a high scintigraphic probability of pulmonary embolism. The ventilation images were obtained with Kr-81m.

is segmental or not. It is therefore appropriate to describe perfusion defects on the basis of their size (small, moderate or large) instead of their shape, although it should be noted that size may be underestimated (33). Similarly, lobar anatomy is not well defined on the V/Q scan and it is therefore acceptable to describe a defect in terms of its zonal location – upper, mid or lower zones. The pathological basis of the mismatched perfusion defect is that in uncomplicated PE the pulmonary architecture remains intact and ventilation therefore continues normally. If PE is followed by lung infarction, a ventilation defect appears, but it is usually smaller than the perfusion defect because the lung around the periphery of the perfusion defect continues to ventilate. Thus, the diagnostic feature of a pulmonary infarct is an incompletely matched perfusion defect in association with an appropriate radiographic abnormality. The positive identification of a pulmonary infarct on a V/Q lung scan depends on high-quality, multi-projection ventilation imaging, such as achieved with Kr-81m, and is understressed in the literature, probably because of the historical predominant use of single projection Xe-133 imaging.

Many patients with suspected PE have multiple perfusion and ventilation abnormalities on V/Q scintigraphy as a result of coincidental cardiopulmonary disease. The diagnosis of PE on such a background of non-embolic V/Q abnormalities is more difficult. Complete matching of perfusion and ventilation defects is seen in obstructive airways disease, including bronchial asthma. Matching is complete because of efficient hypoxic vasoconstriction, a defence mechanism that prevents pulmonary arterial blood from circulating through non-ventilated lung. Hypoxic vasoconstriction may, nevertheless, be incomplete, in which case a region of lung may be better perfused than ventilated – a so-called *reversed* mismatch. Reversed mismatching is a characteristic feature of several chest diseases, including pleural effusions, lobar pneumonia, collapsed/consolidated lung and gross cardiomegaly (34–36), and is also seen in acute partial bronchial obstruction, in which the chest radiograph is usually normal and in chronic obstructive airway disease (Figure 8.11),

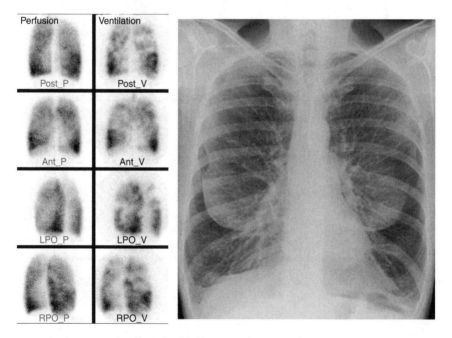

Figure 8.11 Multiple reversed mismatched perfusion defects in a patient with known chronic obstructive airway disease indicating, on scintigraphic criteria, a low probability of pulmonary embolism. The ventilation images were obtained with Kr-81m.

especially in acute exacerbations (37). In these conditions, hypoxic vasoconstriction fails or is incomplete. If the patient is imaged with inert gas or inhales aerosol in the erect posture (as is conventional), pleural effusion typically gives a complete absence of ventilation at the base as a result of lung compression (Figure 8.12). Reduced perfusion is usually visible in the area of compressed lung. If the patient is imaged supine, pleural effusions may produce confusing images as a result of fluid accumulating in the posterior pleural space and attenuating both ventilation and perfusion signals in addition to compressing the lung. In lobar pneumonia, perfusion is maintained, albeit at an abnormally reduced level, but, since the lobe is airless, a ventilation signal is completely absent (Figure 8.13). Lung compression is not evident on the perfusion image unless there is associated collapse (Figure 8.14). Cardiomegaly may give rise to reversed mismatching in the left lower lobe (36). Like pleural effusion, the mechanism is essentially regional lung compression. The effect of cardiomegaly on left lower lobe ventilation is dependent on posture and is greatest in the supine position, when lung compression is maximal. In this position, patients with cardiomegaly develop a physiological right-to-left shunt and this contributes to the orthopnea experienced by these patients. In general, the importance of reversed mismatching has been understated in the literature, particularly regarding lobar pneumonia, which, with high-quality ventilation imaging, can be distinguished from pulmonary infarction. Because it represents physiological right-to-left

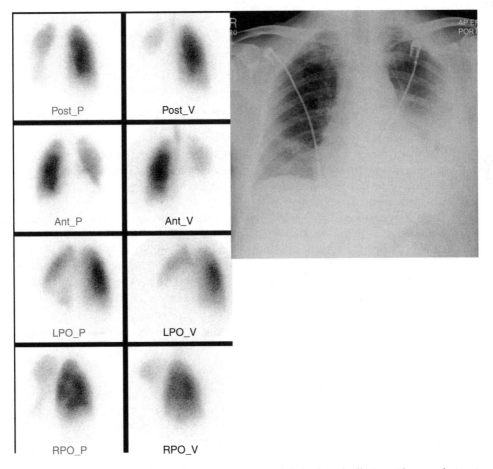

Figure 8.12 Reversed mismatched defect in a patient with left pleural effusion. The ventilation images were obtained with Kr-81m.

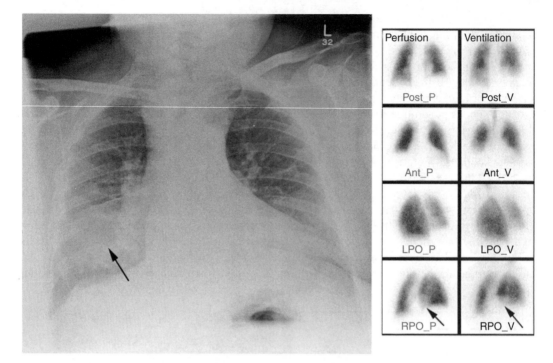

Figure 8.13 Reversed mismatched defect in the right lower zone, corresponding to the air space shadow visible on the chest radiograph (arrow). The ventilation images were obtained with Kr-81m.

shunting, reversed mismatching is an explanation for breathlessness and, as such, is an important finding on V/Q scintigraphy, especially in the patient with suspected pulmonary embolism whose dominant symptom is breathlessness. Single completely matched defects are actually fairly rare and are seen in destructive parenchymal lung diseases, including lung tumours, pulmonary granulomata and pulmonary abscesses.

Because of the complexities of V/Q scan diagnosis against a background of pre-existing or current chest disease, several diagnostic algorithms have been proposed to aid in the interpretation of V/Q lung scans performed for suspected pulmonary thromboembolism (38–49). Notwithstanding its limitations in the detection of small peripheral emboli (50), pulmonary angiography remains the gold standard against which these algorithms have been developed. They are generally based on a comparison of the perfusion and ventilation images and the chest radiograph and express the likelihood of PE on a verbal probability scale: low, intermediate or high. The probability or likelihood that an abnormal scan is due to PE is the positive predictive value of the test, defined as the ratio of true positives to all positives. It is highly dependent on the prevalence of the disease in the patient population studied (51).

The PIOPED study has been the most comprehensive evaluation of the clinical accuracy of V/Q scanning and indeed was followed for many years by modified analyses of the original database with the generation of yet more diagnostic algorithms. Whereas preceding algorithms were described independently of the pre-test clinical likelihood for pulmonary embolism, PIOPED highlighted the impact of the pre-test likelihood on the overall probability of PE. This and the introduction of CT PA have reduced the importance of the details within the published algorithms. Moreover, along with several algorithms preceding it, PIOPED was unfortunately based on ventilation imaging using Xe-133.

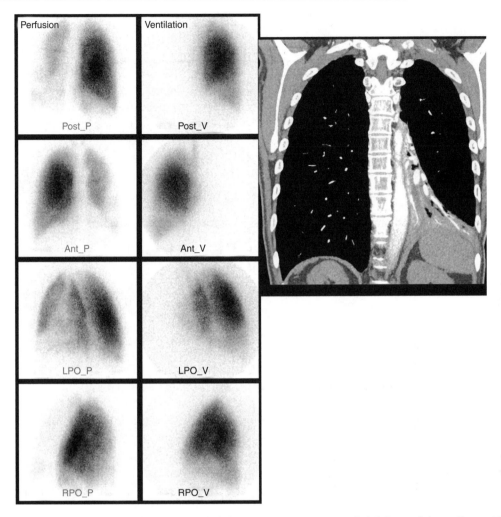

Figure 8.14 Marked reversed mismatched defect seen in a patient with left lower lobe collapse. This finding was confirmed on the CT study. The ventilation images were obtained with Kr-81m.

Pre-test likelihood criteria have changed over recent years, at least in the UK, as a result of successive guidelines published by the British Thoracic Society, in a direction moving away from exclusively objective criteria, such as recent surgery (especially to the abdomen, pelvis and hip), coexisting disease (especially cancer) and immobility towards subjective clinical criteria. Indeed, the latest scheme is based on a points scoring system. Conversely, however, more weight is now attached to the plasma D-dimer assay, an objective criterion.

A normal perfusion scan (Figure 8.15) effectively excludes embolism (likelihood <5%), whatever the ventilation images show (38,39). An abnormal V/Q scan indicating a low probability of pulmonary embolism (Figure 8.16) is one in which the individual perfusion defects are (1) all smaller than 25% of a segment (i.e., subsegmental), regardless of the chest radiographic and ventilation scan appearances, or (2) are matched on the ventilation scan or (3) are accompanied by larger chest radiographic abnormalities. Prominent, non-pulmonary intra-thoracic structures, such as an enlarged hilum, cardiac chamber or aorta (Figure 8.17), are sometimes described as giving matched defects but their origins are usually obvious, readily confirmed from the chest radiograph,

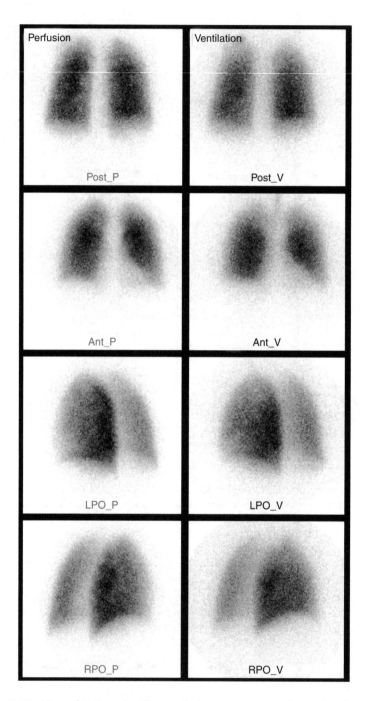

Figure 8.15   Normal V/Q study. The ventilation images were obtained with Kr-81m.

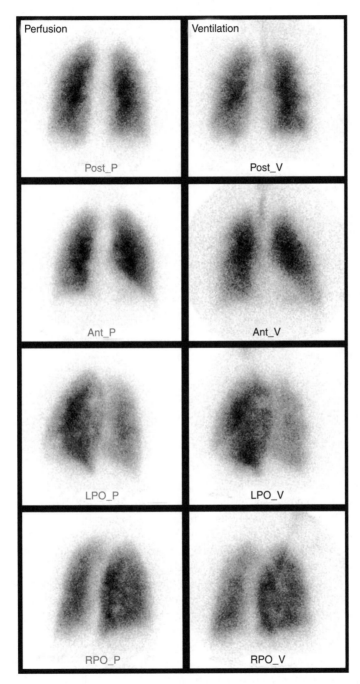

Figure 8.16 V/Q study showing small matched and mismatched defects that on scintigraphic criteria carry a low probability of pulmonary embolism. No embolus was identified on a subsequent CT PA. The ventilation images were obtained with Kr-81m.

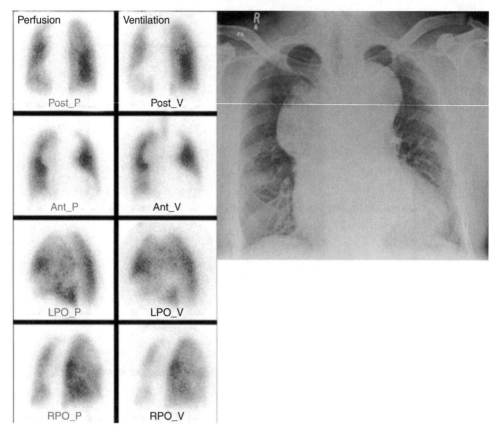

Figure 8.17　V/Q study was performed on a patient with thoracic aortic aneurysm and cardiomegaly. The ventilation images were obtained with Kr-81m.

and should not be described as 'defects'. A V/Q scan indicating a high probability of PE is one in which there are two or more perfusion defects, not matched by corresponding ventilation defects or chest radiographic abnormalities, including at least one of moderate or large size (Figure 8.10). In the appropriate clinical setting, a high-probability V/Q scan indicates a probability of PE exceeding 90%. If the mismatched perfusion defects resolve within days or weeks, the probability of recent embolism is higher.

An intermediate probability V/Q scan, also described, unsatisfactorily, as an indeterminate scan, is simply an abnormal scan that does not fit into the low- or high-probability categories. In general, V/Q scans indicating an intermediate probability of PE have been described in the literature as showing (1) a single unmatched perfusion defect of at least moderate (segmental) size (Figure 8.18), (2) perfusion defects which, although matched, correspond in size and shape to an area of consolidation on the chest radiograph (and may, therefore, represent infarction – so-called triple match) or (3) perfusion defects in areas of severe obstructive lung disease (Figure 8.19), pulmonary oedema or pleural effusion. Good-quality ventilation imaging has the potential to reduce the number of scans described as intermediate, especially on the basis of the criteria in (3) above when the perfusion abnormalities should be seen, on multiple projection ventilation imaging, to be matched by or smaller than, the corresponding ventilation defects and so be appropriately categorised as 'low probability'.

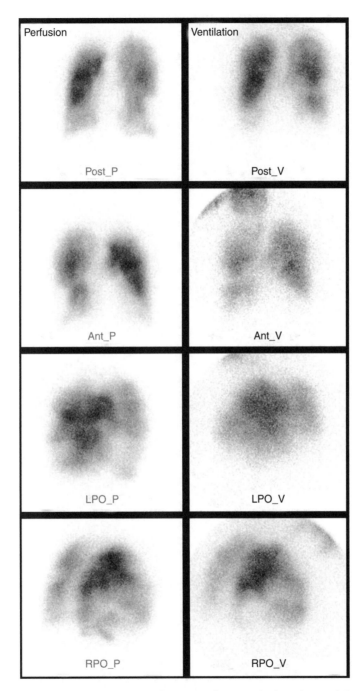

Figure 8.18 V/Q study showing a single, moderate-sized unmatched perfusion defect in the left lower lobe, indicating an intermediate probability of pulmonary embolism. The distribution of perfusion is otherwise patchy but generally matched by the distribution of ventilation, as depicted with Kr-81m.

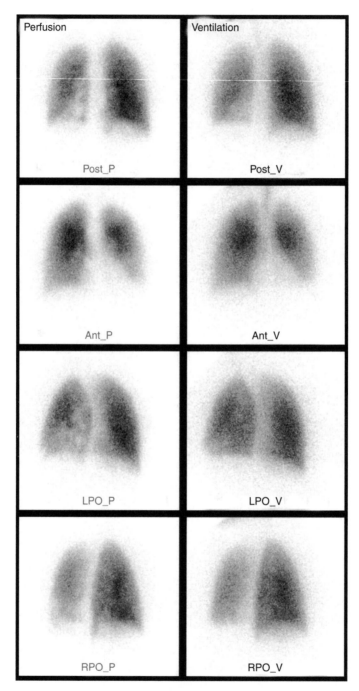

Figure 8.19 V/Q mismatched, matched and reversed mismatched defects were identified on this study on an elderly lady. The appearances carry an intermediate probability of pulmonary embolism. No emboli were identified on subsequent CT PA.

Unmatched perfusion defects may be the result of previous unresolved PE and, if this is suspected, it may be helpful to repeat the scan after an interval of about 3 weeks. Complete (Figure 8.20) or partial resolution (Figure 8.21) of the perfusion defect supports recent PE. Pulmonary emboli resolve at variable rates, broadly dependent on the patient's age and fitness. In young, fit patients, the scan can be repeated within about 1 week, although in older patients at least 3 weeks is appropriate. A follow-up study is essential even when the scan indicates a high probability of embolism, for two reasons: first, because unresolved PE is probably not uncommon, and second, to establish a new baseline in the event of incomplete resolution. It is usually worth taking the trouble to search for previous V/Q scans for comparison with the current study.

Within nuclear medicine reporting practice, the probability-stratification approach, with its specified criteria, is almost exclusive to V/Q scintigraphy performed for suspected PE. The importance of the pre-test likelihood of the disease in defining overall probability was brought out by the PIOPED study (38), in which it was shown that the incidence of abnormal pulmonary angiography was greater, in all scintigraphic probability categories, when the pre-scan clinical likelihood of pulmonary embolism was high compared with when it was it low. This means that the V/Q scan can be regarded as a screening test that increases the pre-test likelihood of embolism, decreases it or leaves it unchanged. Thus, a patient without risk factors for PE who presents with sudden onset of pleuritic chest pain and is deemed to have a low clinical likelihood of embolism and who then has a V/Q scan indicating a low probability of embolism on scintigraphic criteria can be deemed to have a post-V/Q scan likelihood that is even lower and which for clinical purposes rules out the need for anticoagulation. Conversely, a patient with a risk factor for PE, such as recent surgery, cancer or history of previous DVT or PE, who then has a low-probability V/Q scan, retains an overall likelihood of embolism in the region of 10–30% or even higher (52). It is important to appreciate that the scintigraphic criteria for a high-probability scan, although highly specific, had a sensitivity for PE in the PIOPED study of only about 40%. This implies that 60% of patients with current PE have scintigraphic appearances that carry only a low or intermediate probability of PE (Figure 8.22).

Hull *et al.* (46) suggested an even higher incidence of PE (40%) in patients with low-probability scans. However, by combining the V/Q scan with leg imaging for the simultaneous diagnosis of DVT, they found that many of their patients had DVT and therefore an objective risk factor, which is accepted to raise the overall probability of a scintigraphically low-probability scan to levels approaching 40%. In contrast, patients with low-probability V/Q scans who had no evidence of DVT and were not anticoagulated had a very low incidence of recurrent thromboembolism on follow-up. Imaging the leg veins effectively shifts the clinical risk factor status.

In the context of the patient with suspected pulmonary embolism, an important function of the chest radiograph, apart from providing anatomical landmarks, is to avoid missing pulmonary infarction. A matched defect without a corresponding radiographic abnormality is described as having a low probability of pulmonary embolism, although such defects are rarely completely matched. It has been suggested that a corresponding radiographic abnormality should move the V/Q scan into the intermediate category because it increases the likelihood of infarction. Partial mismatching typical of infarction with an appropriate radiographic abnormality further increases the likelihood. An important question that remains unanswered is how often an infarct gives a completely matched defect. If uncommon, the matched defect could be relegated to low probability, irrespective of the chest radiograph.

Further features on V/Q scintigraphy that give rise to difficulties are *symmetrical* unmatched perfusion defects of moderate size, multiple unmatched but small perfusion defects and unmatched perfusion defects of moderate size not clearly seen on any projection to extend to the periphery of the lung (the so-called stripe sign) (Figure 8.23). A solitary moderate-sized unmatched perfusion defect indicates a likelihood of embolism of 30–50% (43,53,54). In a patient with a risk factor

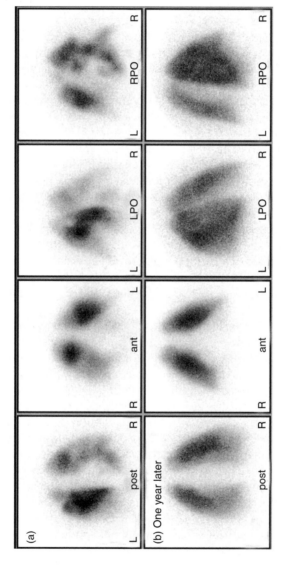

Figure 8.20 Perfusion images showing almost complete resolution of defects 1 year (B) after initial diagnosis of pulmonary embolism (A).

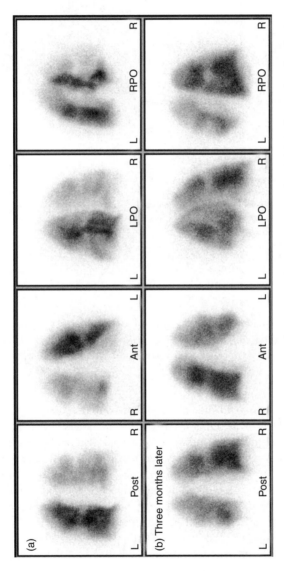

Figure 8.21 Perfusion images showing partial resolution of defects 6 months (B) after initial diagnosis of pulmonary embolism (A).

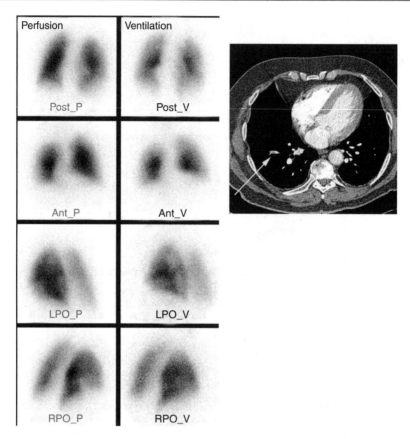

Figure 8.22   V/Q study showing small matched and mismatched perfusion defects that, on scintigraphic criteria, indicate a low probability of pulmonary embolism. A small embolus, identified in a branch of the right lower lobe pulmonary artery (arrow), does however correspond to a small mismatched defect.

for PE, however, this finding would indicate a higher overall probability. On the other hand, if the patient is known to have a medium-sized arteritis or is a smoker and the unmatched perfusion defect involves an entire lung with a normal contralateral lung, clearly the diagnosis of PE would be considerably less certain. Unmatched perfusion defects that are symmetrical do not carry a high probability because thrombi randomly embolize into the lung. Multiple unmatched but sub-segmental perfusion defects are unlikely to be due to PE since, after multiple emboli, at least one would be expected to produce a defect of segmental size. Furthermore, multiple unmatched sub-segmental perfusion defects are seen in primary pulmonary hypertension, Eisenmenger's syndrome and veno-occlusive disease (see below). The 'stripe' sign does not carry the diagnostic weight of a defect that clearly interrupts the normal contour of the lung (55).

DIFFERENTIAL DIAGNOSIS OF MISMATCHING ON V/Q SCANS

There are several diseases other than PE in which the V/Q scan may show mismatched perfusion abnormalities. A mismatched defect indicates pulmonary vascular disease, which usually, although not always, is due to pulmonary embolism.

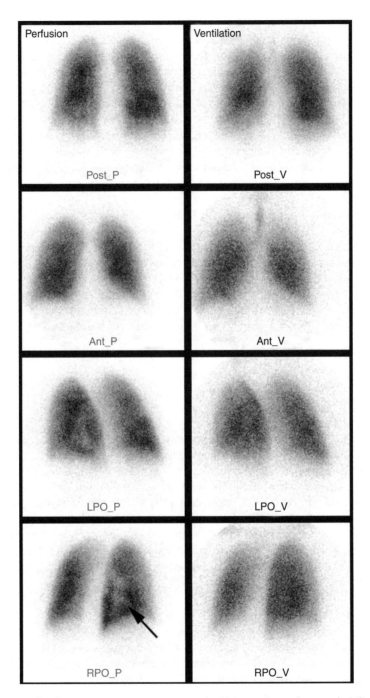

Figure 8.23 V/Q study showing a 'stripe' sign (arrow). This carries a low probability of pulmonary embolism. The ventilation images were obtained with Kr-81m.

Pulmonary hypertension

V/Q scintigraphy in primary pulmonary hypertension may be normal or show multiple small, usually symmetrical and peripheral, unmatched perfusion defects in both lungs (56–62). The appearances are completely different from those in chronic unresolved PE. Wilson *et al.* (61) noted that patients with normal scans were predominantly young women, whereas there was an equal sex distribution in those with multiple perfusion defects. This observation is consistent with a later study by Rich *et al.* (60), who correlated the perfusion scan with lung histology. Their category of plexogenic hypertension was seen in women and associated with a normal scan, while their histological microthrombotic category was seen in both sexes and was associated with multiple small defects, which seems to correspond to Wilson's group with a similar perfusion pattern. The concept that this latter form of primary pulmonary hypertension arises from previously unrecognised microthrombosis is attractive but not established. Nor is it clear whether the microthrombus arises *in situ* or is embolic.

Veno-occlusive disease is considered a third subtype of primary pulmonary hypertension, but is much less common than the other two types. It gives V/Q scans with multiple scattered mismatched perfusion defects (56,63). V/Q lung scan findings in Eisenmenger's syndrome are similar to those in a proportion of patients with primary pulmonary hypertension, consisting of multiple small sub-segmental defects of perfusion with normal ventilation images (56). Pulmonary venous hypertension, particularly if secondary to mitral valve disease, is associated with reversal of the normal gravitational distribution of pulmonary blood flow. This may take on an element of irreversibility so that, even when the patient is injected supine, increased flow to the upper zones is apparent (56).

Pulmonary vasculitis

In systemic lupus erythematosus (SLE), pulmonary vasculitis is characterized by an arteritis involving small vessels. Loss of volume in the bases is seen on radiography and pulmonary function testing. V/Q lung scanning shows 'small lungs' but no mismatching unless the patient also has superimposed pulmonary embolic disease (56); this is more common in SLE than in the general population because of an association between thromboembolism and autoantibodies, such as anti-cardiolipin antibody. In polyarteritis nodosa and Wegener's granulomatosis, there is an inflammatory arteritis of small- to medium-sized vessels. V/Q scintigraphy may show focal matched defects (Figure 8.24) or appearances typical of infarction, with defects of perfusion larger than corresponding ventilation defects. Takayasu's arteritis affects medium-sized and large arteries of the pulmonary vasculature and may give V/Q scans indistinguishable from PE (56,64).

Bronchogenic carcinoma

Depending on its anatomical location, carcinoma of the bronchus may selectively compromise a major pulmonary artery, giving rise to the characteristic finding of a completely non-perfused lung or lobe with variable preservation of ventilation (Figure 8.25).

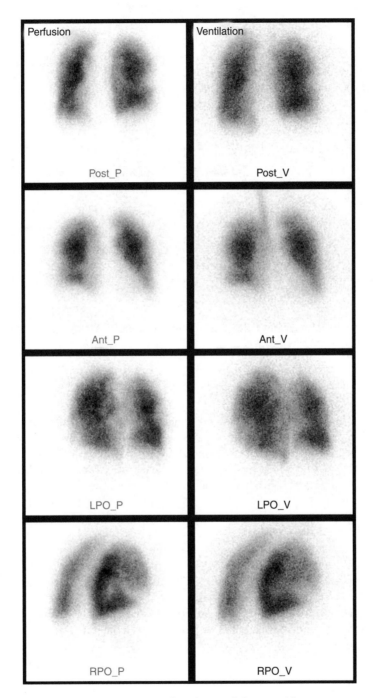

Figure 8.24 Multiple matched and mismatched perfusion defects visible in a patient with large vessel vasculitis. The ventilation images were obtained with Kr-81m.

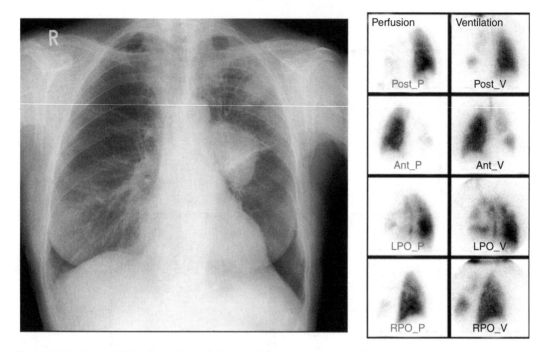

Figure 8.25 Large V/Q mismatched defects visible in a patient with lung carcinoma. The ventilation images were obtained with Kr-81m.

Congenital vascular anomalies

Pulmonary embolism is rare in childhood and, unless a risk factor is present such as long-term central venous lines, unmatched perfusion defects are more likely to be due to sequestered lobes or segments, congenital anomalies of the pulmonary artery (Figure 8.26) and previous surgery for congenital cardiovascular anomalies. Caution is occasionally required in this last setting with regard to the venous site used for injecting the MAA.

Pulmonary interstitial fibrosis

Chronic lung disease with predominant emphysema may, by obliteration of alveolar septae, be associated with mismatched perfusion abnormalities, in a clearly non-segmental distribution, that are not completely matched on ventilation imaging (Figure 8.27). Chronic mycobacterial infection may do the same. The effects of fibrosing alveolitis, which usually involves the upper zones symmetrically, may be similar, giving rise to symmetrical bilateral mismatched, poorly defined perfusion defects (65).

Bullous lung disease

Bullae may occasionally retain some ventilation, albeit reduced, but receive no pulmonary blood supply, and may therefore give large poorly defined incompletely matched perfusion abnormalities (66). They are, however, usually evident on chest radiography and are clearly non-segmental.

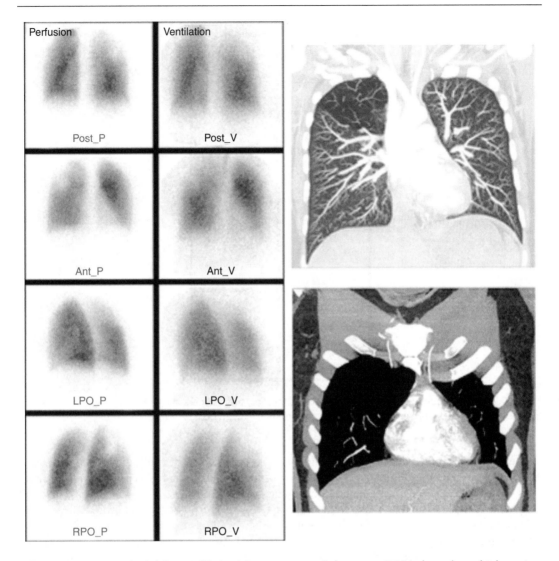

Figure 8.26 A matched defect visible in right upper zone. Subsequent CT PA shows bronchial atresia.

Chronic thromboembolic pulmonary hypertension

Although acute pulmonary embolism is common and incomplete resolution probably not uncommon, chronic thromboembolic pulmonary hypertension (CTEPH) is rare, complicating less than 1% of acute PE (see Chapters 18 and 25). Repeated embolism without intervening clot lysis may lead to CTEPH with all its clinical and radiographic manifestations. Sometimes there is a recognized source of emboli such as a ventriculo-peritoneal shunt or an underlying predisposition to venous thrombosis, but most patients present with no relevant past history. The chest radiograph shows cardiomegaly and right-sided chamber dilatation. The central pulmonary arteries are large and abrupt 'cut-off' is common (67,68). Peripheral pulmonary vessels are disorganized rather than simply tapered. Although pulmonary vascular changes are more common than in acute PE, they may be subtle and can be masked or mimicked by underlying chronic airways obstruction. As

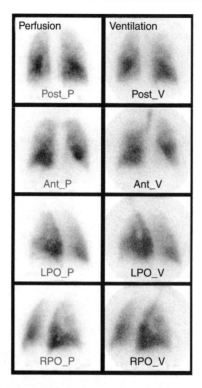

Figure 8.27   V/Q study in a patient with known pulmonary emphysema showing bilateral non-segmental matched defects in the upper zones. The ventilation images were obtained with Kr-81m.

in acute PE, areas of peripheral oligaemia may be seen and correlate well with areas of reduced vascularity on angiography and hypoperfusion on scintigraphy. Normal or near-normal vascularity does not exclude the diagnosis. Pleural thickening, pleural effusions, plate atelectasis and small peripheral foci of consolidation are common, albeit non-specific, associations of CTEPH.

V/Q lung scintigraphy in CTEPH shows multiple segmental mismatched perfusion defects indistinguishable from high-probability scans in acute PE (57–59). The appearances remain unchanged on sequential imaging unless there are new episodes of embolism. It is not uncommon to find patients referred for V/Q scintigraphy for the first time with suspected acute PE who show mismatched perfusion defects that do not resolve on follow-up scans performed several weeks later. This is sometimes loosely referred to as chronic PE. The true incidence of patients with high probability lung scans who have non-resolving defects and no previous V/Q scans is not clearly known but this finding does not appear to be unusual, especially in nuclear medicine departments in which patients with acute embolism are routinely followed up. In other words, unresolved PE may be fairly common but CTEPH is uncommon because failure of acute PE to resolve completely does not necessarily lead to CTEPH. The combination of a plain radiograph suggesting pulmonary hypertension and a V/Q scan with multiple mismatched perfusion defects is diagnostic of CTEPH.

CONCLUSION

V/Q lung scintigraphy still offers a significant amount of information and remains a viable option in the diagnostic pathway of PE, CTEPH and for the assessment of physiological characteristics in the management of a range of lung and pulmonary vascular diseases. Although CTPA has largely replaced V/Q lung scintigraphy in the acute setting, indications in the context of dose reduction remain very much in place today.

REFERENCES

1. Knipping HW, Bolt W, Venrath H, *et al.* Eine neue Methode zur Prufung der Herz and Lungenfunftion: die regionale Funktionanalyse in der Lungen- und Herzlinik mit Hilfe des radioactiven Edelgases Xenon-133. *Dtsch Med Wochenschr* 1955; **80**:1146.
2. Wagner HN Jr, Sabiston DC Jr, McAfee JG, *et al.* Diagnosis of massive pulmonary embolism in man by radioisotope scanning. *N Engl J Med* 1964; **271**:377–84.
3. Robinson DS, Cunningham DA, Dave S, *et al.* Diagnostic value of lung clearance of 99 mTc DTPA compared with other non-invasive investigations of *Pneumocystis carinii* pneumonia in AIDS. *Thorax* 1991; **46**(10):722–726.
4. Clarke-Pearson DL, Coleman RE, Seigel R, *et al.* Indium-111 platelet imaging for the detection of deep vein thrombosis in patients without symptoms after surgery. *Surgery* 1985; **98**(1):98–104.
5. Carretta RF, DeNardo GL, Janshalt AL, Rose AW. Early diagnosis of venous thrombosis using ^{125}I-fibrinogen. *J Nucl Med* 1977; **18**(1):5–10.
6. Kanke M, Khaw BA, Matsueda G, *et al.* Comparison of two kinds of monoclonal antibodies to detect clots in the pulmonary artery. *J Nucl Med* 1986; **27**:923.
7. Som P, Oster ZH, Zamora PO, *et al.* Radioimmunoimaging of experimental thrombi in dogs using Tc-99m labelled antibody fragments reactive with human platelets. *J Nucl Med* 1986; **27**:1315–20.
8. Taillefer R, Edell S, Innes G, *et al.* Acute thromboscintigraphy with 99mTc-apcitide: results of the phase 3 multicenter clinical trial comparing 99mTc-apcitide scintigraphy with contrast venography for imaging acute DVT. Multicenter Trial Investigators. *J Nucl Med* 2000; **41**:1214–23.
9. Baidoo KE, Knight LC, Lin KS, *et al.* Design and synthesis of a shortchain bitistatin analogue for imaging thrombi and emboli. *Bioconjug Chem* 2004; **15**:1068–75.
10. Weiss CR, Scatarige JC, Diette GB, *et al.* CT pulmonary angiography is the first-line imaging test for acute pulmonary embolism: a survey of US clinicians. *Acad Radiol* 2006; **13**(4):434–446.
11. *Making the Best Use of Clinical Radiology Services: Referral Guidelines*, 6th edn. Royal College of Radiologists, London, 2007.
12. Taplin GV, MacDonald NS. Radiochemistry of macroaggregated albumin and newer lung scanning agents. *Semin Nucl Med* 1971; **1**:132–.
13. Heck LL, Duley JW. Statistical considerations in lung imaging with Tc-99m albumin particles. *Radiology* 1974; **113**:675–9.
14. Administration of Radioactive Substances Advisory Committee. *Notes for Guidance on the Clinical Administration of Radiopharmaceuticals and Use of Sealed Radioactive Sources*. Health Protection Agency, Didcot, 2006.
15. Ciofetta G, Piepsz A, Roca I, *et al.* Guidelines for lung scintigraphy in children. *Eur J Nucl Med Mol Imaging* 2007; **34**:1518–26.
16. Hughes JMB, Glazier JB, Maloney JE, West JB. Effect of lung volume on the distribution of pulmonary blood flow in man. *Resp Physiol* 1968; **47**:58–72.
17. Whyte MKB, Peters AM, Hughes JMB, *et al.* Quantification of right-to-left shunt at rest and on exercise in patients with pulmonary arteriovenous malformations. *Thorax* 1992; **47**:790–6.
18. Mason GR, Uszler JM, Effros RM, *et al.* Rapidly reversible alterations of pulmonary epithelial permeability induced by smoking. *Chest* 1983; **83**(1):6–11.
19. Jones JG, Minty BD, Lawler P, *et al.* Increased alveolar epithelial permeability in cigarette smokers. *Lancet* 1980; **i**(8159):66–8.
20. Sundram FX. Clinical studies of alveolar-capillary permeability using technetium-99mDTPA aerosol. *Ann Nucl Med* 1995; **9**(4):171–8.
21. Ruparelia P, Cheow HK, Evans JW, *et al.* Pulmonary elimination of inhaled ^{99m}Tc-sestamibi radioaerosol is delayed in healthy cigarette smokers. *Br J Clin Pharmacol* 2008; **65**:611–4.
22. Diffey BL, Gibson CJ, Scott LE. A new technique for xenon-133 ventilation imaging in the diagnosis of pulmonary embolism. *Br J Radiol* 1986; **59**:1179–84.
23. Nimmo MJ, Merrick MV, Millar AM. A comparison of the economics of xenon 127, xenon 133 and krypton 81m for routine ventilation imaging of the lungs. *Br J Radiol* 1985; **58**:635–6.

24. Peters AM, Gordon I, Kaiser AM, *et al*. Spontaneous abrupt changes in the distribution of ventilation scintigraphy. *Br J Radiol* 1988; **62**:536–43.

25. Weiner C, McKenna WJ, Myers MJ, *et al*. Lung ventilation is reduced in patients with cardiomegaly in the supine but not in the prone position. *Am Rev Resp Dis* 1990; **141**:150–5.

26. Burch WM, Sullivan PJ, McLaren CJ. Technegas – a new ventilation agent for bone scanning. *Nucl Med Commun* 1986; **7**:865–71.

27. James JM, Lloyd JJ, Leahy BC, *et al*. Tc-99m Technegas and krypton-81m ventilation scintigraphy: a comparison in known respiratory disease. *Br J Radiol* 1992; **65**:1075–82.

28. West JB. Uptake and delivery of the respiratory gases. In West JB (ed), *Physiological Basis of Medical Practice*. Williams & Williams, Baltimore, 1985, pp. 546–71.

29. O'Doherty MJ, Peters AM. Pulmonary Tc-99m-DTPA areosol clearance as an index of lung injury. *Eur J Nucl Med* 1997; **24**:81–7.

30. Lemb M, Oei TH, Sander U. Ventilation–perfusion lung SPECT in the diagnosis of pulmonary thromboembolism (PTE) using Technegas. *Eur J Nucl Med* 1989; **14**:442– (abstract).

31. McCauley E, Mackie A. Breast milk activity during early lactation following maternal 99Tcm macroaggregated albumin lung perfusion. *Br J Radiol* 2002; **75**:464–6.

32. Mountford PJ, Coakley AJ. A review of the secretion of radioactivity in human breast milk: data, quantitative analysis and recommendations. *Nucl Med Commun* 1989; **10**:15–27.

33. Morrell NW, Nijran KS, Jones BE, Biggs T, Seed WA. The underestimation of segmental defect size in radionuclide lung scanning. *J Nucl Med*. 1993; **34**:370–4.

34. Cunningham DA, Lavender JP. Fr-81m ventilation scanning in chronic obstructive airways disease. *Br J Radiol* 1981; **54**:110–6.

35. Carvalho P, Lavender JP. The incidence and etiology of the ventilation perfusion reverse mismatch defect. *Clin Nucl Med* 1989; **14**:571–6.

36. Alexander MSM, Peters AM, Cleland J, Lavender JP. Impaired left lower lobe ventilation in patients with cardiomegaly: an isotope study of mechanisms. *Chest* 1992; **101**:1189–93.

37. Lavender JP, Irving H, Armstrong JD. Kr-81m ventilation scanning: acute respiratory disease. *Am J Roentgenol* 1981; **136**:309–16.

38. The PIOPED Investigators. Value of the ventilation/perfusion scan in acute pulmonary embolism. Results of the prospective investigation of pulmonary embolism diagnosis (PIOPED). *JAMA* 1990; **263**:2753–2759.

39. Stein PD, Woodard PK, Weg JG, *et al*. Diagnostic pathways in acute pulmonary embolism: recommendations of the PIOPED II Investigators. *Radiology* 2007; **119**(12); 1048–55.

40. Sostman HD, Stein PD, Gottschalk A, *et al*. Acute pulmonary embolism: sensitivity and specificity of ventilation-perfusion scintigraphy in PIOPED II study. *Radiology* 2008; **246**(3):941–6.

41. McLean RG, Carolan M, Bui C, *et al*. Comparison of new clinical and scintigraphic algorithms for the diagnosis of pulmonary embolism. *Br J Radiol* 2004; **77**(917):372–376.

42. Miniati M, Monti S, Bauleo C, *et al*. A diagnostic strategy for pulmonary embolism based on standardised pretest probability and perfusion lung scanning: a management study. *Eur J Nucl Med Mol Imaging* 2003; **30**(11):1450–6.

43. Spies WG, Burstein SP, Dillchan GL, *et al*. Ventilation–perfusion scintigraphy in suspected pulmonary embolism: correlation with pulmonary angiography and refinement of criteria for interpretation. *Radiology* 1986; **159**(2):383–90.

44. Hull RD, Hirsch J, Carter CJ, *et al*. Pulmonary angiography, ventilation lung scanning and venography for clinically suspected pulmonary embolism with abnormal perfusion lung scan. *Ann Intern Med* 1983; **98**:891–9.

45. Hull RD, Hirsch J, Carter CJ, *et al*. Diagnostic value of ventilation perfusion lung scanning in patients with suspected pulmonary embolism. *Chest* 1985; **88**:819–28.

46. Hull RD, Raskob GE, Coates G, *et al*. A new noninvasive management strategy for patients with suspected pulmonary embolism. *Arch Int Med* 1989; **149**:2549–55.

47. Wells PS, Ginsberg GS, Anderson DR, *et al*. Use of a clinical model for safe management of patients with suspected pulmonary embolism. *Ann Intern Med* 1998; **129**(12):997–1005.

48. Kearon C, Ginsberg JS, Douketis J, *et al*. An evaluation of D-dimer in the diagnosis of pulmonary embolism: a randomized trial. *Ann Intern Med* 2006; **144**(11):812–21.

49. Gottschalk A, Stein PD, Sostman HD, *et al*. Very low probability interpretation of V/Q lung scans in combination with low probability objective clinical assessment reliably excludes pulmonary embolism: data from PIOPED II. *J Nucl Med* 2007; **48**(9):1405–7.

50. Diffin DC, Leyendecker JR, Johnson SP, *et al*. Effect of anatomic distribution of pulmonary emboli on interobserver agreement in the interpretation of pulmonary angiography. *Am J Roentgenol* 1998; **171**(4):1085–9.
51. McNeil BJ. Ventilation perfusion studies and the diagnosis of pulmonary embolism: concise communication. *J Nucl Med* 1980; **21**:319–23.
52. Bone RC. The low probability lung scan: potentially lethal reading. *Arch Int Med* 1993; **153**: 2621–2.
53. Gray HW. The single perfusion abnormality: *Quo vadis? Nucl Med Commun* 1991; **12**:377–9.
54. Edeburn GF, McNeil BJ. A single moderate-sized segmental V/Q mismatc: moderate probability for pulmonary embolus. *J Nucl Med* 1986; **27**(4):568–.
55. Sostman HD, Gottschalk A. Prospective validation of the stripe sign in ventilation–perfusion scintigraphy. *Radiology* 1992; **184**(2):455–9.
56. Lavender JP, Finn JP. V/Q patterns in nonthromboembolic lung diseases. In Loken MK (ed). *Pulmonary Nuclear Medicine*. Appleton & Lange, Norwalk, CT, 1987, pp. 103–31.
57. Worsley DF, Palevsky HI, Alavi A. Ventilation–perfusion lung scanning in the evaluation of pulmonary hypertension. *J Nucl Med* 1994; **35**(5):793–6.
58. Lisbona R, Kreisman H, Novales-Diaz J, *et al*. Perfusion lung scanning: differentiation of primary from thromboembolic pulmonary hypertension. *Am J Roentgenol* 1985; **144**:27–30.
59. Powe JE, Palevsky HI, McCarthy KE, *et al*. Pulmonary arterial hypertension: value of perfusion scintigraphy. *Radiology* 1987; **164**:727–30.
60. Rich S, Pietra GG, Kieras K, *et al*. Primary pulmonary hypertension: radiographic and scintigraphic patterns of histologic subtypes. *Ann Intern Med* 1986; **105**:449–502.
61. Wilson AG, Harris CN, Lavender JP, *et al*. Perfusion lung scanning in obliterative pulmonary hypertension. *Br Heart J* 1973; **35**:917–30.
62. Fukuchi K, Hayashida K, Nakanishi N, *et al*. Quantitative analysis of lung perfusion in patients with primary pulmonary hypertension. *J Nucl Med* 2002; **43**(6):757–61.
63. Thadani V, Burrow C, Whitaker W, *et al*. Pulmonary veno-occlusive disease. *Q J Med* 1975; **173**:133–59.
64. Shlomai A, Hershko AY, Gabbay E, Ben-Chetrit E. Clinical and radiographic features mimicking pulmonary embolism as the first manifestation of Takayasu's arteritis. *Clin Rheumatol* 2004; **23**(5):470–2.
65. Strickland NH, Hughes JMB, Hart DA, *et al*. Cause of regional ventilation–perfusion mismatching in patients with idiopathic pulmonary fibrosis. *Am J Roentgenol* 1993; **161**:719–25.
66. Cunningham DA, Mitchell DM. Well ventilated bullae: a potential confusion on ventilation/perfusion scanning. *Br J Radiol* 1991; **64**:56–60.
67. Hasegawa I, Boiselle PM, Hatabu H. Bronchial artery dilatation on MDCT of patients with acute pulmonary embolism: comparison with chronic or recurrent pulmonary embolism. *Am J Roentgenol* 2004; **182**(1):67–72.
68. Schmidt HC, Kauzcor HU, Schild HH, *et al*. Pulmonary hypertension in patients with chronic thromboembolism: chest radiograph and CT evaluation before and after surgery. *Eur Radiol* 1996; **6**(6):818–25.

CHAPTER 9

MRI and MRA of the Pulmonary Vasculature

Hans-Ulrich Kauczor[1], Peter M.A. van Ooijen[2], Edwin J.R. van Beek[3] and Matthijs Oudkerk[2]

[1]Department of Diagnostic Radiology, University Hospital Heidelberg, Heidelberg, Germany
[2]Department of Radiology, Academic Medical Center Groningen, Groningen, The Netherlands
[3]Department of Radiology, Carver College of Medicine, Iowa City, USA

INTRODUCTION

Since the introduction of magnetic resonance imaging (MRI) in the late 1970s, the ongoing breakthroughs in this technique have resulted in a versatile modality that offers strong potential for a multitude of evaluation and diagnostic capabilities. Many aspects of the pulmonary circulation have been investigated with MRI, such as pulmonary embolism (PE) (1–8), including clot age determination (4,5), pulmonary hypertension (5,8), blood flow quantification and vessel distensibility (8,9), concomitant deep vein thrombosis (DVT) (10) and congenital abnormalities (11). In addition, therapy monitoring and patient follow-up procedures after elective surgery or anticoagulant treatment can be easily performed non-invasively and may be repeated as often as required (3,4).

Furthermore, fast MRA high spatial or temporal resolution promises to be an alternative for the morphological assessment of the pulmonary vascular tree and the circulatory system with the recent development of state-of-the-art MR angiographic (MRA) techniques and breath-hold scan times (12,13). The routine administration of contrast agents has been recommended to enhance further the pulmonary vasculature and parenchymal signal (14–16).

High-resolution MR pulmonary angiography (MRPA), like other MRI techniques applied to the thorax, requires special attention for the following issues:

- Imaging in the presence of respiratory and cardiac motion (17,18).
- Signal loss from the large magnetic field inhomogeneities present in the thoracic region (extensive air/tissue interfaces). Susceptibility differences lead to irreversible dephasing of the MR signal.
- Limited signal-to-noise ratio (SNR). Poor SNR often requires a longer imaging time, usually improved by averaging multiple acquisitions and consequently image quality could once more be compromised by motion.

Two features in new MRI hardware have jointly made it possible to improve the quality of two-dimensional (2D) and three-dimensional (3D) MRPA. The strength and speed of the gradient system and signal reception using multiphase-array coil technology have provided a several-fold improvement in data encoding speed and volume coverage.

The MR gradient system is the most influential component for imaging of the pulmonary vascular anatomy with good image quality and good coverage. Recent MRI systems have imaging gradients with stronger peak gradient amplitudes ($>40\,$mT/m) and faster rise times ($200\,$mT/m/ms). This results in the following improvements:

- Markedly increased data collection speed by making shorter repeat times (TR) possible; hence fast MRA protocols and high-resolution morphological imaging can be performed in breath-hold imaging times, together with good flexibility for balancing acquisition speed, SNR and resolution per unit time.
- Echo times in the sub-millisecond range may be used, suppressing the effects of magnetic field inhomogeneities in gradient echo (GRE) techniques.
- The execution of gradient events outside the acquisition window can be improved, providing better data sampling efficiency with lower acquisition bandwidths (reduced receiver sampling rates) and increased SNR.

However, increased speed can diminish the SNR in the final image by an increase in acquisition bandwidth (large acquisition bandwidths produce noisier images). Fortunately, recently introduced technologies, such as parallel imaging and multiphase-array coils, increase spatial and/or temporal resolution without a substantial loss of SNR. The breakthrough in MRPA has been possible with a combination of these two features with the application of contrast agents for the generation of increased SNR.

MR SIGNAL FORMATION

Spin echo and gradient echo readouts

A receiver coil acquires the MR signal from transverse magnetization generated after the longitudinal magnetization component stored along the main magnetic field is perturbed by radiofrequency (RF) excitation. This transverse magnetization component can be read either in the form of a spin echo (SE) or a gradient recalled echo.

In a simple SE readout, a 90° RF excitation converts all the longitudinal magnetization available to transverse magnetization and is immediately followed by a 180° RF refocusing pulse to produce a spin echo (Figure 9.1a). A gradient echo readout can collect the MR signal after the application of the 90° RF excitation, but it requires that a bipolar readout imaging gradient be applied to diphase and consequently rephrase the transverse magnetization to form an echo (Figure 9.1b).

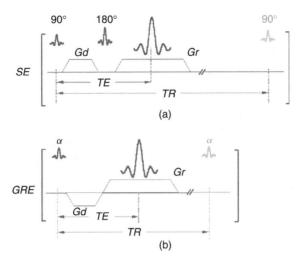

Figure 9.1 Signal formation in MRI. (a) A spin echo requires the application of a 90° RF excitation followed by a refocusing 180° RF pulse to form an echo. (b) The formation of an echo using a GRE readout requires the application of a dephasing gradient that is cancelled by a rephasing gradient to form an echo. The echo formed in SE readouts is insensitive to signal loss from magnetic field inhomogeneities and magnetic susceptibility changes with TE selected to coincide at twice the time interval between the 90°–180° RF pair, in contrast to GRE readouts. Gd, dephasing gradient; Gr, rephasing gradient; TR, repeat time; TE, echo time; α, flip angle/RF excitation angle.

Sensitivity of spin echo and gradient recalled echo imaging to magnetic field inhomogeneities

Both 2D and 3D acquisitions using SE techniques are virtually insensitive to signal loss from field inhomogeneities (immunity to spin dephasing across a voxel, a volume element), losses that mainly arise from differences in the magnetic susceptibility between tissues. Imaging in the thorax and specifically lung parenchyma is especially problematic because of the extensive interfaces between tissue/water and air. The use of scans using SE readouts is optimal in this case. Gradient echo techniques do not share this immunity to field inhomogeneities and are regarded as less adequate for imaging the lung parenchyma.

Two-dimensional GRE techniques present greater sensitivity to signal loss (intravoxel dephasing) than their counterpart 3D GRE scans. Therefore, the latter are selected more often for imaging the pulmonary vasculature. The effect of field inhomogeneities in GRE is voxel dependent and the results are improved with small voxels. Therefore, in addition to the use of the shortest TE possible and a 3D scan, data acquisition should proceed with the largest matrix size available and a large number of sections, all within SNR limits and scan time. These considerations minimize the intravoxel dephasing, making GRE techniques compare more closely to SE techniques, and provide a fast alternative to imaging in the thoracic region.

Signal manipulation and image contrast

In conventional SE imaging, proton-density, T1- and T2-weighted images are acquired by setting a specific repetition time (TR) and echo time (TE). Proton-density weighting may be acquired by using long TR and short TE. T2 weighting is adjusted by lengthening TE. Intermediate values of TR with short TE produce T1-weighted images. The rigid $90°-180°$ combination in conventional SE readouts slows the longitudinal magnetization recovery, restricting the maximum possible signal that may be requested for a particular TR. Imaging techniques using GRE readouts, on the other hand, can modify the RF excitation or flip angle ($\leq 90°$, partial flip angle imaging) to produce optimal signal strength for a specific tissue at a fixed TR value. The flexibility of GRE techniques to use partial flip angles provides proton density, T1-, T2-, T2*- and T1/T2-weighted images with short TR settings that makes it more compatible for breath-hold imaging.

It is important to note that recently introduced scans using SE readout variants, referred to as fast SE, make them competitive with GRE scans for fast imaging in the thorax with good SNR and resolution and single-shot imaging capabilities. Fast SE techniques make use of multiple refocusing $180°$ RF pulses after the initial $90°$ RF excitation and are discussed in more detail below.

MR DATA ACQUISITION

The k-space matrix

The acquired MR signal is sorted into a matrix of discrete points that has been termed the k-space matrix (Figure 9.2). The k-space is defined as the spatial frequency domain and it contains the spatial frequencies that represent the number of sinc wave cycles per unit length of an object. An inverse discrete fast Fourier transform (IFFT) is applied to this matrix to produce an anatomical image. The k-space matrix can be multidimensional, e.g., to resolve an object in three dimensions a 3D k-space matrix is collected and processed.

Relation between k-space and image signal and contrast

Thr k-space contains information that provides all spatial frequencies acquired to form the complete image and not only a portion. However, the information in the central portion and that towards the edges of the k-space matrix defines completely different image features. The central portion of

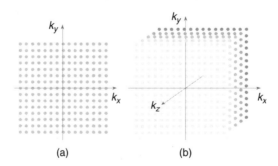

(a)   (b)

Figure 9.2   The k-space matrix denotes the spatial-frequency domain. The digitized MR signal is stored in this domain into a 2D (a) or a 3D (b) array of points to reconstruct a 2D or a 3D representation of the object after the application of an inverse fast Fourier transform (FFT). The time interval between phase encoding steps (in-plane and along the section select phase encoding directions) is usually associated with TR, the repetition time of the MRI experiment. In general, all points along the readout (frequency encoding) direction (k_x) are collected for each MR signal reception event. k_x, Frequency encoding direction; k_y, in-plane phase encoding direction; k_z, section select phase encoding direction.

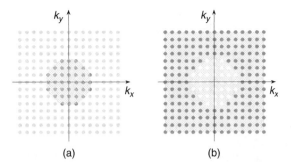

(a) (b)

Figure 9.3 Each portion of k-space has different weightings in the image domain. (a) The centre of k-space (low spatial frequencies) mostly contains information about the resulting image contrast. (b) On the other hand, the edges of k-space are associated with edge information and, therefore, are linked to image resolution. Objects that are very small (on the order of a pixel or a voxel in 2D and 3D, respectively) contain energy that is spread over all k-space points. k_x, Frequency encoding direction; k_y, in-plane phase encoding direction.

the k-space matrix (low spatial frequencies) relates to the contrast between tissues (Figure 9.3a). Data points towards the edges of the k-space matrix (high spatial frequencies) characterize the smaller details and edge information in the image (Figure 9.3b).

Hence the knowledge of the contribution of each portion of the k-space matrix to the resulting image is important and has many practical implications with respect to image contrast, SNR and resolution, especially in magnetization-prepared GRE acquisitions and acquisitions occurring during the transient T1 shortening induced in the blood pool with dynamic contrast injections as in contrast-enhanced MRPA.

2D and 3D imaging times

The time-varying MR signal received is digitized to form a row of data (frequency encoding process, 1D encoding). In general, to resolve a 2D or 3D acquisition the MR signal must be repeatedly acquired and phase-encoded accordingly to form an image or a volume data set. Assuming that a single in-plane phase encoding step is acquired per TR, the time necessary to encode a 2D image is determined by

$$\text{Acquisition time 2D} = (N_y \times \text{TR})N_{acq} \tag{9.1}$$

where N_y indicates the number of in-plane phase encoding steps and N_{acq} the number of signal averages performed. An extra phase encoding is required to resolve sections in a 3D acquisition. Defining the number of sections 3D partitions as N_z, the acquisition time is given by

$$\text{Acquisition time 3D} = (N_y \times \text{TR})N_z N_{acq} \tag{9.2}$$

The time to acquire a 3D data set amounts to that of a 2D acquisition weighted by the number of sections desired. The imaging time for 2D and 3D acquisitions is the same if the number of sections acquired is identical. The 3D acquisitions present an additional advantage: if all imaging parameters are kept the same (TR, TE, flip angle) as in its counterpart 2D technique, the SNR of 3D acquisitions increases as the square root of the number of partitions collected.

Equations (9.1) and (9.2) only represent the imaging time in the very general case. The scan time for the 2D and 3D techniques can be shortened appropriately depending on specific phase encoding strategies (see below). Shortening the scan time makes it possible to collect data using breath-holds and eliminate some of the detrimental effects that respiratory motion produces on 2D and 3D images.

Motion sensitivity of 2D and 3D imaging

Three-dimensional acquisitions are most appealing for thoracic and pulmonary vascular imaging because of their SNR possibilities and reduced sensitivity to field inhomogeneities. However, 3D acquisitions present a serious drawback with respect to motion artefacts. Each section of a 2D acquisition is independent of the others acquired, whereas in 3D, sections are reconstructed after the data acquisition has been completed (slice-select phase encoding). Thus, for 3D acquisitions the motion artefacts propagate across the entire data set whereas in 2D they will remain constrained to the slices where motion occurred. Therefore, imaging planes and phase encoding directions must be carefully chosen to minimize ghosting artefacts over the lung parenchyma.

k-Space ordering

Two basic ordering schemes are used most commonly during the filling of k-space: sequential and centric ordering. Additional k-space ordering schemes (e.g., spiral, elliptical ordering) that are important for contrast-enhanced MRPA are discussed below.

Sequential ordering is standard in most MRI and MRA techniques used. Denoting N_y as the number of in-plane phase encoding lines chosen for screening a 2D imaging strategy, k-space is acquired from its most negative value of the phase encoding table, $-N_y/2$, and increases linearly towards the most positive value, $N_y/2 - 1$ (Figure 9.4a). This is equivalent to first filling the negative high spatial frequency information, traversing through the centre of k-space during the middle of the acquisition and ending up collecting the positive higher spatial frequencies. The

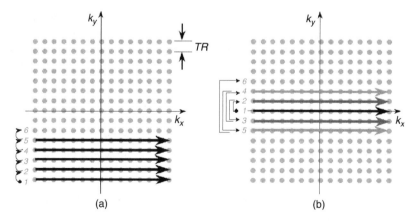

(a)   (b)

Figure 9.4 Sequential and centric phase encoding schemes. (a) With a sequential phase encoding order, the phase encoding table scans k-space linearly from its most negative value as defined by the maximum number of lines collected, N_y, to its most positive value. The centre of k-space is acquired during the middle of the scan. (b) During centric phase encoding ordering, data are collected starting from the centre of k-space and the phase encoding table values toggle about this point to collect the positive and negative values of k-space one at the time. The arrows between k-space lines indicate the succession of the lines collected. k_x, Frequency encoding direction; k_y, in-plane phase encoding direction; TR, repetition time.

centre of k-space may be acquired asymmetrically in some techniques to manipulate the image contrast more adequately, e.g., with partial Fourier scanning and contrast-enhanced MRPA.

Centric ordering first encodes the centre of k-space before toggling back and forth between negative and positive phase encoding values to collect the number of N_y lines set (Figure 9.4b). Thus, the first view acquired is 0, continuing to collect phase encoding lines 1,−1, 2,−2, and so forth until reaching the highest spatial frequencies (set $N_y/2$). This scheme is used specifically to ensure that image contrast, e.g., as set by a magnetization preparation scheme, can be obtained in the reconstructed image virtually independent of sequence scanning parameters. The scheme has also been used for scans that commence data collection when a particular condition is reached and the contrast that develops should be encoded at that particular moment, as 'smart preparation' or 'care bolus' in contrast-enhanced MRPA.

k-Space segmentation is a concept that is associated with shorter scan times and corresponds to one of the many concepts that are used exclusively in fast MRI, particularly for fast SE scans. In essence, k-space segmentation is a data collection strategy that is mainly used to fit in two particular situations:

- To share a contrast that is prepared among several lines of data collected. This is used to improve the quality of magnetization-prepared GRE scans. It serves the purpose of eliminating the time required to repeat particular events, such as a presaturation band or a pause between a string of RF excitations executed very rapidly, that would be applied for each phase encoding line.
- To collect more data that are to be synchronized with a specific physiological event, e.g., data collection during systolic or diastolic events, by lowering the time resolution of the dynamic event encoded but making it possible to collect breath-hold cine acquisitions by virtue of the time reduction involved.

The time-saving factor involved during k-space segmentation can only be envisioned with the above situations. When this is the case, this accounts for a reduction in scanning time that is proportional to the number of lines collected. k-Space segmentation is usually performed in a sequential interleaved fashion (Figure 9.5), that is, to collect lines as in the sequential ordering case (see above) but with phase encoding jumps equal to the number of shots that must be performed to fill the number of phase encoding lines of the matrix size chosen. The sequential interleaved order reduces ghosting artefacts that can appear from the step-like changes in amplitude or phase in the raw data between the lines encoded by each echo.

This strategy has been used in 2D and 3D MRPA in scans that necessitate the elimination of signal from unwanted structures with a time-efficient scheme, such as the use of saturation bands to suppress venous or arterial components. k-Space segmentation is also used to produce breath-hold scans that synchronize data collection with a specific phase of the cardiac cycle, e.g., to maximize contrast between an embolus and blood when blood inflow effects are at a maximum during systole or minimize flow dephasing effects in diastole.

Shortening the data collection time

Rectangular field-of-view (RecFOV) makes it possible to increase the resolution per unit time or maintain resolution with shorter scanning when an object does not fill the entire view along the in-plane phase encoding direction for a predefined FOV. The decrease in imaging time possible is performed by scaling down the original number of in-plane phase encoding lines by the ratio between the extent of the object along the in-plane phase encoding direction and the predefined FOV. During scanning, the phase encoding gradients are amplified accordingly by this ratio while the image is compressed after the IFFT is performed to produce the correct aspect ratio.

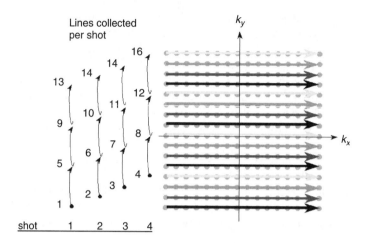

Figure 9.5   With k-space segmentation, a limited number of lines that share similar contrast characteristics are collected in rapid succession and placed in the raw data matrix. The pattern displayed is a sequential interleaved. In this example, k-space is composed of a 16 × 16 matrix and four shots collecting four k-space lines each were chosen to encode the matrix. The lines are encoded in sequential order, e.g., 1, 5, 9, 13 for the first shot. If cardiac synchronization is used, four heart cycles are required to fill the entire matrix. The curved arrows between k-space lines indicate the succession of the lines collected. k_x, Frequency encoding direction; k_y, in-plane phase encoding direction.

For both 2D and 3D measurements, the acquisition time can be nearly halved by collecting half of the k-space data and using several post-processing algorithms to recover the complete resolution (Figure 9.6). This is known as partial Fourier imaging (19–21). This is possible because of the conjugate symmetry of the Fourier transform that permits recreation of the k-space portion that was not acquired. Partial Fourier imaging along the in-plane phase encoding direction (Figure 9.6a) or along the frequency encoding direction (Figure 9.6b) can be used effectively to decrease the scan time without a decrease in resolution. The first option is more widely known and used, consisting of decreasing the number of scanned k-space lines. Partial Fourier imaging along the frequency encoding is particularly useful for shortening TR in MRPA scans by collecting only a partial number of points, therefore shortening the readout window and consequently TR. In this case, the time saving will be greater with lower readout bandwidths.

Partial Fourier imaging applied to GRE techniques with very short echo times (TE <2 ms) can be attempted for MRPA without major artefacts. Phase cancellation from out-of-phase water–fat condition distorts the phase estimate but this is not a problem for imaging the pulmonary vasculature, as there is minimal contribution from fat signal in the lungs. Partial Fourier imaging has a small drawback with respect to SNR, generating images that can be noisier by a factor of $\sqrt{2}$ (at most, half of the phase encoding steps are acquired as compared with full k-space coverage). Several partial Fourier algorithms have also been devised that are more robust for reconstructing images generated with GRE techniques. The main difference between the available partial Fourier algorithms is the sensitivity of the reconstructed image magnetic field inhomogeneities and flowing blood (22).

In general, the conventional data encoding process collects a rectangle or a rectangular volume of data points to form a 2D or 3D k-space data set, respectively. However, isotropic resolution data sets for 2D images or 3D volumes are produced by collecting all data points to conform to the area of an ellipse or an ellipsoidal volume in the k-space domain, respectively, with the appropriate radius as required by the FOV in each axis. For scans in which the FOV in all encoding directions

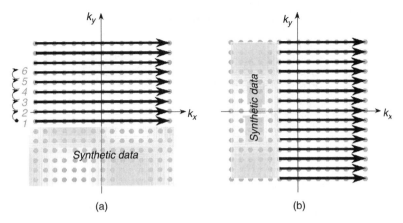

Figure 9.6 Partial Fourier acquisition of k-space. Ideally, only half of the k-space data are necessary to reconstruct an image without any loss in resolution. (a) Partial Fourier along the in-plane phase encoding direction. (b) Partial Fourier along the frequency encoding direction. Both strategies are useful to decrease imaging time, decreasing the number of lines or the TR used for imaging, respectively. (c) MIP image of a 3D MRPA scan collected with an echo asymmetric in the frequency encoding direction. (d) MIP image with the data processed with partial Fourier along the frequency encoding direction. Echo asymmetry was approximately 31% (40 points rather than 128 points collected before the echo for a 256-point readout). The resolution enhancement is not as apparent on the MIP as compared with the original sections. There is an SNR penalty (maximum loss of $\sqrt{2}$) and also fidelity in the reconstruction depending on the particular partial Fourier algorithm selected. k_x, Frequency encoding direction; k_y, in-plane phase encoding direction.

and the number of data points collected are the same, the data conform to a circle or a sphere in k-space for 2D and 3D imaging, respectively, with a diameter equal to the scanned imaging matrix.

The statement above suggests that the edges of k-space for a rectangular area or a rectangular volume of k-space data do not necessarily contribute actively in the resolution of the reconstructed images (unless the data are interpolated by zero filling to a higher matrix size; see below). Therefore, the time necessary to acquire the edges of k-space can be spared. The potential time savings are represented by the ratio between the area or volume to be encoded and that covered in the conventional case. For example, a cubic volume can be encoded using a cylinder or a sphere of k-space data (Figure 9.7) to cut the imaging time by approximately 21% and 48%, respectively.

Cylindrical acquisitions are straightforward to implement for 3D imaging and require a predetermined filling pattern that will depend only on the acquisition strategy used, e.g., normal or contrast-enhanced imaging. Although the time saving is greater if an ellipsoid is encoded, it is impossible to describe an adequate k-space trajectory with conventional signal readouts (remember that there is no inherent time saving with a conventional frequency encoding as it is possible to collect any arbitrary number of points). Therefore, special 3D k-space trajectories have been formulated that employ time-varying imaging gradients during data collection (stack of spirals, cones, etc.) (23).

The utilization of interpolation to produce isotropic voxels (cubic volume elements), despite the size of the k-space data collected, has been advantageous for MRA to improve the overall display of vascular structures, especially for small vascular branches. Interpolation can be performed in the image domain but it is more efficient and is more beneficial when it is performed using the raw data directly. The best interpolation possible is known as sinc interpolation. This is accomplished by placing the original raw data collected into a larger 2D or 3D matrix (reconstruction matrix) and zero-filling those k-space values that have not been collected (most commonly the outer edges

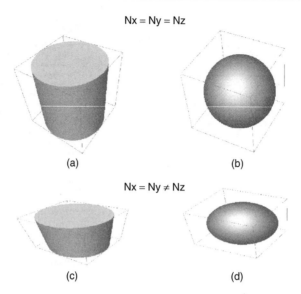

$N_x = N_y = N_z$

(a)   (b)

$N_x = N_y \neq N_z$

(c)   (d)

Figure 9.7   Reducing the scan time is important for scanning patients with documented PE and essential if breath-hold imaging is performed. Time saving is practical for 3D imaging. Using a cylindrical coverage (a) or a sphere (b), the scan time can be reduced by 21 and 48%, respectively, compared with a cubic data set (time saving proportional to the ratio between the volumes scanned and that of a cube). (c) and (d) show the cases for 3D when the number of points along the k_z axis is different from k_x and k_y. There is no loss in resolution in either case. N_x, N_y and N_z define the number of points collected along each k-space direction.

of k-space) prior to image reconstruction using the IFFT. The improved vascular presentation is appreciated mostly in regions where the vessel would otherwise display a clear staircase pattern with the original reconstruction matrix (Figure 9.8).

There is an additional advantage to interpolation by zero-filling, that is, it can compensate for some of the signal loss that may arise from intravoxel phase cancellation (reducing the phase dispersion caused by flow dephasing or field inhomogeneities across a smaller reconstructed voxel) (24). This property is clearly desirable for MRPA because it helps to reduce the dephasing occurring from magnetic field susceptibility differences.

Sinc interpolation is becoming increasingly popular for producing 3D image data sets with isotropic voxels without the need to increase the acquisition time, especially for breath-hold examinations. The reconstructed resolution will not be higher than that of the originally collected raw data. Nonetheless, when conventional encoding is performed (a cubic data set), the k-space values at the edges of the raw data can now help to improve the resolution. Interpolation requires additional memory to perform the computation and storage space for a larger data set.

Spiral encoding of k-space trajectories is becoming increasingly popular (Figure 9.9) (25) and has already been applied to the pulmonary vasculature (26). Spiral encoding describes a spiral trajectory through k-space using two gradients oscillated in tandem in the imaging plane. Spiral scanning is intrinsically flow compensated (the centre of k-space is collected first) and reduces many of the blurring and displacement artefacts when visualizing flowing blood. Additionally, the gradient moments of a spiral trajectory are small near the origin of k-space, smoothly varying and circularly symmetric over k-space. Rewinding is inherent in a spiral trajectory and does not require the extreme hardware requirements to achieve short TE. Acquisition is approximately 27% faster than with standard spin warp encoding (time savings are proportional to the area ratio between a square and a circle).

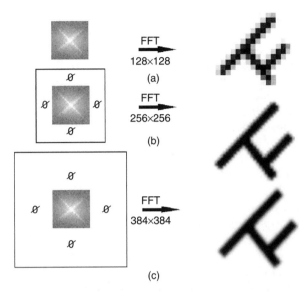

Figure 9.8 Improvements in the vascular display using raw data interpolation by zero filling. The process depicted considers zero filling of the raw data to a larger matrix and the application of an inverse Fourier transform to produce the interpolated image with smaller isotropic voxels. Using a raw data set of 128×128 points, a simulated structure is reconstructed showing a staircase pattern (a). After zero filling, the interpolation to a matrix size that is twice (256×256 points) (b) or three times (384×384 points) (c) the original size can produce a much better display of the structure without the necessity for an increased scan time. By using this type of interpolation, the smaller voxels reconstructed can also present less phase dispersion and therefore can regain some signal loss from phase effects that can prevail across the original voxel size.

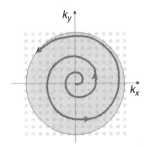

Figure 9.9 Time saving is possible for 2D using a circular coverage of k-space, e.g., using a spiral k-space trajectory. The acquisition is approximately 27% faster than that of a standard spin warp encoding. The trajectory makes it possible for ultrashort TE imaging and it is inherently flow compensated. The gradients are oscillated in tandem to describe the trajectory. k_x, Frequency encoding direction; k_y, in-plane phase encoding direction.

Alternatively, centric or elliptic-centric imaging, where equidistant points are sampled at the same time from k-space centre towards the periphery and filling of the centre of k-space in random order (CENTRA) have been introduced (27). Spiral imaging is very fast, has sufficient SNR and is increasingly often used for time-resolved imaging as it conveniently allows easy k-space undersampling. Both spiral and elliptic-centric trajectories are insensitive to venous superimposition as the acquisition of the k-space centre and, hence, the determination of the image contrast takes place at the beginning of the initial arterial vessel enhancement prior to venous return. On the other hand, they are even more susceptible to missed bolus timing. CENTRA is a robust approach for k-space filling.

Radial imaging, a newly arising imaging technique, allows for very fast imaging and has inherent undersampling properties as central and peripheral parts of k-space are acquired at the same time. An image can be reconstructed from just a few sampled views. However, with too few views acquired there are characteristic reconstruction artefacts, so called streak artefacts, which can only be alleviated with an increased number of sampled views.

Conventional and fast SE techniques

Conventional SE techniques acquire one line of data per TR. Even for a multi-echo SE scan, commonly performed to acquire images at different echo times during the same imaging session, e.g., proton-density and T2-weighted together, a single line of data is collected per image per TR. This can be a lengthy acquisition process when a long TR is required.

Fast SE (FSE) techniques have been conceived to reduce the scanning time without a significant loss in contrast (Figure 9.10) (28,29). Fast SE features the same idea as in multi-echo SE scans but encodes the echoes generated in the same k-space matrix using the concept of k-space segmentation. The decrease in encoding time is specially noted for long T2-weighted scans using long TR. FSE imaging shares the great advantage from conventional SE with respect to insensitivity to magnetic field inhomogeneities and presents, among other things, a better SNR profile than most GRE scans. Although the initial application of RARE was geared to produce heavily T2-weighted images (CSF myelography and urography), the introduction of new imaging hardware and the addition of partial Fourier data collection and reconstruction permit snapshot scans with good

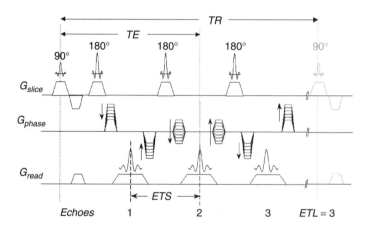

Figure 9.10 Fast SE imaging. A 90° RF excitation pulse is followed by a string of 180° refocusing RF pulses that are closely spaced. One echo is generated for each 180° RF pulse applied. The separation between the 180° or the echoes is known as the echo train spacing or ETS. The signal of the echo train generated decays with the T2 relaxation of the tissues imaged. The echoes are usually encoded in k-space using a sequential interleaved trajectory (see Figure 9.5). The echo that coincides with the centre of k-space determines mainly the image contrast. In this example, three echoes are collected. The second echo weights the resulting image contrast. The scan time is one-third of that for a conventional SE readout. TR is defined as the total time necessary per shot. N_y, number of in-plane phase encoding lines; $N_{shot} = N_y/ETL$, number of shots; G_{read}, readout gradient; G_{phase}, in-plane phase encoding; G_{slice}, section select gradient; ETL, echo train length; ETS, echo train spacing.

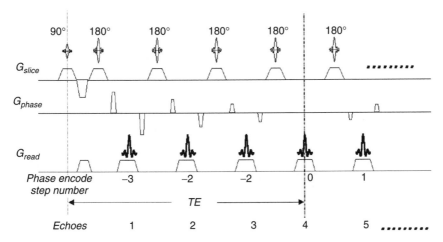

Figure 9.11 HASTE (half Fourier acquisition with Turbo SE) imaging. Partial Fourier encoding is applied to shorten the scan time by half. The contrast is defined by the echo that is made to coincide with the centre of k-space (the fourth echo in the diagram). The echo train length (ETL) is equal to the number the number of in-plane phase encoding steps, N_y. The TR is infinite because of the single shot nature of the scan. G_{read}, readout gradient; G_{phase}, in-plane phase encoding; G_{slice}, section select gradient; ETL, echo train length; ETS, echo train spacing.

SNR and sub-second imaging times. This has made it possible to incorporate the use of HASTE (Half Fourier Acquisition Single shot Turbo spin Echo) imaging (Figure 9.11) (30). HASTE has been used in many applications but its major asset is the short scanning time, making it possible to collect images in uncooperative patients and scan in the thorax without the necessity for breath-holding. Because the image is collected under a long echo train decaying with T2, blurring along the in-plane phase encoding is generally observed for tissues with short T2 relaxation times. The amount of blurring is dictated by the T2 relaxation time of each tissue with respect to the length of the acquisition.

Gradient recalled echo imaging

GRE imaging offers a variety of tissue contrast possibilities that can be generated in the same imaging time without changing TR, the opposite to what is generally possible with SE readouts. Proton-density, T1-, T2- and T1/T2-weighting are possible depending on the strength and state of the transverse and longitudinal magnetization components for a particular T1 and T2 and a choice of TR and RF excitation angle.

There are two major distinctions between GRE sequences, depending on the state of the longitudinal and transverse magnetization. Steady-state incoherent (SSI) GRE techniques refer to those techniques in which only the longitudinal magnetization is used during the acquisition. Techniques that combine both longitudinal and transverse magnetization components to generate the signal are referred to as steady-state coherent (SSC) GRE techniques.

In SSI GRE techniques, the signal contribution to the image formation comes exclusively from longitudinal magnetization recovered between two successive RF excitations. The acronym FLASH (Fast Low Angle SHot) has been used extensively (other acronyms are RF-spoiled GRASS or SPGR, spoiled Gradient Recalled Acquisition in the Steady State) [see Haacke and Frahm (31) for a summary of all abbreviations used by system manufacturers for most techniques clinically available]. Figure 9.12 illustrates a typical 3D FLASH sequence diagram. The signal intensity

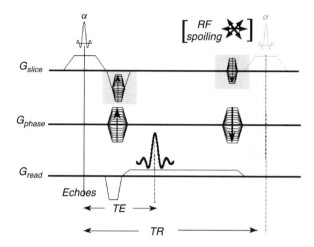

Figure 9.12 Diagram of a 3D SSI GRE imaging technique primarily referred to as FLASH (fast low angle shot) imaging. The use of RF spoiling (changing the phase of the RF angle per phase encoding step) in conjunction with rewinder phase encoding tables after reading the signal is effective for producing signal that is weighted by only the longitudinal magnetization component during steady-state conditions. FLASH is also known as RF-spoiled gradient recalled acquisition in the steady-state (RF-spoiled GRASS).

for SSI GRE techniques assumes no contribution from transverse magnetization prior to each RF excitation to the signal formation, resulting in a very well known expression:

$$S = \frac{M_0 \sin\alpha (1 - E1) E2^*}{1 - \cos\alpha E1} \tag{9.3}$$

where α is the RF flip angle, $E1 = \exp(-TR/T1)$ and $E2^* = \exp(-TE/T2^*)$. This expression is important for setting the optimal imaging parameter corresponding to a specific T1 relaxation time.

For sufficiently small flip angles and short TR, the image contrast is predominantly proton-density weighted ($S \sim M_0\sin\alpha$); otherwise, T1 contrast can develop at larger flip angles. T2* weighting can only be generated by lengthening TE, making the image more sensitive to signal loss from susceptibility changes between air/tissue interfaces (or within a blood clot). Figure 9.13 illustrates the signal behaviour for various T1 relaxation values and TR. For SSI GRE imaging applied at a particular TR, the maximum signal can be obtained by choosing the RF excitation at the optimal angle, usually referred to as the Ernst angle or α_E (E tref). The Ernst angle is given by

$$\alpha_E = \cos^{-1}(E1) \tag{9.4}$$

At α_E (E tref), the signal will be

$$S\alpha_E = \sqrt{\frac{1 - E1}{1 + E1}} \tag{9.5}$$

which is roughly proportional to $\sqrt{(TR/2T1)}$. For a fixed TR, the Ernst angle decreases as T1 increases and, vice versa, a decrease in T1 will increase the Ernst angle. Figure 9.13d illustrates the signal behaviour for a fixed T1 and a varying TR, indicating that higher flip angles are necessary to obtain the optimal signal at longer TR. Maximum contrast between two tissues occurs at a flip

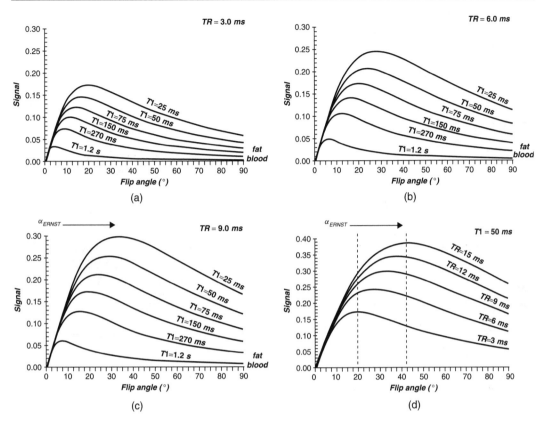

Figure 9.13 Signal intensity behaviour for SSI GRE techniques (FLASH imaging). Simulations performed for different values of TR for several T1 relaxation values as a function of flip angle: (a) TR = 3.0 ms, (b) TR = 6.0 ms and (c) TR = 9.0 ms. Note in (c) the arrow indicating that the Ernst angle, the RF excitation that produces optimal SNR, increases as the T1 relaxation decreases at a fixed TR. In (d), a fixed T1 of 50 illustrates that optimal SNR is met at increasing RF flip angles with longer TRs. T1 relaxation values considered were 25, 50, 75, 150, 270 and 1200 ms. The longest values correspond to the T1 relaxation of fat and blood, respectively. Short T1 relaxation values were chosen to illustrate the enhancement possible when using paramagnetic and superparamagnetic contrast agents to enhance the signal of blood.

angle different than the Ernst angle. All the above equations are necessary to calculate the optimal excitation for contrast-enhanced MRA scans.

Generally, GRE sequences for MRPA will refer to the application of SSI GRE techniques. A magnetization preparation (MP) period prior to a short TR SSI GRE sequence (a FLASH sequence), as depicted in Figure 9.14, can modify effectively the initial longitudinal magnetization to produce an image with improved contrast with sub-second SSI GRE acquisitions. This technique is known as turboFLASH imaging (32).

Increased T1 weighting is possible after the application of an inversion pulse (Figure 9.14a). A T2 magnetization preparation scheme or magnetization transfer pulses can also be applied (Figure 9.14b and 9.14c, respectively). A special preparation that has been increasingly used in later years for many techniques is referred to as a black blood preparation or PRESTO, illustrated in Figure 9.14d (33). The methodology of MP SSI GRE scans has been applied effectively for the detection of pulmonary emboli for 2D and 3D scans. Additionally, the T1-weighted turboFLASH sequence is generally used for timing the delivery of contrast material in contrast-enhanced MRPA scans.

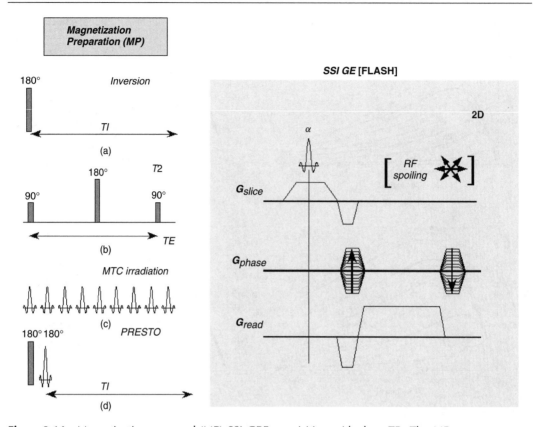

Figure 9.14 Magnetization prepared (MP) SSI GRE acquisition with short TR. The MP stage may consist of a simple 180° pre-inversion pulse (inversion–recovery) to provide strong T1-weighting (a). A 90°x–180°y–90°x driven equilibrium pulse scheme produces T2-weighting (b). A long train of RF pulses can be used to augment the magnetization transfer contrast (MTC) and accentuate signal attenuation in tissues with higher density of bound water molecules (c). A black blood preparation can be used (d). This executes a non-selective inversion over the entire imaging volume immediately followed by a selective inversion to restore full magnetization in the imaging slice. For (d), imaging is performed after a suitable delay time (inversion time of blood, TI = T1 × ln 2 ≈ 800 ms) that permits the inflow of initially inverted blood into the imaging region and procures a null longitudinal magnetization to render blood black. This MP is known as a PRESTO preparation and is used in a multitude of imaging scenarios to help eliminate the signal from blood while maintaining a high SNR for stationary tissues. FLASH, fast low angle shot; TE, echo time; TI, inversion time; G_{slice}, slice selection gradient; G_{phase}, phase encoding gradient; G_{read}, frequency encoding gradient; α, RF flip angle.

A transient behaviour develops, related to the approach to the steady-state, between the prepared longitudinal magnetization and the signal obtained during the application of the string of RF excitations that is used to form the signal. During this transient, the signal can be encoded. The equation that drives the signal evolution of different magnetization preparation SSI experiments is

$$M_0 \sin\alpha [M_s + (M_t - M_s)r^{n-1}] \qquad (9.6)$$

for $n \geqslant 1$, in which the term M_t is directly related to the state of the magnetization after the application of the particular RF scheme that will encode the desired contrast (T1, T2, diffusion weighting, etc.). Equation 9.7 indicates some useful values for M_t:

$$M_t = 1 \tag{9.7a}$$

$$M_t = (1 - 2E_{TI}) \tag{9.7b}$$

where $E1 = \exp(-TR/T1)$, $r = E1\cos\alpha$, $M_s = (1 - E1)/(1 - r)$, $E_{TI} = \exp(-TI/T1)$, $E_{TW} = \exp(-TW/T1)$ and $q = E_{TW}\cos\alpha$. Equation (9.7a) demonstrates that the longitudinal magnetization starts from M_0 for a sample 2D SSI GRE scan that collects data during the approach to the steady state. Equation (9.7b) is the typical signal received when the MP is an inversion pulse where TI is the inversion time to the start of data collection.

The approach to the steady state produces different signal strengths during data encoding. This introduces a filter function that can affect the resolution and the appearance of each tissue depending on their size relative to the imaging FOV and the specific pattern utilized to fill k-space. The filter function is complex but may be regarded as a high-pass filter that enhances sharp features such as edges and tissue boundaries. Edge enhancement is more prominent with an inversion pulse used for the magnetization preparation, which is important for morphological imaging and for detection of pulmonary emboli.

Parallel imaging

Since its introduction in the late 1990s (34,35) parallel imaging has revolutionized MRA. The technical prerequisites for parallel imaging are coil systems with multiple coil elements providing spatially differing sensitivity profiles, allowing for acquisition of data with all coil elements simultaneously. Parallel imaging systemically under-samples the k-space and thus reduces the acquisition time (36). The images are reconstructed from the under-sampled data set either in the image domain using the known sensitivity profiles (SENSE) or in the k-space domain using reconstruction weights (GRAPPA). GRAPPA seems to be somewhat superior as it is less susceptible to patient motion and aliasing artefacts, which are more common for MRA with a limited FOV in the right–left direction (37).With a typical acceleration factor of 2, every second line in k-space is skipped, which leads to a reduction in scan time of approximately 50% (38). This reduced acquisition time can also be traded for higher spatial resolution, resulting in a voxel size of $1.2 \times 1.0 \times 1.6$ mm requiring an acquisition period and also a breath hold of 20–30 s. The trade-off which the user has to accept for the reduction in scan time or the higher spatial resolution is a decreased SNR, which is inversely proportional to the square root of the acceleration factor times a geometry factor that is mainly determined by the coil design (34). Due to the higher available SNR, contrast-enhanced MRA is well suited for the application of parallel imaging. In the case of an acceleration factor of 2, the best available yielding signal is 71% of the original signal. Although an acceleration factor of 3 seems to be acceptable for the renal arteries (39), an acceleration factor of 2 is usually recommended for the pulmonary arteries. It should be noted that backfolding artefacts in the centre of the image can appear if acceleration factors of 2 are used in a coronal acquisition. To overcome this problem, patients are scanned with their arms above their heads, which may cause discomfort in some patients (36).

All vendors now offer multi-element array coils which allow parallel imaging with acceleration factors of at least 2 in the right–left phase-encode direction. Parallel imaging with a factor of 2 can be used in anterior–posterior phase-encode direction when a separate spine and body coil are used. Recent developments comprise multi-element body coils with up to 32 elements, which further enable faster imaging with higher acceleration factors of at least 3 in the phase-encoding direction. Apart from the good signal (despite the shortened acquisition time), the combination of 3 T and parallel imaging results in additional benefits for MRA. The doubled SNR at 3 T offers enough SNR for increasing the spatial resolution in combination with higher factors of parallel imaging, e.g., factor 4, without a visible degradation in image quality. MRA sequences are largely unaffected by the typical dielectric artefacts and increased susceptibility at 3 T. Whereas the increase of SNR at 3 T is desirable for parallel imaging, the four-fold increase in the specific absorption rate (SAR) is an undesired characteristic of 3 T imaging. Due to the reduced overall number of excitations that are needed when only a fraction of k-space is read out with parallel imaging, the SAR can be reduced and hence imaging limitations can be avoided. In return, however, as fewer pulses are applied in a shorter time, the stimulation threshold may be surpassed. Thus, parallel imaging helps effectively in reducing the SAR but choosing the shortest TR is not recommended due to the above-mentioned limitations.

With the use of parallel imaging and its decrease in image acquisition time, timing of the contrast administration becomes even more crucial, in particular with centric k-space filling. It seems that the contamination of image quality by venous signal decreased when centric approaches and parallel imaging were combined and image acquisition was timed correctly. As parallel imaging leads to a decrease in the SNR, the application of novel contrast agents may be beneficial and a variety of new agents have been applied, including 1 M gadobutrol (Bayer Schering), the high-relaxivity gadobenate dimeglumine (Bracco) and the intravascular protein-binding gadofosveset (Bayer Schering). These seem to offer better enhancement during the first pass of the contrast agent in the body, which may not necessarily hold true for the pulmonary arteries, and further research needs to focus on their potential benefits for MRPA. By the combination of the latest technical developments, such as 32-channel chest coil, 3 T field strength, high-relaxivity contrast agent, acceleration factor of 6 and the acquisition of isotropic ($1 \times 1 \times 1$ mm) voxels, the entire pulmonary circulation can now be covered in less than 20 s (40).

MR PROPERTIES OF LUNG PARENCHYMA, BLOOD AND BLOOD CLOTS

Three tissue MR parameters have been predominantly used to produce the differentiation between tissues: the proton density, the T1 relaxation time (rate of recovery of the longitudinal magnetization) and the T2 relaxation time (rate of decay of the transverse magnetization). Only the last two can be exploited adequately to provide the necessary differentiation between blood and blood clots. The water distribution and relaxation times of lung parenchyma are difficult to quantify due to the cyclic alteration of blood flow through the vessels, cardiac output, vascular permeability and changes in position and inflation during respiration. There is a large difference in the amount of blood present proportional to lung tissue and interstitial fluid in the least dependent areas when compared with that seen in the lower zones of the lung where the vasculature is distended with blood.

The composition of the lung is gravity dependent and this contributes to the complexity of the data interpretation. The various perfusion zones help create a continuous change in the lung composition from the least dependent to the most dependent areas. Thus, the proton density and relaxation parameters are related to the proportion of blood in relation to air, lung tissue and interstitial fluid and differences should be expected depending on the measurement site. A more detailed description of the magnetic properties of lung parenchyma has been compiled by Cutillo (41).

The MR signal of blood is proportional to its proton density, which is similar to that of other tissues and constituents. The relaxation times in blood have been found to be a linear function of the haematocrit (H). This is a direct consequence of the fast exchange occurring between the intracellular and extracellular water due to the random passage of water molecules, particularly between the plasma and the red blood cells (RBCs) (42–44). The relaxation rates of blood, R_{blood},

Table 9.1 Relaxation times for blood and plasma. T2 measurements performed with a Carr–Purcell–Meiboom–Gill sequence using an interpulse spacing of 3 ms

Variable[a]	T1 (ms)	T2 (ms)
Anticoagulant plasma		
EDTA	1754	455
Citrate	1786	526
Heparin	1563	455
Blood		
EDTA	1124	181
Citrate	1042	222
Heparin	1064	182

[a]EDTA, sodium ethylenediaminetetraacetate; citrate, sodium citrate. Adapted from Reference 42.

depend predominantly on the relaxation rates of the RBCs, $1/f_c$ and the plasma, $1/f_p$, weighted by the relative population of protons existing in each environment, f_c and f_p, respectively (see Table 9.1). This may be reflected in:

$$R_{blood} = \frac{f_c}{T_c} + \frac{f_p}{T_p}$$
$$= \frac{H}{T_c} + \frac{1-H}{T_p}$$
$$= \frac{1}{T_c} + H\left(\frac{1}{T_c} + \frac{1}{T_p}\right) \tag{9.8}$$

Paramagnetic relaxation effects are usually not seen in most tissues. Blood is an exception in that its properties are strongly coupled to the presence of haemoglobin (Hb) in the RBCs and its oxidation states. Hence the relaxation in whole blood is similar to that of an Hb solution, despite the effects of membrane exchanges and of plasma proteins (45,46). Haemoglobin binds free O_2 to form oxyhaemoglobin (oxyHb) when the O_2 binds to the haem iron in its reduced ferrous state (Fe^{2+}). Haemoglobin alternates between oxyhaemoglobin and deoxyhaemoglobin (deoxyHb) as the oxygen is exchanged between the RBCs in the lung and capillaries.

When the blood is exposed to certain drugs or oxidizing agents *in vitro* or *in vivo*, the ferrous iron (Fe^{2+}) of the molecule is converted into ferric iron (Fe^{3+}), forming methaemoglobin (metHb). In the circulation, some oxidation of deoxyHb occurs, transforming a portion of the deoxyHb into metHb. Nevertheless, an enzymatic system in the RBCs, NADH methaemoglobin reductase (NADH is the reduced form of nicotinamide adenine dinucleotide), converts the metHb into deoxyHb again. With continued oxidative denaturation, metHb is further reduced to derivatives known as hemichromes.

In blood, the paramagnetic properties are confined to the RBCs. DeoxyHb and metHb are paramagnetic because they contain unpaired electrons, whereas oxyHb is not, given that the haem iron electron spin is cancelled by the oxygen electron spin. Hemichromes do not have unpaired electrons like metHb, so the molecule is not paramagnetic.

The paramagnetism of deoxyHb and metHb can affect the relaxation times in two ways. The first is seen in deoxyHb and metHb and it manifests itself as shortening of the T2 relaxation time, a consequence of the presence of increased magnetic field inhomogeneities. This is caused by the concentration of Hb in RBCs, which produces microscopic magnetic field inhomogeneities that increase the dephasing effects of diffusing molecules between the RBC interior and the extracellular plasma (43–46). Even with the use of SE readouts, the effect is marked because water molecules diffuse to regions with very different magnetic field strengths within small distances between RF excitations that increases phase dispersion, even more when the field inhomogeneities are not static, as in this case.

The dependence of T2 has been investigated using a Meiboom–Gill–Carr–Purcell pulse sequence (Table 9.1). This provided an estimate for the mean residence time of water inside the RBC of about 10 ms (43). The T2 shortening and susceptibility effects (comprised under T2*) are better seen with GRE imaging techniques (47), producing major signal attenuation with increasing echo times, illustrating the magnitude of the field inhomogeneities present. The T2 relaxation enhancement increases as the square of the local field gradient and it has been demonstrated to be as much as 1.6 times stronger for intracellular metHb than for extracellular deoxyHb (46). Biological field gradients are caused by the heterogeneity in magnetic susceptibility and are directly proportional to the applied main magnetic field. The T2 relaxation of RBC lysates does not change with different magnetic field strengths because the susceptibility effects once present when RBCs were intact are eliminated.

On the other hand, the direct magnetic interaction between the water protons with unpaired electron spins reduces the T1 relaxation time, as in the case of metHb (distances between Hb and water molecules are well within 3 Å). This effect is not possible in deoxyHb because the water molecules cannot approach the haem iron closely enough to make an important contribution to proton relaxation enhancement. Much of the T1 relaxation enhancement is also due to the electron spin relaxation time of metHb, which is closer to the Larmor frequencies used in MRI (45). Table 9.2 summarizes the changes in the relaxation times for the different stages of oxidation of blood as compared with intact blood.

The proportion of fibrin, platelets, RBCs and other components varies for each clot and over time as Hb progresses from its oxygenated state to deoxyHb, to metHb and finally to hemisiderin. Acute intracerebral haemorrhage contains blood at varying stages of clot formation and retraction and the effects on the relaxation times are depicted in Table 9.3, showing the form of haemoglobin that prevails for each clot formation stage. The relaxation rates for blood and plasma before and after clotting are summarized in Table 9.4. These are the relaxation times that must be taken into account when defining the sensitivity of a specific MRI technique to clot detection within a vessel.

Improved contrast between blood and thrombi can be obtained by taking advantage of blood motion itself. Blood flow has been exploited extensively to form the basis of conventional time-of-flight (TOF) and phase-contrast MRA evaluations (see below). In essence, in TOF MRA techniques stationary tissue will remain with a relatively low signal whenever the signal enhancement possible by flowing blood into the imaging section is high. In phase-contrast MRA, the phase that can be accumulated from moving blood (essentially the phase is made proportional to

Table 9.2 Relative change in the relaxation times of blood for different stages in the oxidation process[a]

Stages[a]	T1	T2
Intact RBC with oxyHb	=	=
Intact RBC with deoxyHb	=	≪
Intact RBC with metHb	≪	≪
Free metHb	≪	>
Haemosiderin	=	≪

[a]Symbol > indicates prolongation of relaxation time, ≪ indicates marked shortening, = indicates no change.
Adapted from Reference 103.

Table 9.3 Appearance of haemorrhage at different stages of clot formation. Signals in T1- and T2-weighted scans as compared against white matter

Stage	Time	Comp[a]	Haemoglobin	T1	T2
Hyperacute	≤ 24 h	Intra	OxyHb	Low	High
Acute	1–3 d	Intra	DeoxyHb	Isointense	Low
Subacute					
Early	3+ d	Intra	MetHb	High	Low
Late	7+ d	Extra	MetHb	High	Mildly high
Chronic					
Centre	14+ d	Extra	Hemichromes	Medium	Medium
Rim		Intra	Haemosiderin	Low	Low

[a]Comp = composition/intracellular/extracellular.
Adapted from Reference 45.

Table 9.4 Relaxation times for blood and plasma before and after clotting. T2 measurements performed with a Carr–Purcell–Meiboom–Gill sequence using an ETS spacing of 3 ms

	T1 (ms)	T2 (ms)
Plasma		
Before clotting	1639	500
Unretracted clot	1724	500
Retracted clot	1667	208
Blood		
Before clotting	1250	182
Unretracted clot	1205	172
Retracted clot	833	95

Adapted from Reference 42.

flow velocity) is the mechanism that provides contrast while stationary signal will have a zero contribution to the formation of the vascular image. This can be performed with both SE and GRE techniques, but most MRA used today falls into the latter category. In both TOF and phase-contrast techniques, the signal from thrombi can be low but the range of signal variability depending on the age of blood clots (variable T1 relaxation values; see above) will modulate the contrast possible with TOF MRA.

Other methodology has also been exploited, mostly with the use of techniques using SE readouts. Blood motion can provide negative contrast, that is, provide an image in which blood will have no signal whereas surrounding tissues will have higher signal intensities. These techniques fall into what has been referred to as black blood MRA. Thrombi can be rendered bright against the darker signal from blood.

CONTRAST-ENHANCED MRPA

Basic considerations

The improvement in acquisition speed that is possible with faster MRI gradient hardware usually requires additional help to improve the SNR and image contrast. Therefore, contrast agents affecting the characteristic relaxation time of blood have shown a positive impact for fast MRPA and MRA in different regions in the body. The T1 relaxation of blood can be shortened with the intravenous administration of paramagnetic contrast agents (gadolinium Gd^{3+} chelates) and ultra-small iron oxide particles (USPIOs). When present at the right concentration, the T1 relaxation time of blood can drop to values below 50 ms and produce results that are virtually independent of flow for any MRA acquisitions (substantially shorter than the T1 relaxation time exhibited by fat, approximately 270 ms). The T2 relaxation time of blood also changes, remaining shorter than the T1 relaxation time. The dynamic T1 shortening experienced in the presence of a paramagnetic contrast medium, $T1_{blood}(t)$, can be modelled in relation to the concentration of the contrast medium in time according to

$$\frac{1}{T1_{blood}(t)} = \frac{1}{T1_{blood}} + R1_{Gd} \cdot [Gd](t) \tag{9.9}$$

where at 1.5 T the relaxivity of pure blood, $T1_{blood}$, is approximately 1200 ms and the relaxivity of Gd-DTPA, $R1_{Gd}$, is approximately 4.5 s^{-1} $mmol^{-1}$. The concentration of Gd-DTPA, indicated by [Gd], depends on the dose and how it is being administered during image acquisition. There is a similar equation for the T2 relaxation of blood.

Contrast-enhanced MRPA can be performed in two modalities, using acquisitions that take place during the transient T1 relaxation effects in blood after a bolus injection of a contrast agent or during steady-state conditions using intravascular contrast agents. In routine application, MRPA is mainly performed during dynamic contrast injections. Assuming a one-compartment model, the concentration of the contrast agent can be related to the rate of contrast injection and the cardiac output as follows (48,49):

$$[Gd] = \frac{\text{rate of Gd injection in mol/s}}{\text{cardiac output in L/s}} \tag{9.10}$$

where [Gd] denotes the steady-state concentration of Gd-DTPA that is expected when the injection time is long enough that no variations in concentration occur during the MRPA acquisition. The T1 relaxation values for blood of 36 and 18 ms for 1 and 2 mL/s injections for a typical cardiac output of 5 L/min, respectively. Under realistic imaging conditions, these relaxation values are adequately supported by commercial imaging hardware for the resolution that is necessary for the evaluation of the MRPA for full lung coverage (approximately 5 mm^3 voxels). Injection rates greater than 4 mL/s may not yield better MRPA quality. Shortening TR is only possible to a certain extent, given that the readout window directly affects the SNR and resolution possible for the available gradient amplifier. The RF excitation must be kept below the maximum output of the RF amplifier and RF exposure limits to the patient.

With the T1 relaxation times expected in blood after the administration of contrast, optimal imaging parameters can be computed using the signal for FLASH imaging (SSI GRE imaging, equation 9.3). This assumes that the T1 relaxation is maintained constant during the entire scan time. The signal intensity plots illustrated in Figure 9.13 provide the characteristic signal behaviour for FLASH imaging for short TR scans, as currently implemented in advanced 3D MRPA protocols with the range of T1 relaxation times expected for contrast-enhanced scans.

Considerations for breath-hold capabilities

Evaluation of the patient's breath-hold ability should be performed prior to every examination. It could be done using a sagittal or a coronal imaging plane to generate images at a rate of one per second that demonstrate the diaphragmatic position. Patients who are short of breath will not be able to produce images with adequate resolution to review arteries effectively beyond fourth-order branches of the pulmonary tree. Studies have shown that adequate resolution for evaluation is possible if breath-holds are held consistent at least for half of the scan time, preferably during the centre of the data acquisition (sequential scanning) (49). A breath-hold time of less than 17 s has been appropriate for all patients with good image quality for the assessment (50). In most contrast-enhanced MRPA clinical studies, breath-hold fast 3D GRE scans acquired during the first pass of a Gd-DTPA contrast bolus have been used (51–55).

Imaging protocols varied with respect to acquisition orientation (sagittal, transverse, coronal or double oblique volumes). Coronal and sagittal orientations are most often used for assessing PE. Coronal imaging is preferred if a single contrast injection is performed and provides a 3D volume with predominant enhancement of the pulmonary arteries (Figure 9.15a). The image quality is comparable to state-of-the-art computed tomography (CT) (Figure 9.15b). Breath-holds have ranged between 15 and 30 s with imaging parameters tailored to obtain results that take into account the patient's breath-hold ability (56).

Coronal scanning with short breath-hold acquisitions may prove ineffective for PE detection at sub-segmental level unless both lungs are entirely covered with appropriate spatial resolution (voxels <5 mm³). It is also important in coronal scanning that the in-plane phase encoding loop is scanned faster than the section select phase encoding loop. This can reduce ghosting from heart motion whenever all in-plane phase encoding lines are acquired in less than one cardiac cycle.

Shorter breath-holds with satisfactory spatial resolution necessitate that each lung be scanned separately. However, the reduction of the acquisition time can be traded off to increase spatial resolution by two sagittal slabs. As a drawback of the sagittal set-up two contrast injections must be administered (57). The sequential acquisition of two sagittal slabs covering the right and left lung

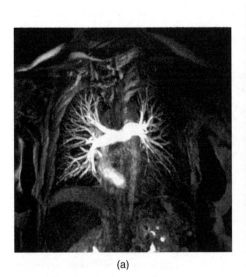
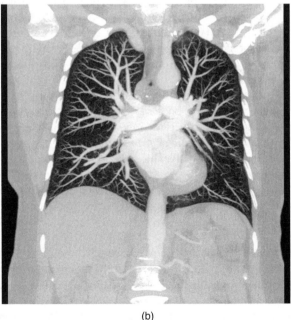

(a)   (b)

Figure 9.15   Contrast-enhanced MRA of the pulmonary vasculature acquired in coronal orientation (a) and CT (b) for comparison: exclusion of acute PE.

separately has been used employed successfully in patients suffering from chronic thromboembolic pulmonary hypertension (58).

Contrast-enhanced 3D MRPA makes use of the shortest TR that it is possible by the MRI gradient hardware in order to generate the desired resolution within a prescribed, short imaging time. Nonetheless, satisfactory SNR is the parameter that modulates the appropriate choice for TR and readout acquisition bandwidths that are employed for all MRPA protocols. Typical TR and TE values range between 2.4 and 5 ms and 0.9 and 3.0 ms, respectively, for fast MRI gradient hardware. A short TR allows for short breath hold acquisitions. A short TE minimizes background signal and susceptibility artefacts. Readout acquisition bandwidths have been set, in general, to less than 900 Hz/pixel.

The readout flip angle is chosen according to the expected concentration (T1 relaxation induced) of the contrast medium in blood during the scanning time and calculated according to the optimal flip angle equation for FLASH imaging (Ernst angle, equation 9.4). Flip angle values that have been used have ranged between 15 and 60°. Higher flip angles tend to be chosen for scans with longer TR or higher contrast concentration or both. The RF amplifier and heat exposure limits on patients (SAR) may limit the application of short RF excitations that are required for short TR sequences.

Contrast administration

The contrast arrival time at the pulmonary vasculature and the pulmonary circulation time (transit time between arterial and venous phase) are very short. The selective visualization of the pulmonary arteries alone without any venous overlay is challenging. Figure 9.16 illustrates the course of signal enhancement for different vascular compartments in the cardiothoracic circulatory system after a short bolus of contrast. From these curves, several parameters can be calculated. The time of arrival of contrast to the pulmonary arteries (PA), lung parenchyma (PP), pulmonary veins (PV) and descending aorta (Ao) can be seen. The transit time through the pulmonary circuit (τ) can be derived from the difference between the PA and PV intensity curves. The bolus dispersion time (T_{bd}), that is, the associated expansion of the bolus shape during the time it remains in the pulmonary circulation, can be calculated. The enhancement speed recorded in the pulmonary artery (E_{rt}), has been set as the time elapsed from the start of enhancement and half the intensity is reached (Table 9.5).

The transit time τ is very short, approximately 3.6 s, and remains fairly constant in all patients. Similar values have been recorded by other investigators using dynamic contrast enhanced scans with high temporal resolution (15,59). It is also important to note that the bolus can spread considerably depending on the condition of the patient, with recorded values between 4.98 and 20.25 s (mean 8.71 s). The speed of enhancement in the pulmonary artery, E_{rt}, also has a large variation with a range of 0.5–5.2 s (mean 2.10 s). The effect of these parameters on MRPA image quality has not been yet correlated adequately. In general, studies that have a short time of arrival to the PA with small E_{rt} and T_{bd} provide the best enhancement in the MRPA, where in vascular obstruction, e.g., massive pulmonary embolism, the transit time can be substantially prolonged (Figure 9.17).

Contrast is generally administered through an intravenous catheter placed in the antecubital vein. A long bolus will extend the plateau during which the acquisition is to be performed. Excellent results for MRA and MRPA have been reported using a fixed dose of contrast of 40 mL (approximately a double dose of contrast). Single dose injections (approximately 20 mL) have also been reported to produce good results for either coronal (13) or sagittal data collection strategies (60) when timing is optimal and sequence parameters are tuned accordingly (Figure 9.18). Hany *et al.* (60) have determined that a double dose of contrast (0.2 mmol/kg) is optimal for any MRA examination (dose ranging between single dose and quadruple dose).

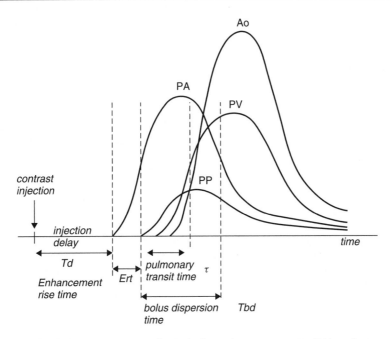

Figure 9.16 Typical enhancement curves through the pulmonary artery (PA), pulmonary parenchyma (PP), pulmonary vein (PV) and aorta (Ao) after the injection of a short bolus of contrast. T_d indicates the time between the start of injection and the instance that enhancement in PA appears. The enhancement rise time, E_{rt}, is defined between T_d and half the maximum intensity at PA. The bolus dispersion time, T_{bd}, is calculated as the full width at half-maximum of the PA curve. The transit time through the pulmonary circuit, ϑ, is the time interval between one half of the maximum enhancement recorded at PA and PV.

Table 9.5 Circulation times from the injection site to and through the pulmonary vasculature quantified using a 3D dynamic contrast-enhanced scan with a time resolution of 1 s[a]

Circulation parameter (55 patients, mean age = 50.2 years)	Time (s)
Arrival time to PA	5.00
Arrival time to 1/2 intensity at PA	6.99
Arrival time to 1/2 intensity at PP	9.69
Arrival time to 1/2 intensity at PV	10.60
Arrival time to 1/2 intensity at Ao	13.08
Enhancement rise time (E_{rt})	2.10
Pulmonary transit time (t)	3.60
Bolus dispersion time (T_{bd})	8.71
Maximum E_{rt}	0.50
Minimum E_{rt}	5.20
Maximum T_{bd}	20.25
Minimum T_{bd}	4.98

[a]Contrast injection was performed at the antecubital vein using a power injector delivering a short bolus of contrast with 8 mL at a rate of 4 mL/s flushed with 20 mL of saline at a rate of 2 mL/s. All values represent averages over data collected on 55 patients and measured at two different sites in each data set. Thirteen patients presented PE by conventional pulmonary angiography. PA, descending pulmonary arteries; PV, Pulmonary veins; PP, posterior pulmonary parenchyma; Ao, descending aorta.

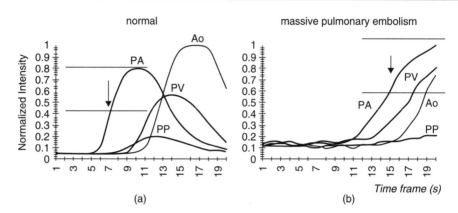

Figure 9.17   Representative signal intensity curves in the descending pulmonary artery (PA), pulmonary vein (PV), posterior pulmonary parenchyma (PP) and the descending Aorta (Ao). (a) Normal patient. (b) Patient with large thrombi lodged in both descending pulmonary arteries. The dynamic acquisition was performed with a time resolution of 1 s after the injection of an 80 mL bolus of Gd-DTPA at a rate of 4 mL/s and flushed with 20 mL of saline at a rate of 2 mL/s.

Injection flow rates are set to 2 mL/s although variable rates have been reported to produce a greater enhancement during the collection of the central k-space lines whenever a limited amount of contrast agent is used. An injection scheme with a flow rate of 2 mL/s results in a mean transit time of the contrast agent through the pulmonary circulation of 14 s; and it is reduced to 9 s using an injection speed of 4 mL/s. The administration of a saline flush, minimum 20 mL injected at the same flow rate, at least 2 mL/s, immediately after the administration of the contrast agent is strongly recommended to achieve a compact bolus profile (61). The saline chaser will ensure that the whole amount of contrast medium contributes to vessel opacification.

Several general points should be considered:

- A single dose of contrast delivered over a shorter period than the duration of the MRPA acquisition produces constant signal enhancement during the entire scan time (Figure 9.18a).
- A double dose of contrast delivered during the same time produces twice the signal enhancement (Figure 9.18c).
- A single dose of contrast delivered for a longer time produces a constant enhancement during the acquisition but part of the contrast is misused (Figure 9.18b).
- A double dose delivered for a shorter time provides more vascular enhancement but over a smaller portion of k-space (Figure 9.18d).

In Figure 9.18a–c, the signal is uniform for all k-space values and consequently no filtering artefacts (blurring or edge enhancement) will be present in the reconstructed images. Figure 9.18d requires special consideration of the way in which k-space is encoded to produce the least amount of filtering artefacts while achieving appropriate vascular contrast between pulmonary arteries and veins. Variable contrast delivery flow rates have been proposed, enabling contrast to appear for all k-space values but with a higher concentration during the collection of the centre of k-space. Under real conditions, the contrast washout period can be elongated, providing a buffering effect. This varies depending on physiology and patient condition.

Precise differentiation between pulmonary arteries and veins depends on the concentration of the contrast agent in each compartment at the time the centre of k-space is acquired. The time at which peak enhancement occurs in each vascular compartment is not fixed and can vary enormously

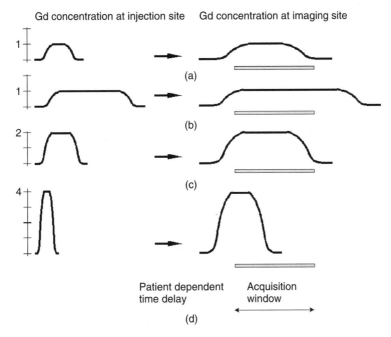

Gd concentration at injection site   Gd concentration at imaging site

(a)

(b)

(c)

Patient dependent   Acquisition
time delay   window

(d)

Figure 9.18 Contrast concentration curves in the pulmonary arteries following a bolus of contrast with four different delivery strategies. (a), (c) Timings administration that can be produced during the acquisition of a contrast-enhanced MRPA acquisition in the pulmonary vasculature of a contrast-enhanced MRPA protocol during and after the administration of a bolus of contrast with optimal use of the contrast whether it is applied as single dose or double dose. (b) The case where contrast is wasted, in contrast to (d), where portions of k-space are acquired without contrast and therefore artefacts will be present in the reconstructed data (smoothing or edge enhancement). The choice of k-space ordering scheme.

in patients referred for MRPA. Four different strategies for contrast delivery and scanning are therefore possible:

- best guess technique
- test bolus technique
- automated bolus detection
- MR fluoroscopy.

Of these, only the first two have been reported for MRPA. The best guess technique considers an educated guess as to what the contrast arrival time may be between the injection site and the pulmonary arteries. This is difficult to determine from the patient condition alone because the arrival time can change substantially when emboli or pulmonary arterial hypertension are present. In general, guessing yields sub-optimal results and provides a wide spectrum of enhancement patterns between the pulmonary arteries and veins. The estimated contrast travel time should be taken as the average arrival time to the pulmonary artery, which is approximately 5 s from an injection in the antecubital vein. As such, a test bolus examination or a care bolus procedure is strongly recommended, in particular in patients with suspected PE or pulmonary hypertension.

A test bolus injection, using 1–3 mL of contrast, is only required in routine practice if an automated bolus detection is not available. A dynamic 2D T1-weighted scan with a time resolution of 1 s is usually employed to determine the arrival time at the main pulmonary arteries. This involves an additional scanning time and analysis of the contrast enhancement time course, but the results are more consistent and generally lead to optimal enhancement of the pulmonary arteries. However, it must be considered that the injection delay may change between the test scan and the MRPA. In the event that sequential k-space encoding is used and the centre of k-space is collected in the middle of the acquisition time, the timing of contrast prior to scanning can be calculated as (62)

$$\text{Imaging delay} = \text{estimated contrast travel time} + (\text{injection time}/2) - (\text{imaging time}/2) \quad (9.11)$$

Note that if the injection time is the same as the imaging time, the imaging delay is equal to the estimated contrast travel time. For the test bolus technique, the estimated contrast travel time is taken as the moment when contrast appears in the pulmonary artery.

Guessing or data analysis prior to scanning can be offset using real-time monitoring of the arrival of contrast at the pulmonary arteries with an automated bolus detection scheme and trigger (63,64) or an operator-dependent scan trigger using MR fluoroscopy (65). With automated bolus detection and triggering, the operator places a small measuring voxel in the main pulmonary artery to detect the signal changes induced by the passage of the contrast. The signal from the voxel is processed in real time and decisions are made after setting a suitable threshold over the background signal. Upon detection, the MRPA scan starts data collection automatically or the operator is alerted to start the scan manually. MR fluoroscopy collects instead an entire image in any desired plane to monitor the contrast arrival from which breath-hold and start of scan are instructed. MR fluoroscopy may be more reliable for MRPA as there is no need for positioning the measuring voxel to detect the contrast and it eliminates any failure of detection if the monitor voxel does not appear correctly positioned at all times because of breathing. Both schemes require that the operator delivers the instruction conveniently to the patient (which may be difficult in some cases). Centric or elliptical ordering of k-space should be used in these cases.

For sequential encoding, a variable flow rate can yield greater enhancement during the centre of k-space. For a centric ordering scheme, encoding should start whenever contrast arrives at the pulmonary artery while the contrast is delivered at a constant flow rate. Most important is the speed at which the central portion of k-space is encoded (in the $k_y - k_z$ plane) that determines the separation between arterial and venous enhancement and the filtering artefacts that occur along both phase encoding directions.

Scan choice is dependent on the size of the central k-space data, which is related to the encoded matrix ($k_y - k_z$ plane, number of sections and in-plane phase encoding steps chosen). There are two set-ups that can be envisioned: scanning the in-plane phase encoding steps inside the section select phase encoding loop or the other way round. Considering that the same number of points around the centre of k-space are scanned, the resulting pattern for each one of these ordering schemes is illustrated in Figure 9.19a and b, respectively. The best representation of the contrast encoded and the milder filtering effects occur in the case of Figure 9.19b, performing the acquisition using the 'faster' loop in the direction of the smaller amount of phase encoding steps. This ordering scheme should be used for either sagittal or coronal orientation set-ups. However, increased ghosting laterally can occur for coronal MRPA, which may be unacceptable for a good evaluation and, therefore, the reversed looping of Figure 9.19a is generally used.

Elliptical encoding provides the best compromise (Figure 9.19c). Symmetrical weighting of the contrast enhancement curve in the $k_y - k_z$ plane is possible with the same k-space area scanned as in Figure 9.19a and b. Both phase encodings are played such that k-space is accessed from its centre in a spiral fashion. This scheme also produces the best venous suppression possible, minimum amount of filtering (equal weighting in both directions) and ghosting evenly distributed along both phase encoding directions.

Elliptical encoding can yield a higher degree of venous suppression and artefact reduction whenever the E_{rt} time (enhancement rate) and the bolus dispersion time are short, as determined

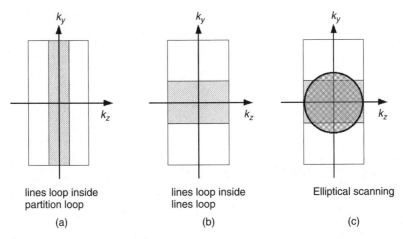

Figure 9.19 Shape of the k-space area covered in the k_y-k_z plane by different phase encoding strategies for the same time interval during the center of k-space. (a) In-plane phase encoding steps acquired in the inner most loop, inside the slice select phase encoding loop. (b) Reversed loop as in (a), with the slice select phase encoding in the inner most loop. (c) Elliptical encoding collecting both phase encoding steps with symmetrical weighting in both k_y and k_z. It is the optimal ordering scheme for any 3D MRPA acquisition as the contrast enhancement signal distribution is weighted equally in all directions in the k_y-k_z plane and provides the highest degree of suppression between arterial and venous structures with short transit times and good artifact equilibration along both phase encoding directions.

from a test bolus scan. However, for a short bolus of contrast, sequential encoding represents the best choice because the acquisition window can be twice as long in comparison with any centric ordering scheme.

DISPLAY AND EVALUATION OF MRPA

The evaluation of vascular data sets of patients with suspected PE can be a difficult task because of the extent and complexity of the pulmonary vascular tree. Furthermore, the evaluation can be hampered with data sets that are not free from artefacts (blurring in non-cooperative patients or ghosting from blood pulsation) or present poor vascular enhancement (wrong timing for contrast-enhanced scans). Several image post-processing tools can be used, including multiplanar reformation (MPR), maximum intensity projections (MIP) (Figure 9.20) and standard 3D workstations. A suitable combination of these image post-processing tools permits the evaluation of all branches for the eventual detection of thrombi in PE.

Other image presentation and post-processing techniques for MRA have been reviewed in detail by Siebert (66), but they have not been analyzed for MRPA. It is important to note that 3D image post-processing routines only make sense for an improved evaluation and display of the MRPA data when the SNR, contrast and resolution are adequate.

Multiplanar reformation (MPR)

Multiplanar reformation is an excellent tool for evaluation that is simple to use and effective for intraluminal vessel inspection. MPR permits the reformation of double oblique planes along any particular vessel path, making it possible to localize intraluminal defects directly. Three planes

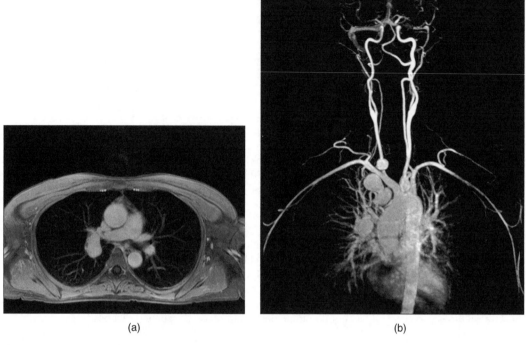

Figure 9.20   Transaxial source image and maximum intensity projections (MIP) in a patient with aneurysms of pulmonary and systemic arteries in Takayasu's disease.

are most often visualized at once, e.g., the target orientation along a vessel and two adjunct perpendicular views. It is common to produce a reformatted image with a thicker slice than that set by the voxel dimensions. This helps to visualize longer vessel sections (in cases with vessel tortuosity) without hiding intraluminal defects completely through partial volume effects. Multiplanar reformations can be time consuming, as it is necessary to inspect every arterial branch separately. Thrombus visualization is also highly dependent on its location within a vessel. Cases that are fairly easy to document conform to those where thrombi are completely surrounded by bright blood. Experience is binding for the detection of thrombi lying against a vessel wall (partial narrowing or constriction) or when complete vessel cut-off occurs (requiring good knowledge of the pulmonary anatomy). The latter two can be problematic because a thrombus can be easily missed when the signal is similar to that of the darker lung parenchyma (especially with contrast-enhanced scans using a high contrast dosage at high flip angles). In any case, the review is significantly facilitated when using an MPR platform that is highly interactive, fast and provides adequate localization freedom.

Maximum intensity projection (MIP) and volume rendering

The most commonly used and widely available technique for vascular visualization is MIP. The concept behind MIP is straightforward. The MIP algorithm projects rays through voxels of a volume data set and forms an image that has the signal intensity of those voxels that contain the highest intensity values encountered along the casting ray. Another technique that provides a higher degree of control over the display of the MRPA is volume rendering. Volume rendering assigns particular properties to voxels, such as opacity, colour and brightness (among others that are definable). These properties are later selectively added to form the rendered image along a specific view. With volume rendering a voxel can be made completely opaque whenever the opacity value assigned is one or, otherwise, completely transparent if the values make it possible to distinguish overlapping vessels or to enhance features that may be hidden within a vessel, e.g., a thrombus. The volume rendering process is more computationally expensive than MIP and requires faster processing hardware for interactive display.

To demonstrate the main difference between MIP and volume rendering, simulated vessels (software generated) are used that contain different thrombi shapes in similar locations as demonstrated in pulmonary arteries of patients with proven PE. The simulated vessels are constructed from the different cross-sections illustrated in Figure 9.21. The vessel lumen has been assigned a value of 100% with emboli and background at 20% and zero, respectively. Two cases account for the signal of an intact vessel or a completely occluded one (Figure 9.21a and e). Three cases are of interest for the visualization:

- a cylindrical embolus completely contained and in the centre of the vessel lumen (Figure 9.21b)
- a small cylindrical embolus placed near to the vessel wall (Figure 9.21c)
- an irregular embolus obstructing half of the vessel lumen (Figure 9.21d).

As noted in Figures 9.22–9.24, MIP has major drawbacks compared with volume rendering techniques. Completely intraluminal defects or small emboli relative to the vessel lumen will not be displayed in an MIP image. It is clear that the only instance where MIP demonstrates the unequivocal presence of an embolus will be when this is larger than half of the vessel lumen and with the condition that a large area is attached to the lumen wall. If this is the case, part of the casting rays will pass through the embolus without touching the lumen with higher signal intensity (see Figure 9.24 with viewing angles at 60° and 120°). Volume rendering, in contrast, can show any intraluminal defect independent of size and location of the thrombi. Because the properties of the voxels can be changed at will, the embolus can be extracted from the histogram of intensities and its brightness and opacity enhanced so that it appears brighter than the vessel lumen itself.

Unfortunately, the single vessel display does not correspond to reality because features and other vessels do not overlap in the reconstruction, especially when vessel information is abundant, as in the case of MRPA. In practice, finding thrombi will be a more realistic task towards the peripheral pulmonary vasculature, where vessel overlap is less likely to occur. There is another situation where MIP can fail completely. Such is the case when the reconstructed vessel cannot rotate on its axis, e.g., a horizontal vessel viewed in a coronal rotation where the casting rays always pass through the bright vessel and the embolus.

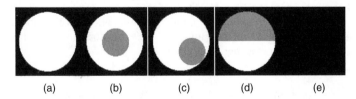

Figure 9.21 Cross-sections of several vessels used to compare the resulting images formed by MIP and volume rendering. (a) Plain vessel; (b) embolus completely embedded within the vessel lumen; (c) small embolus closer to the vessel wall; (d) embolus attached to the vessel wall obstructing one half of the vessel lumen; (e) vessel completely occluded. The signal intensity for the vessel was set to 100% while emboli and background are approximately 20% and zero, respectively.

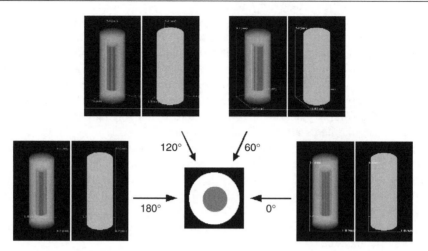

Figure 9.22 Comparison between MIP and volume rendering for an embolus completely embedded and centred within the vessel lumen. Projections from all angles demonstrate the same images given the symmetry of the set-up. Images to the left and right of each comparison correspond to volume rendering and MIP, respectively. The embolus can be appreciated with the opacity setting used for volume rendering while it is completely masked with MIP.

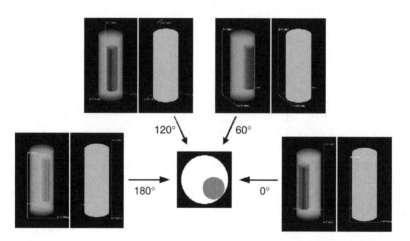

Figure 9.23 Comparison between MIP and volume rendering for a small diameter embolus completely embedded within the vessel but close to the vessel wall. Images to the left and right of each comparison correspond to volume rendering and MIP, respectively. The embolus can be appreciated with the opacity setting used for volume rendering while it is still completely masked with MIP. Note that the intensity of the embolus for the rendered projections at 0° and 180° differ to illustrate the shorter distance between the observer and the embolus for the former.

MIP presents some additional serious drawbacks. Because a single value is recorded along the casting ray, MIP cannot provide depth information, resulting in a loss in the spatial position of individual vessels along the casting ray. MIP obscures features that have lower intensity (as illustrated in Figures 9.22 and 9.24), as is the case of intraluminal pulmonary emboli. A partial solution to these two issues has been the cine viewing of the processed images at different angles. Another solution has been 'sliding' thin slab MIPs through the entire vascular data set. A 'sliding'

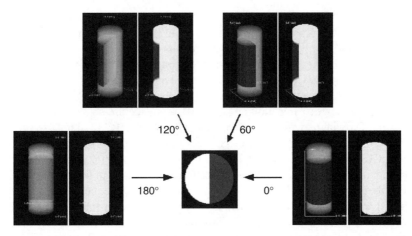

Figure 9.24 Comparison between MIP and volume rendering for an embolus occluding half of the vessel lumen. This is the only case where MIP can demonstrate the presence of an embolus. In order to appreciate the embolus, several projections must be reconstructed and played in a cine loop to illustrate the defect. Note that the size of the signal void is smaller than the size of the embolus because information is masked. Images to the left and right of each comparison correspond to volume rendering and MIP, respectively. The embolus can be appreciated with the opacity setting used for volume rendering while it is completely masked with MIP.

MIP can provide enough vascular coverage to ease the integration of all the vascular information as it is played in the cine loop while it provides a better chance for the detection of intraluminal emboli. More peripheral emboli are easy to detect with both volume rendering and MIP.

Optimal visualization can also be difficult because of the signal variability between data sets. Contrast enhancement differences will always be present between arteries and veins but also from the existence of atelectasis, pneumonia, haemorrhage, pleural effusion and tumours that can overlap during the formation of suitable images that provide a global visualization of the entire vascular structure. A targeted reconstruction or structure segmentation is therefore appropriate.

Combining multiplanar reformation and vascular visualization

Multiplanar reformation can also be combined with volume rendering (or MIP) with the incorporation of 'clipping' planes in the 3D vascular volume to demonstrate any pulmonary vessel branch in relation to its surroundings. Clipping planes are double oblique planes that cut into the volume to stop the rendering process at the surface defined by the plane. In this way, a thrombus lodged inside a pulmonary vessel can be accompanied with all the surrounding vascular information for improved visualization.

The observer viewing angle can be adjusted with the clipping plane held constant to permit other views of the vascular territory. The number of clipping planes that can be applied is virtually unlimited (but software dependent). Clipping planes can also be used to eliminate interference from unwanted structures during the volume rendering process.

DYNAMIC CONTRAST-ENHANCED MRPA

An alternative approach for MRA of the pulmonary vasculature is to optimize the MR sequence for high temporal resolution and to apply it as a multiphasic acquisition (67–69). Imaging begins before arrival of the contrast agent and continues for as many volume frames as clinically necessary. In time-resolved MRPA, the scan time for the individual 3D data set is substantially reduced, e.g., to less than 5 s. The rationale is three-fold. First, patients with severe respiratory disease and very limited breath-hold capabilities can be examined. Second, the arterial–venous discrimination is improved. This allows for characterization of vascular territories, especially in congenital anomalies and shunts. Third, time-resolved multiphasic contrast-enhanced (CE) MRPA is independent of the bolus timing, since the contrast injection and the MR sequence are started simultaneously (70).

Departing from 2D dynamic MRPA concepts, the 3D time-resolved volumetric imaging concept (3D TRICKS, 3D time-resolved imaging of contrast kinetics) has also been applied for dynamic MRPA (68). TRICKS involves the use of temporal interpolation, whereby the low spatial-frequency data within the centre of k-space are sampled more frequently than are the higher spatial frequency data, located further peripherally This method shared high spatial frequency data between adjacent frames, such that a full k-space complement is available for each individual frame. This technique provides images with sufficiently high through-plane spatial resolution. Several variations have been developed and are currently used, such as projection reconstruction, TRICKS, CE timing robust angiography (CENTRA), TR echo shared angiographic technique (TREAT) and TR angiography with interleaved stochastic trajectories (TWIST) (71). Using these techniques in conjunction with cardiac triggering, the passage of contrast through the pulmonary vasculature can be observed with good temporal resolution (2 s) in order to detect the selective enhancement of arteries and veins with good spatial resolution (72). To maintain both good spatial and good temporal resolution, k-space filling is performed in a segmented fashion (k-space segmentation using blocks of contiguous data) and k-space data are shared between the volumes encoded. Depending on the set-up, the centre of k-space can be updated at reasonable time resolution while high k-space lines are shared between several data sets using time interpolation with a sliding acquisition window that updates these values at lower speed. Using this methodology, good temporal and spatial resolution can be obtained with low readout bandwidths and using MRI scanners with slower imaging gradients. Wielopolski *et al.* (57) applied a similar k-space sharing concept to a 3D scan making use of a faster gradient hardware. The implementation was based on an ultrashort FLASH TR/TE sequence (TR/TE = 1.7/0.8 ms) covering the entire thorax with a time resolution of one volume per second with a short sliding window of 1.5 s together with a low resolution MRPA, with $2.6 \times 2.6 \times 9$ mm voxel sizes. Advanced imaging techniques integrate a view-sharing approach to achieve a temporal resolution of 3.3 s for a 3D dataset with a relatively high spatial resolution of e.g., $1.3 \times 1.8 \times 3$ mm. This allows for volumetric assessment of perfusion of the entire lung parenchyma (Figure 9.25) and easy depiction of perfusion deficits due to vascular obstruction (Figure 9.25) or hypoxic vasoconstriction (Figure 9.26).

Alternative approaches focus on sub-second temporal imaging while compromising on through-plane resolution. Finn *et al.* (73) used a partial Fourier scheme of 80% in the in-plane phase encoding direction and only 62.5% of the full k-space vector in the slice-select direction. They achieved a volume acquisition time of 800 ms and rather recommended acquisition in a second plane with a second injection of contrast if the first imaging plane yielded inconclusive results with regard to separation of overlying vessels in the absence of off-axis reconstructions.

Image artefacts in contrast-enhanced MRPA

Two types of artefacts can be distinguished: those that are derived from physiological conditions (such as breath-holding and blood pulsation) and those that are coupled to the change in concentration of the contrast agent during data acquisition. Poor breath-holding can produce inadequate results for high order branches but the resulting MRPA can still have diagnostic quality for the vessels with larger diameter (Figure 9.27). The reason for this is that vessel display has a direct

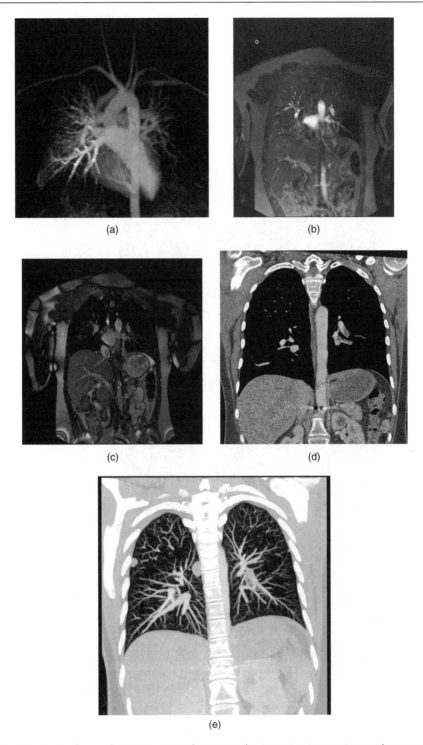

(a)

(b)

(c)

(d)

(e)

Figure 9.25 Contrast-enhanced MRPA acquired in coronal orientation in a patient with acute pulmonary embolism: all images show the embolus in the left lower lobe artery. (a) Coronal MIP also showing rarefication of pulmonary artery branches in the left lower lobe; (b) coronal source image showing the perfusion defect in the left lower lobe; (c) white-blood non-enhanced image acquired during free breathing; (d) coronal MPR of CT; (e) coronal MIP of CT also showing pleural metastases.

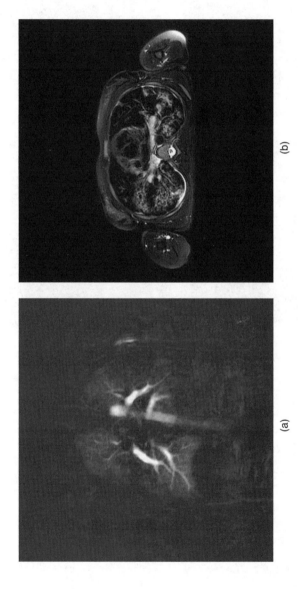

(a)

(b)

Figure 9.26 Patient with cystic fibrosis showing multiple perfusion defects due to hypoxic vasoconstriction in contrast-enhanced MRA (a) and enhancing inflammatory changes with bronchiectasis in both lungs demonstrated by fat-suppressed T1weighted volume-interpolated GRE (b).

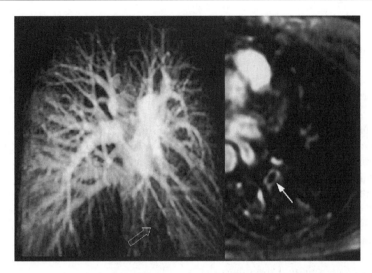

Figure 9.27   Images corrupted with blurring from poor breath-holding. Vessels towards the periphery are completely blurred and the scan may be considered non-diagnostic. In this case, an embolus appearing in the left descending pulmonary artery can be seen clearly with MPR (b) despite blurring (arrow), providing a positive result for the detection of PE. The block arrow points at a region with a clear lack of vascular enhancement demonstrated by MIP (a).

link to the speed that is used to acquire the centre k-space lines. Therefore, it is possible to affirm that the presence of thrombus can be confirmed with a good degree of confidence to the third-order branches with poor breath-holds. Even dyspneic patients who present with emboli in the larger vessels can be diagnosed with contrast-enhanced MRPA.

Ghosting can arise from blood pulsation during the acquisition. The superimposition of ghosted vessels over others can produce signal voids (signal cancellation) that can be confused with a thrombus. Careful review along both phase encoding directions with multiplanar reformatting can indicate the presence of such an artefact. Ghosting is mainly present because the acquisition is not synchronized with the cardiac motion.

Ghosting artefacts can arise from two different origins, one related exclusively to variations in the signal intensity of blood during the acquisition and the other associated with changes in the phase of the signal. Both effects are intensified with high signals produced by the contrast-enhanced blood. Since MRPA sequences do not use flow compensation to achieve speed, there will be some variation in the phase of the signal from blood pulsation.

Artefacts related to contrast agents depend on the concentration of the contrast agent during the course of the acquisition. These artefacts tend to disappear since the concentration during the entire acquisition remains constant. Therefore, there will be no special weighting associated for each portion of k-space scanned.

Contrast agents induce a T2 and T2* shortening in blood which can result in unwanted signal loss. The TE of the MRPA acquisition is chosen such that it is several-fold shorter than the T2* relaxation of the contrast-enhanced blood. However, the contrast concentration can be so high that the T2* shortening is comparable to TE, resulting in a decrease in signal intensity in the vessel. This can be noted in the majority of cases in the subclavian vein, which is close to the point where the contrast agent is injected. The local dephasing that is produced can also affect the signal of surrounding tissues and other vessels. This void can be misinterpreted as a possible stenosis or thrombus and can be better appreciated on the original sections of the MRPA.

Good contrast timing is required to form an arterial MRPA only data set. To achieve good vessel selectivity with short circulation times between arteries and veins, there should always be a sharp peak T1 relaxation shortening occurring at different positions in k-space. The T1 relaxation shortening occurs during a brief period of the acquisition and has a Gaussian-like shape over a small portion of k-space. When the Gaussian curve (maximum T1 relaxation shortening) occurs during the collection of the edges of k-space, ringing and edge enhancement are produced in the image of the vessel. This edge enhancement produces a darkening of the vessel centre that may be confused with an embolus if the signal characteristics of the MRPA scan are not known for the chosen imaging parameters. Blurring (or vessel smoothing) occurs when the maximum T1 relaxation occurs only during the centre of k-space, creating an effect that is similar to a low-pass filter.

Saturation can occur, which manifests itself as a local or global signal intensity decrease, when a stenosis or a thrombus restricting blood flow is present. Mixing of contrast-enhanced blood with normal blood can be slower and therefore a longer T1 relaxation time will occur compared with other vessels where contrast may be more concentrated. Saturation occurs more often with the use of a short contrast bolus. This indicates that the flip angle chosen is too high for the concentration of contrast expected. Luckily, in cases of saturation, the blood T1 relaxation values have remained shorter than that of surrounding thrombus.

High venous signal is a by-product of wrong contrast timing, indicating that the centre of k-space was acquired after most of the contrast had already passed through the pulmonary arterial system. Artefacts in the arteries are not likely to appear because there is always some residual contrast during the entire length of the scan that provides T1 relaxation enhancement for the arteries.

Intravascular contrast agents

Dynamic injections provide a single chance to obtain fast breath-hold MRPA with good image quality. To overcome this constraint and enhance the limited resolution and SNR possible with ultra-fast breath-hold acquisitions, a variety of intravascular contrast agents have been investigated that produce steady-state T1 relaxation effects in blood similar to those with gadolinium complexes during dynamic injections. The time that these new contrast agents remain in blood varies, depending on the size of the molecule and its excretion metabolism, ranging between 20 min to several hours. Studies already performed on animals have produced a continuous several-fold enhancement of pulmonary vessels and pulmonary parenchyma (74–76). When the contrast agent is confined to the blood compartment, a steady-state condition for the T1 and T2 relaxation values is achieved, which makes the design independent of all considerations of k-space scanning exposed earlier. Some intravascular contrast agents have become available recently (Figure 9.28), whereas others are still not available outside clinical trials (77,78).

The use of blood pool agents allows for a combination of 3D perfusion MRI of the lung and MRPA with a single injection whereas with conventional extracellular contrast agents a combined imaging approach would require repeated injections eventually exceeding the clinically approved dose. Blood pool agents were investigated for the detection of pulmonary emboli in a pig model with autologous thrombi. This technique achieved a higher SNR of the lung parenchyma than the use of conventional extracellular contrast agents (79). Additionally, with blood pool MR contrast agents, alternative imaging techniques, such as navigator gated MRA, might be realized for MRPA, which cannot be used with conventional extracellular MR contrast agents (80). The use of ultra-small particles of iron oxide (USPIO) permits imaging of the pulmonary vasculature with continuous breathing due to the longer presence of the contrast agent in the blood, which allows the use of navigator echoes for respiratory triggering. This is of importance in the investigation of pulmonary embolism where the patients can have problems with holding their breath for long enough to obtain sufficient image quality. It also allows longer acquisition times for higher

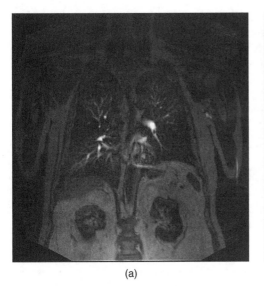
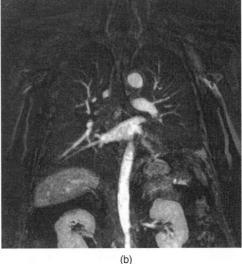

(a)   (b)

Figure 9.28   MRPA enhanced with a blood pool contrast agent, intravascular protein-binding gadofosveset (Bayer Schering). Clear delineation of the embolus in the left lower lobe artery shown in the arterial phase (a), less clear on the equilibrium image (b).

resolution and cardiac triggering, which improves the image quality further by avoiding motion artefacts from the heart. Due to the prolonged imaging window, blood pool agents further permit dual imaging of pulmonary embolism and detection of the source of the emboli. As a drawback, blood pool contrast agent types equally enhance arteries and veins during the steady-state phase (Figure 9.28b).

NON-CONTRAST-ENHANCED MRPA

Critically ill patients will not even tolerate a short breath-hold time of 5–10 s for CE-MRPA. The same is true for CT angiography; and its imaging results might also be sub-optimal. For these patients. free-breathing real-time imaging techniques based on SSFP – also called balanced fast-field echo or fast imaging using steady-state acquisition – are available (81,82). The whole chest can be covered in all three orientations in less than 180 s with 50% overlapping of the slices due to an acquisition time per image of approximately 0.4–0.5 s. This approach allows for a lobar and segmental evaluation of the pulmonary arteries. Real-time MRI showed a high specificity (98%) and sensitivity (89%) in a study of patients with acute PE with 16-slice MDCT serving as the reference modality (81).

A technique that may offer an alternative to breath-hold imaging is navigator-gated MRI, in which imaging is performed during free breathing. The navigator was first described in 1989 by Ehman and Felmlee (83), and it has been used primarily to image blood vessels which are subject to respiratory and cardiac motion, particularly the coronary arteries (84). This method has rarely been used for pulmonary imaging (85). With the advent of faster gradient systems and continued development of SSFP, it has become possible to perform rapid 3D imaging. The faster gradient systems allow for reduced repetition times, making SSFP practical. Further, the refocusing nature of SSFP, as opposed to the standard spoiled gradient echo technique, allows for both a higher flip angle and many more views per segment before significant signal decay. In a study in healthy volunteers, a breath-hold SSFP sequence was compared with a navigator gated SSFP.

Both sequences resulted in a comparable image quality with the same SNR level; however, no analysis was performed regarding vessel conspicuity on a segmental level. Image acquisition was approximately 29 s for the breath-hold and 180 s for the navigator technique (86). Therefore, in critically ill patients this technique may be worth trying as an alternative.

Magnetization-prepared gradient recalled echo imaging

Magnetization-prepared GRE acquisitions can detect thrombi using a non-selective inversion pulse prior to a short TR GRE readout module (87,88). Using a 3D acquisition scheme, resolution and SNRs can be enhanced to provide 3D multiplanar reformation capabilities for arterial lumen inspection. The technique proved sensitive for the detection of some thrombi, as it provided a positive high contrast against suppressed blood. Moody *et al.* (89) revisited this concept using a single-shot 2D MP GRE approach in patients with proven pulmonary emboli, concluding positively on the sensitivity of the approach.

The choice on the inversion time makes this black blood imaging possible. Nonetheless, it is possible to suppress the signal from thrombi instead by using a short inversion time to make the signal from surrounding blood bright. A comparison for different inversion times is illustrated in Figure 9.29. The use of a T2 or magnetization transfer preparation can produce a similar effect by

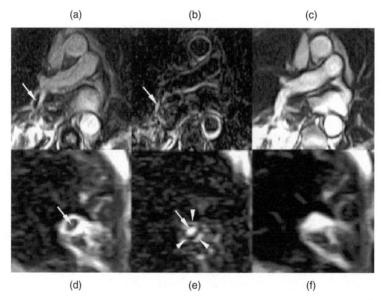

Figure 9.29 Acute pulmonary embolus in the right descending pulmonary artery may be depicted with different signal intensities depending on the imaging parameters chosen for a single-shot magnetization prepared (MP) 2D GRE scan. In this case, an inversion pulse and a delay are used as magnetization preparation prior to image acquisition. (a) Without an inversion pulse a proton density weighted image is generated with no discernible contrast between thrombus and blood. (b) Choice of a short inversion time suppresses the signal from the embolus (arrow) while moderate signal is maintained for surrounding blood. (c) Inversion time tuned to suppress the signal from blood demonstrates a bright clot (arrow). Small arrowheads in (c) point to unsuppressed signal from the vessel wall and high-spatial frequency artefacts from remnant signal from blood. (d)–(f) correspond to views perpendicular to those shown in (a)–(c). The 2D MP GRE acquisition used TR/TE/α = 3.5 ms/1.6 ms/10°, 8 mm slice thickness and a 3.3 × 3.0 mm in-plane resolution. Body phased array coil acquisition.

suppressing the signal from the thrombus (shorter T2 than blood and higher magnetization transfer coefficient) while maintaining a high signal for blood.

The inversion-based MP GRE technique can be problematic for the detection of clot in small vessels for three reasons:

- Vessel walls are not suppressed and the signal remains in peripheral small vessels because of partial volume effects.
- A long string of low flip angle RF pulses (typically 80–128) after a single magnetization preparation can suppress the blood signal only in the larger vessels (poor suppression of high spatial frequencies during signal encoding typically forming the signal of small vessels). The remnant signal in the vessel wall can be seen in Figure 9.29 (90).
- The SNR for MP GRE approaches is usually low because of the low RF excitation readout used to maintain the prepared contrast.

Advantages to the 2D and 3D MP GRE techniques include blood flow-independent results, a drawback often found with non-contrast-enhanced MRA techniques (conventional TOF MRA) for obtaining a high blood signal with a slow flow. Both SE and fast MP GRE approaches have a limited scope for PE detection and may only identify intraluminal abnormalities up to fourth-order branches reliably. The incorporation of negative contrast agents to suppress blood signal (shortening T2 and T2* dramatically) can prove useful for rapid thrombus imaging (91).

CLINICAL EVALUATION OF MRPA FOR PULMONARY EMBOLISM

The number of studies reporting on the use of MRPA for the detection of PE has been constantly growing during recent years. Very early reports mainly focused on the utility of conventional TOF or contrast-enhanced 2D GRE scans, whereas more recent work almost exclusively relies on the use of contrast-enhanced 3D GRE. The latter offers the advantage of its robustness and easy interpretation.

Time-of-flight MRPA

Schiebler *et al.* (92) evaluated 18 patients prospectively with 2D sequential MRPA (TR/TE/α = 6.8–9.8/2.2/20°, 128 × 256 matrix, breath-hold, two averages, sagittal) in conjunction with cardiac-gated SE and cine 2D GRE with spatial modulation of magnetization (SPAMM). The overall sensitivity for the detection of acute pulmonary emboli was 85% (42% for chronic emboli). Confirmation was performed with conventional angiography on eight patients; five received radionuclide ventilation–perfusion (V/Q) scans and six had direct surgical intervention. Another study (93) reported on the accuracy of a similar breath-hold 2D sequential MRPA set-up (TR/TE/α = 6.8–12/(2.2–3.4)/20–30°, 128 × 256 matrix, breath-hold, four averages, sagittal). A sensitivity of 92–100% and a specificity of 62% were reached in 20 patients evaluated prospectively (16 with angiographic correlation, four with known PE). Sostman *et al.* (94) investigated a free-breathing 2D sequential GRE (TR/TE/α = 12/1.8–2.8/30°, 256 × 256 matrix, eight averages, sagittal) in 25 patients. Several levels of expertise were discussed, reporting sensitivities ranging between 43 and 92% and specificities between 67 and 100%. In the expert group, a mean sensitivity of 73% and a specificity of 97% were obtained. Study confirmation was performed using a decision tree involving conventional angiography and radionuclide V/Q scans.

2D contrast-enhanced MRPA studies

Using a multiplanar MRPA set-up with a thick-section magnetization prepared 2D GRE scan (TR/TE/α = 6.5/3.0 ms/12°, inversion time to null blood = 300 ms, 128 × 128 matrix, free breathing) (95), Loubeyre *et al.* (96) imaged 23 consecutive patients with suspected PE. A comparison with pulmonary angiography yielded a sensitivity of 70% and a specificity of 100% only for proximal pulmonary emboli (segmental emboli were completely missed). Shortly afterwards, Bergin *et al.* (97) investigated the accuracy of a 2D interleaved acquisition (TR/TE/α = 113/4.3 ms/70°, 128 × 256 matrix, breath-hold) combined with spiral contrast-enhanced CT angiography in 26 patients with chronic thromboembolic disease. After angiographic and surgical confirmation, MRPA provided a sensitivity of 36% and a specificity of 65% for thrombus detection in the central pulmonary arteries and higher values for segmental branches, reaching a sensitivity of 72% and a specificity of 59%. The poor figures may be attributed to the thickness of the slices utilized (10 mm).

3D contrast-enhanced MRPA studies

The report by Isoda *et al.* (51) may be considered the first clinical experience with breath-hold contrast-enhanced 3D MRPA. The group investigated 13 patients (nine with lung cancer, one metastatic lung tumour, two pulmonary sequestrations, one suspicious PE) with a contrast-enhanced 3D GRE scan (TR/TE/α = 12/5 ms/20°, 16 slices, 100 × 128 matrix, breath-hold 19 s, coronal, test bolus injection). Correlation with conventional angiography revealed a sensitivity of 80%, a specificity of 95% and an accuracy of 95.5% for the detection of segmental artery stenosis or occlusion.

More recent investigations with breath-hold contrast-enhanced 3D MRPA using higher spatial resolution protocols have reported the routine visualization of fifth- to seventh-order branches and have provided data sets that can be reformatted to assess any vessel obstruction caused by emboli with increased accuracy. Meaney *et al.* (54) investigated 30 consecutive patients prospectively (TR/TE/α = 6.5/1.8 ms/40–45°, 32 slices, 128 × 256 matrix, breath-hold 27 s, coronal, fixed injection delay 7–10 s, dose 0.3 mmol/kg Gd-DTPA). Readings by three independent radiologists provided sensitivities of 100, 87 and 75% (mean 87.3%) and specificities of 95, 100 and 95% (mean 96.6%) compared with conventional angiography. The overall score by consensus agreed on a sensitivity of 100% and a specificity of 95%, but without including data from three patients with unreadable MRPAs. Remarkably, good inter-observer agreement with kappa values ranging from 0.57 to 0.83 was demonstrated.

A subsequent study evaluated the accuracy of MRPA in 36 patients with intermediate- or low-probability lung scintigraphy. All patients in this study underwent pulmonary DSA as the gold standard, which demonstrated PE in 13 patients. MRPA diagnosed 12 patients as having PE but missed two cases. This resulted in a sensitivity of 85% and a specificity of 96%. Both missed pulmonary emboli were isolated and subsegmental in location (98).

In the largest study so far, Oudkerk *et al.* assessed the accuracy of MRPA in 141 patients with an abnormal perfusion lung scintigraphy and compared the findings with pulmonary DSA, which was performed in all patients within a few hours (99). 3D contrast-enhanced MRPA detected 27 of 35 cases with confirmed PE, resulting in an overall sensitivity of 77%. The sensitivity for isolated subsegmental, segmental and central/lobar PE was 40, 84 and 100%, respectively. MRPA demonstrated emboli in two patients with a normal angiogram, i.e., the specificity was 98%.

In a more recent study, 89 patients with suspected PE were examined using coronal, axial and sagittal orientated 3D contrast-enhanced MRPA (100). The images were interpreted independently

Table 9.6 Typical current state-of-the-art protocol for MRPA at 1.5 T

TR (ms)	2.4
TE (ms)	0.9
Voxel size (mm)	$1.3 \times 1 \times 1.1$
Scan time (s)	20
Matrix	384×77
FOV (mm)	390×100
Bandwidth (Hz/pixel)	870
PI factor	2–3

by two teams of radiologists. In contrast to the previous studies, patients exhibited different clinical probabilities of having PE and demonstrated a higher PE prevalence of 71%. D-dimer testing, spiral CT, compression venous ultrasound and pulmonary DSA served as the gold standard in this study. Depending on the team of readers, the sensitivity and specificity of contrast-enhanced MRA were highly variable with ranges of 31–71% and 85–92%, respectively.

In the most recently published study, by Kluge *et al.* (81), pulmonary contrast-enhanced MRA was performed in 62 patients with suspected PE. Using parallel imaging, their MRA technique achieved a substantially higher spatial resolution ($0.7 \times 1.2 \times 1.5$ mm) than the previous studies in a short acquisition time of 15 s. With this technique, a sensitivity of 81% and a specificity of 100% were achieved with pulmonary contrast-enhanced MRA compared with 16-slice CTA. A current state-of-the-art protocol is given in Table 9.6.

Lung perfusion defects can appear in many circumstances, but PE can only be diagnosed with high confidence if the thrombus occluding the lumen is visualized after inspection with MPR (Figures 9.25 and 9.30). Another indication that may show during review is a pulmonary branch with a lower signal intensity than others. This sign seldom appears but has been seen with emboli blocking a branch almost entirely, producing a lower concentration of the contrast agent in the vessel with reduced blood flow. This is similar to inadequate bolus timing. Pulmonary perfusion with sufficient temporal resolution (one image per second) has documented regional differences of contrast arrival.

MRI offers a combination of morphological assessment and new aspects of functional imaging, such as pulmonary perfusion. 3D contrast-enhanced MRA can be regarded as a 'one-stop-shop' imaging procedure to investigate both the pulmonary arteries and the deep lower venous system within a single session. This approach is successful since it might detect 17% more cases of thromboembolic disease than with separate examinations (101). In addition, MRPA and MR venography show concordant results with CAT and duplex sonography in more than 90% of patients.

MULTIPHASIC CONTRAST-ENHANCED MRPA

Time-resolved, multiphasic MRPA is particularly advantageous in dyspneic patients with suspected PE, as was demonstrated in a feasibility study studying eight dyspneic patients with known or suspected PE using time-resolved MRPA with an acquisition time of less than 4 s per data set (69). The images allowed the assessment of the pulmonary arterial tree down to the subsegmental level and identified PE in all four subsequently confirmed cases. All patients could hold their breath for at least 8 s, during which time a dataset with an angiogram of the pulmonary arteries could be obtained.

In a more recent study, Ohno *et al.* compared the diagnostic accuracy of time-resolved multiphasic contrast-enhanced MRA with parallel imaging (SENSE) with CTA and ventilation–perfusion

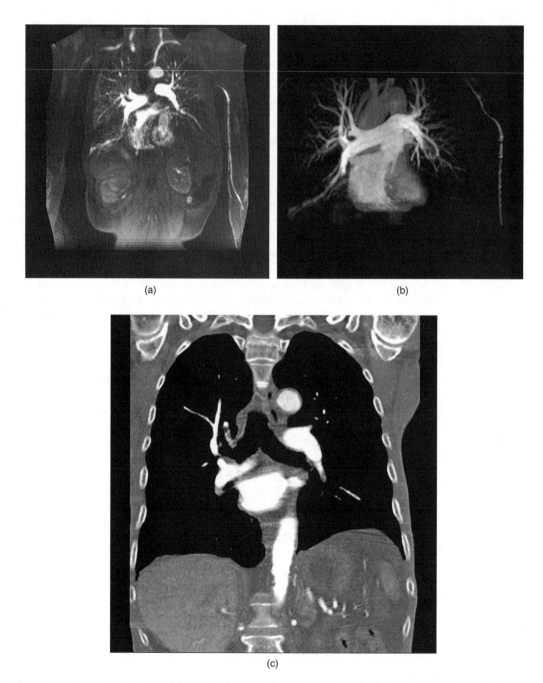

(a)

(b)

(c)

Figure 9.30   Contrast-enhanced MRPA with source image (a) and MIP (b) showing an embolus in the left lower lobe artery and also perfusion defects in both lower lobes. Findings are confirmed by CT (c).

scintigraphy (V/Q scan) in 48 patients with suspected PE (102). Conventional pulmonary DSA served as the gold standard. In this study, time-resolved MRPA had a higher sensitivity [92% vs 83% (CTA) and 67% (V/Q scan)] and specificity [94% vs 94% (CTA) and 78% (V/Q scan)] for the detection of PE than CTA and V/Q scan. Moreover, depending on the temporal resolution, the perfusion of the lung parenchyma can also be evaluated, allowing for the detection of perfusion defects. This technique is also referred to as pulmonary perfusion MRI.

As has been shown in this chapter, pulmonary MR imaging for PE has become increasingly versatile and is now able to be applied for clinical use. Although CT is still the easier access workhorse for PE diagnosis, certain subgroups of patients should be considered, such as pregnant women, those with iodinated contrast allergy or those where ionizing radiation is of particular concern. It is expected that MR imaging will continue to play an increasingly large role in the diagnosis of pulmonary vascular diseases, including PE and pulmonary hypertension.

REFERENCES

1. Alderson PO, Martin EC. Pulmonary embolism: diagnosis with multiple imaging modalities. *Radiology* 1987; **164**:297–312.
2. Kelley M, Carson J, Palevsky H, Schwartz J. Diagnosing PE: new facts and strategies. *Ann Intern Med* 1991; **1** T4:300–6.
3. Moore E, Gamsu G, Webb WR, MS S. Pulmonary embolus: detection and follow up using magnetic resonance. *Radiology* 1984; **153**:471–2.
4. Gamsu G, Hirji M, Moore EH, Webb WR, Brito A. Experimental pulmonary emboli detected using magnetic resonance. *Radiology* 1984; **153**:467–70.
5. White R, Winkler ML, Higgins CB. MR imaging of pulmonary arterial hypertension and pulmonary emboli. *Am J Roentgenol* 1987; **149**:15–21.
6. Posterano R, Sostman H, Spritzer C, Herfkens R. Cine-gradient refocused MR imaging of central pulmonary emboli. *Am J Roentgenol* 1989; **152**:465–8.
7. Moser K. Pulmonary vascular obstruction due to embolism and thrombosis. In Weir EK, Reeves JT (eds), *Pulmonary Vascular Physiology and Pathophysiology*. Lung Biology in Health and Disease, Vol. **38**. Marcel Dekker, New York, 1989.
8. Bogren HG, Klipstein RH, Mohiaddin RH, *et al*. Pulmonary artery distensibility and blood flow patterns: a magnetic resonance study of normal subjects and of patients with pulmonary arterial hypertension. *Am Heart J* 1989; **118**:990–9.
9. Mohiaddin RH, Paz R, Theodonopoulos S, *et al*. Anatomic and flow MR imaging of pulmonary arteries in patients following single lung transplantation. *Radiology* 1990; **177**(Suppl.):139.
10. Spritzer CE, Sostman HD, Wilkes DC, Coleman RE. Deep venous thrombosis: experience with gradient-echo MR imaging in 66 patients. *Radiology* 1990; **177**:235–41.
11. Gomes AS, Lois JF, Williams RG. Pulmonary arteries: MR imaging in patients with congenital obstruction of the right ventricular outflow tract. *Radiology* 1990; **174**:51–7.
12. Kauczor HU. Contrast-enhanced magnetic resonance angiography of the pulmonary vasculature. A review. *Invest Radiol* 1998; **33**:606–17.
13. Bongartz G, Boos M, Scheffler K, Steinbrich W. Pulmonary circulation. *Eur Radiol* 1998; **8**:698–706.
14. Hatabu H. MR pulmonary angiography and perfusion imaging: recent advances. *Semin Ultrasound CT MR* 1997; **18**:349–61.
15. Hatabu H, Gaa J, Kim D, *et al*. Pulmonary perfusion: qualitative assessment with dynamic contrast-enhanced MRI using ultra-short TE and inversion recovery turbo FLASH. *Magn Reson Med* 1996; **36**:503–8.
16. Amundsen T, Kvaerness J, Jones RA, *et al*. Pulmonary embolism: detection with MR perfusion imaging of lung – a feasibility study. *Radiology* 1997; **203**:181–5.
17. Axel L, Summers RM, Kressel HY, Charles C. Respiratory effects in two-dimensional Fourier transform MR imaging. *Radiology* 1986; **160**:795–801.
18. Lewis CE, Prato FS, Drost DJ, Nicholson RL. Comparison of respiratory triggering and gating techniques for the removal of respiratory artefacts in MR imaging. *Radiology* 1986; **160**:803–10.
19. Liang ZP, Boada FE, Constable RT, *et al*. Constrained reconstruction methods in MR imaging. *Rev Magn Reson Med* 1992; **4**:67–185.

20. McGibney G, Smith MR, Nichols ST, Crawley A. Quantitative evaluation of several partial Fourier reconstruction algorithms used in MRI. *Magn Reson Med* 1993; **30**:51–9.

21. Haacke E, Lindskog E, Lin W. Partial-Fourier imaging. A fast, iterative, POCS technique capable of local phase recovery *J Magn Reson* 1991; **92**:126–44.

22. Haacke EM, Masaryk TJ, Wielopolski PA, *et al.* Optimizing blood vessel contrast in fast three-dimensional MRI. *Magn Reson Med* 1990; **14**:202–21.

23. Irarrazabal P, Nishimura DG. Fast three dimensional magnetic resonance imaging. *Magn Reson Med* 1995; **33**:656–62.

24. Parker DL, Du YP, Davis WL. The voxel sensitivity function in Fourier transform imaging: applications to magnetic resonance angiography. *Magn Reson Med* 1995; **33**:156–62.

25. Meyer CH, Hu BS, Nishimura DG, Macovski A. Fast spiral coronary artery imaging. *Magn Reson Med* 1992; **28**:202–13.

26. Du J, Bydder M. High-resolution time-resolved contrast-enhanced MR abdominal and pulmonary angiography using a spiral-TRICKS sequence. *Magn Reson Med* 2007; **58**:631–35.

27. Willinek WA, Gieseke J, Conrad R, *et al.* Randomly segmented central k-space ordering in high-spatial-resolution contrast-enhanced MR angiography of the supraaortic arteries: initial experience. *Radiology* 2002; **225**:583–8.

28. Melki PS, Jolesz FA, Mulkern RV. Partial RF echo planar imaging with the FAISE method. I. Experimental and theoretical assessment of artefact. *Magn Reson Med* 1992; **26**:328–41.

29. Melki PS, Jolesz FA, Mulkern RV. Partial RF echo-planar imaging with the FAISE method. II. Contrast equivalence with spin-echo sequences. *Magn Reson Med* 1992; **26**:342–54.

30. Stehling MK, Holzknecht NG, Laub G, *et al.* Single-shot T1- and T2-weighted magnetic resonance imaging of the heart with black blood: preliminary experience. *Magma* 1996; **4**:231–40.

31. Haacke EM, Frahm J. A guide to understanding key aspects of fast gradient-echo imaging. *J Magn Reson Imaging* 1991; **1**:621–4.

32. Haase A, Matthaei D, Bartkowski R, Duhmke E, Leibfritz D. Inversion recovery snapshot FLASH MR imaging. *J Comput Assist Tomogr* 1989; **13**:1036–40.

33. Edelman R, Chien D, Kim D. Fast selective black blood MR imaging. *Radiology* 1991; **181**:655–60.

34. Pruessmann KP, Weiger M, Scheidegger MB, Boesiger P. SENSE: sensitivity encoding for fast MRI. *Magn Reson Med* 1999; **42**:952–62.

35. Griswold MA, Jakob PM, Chen Q, *et al.* Resolution enhancement in single-shot imaging using simultaneous acquisition of spatial harmonics (SMASH). *Magn Reson Med* 1999; **41**:1236–45.

36. Oosterhof T, Mulder BJ. Magnetic resonance angiography for anatomical evaluation of the great arteries. *Int J Cardiovasc Imaging* 2005; **21**:323–4.

37. Blaimer M, Breuer F, Mueller M, *et al.* SMASH, SENSE, PILS, GRAPPA: how to choose the optimal method. *Top Magn Reson Imaging* 2004; **15**:223–36.

38. Sodickson DK, Griswold MA, Jakob PM, Edelman RR, Manning WJ. Signal-to-noise ratio and signal-to-noise efficiency in SMASH imaging. *Magn Reson Med* 1999; **41**:1009–22.

39. Michaely HJ, Herrmann KA, Kramer H, *et al.* High-resolution renal MRA: comparison of image quality and vessel depiction with different parallel imaging acceleration factors. *J Magn Reson Imaging* 2006; **24**:95–100.

40. Nael K, Michaely HJ, Kramer U, *et al.* Pulmonary circulation: contrast-enhanced 3.0-T MR angiography – initial results. *Radiology* 2006; **240**:858–68.

41. Cutillo A. *Application of Magnetic Resonance to the Study of the Lung*. Futura Publishing, Armonk, NY, 1996.

42. Blackmore CC, Francis CW, Bryant RG, Brenner B, Marder VJ. Magnetic resonance imaging of blood and clots in vitro. *Invest Radiol* 1990; **25**:1316–24.

43. Bryant RG, Marill K, Blackmore CC, Francis CW. Magnetic relaxation in blood and blood clots. *Magn Reson Med* 1990; **13**:133–44.

44. Fullerton GD. Physiologic basis of magnetic relaxation. In Stark DD, Bradley WG (eds), *Magnetic Resonance Imaging*, 2nd edn. Mosby Year Book, St Louis, MO, 1992, pp. 88–108.

45. Brooks RA, Di Chiro G. Magnetic resonance imaging of stationary blood: a review. *Med Phys* 1987; **14**:903–13.

46. Gomori JM, Grossman RI, Yu-Ip C, Asakura T. NMR relaxation times of blood: dependence on field strength, oxidation state and cell integrity. *J Comput Assist Tomogr* 1987; **11**:684–90.

47. Edelman RR, Johnson K, Buxton R, *et al.* MR of hemorrhage: a new approach. *AJNR Am J Neuroradiol* 1986; **7**:751–6.

48. Prince MR. Body MR angiography with gadolinium contrast agents. *Magn Reson Imaging Clin N Am* 1996; **4**:11–24.

49. Maki JH, Prince MR, Londy FJ, Chenevert TL. The effects of time varying intravascular signal intensity and k-space acquisition order on three-dimensional MR angiography image quality. *J Magn Reson Imaging* 1996; **6**:642–51.

50. Oudkerk M, de Bruin HG, Wielopolski PA, *et al*. PE detection using contrast-enhanced, breath-hold 3 D magnetic resonance angiography. In Oudkerk M, Edelman RR (eds),. *High-Power Gradient MR Imaging. Advances in MRI II*. Blackwell Science, Berlin, 1997, pp. 78–86.

51. Isoda H, Ushimi T, Masui T, *et al*. Clinical evaluation of pulmonary 3D time-of-flight MRA with breath holding using contrast media. *J Comput Assist Tomogr* 1995; **19**:911–9.

52. Wielopolski P, Hicks S, Obdeijn A, Oudkerk M. PE Detection using contrast-enhanced, breath-hold 3D magnetic resonance angiography: preliminary experience. *Proc Int Soc Magn Reson Med* 1996; **2**:705.

53. Steiner P, McKinnon GC, Romanowski B, *et al*. Contrast-enhanced, ultrafast 3D pulmonary MR angiography in a single breath-hold: initial assessment of imaging performance. *J Magn Reson Imaging* 1997; **7**:177–82.

54. Meaney JF, Weg JG, Chenevert TL, *et al*. Diagnosis of pulmonary embolism with magnetic resonance angiography. *N Engl J Med* 1997; **336**:1422–7.

55. Leung DA, Debatin JF. Three-dimensional contrast-enhanced magnetic resonance angiography of the thoracic vasculature. *Eur Radiol* 1997; **7**:981–9.

56. Gay S, Sistrom C, Holder C, Suratt P. Breath-holding capability of adults: implications for spiral computed tomography, fast-acquisition magnetic resonance imaging and angiography. *Invest Radiol* 1994; **29**:848–51.

57. Wielopolski PA, Oudkerk M, Hicks SG, Berghout A. Breath-hold 3D MR pulmonary angiography after contrast material administration in patients with pulmonary embolim: correlation with conventional pulmonary angiography. *Radiology* 1996; **201**(Suppl):2.

58. Oberholzer K, Romaneehsen B, Kunz P, *et al*. Contrast-enhanced 3D MR angiography of the pulmonary arteries with integrated parallel acquisition technique (iPAT) in patients with chronic-thromboembolic pulmonary hypertension CTEPH-sagittal or coronal acquisition? Rofo Fortschr Geb Rontgenstr. *Neuen Bildgeb Verfahren* 2004; **176**:605.

59. Wang Y, Jonston DL, Breen JF, *et al*. Dynamic MR digital subtraction angiography using contrast enhacement, fast data acquisition and complex subtraction. *Magn Reson Med* 1996; **36**:551–6.

60. Hany TF, Schmidt M, Davis CP, Gohde SC, Debatin JF. Diagnostic impact of four postprocessing techniques in evaluating contrast-enhanced three-dimensional MR angiography. *AJR Am J Roentgenol* 1998; **170**:907–12.

61. Schoenberg SO, Knopp MV, Prince MR, Londy F, Knopp MA. Arterial-phase three-dimensional gadolinium magnetic resonance angiography of the renal arteries. Strategies for timing and contrast media injection: original investigation. *Invest Radiol* 1998; **33**:506–14.

62. Maki JH, Prince MR, Chenevert TC. Optimizing three-dimensional gadolinium-enhanced magnetic resonance angiography. Original investigation. *Invest Radiol* 1998; **33**:528–37.

63. Foo TK, Saranathan M, Prince MR, Chenevert TL. Automated detection of bolus arrival and initiation of data acquisition in fast, three-dimensional, gadolinium-enhanced MR angiography. *Radiology* 1997; **203**:275–80.

64. Ho VB, Foo TK. Optimization of gadolinium-enhanced magnetic resonance angiography using an automated bolus-detection algorithm (MR SmartPrep). Original investigation. *Invest Radiol* 1998; **33**:515–23.

65. Wilman AH, Riederer SJ, Huston J, III, Wald JT, Debbins JP. Arterial phase carotid and vertebral artery imaging in 3D contrast-enhanced MR angiography by combining fluoroscopic triggering with an elliptical centric acquisition order. *Magn Reson Med* 1998; **40**:24–35.

66. Siebert JE. Image presentation and post-processing. In Potchen EJ, Haacke EM, Siebert JE, Gottschalk A (eds). *Magnetic Resonance Angiography, Concepts and Applications*. Mosby Year Book, St Louis, MO, 1993, Chapter 11, pp. 220–45.

67. Fink C, Ley S, Kroeker R, Requardt M, Kauczor HU, Bock M. Time-resolved contrast-enhanced three-dimensional magnetic resonance angiography of the chest: combination of parallel imaging with view sharing (TREAT). *Invest Radiol* 2005; **40**:40–8.

68. Korosec FR, Frayne R, Grist TM, Mistretta CA. Time-resolved contrast-enhanced 3D MR angiography. *Magn Reson Med* 1996; **36**:345–51.

69. Goyen M, Laub G, Ladd M, *et al*. Dynamic 3D MR angiography of the pulmonary arteries in under four seconds. *J Magn Reson Imaging* 2001; **13**:372.

70. Schoenberg SO, Bock M, Floemer F, *et al*. High-resolution pulmonary arterio- and venography using multiple-bolus multiphase 3D-Gd-MRA. *J Magn Reson Imaging* 1999; **10**:339–46.

71. Lohan D, Krishnam M, Tomasian A, Saleh R, Finn P. Time-resolved MR angiography of the thorax. *Magn Reson Imaging Clin N Am* 2008; **16**:235–48.

72. Peters DC, Korosec FR, Frayne R, Grist TM, Mistretta CA. Cardiac-gated contrast-enhanced time-resolved 3D imaging of the pulmonary arteries. *Proc Int Soc Magn Reson Med* 1997; **3**:1859.

73. Finn JP, Baskaran V, Carr JC, *et al.* Thorax: low-dose contrast-enhanced three-dimensional MR angiography with subsecond temporal resolution – initial results. *Radiology* 2002; **224**:896–904.

74. Bàck J, Kaufmann F, Felix R. Comparison of gadolinium-DTPA and macromolecular gadolinium-DTPA polylysine for contrast-enhanced pulmonary time-of-flight magnetic resonance angiography. *Invest Radiol* 1996; **31**:652–7.

75. Frank H, Weissleder R, Bogdanov AJ, Brady T. Detection of pulmonary emboli by using MR angiography with MPEG-PL-GcDTPA: an experimental study in rabbits. *Am J Roentgenol* 1994; **162**:1041–6.

76. Li KC, Pelc LR, Napel SA, *et al.* MRI of pulmonary embolism using Gd-DTPA-polyethylene glycol polymer enhanced 3D fast gradient echo technique in a canine model. *Magn Reson Imaging* 1997; **15**:543–50.

77. Lauffer RB, Parmelee DJ, Dunham SU, *et al.* MS-325: albumin-targeted contrast agent for MR angiography. *Radiology* 1998; **207**:529–38.

78. Grist TM, Korosec FR, Peters DC, *et al.* Steady-state and dynamic MR angiography with MS-325: initial experience in humans. *Radiology* 1998; **207**:539–44.

79. Fink C, Ley S, Puderbach M, *et al.* 3D pulmonary perfusion MRI and MR angiography of pulmonary embolism in pigs after a single injection of a blood pool MR contrast agent. *Eur Radiol* 2004; **14**:1291–6.

80. Abdolmaali N, Hietschold V, Appold S, Ebert W, Vogl T. Gadomer-17-enhanced 3D navigator-echo MR angiography of the pulmonary arteries in pigs. *Eur Radiol* 2002; **12**:692–7.

81. Kluge A, Luboldt W, Bachmann G. Acute pulmonary embolism to the subsegmental level: diagnostic accuracy of three MRI techniques compared with 16-MDCT. *AJR Am J Roentgenol* 2006; **187**:W7–14.

82. Kluge A, Muller C, Hansel J, Gerriets T, Bachmann G. Real-time MR with TrueFISP for the detection of acute pulmonary embolism: initial clinical experience. *Eur Radiol* 2004; **14**:709–18.

83. Ehman RL, Felmlee JP. Adaptive technique for high-definition MR imaging of moving structures. *Radiology* 1989; **173**:255–63.

84. Spuentrup E, Bornert P, Botnar RM, *et al.* Navigator-gated free-breathing three-dimensional balanced fast field echo (TrueFISP) coronary magnetic resonance angiography. *Invest Radiol* 2002; **37**:637–42.

85. Wang Y, Rossman PJ, Grimm RC, *et al.* 3D MR angiography of pulmonary arteries using real-time navigator and magnetization preparation. *Magn Reson Med* 1996; **36**:579–87.

86. Hui BK, Noga ML, Gan KD, Wilman AH. Navigator-gated three-dimensional MR angiography of the pulmonary arteries using steady-state free precession. *J Magn Reson Imaging* 2005; **21**:831–5.

87. Wielopolski P, Haacke E, Adler L. Three-dimensional pulmonary vascular imaging. In Potchen EJ, Haacke EM, Siebert JE, Gottschalk A (eds), *Magnetic Resonance Angiography, Concept and Applications*. Mosby Year Book, St Louis, MO, 1993, Chapter 12, pp. 246–77.

88. Wielopolski P, Haacke EM, Adler LP. Evaluation of the pulmonary vasculature with three-dimensional magnetic resonance techniques. *Magma* 1993; **1**:21–34.

89. Moody AR, Liddicoat A, Krarup K. Magnetic resonance pulmonary angiography and direct imaging of embolus for the detection of pulmonary emboli. *Invest Radiol* 1997; **32**:431–40.

90. Wielopolski PA, Haacke E, Adler LP. Three-dimensional MR imaging of the pulmonary vascular system. In Cutillo AG (ed), *Application of Magnetic Resonance to the Study of the Lung*. Futura Publishing, Armonk, NY, 1996, Chapter 11, pp. 341–65.

91. Thakur ML, Vinitski S, Mitchell DG, *et al.* MR imaging of pulmonary parenchyma and emboli by paramagnetic and superparamagnetic contrast agents. *Magn Reson Imaging* 1990; **8**:625–30.

92. Schiebler ML, Holland GA, Hatabu H, *et al.* Suspected pulmonary embolism: prospective evaluation with pulmonary MR angiography. *Radiology* 1993; **189**: 125–31.

93. Grist TM, Sostman HD, MacFall JR, *et al.* Pulmonary angiography with MR imaging: preliminary clinical experience. *Radiology* 1993; **189**:523–530.

94. Sostman HD, Layish DT, Tapson VF, *et al.* Prospective comparison of helical CT and MR imaging in clinically suspected acute pulmonary embolism. *J Magn Reson Imaging* 1996; **6**:275–81.

95. Revel D, Loubeyre P, Delignette A, Douek P, Amiel M. Contrast-enhanced magnetic resonance tomoangiography: a new imaging technique for studying thoracic great vessels. *Magn Reson Imaging* 1993; **11**:1101–5.

96. Loubeyre P, Revel D, Douek P, *et al.* Dynamic contrast-enhanced MR angiography of pulmonary embolism: comparison with pulmonary angiography. *AJR Am J Roentgenol* 1994; **162**:1035–9.

97. Bergin CJ, Sirlin CB, Hauschildt JP, *et al.* Chronic thromboembolism: diagnosis with helical CT and MR imaging with angiographic and surgical correlation. *Radiology* 1997; **204**:695–702.

98. Gupta A, Frazer C, Ferguson J, *et al.* Acute pulmonary embolism: diagnosis with MR angiography. *Radiology* 1999; **210**:353–9.

99. Oudkerk M, van Beek E, *et al.* Comparison of contrast-enhanced magnetic resonance angiography and conventional pulmonary angiography for the diagnosis of pulmonary embolism: a prospective study. *Lancet* 2002; **359**:1643–7.

100. Blum A, Bellou A, Guillemin F, Douek P, Laprevote-Heully M, Wahl D. Performance of magnetic resonance angiography in suspected acute pulmonary embolism. *Thromb Haemost* 2005; **93**:503–11.

101. Obernosterer A, Aschauer M, Portugaller H, Koppel H, Lipp RW. Three-dimensional gadolinium-enhanced magnetic resonance angiography used as a 'one-stop shop' imaging procedure for venous thromboembolism: a pilot study. *Angiology* 2005; **56**:423–30.

102. Ohno Y, Higashino T, Takenaka D, *et al.* MR angiography with sensitivty encoding (SENSE) for suspected pulmonary embolism: comparison with MDCT and ventilation–perfusion scintigraphy. *AJR Am J Roentgenol* 2004; **183**:91–8.

103. Gomori JM, Grossman RI, Goldberg HI, Zimmerman RA, Bilaniuk LT. Intracranial hematomas: imaging by high-field MR. *Radiology* 1985; **157**:87–93.

CHAPTER 10

Pulmonary Angiography: Technique, Indications and Complications

Marjolein van Loveren[1], Edwin J.R. van Beek[2] and Matthijs Oudkerk[1]

[1]Department of Radiology, University Medical Center Groningen, University of Groningen, Groningen, The Netherlands
[2]Department of Radiology, Carver College of Medicine, Iowa City, USA

INTRODUCTION

Pulmonary angiography has developed over a period of nearly 80 years. It has proven its superior diagnostic accuracy in the assessment of patients with clinically suspected pulmonary embolism (PE) and has gained widespread acceptance as the reference method. Nevertheless, its invasive nature has led to the investigation of many non-invasive techniques and computed tomographic pulmonary angiography (CTPA) is now considered the standard for the diagnosis of PE, as described in Chapter 7. In this chapter, the main technique, interpretation and complications of pulmonary angiography will be described. It is our firm belief that, when using the described precautions, pulmonary angiography is safe enough to remain an important final diagnostic test in the management of selected patients with suspected PE, such as those where non-invasive methods are not interpretable or not acceptable and in those in whom intervention procedures are a consideration.

HISTORY OF TECHNIQUE

Forssmann is credited with the first successful introduction of a catheter into the right atrium when he performed an experiment on himself in 1929 (1). Subsequently, he was able to visualize the right heart chambers and the pulmonary artery using a 20% sodium iodide solution in dogs (1). It took nearly another 25 years before Bolt and co-workers were able to perform selective pulmonary angiography, i.e., with catheter position through the heart into the pulmonary artery (1).

Several advances were essential in the development of pulmonary angiography as it is being performed today. To name a few: the development of safe catheter introduction by Seldinger, the development of rapid imaging equipment (film changers) followed by the progressive improvements in digital subtraction angiography, the introduction of the pigtail catheter, the development of ever safer contrast agents and catheter and guide-wire materials. These improvements have led to pulmonary angiography being a relatively safe procedure. In fact, this increased safety is supported by data in the literature. Studies which were published during the period 1960–1980 (2–5) showed an average complication rate of 2.1%; in those that were published during 1980–1999 (6–11) this rate declined to only 0.62%. Nowadays the complication rate is estimated to be as low as 0.03% and 0.3–0.5% fatal and non-fatal complications, respectively (12).

INDICATIONS/CONTRAINDICATIONS

Catheter pulmonary angiography was, for a long time, the 'gold standard' technique for PE diagnosis and has the advantage of providing haemodynamic information at the same time. Nevertheless, due to the misconception of patient risks and with the development and growing availability of non-invasive diagnostic imaging tests [e.g., CTPA, ventilation perfusion imaging and even magnetic resonance imaging (MRI)], the role of pulmonary angiography in diagnosing PE waned quickly. Also, the expertise of the radiologist is declining, so that performing a pulmonary angiography has become a state-of-the-art procedure available in a decreasing number of centres.

As a result of the aforementioned, currently pulmonary angiography is reserved for the few patients in whom interventions are considered (see Chapters 25 and 26) and in those with a high clinical probability of PE and exclusively non-diagnostic test results (12–17). It should be obvious that pulmonary angiography can only be performed in an experienced clinic, usually a tertiary referral centre.

Contraindications for pulmonary angiography have declined over the years. No absolute contraindications currently exist, although several relative contraindications should be noted (Table 10.1). Some extra measures may be required to reduce the risks in these patients:

1. Allergy to iodine-containing contrast agents: with a previously documented allergic reaction to contrast agents, patients should have prophylactic steroids and antihistamines prior to the procedure.
2. Impaired renal function: the present contrast agents and the use of digital subtraction angiography have resulted in less nephrotoxicity and the ability to use less contrast agents. Hence impaired renal function is no longer considered an absolute contraindication. Nevertheless, renal function should be monitored in these patients following angiography and dialysis equipment

Table 10.1   Relative contraindications for pulmonary angiography

Documented previous iodinated contrast allergy
Renal failure
Congestive heart failure
Ventricular ectopy or left bundle branch block
Severe pulmonary hypertension (mean PAP >40 mmHg)
Right-sided endocarditis
Anticoagulated state or thrombocytopenia
Pregnancy

should be available if one is to perform angiography in these patients. In patients who suffer from severe renal insufficiency prior to angiography, dialysis should be scheduled following the procedure.

3. Left bundle branch block: this is not a contraindication, but extra care must be taken. During passage of the catheter through the right heart, a total ventricular block may develop. Hence it is advised that a pacemaker is on stand-by during the procedure.

4. Severe congestive heart failure: this increases the risks of complications, largely as a result of volume overload during the injection of contrast agent. It is advised that patients should preferably be treated for their heart failure during 24 hours prior to angiography. If this is insufficient or not feasible, angiography should be undertaken using an amended contrast injection scheme consisting of a longer duration of linear rise, reduced amounts of contrast and more selective catheterization.

5. Severe pulmonary hypertension (mean pulmonary artery pressure >40 mmHg): this situation increases the risks of complications, but with the reduced amounts of contrast and longer duration of linear rise this is well within reasonable limits. Several studies have reported on the safety of pulmonary angiography in large patient groups with pre-existing pulmonary hypertension (8,18,19). Furthermore, as described in Chapter 25, pulmonary angiography still forms an essential part of the work-up and planning for patients considered for thromboendarterectomy.

6. Right-sided endocarditis: this poses the risk of septicaemia and septic embolism during catheter manipulation. Pulmonary angiography should be carried out if other diagnostic techniques have failed to offer an adequate diagnosis and the bleeding risks are deemed too large.

7. Anticoagulated state or thrombocytopenia: these are mainly of concern for haematomas at the puncture site. In patients who are heparinized while awaiting angiography, the heparin pump should be stopped once the patient is prepared in the angiography suite. If pulmonary emboli are proven, the pump can be restarted and aPTT monitoring will be required to assess the need for additional heparin administration. In patients with thrombocytopenia between 30×10^{12} and 100×10^{12}/L, no additional measures are required. For those with thrombocytopenia of less than 30×10^{12}/L, a donation of 6–12 units of thrombocytes may be required if bleeding at the puncture site cannot be controlled within 20–30 minutes.

8. Pregnancy is not an absolute contraindication (as discussed in Chapter 16). However, lead shielding of the abdomen, the preferential use of the brachial route and radiation hygiene are advised.

Albeit that these contraindications are relative, they are usually part of the decision not to perform pulmonary angiography. However, the general condition of the patient is mostly the deciding factor, as demonstrated in two studies where pulmonary angiography could not be performed in 10–20% of patients who were scheduled for the procedure (6,9).

PATIENT MONITORING DURING PROCEDURE

Patients who are entering an angiography suite to undergo pulmonary angiography need to be monitored, and at the same time several items should be available at all times. First, it is imperative that oxygen can be obtained freely, since many patients are suffering from hypoxaemia. An oxymeter may be useful, but is not essential since it has relatively little influence on patient management at the time of angiography. Second, an automated blood pressure and pulse measurement device is advised, which can do rapid readings, i.e., one reading per minute, during the procedure.

The use of electrocardiography during the procedure is debatable. Rhythm disorders do occur during passage of the catheter through the right heart chambers (as described below). However, if electrocardiography prior to the procedure does not show a left bundle branch block or ventricular extrasystoles, one could decide to leave the electrocardiography monitoring and rely on blood pressure, pulse and oxymeter readings only.

COMPLICATIONS

Complications of pulmonary angiography can be divided into two main categories relative to the performance of pulmonary angiography, with a number of subcategories:

1. Complications of catheter placement, which include puncture site difficulties, pulmonary embolism (PE) from pelvic/caval thrombus, vessel/cardiac injury or perforation and cardiac arrhythmias.
2. Complications of contrast injection, which include iodinated contrast related issues and cardiopulmonary alteration (due to contrast load).

Although this list is certainly not inclusive of every possible complication, it serves as a basis for discussion.

Complications of catheter placement

Puncture site complications

Pulmonary angiography is most often performed through the femoral vein. At the site of catheter insertion, complications such as infection, haemorrhage, thrombosis and arteriovenous fistula (AVF) formation can occur. In general, access site complications are relatively rare and consist mostly of haematomas. Note that due to the acute character of haematomas they are more easily detected than complications such as thrombosis, infection or even AVF, which needs long-term follow-up to record.

Pulmonary embolism from pelvic/caval thrombus

Most pulmonary emboli originate in the venous system of the legs, pelvis and inferior vena cava (20). Catheter thrombosis must be avoided in all situations, but is particularly dangerous when angiography is performed for pulmonary arteriovenous malformations and in patients with a patent foramen ovale, as a left to right shunt may be sufficiently present to allow systemic embolization with catastrophic consequences (e.g., stroke). If venography is not performed prior to catheter placement from the common femoral vein to the right atrium, thrombus could theoretically be dislodged by catheterization causing PE. Grollman stated in a review in 1992 that he had only rarely encountered unsuspected thrombus in the inferior vena cava during pulmonary angiography and he successfully and safely demonstrated such thrombus by angiography (21). However, he did not routinely perform cavography prior to pulmonary angiography. We and most others agree with this approach (22). In a patient with caval thrombosis, it is possible to catheterize safely around the thrombus. This may be clinically necessary in certain selected cases, such as in patients who require inferior vena cava filter placement or in patients who are considered for thrombolysis; if no other access is available, alternative routes, such as brachial vein or internal jugular vein approach may be used; the internal jugular vein is favoured by most.

Vessel and cardiac injury or perforation

Any time catheterization of a vessel occurs, one must be concerned with intimal injury or even perforation. Injury to the pelvic veins, inferior vena cava or pulmonary artery is theoretically

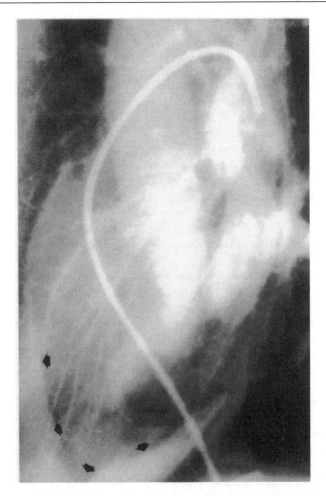

Figure 10.1 Lateral view of the late phase of a pulmonary angiogram using an NIH-type catheter. During passage of the catheter through the heart there was myocardial perforation. There is a persistent contrast collection (arrows) surrounding the cardiac silhouette. Angiography was completed without difficulty and the patient remained asymptomatic.

possible. One of the historical worries with pulmonary angiography was for cardiac perforation (Figure 10.1), which was more common with the straight-configuration and (stiff) guidewires. To reduce this risk, Grollman and co-workers developed the pigtail catheter in 1970 and various modifications in the design have been made since (23,24). Together with the introduction of new catheter and guidewire materials, the rate of cardiac perforation has decreased. Where in the past cardiac perforation rates ranging from 0.4 to 2.1% were described (2,525–27), Hudson *et al.* noted none in their series of 1434 pulmonary angiograms, which were all performed with pigtail catheters (8). Pigtail catheters are not without their own complications. The catheter can become entangled in the chordae tendineae of the tricuspid valve or even become knotted (28).

Cardiac dysrhythmias

Cardiac dysrhythmias occur during the performance of pulmonary angiography either from catheter manipulation or during contrast injection. The latter is uncommon and self-limited, whereas cardiac dysrhythmias during the passage of catheters through the right heart are fairly common and often exacerbated by the use of guidewires.

During passage of the catheter through the right atrium to the tricuspid valve, mechanical stimulation may induce atrial extra-systoles or tachycardia as a result of the development of atrial tachycardia, atrial flutter or atrial fibrillation. In the majority of cases, this is transient and terminates on stopping catheter manipulation. If atrial flutter or fibrillation persists, the rapid ventricular rate may be slowed by use of β-adrenergic blocking agents (e.g., isoptin or metoprolol i.v. – slowly injected 1–5 mg). In rare instances, electrical cardioversion may be indicated.

During manipulation of the catheter in the area of the tricuspid valve, irritation of the wall may cause bundle branch block or bradycardia due to second-degree AV-block or complete AV-block. These conduction disturbances are usually temporary, but if sustained atropine 0.5–1.0 mg i.v. may restore A–V node conduction. With complete AV block that does not spontaneously resolve, temporary transvenous right ventricular pacing is indicated.

Manipulation of the catheter within the right ventricle may irritate the wall, causing ventricular extrasystoles, which are innocent or short bursts of ventricular tachycardia, which usually terminate after cessation of catheter manipulation.

Sustained ventricular tachycardia is a very rare occurrence and requires triggered electrical cardioversion. Ventricular fibrillation may occur, frequently this is self-limited, but if persisting this requires immediate electrical defibrillation (200–400 J).

Crossing the tricuspid valve with the catheter may occasionally induce right bundle branch block, which spontaneously reverts to normal conduction.

In the PIOPED study, there were nine cases of arrhythmia in 1111 patients (0.8%), all of which converted into sinus rhythm spontaneously or promptly responded to medication (29). However, two of the deaths in this series appear to be related, at least in part, to cardiac dysrhythmias encountered at pulmonary angiography. In one of these patients electromechanical dissociation occurred with the catheter in the right ventricle, although no arrhythmia was noted and the mechanism of events was reported to be unclear. The second patient had a catheter in the right ventricle when ventricular tachycardia occurred, which was reverted but respiratory arrest and hypotension occurred soon after and the patient died 24 hours after catheterization. In the series of Hudson et al. consisting of 1434 pulmonary angiograms, eight patients (0.6%) had significant cardiac dysrhythmias requiring treatment (8). In six patients (0.4%), treatment with intravenous lidocaine was successful and pulmonary angiography was completed. In two patients (0.1%), ventricular arrhythmia recurred during each catheter manipulation despite medical therapy and the procedure was selectively discontinued. All of these patients left the angiography suite in sinus rhythm and had no further cardiac rhythm disturbances during 48 hours of follow up.

Overall, although cardiac dysrhythmias appear to occur frequently during catheter manipulation for pulmonary angiography, they are for the most part self-limited and respond well to a pause in catheter manipulation and/or catheter repositioning. Medical treatment appears to be necessary in less than 1% of patients with near 100% favourable response. Although fairly rare, complete heart block has been produced in patients with a pre-existing left bundle branch block when a right block is induced by catheter manipulation.

Complications of contrast injection

Pulmonary angiography requires the use of iodinated contrast material, which carries a small risk for adverse events. Contrast, which is rapidly injected under high power, as with pulmonary angiography, can cause intimal dissection depending on the catheter position. In addition, contrast injection for pulmonary angiography has been associated with some benign dysrhythmias. These complications are discussed above. Additional complications consist mostly of contrast-induced nephrotoxicity and allergic reactions. The latter consist mostly of haemodynamic alterations associated with contrast injection into the pulmonary vascular bed.

For the development of contrast-induced nephrotoxicity, several risk factors may be recognized, including pre-existing renal insufficiency (30,31), contrast volume (32) and the choice of contrast agents. Low osmolar non-ionic agents cause less haemodynamic alterations then high osmolar ionic agents, and are therefore safer in terms of nephrotoxicity and severe contrast media reactions (33). Although most cases of contrast media-associated nephrotoxicity are largely reversible by medical therapy, acute renal failure can lead to significant associated morbidity and mortality (34).

Adverse reactions to the injection of contrast material are well known, albeit less problematic with low-osmolar non-ionic agents, and can be divided into idiosyncratic and non-idiosyncratic reactions (35–37). Idiosyncratic reactions are not dose dependent and are anaphylactoid in nature (i.e., bronchospasm, urticaria, itching and periorbital oedema). Severe idiosyncratic reactions are fairly rare due to the rapid, focal pulmonary arterial injection of contrast, but a few deaths have been reported even with use of low-osmolar non-ionic agents (38,39). Non-idiosyncratic reactions are volume dependent and are the result of chemotoxic or hyperosmolar properties of the contrast (e.g., agent-induced coughing). Where non-idiosyncratic reactions are concerned, probably the most striking advantage of the low-osmolar non-ionic agents has been the reduction of contrast agent-induced coughing during pulmonary angiography (40,41). Prior assessment of patients and appropriate prophylaxis are the main method to diminish adverse reactions. In addition, routine use of low-osmolar non-ionic agents is currently the standard of care. For pulmonary angiography, there are probably only two disadvantages of the non-ionic agents: their reported increased thrombogenicity (which does not appear to be a significant clinical problem) and costs. As far as costs are concerned, there is a clear benefit and this overrides the slight cost increase in the relatively limited number of patients requiring pulmonary angiography.

HAEMODYNAMIC AND RESPIRATORY ALTERATIONS

Patients undergoing pulmonary angiography have been reported to have a variety of haemodynamic alterations, including systemic hypotension, increased pulmonary arterial pressures and cardiopulmonary collapse (42). Systemic hypotension can be due to a number of causes, including idiosyncratic adverse contrast reactions as reported above. Transient hypotension has been reported to occur with contrast injection due to peripheral vasodilation. It has been postulated that these systemic hypotensive reactions may be a reflection of reduced aortic pressure by the temporary decrease in pulmonary blood flow to the left heart. Many patients who are undergoing pulmonary angiography may be dehydrated, resulting in a relative state of hypotension. Obviously this state needs correction if possible, not only from a cardiovascular perspective, but also from one of contrast-associated nephrotoxicity. Finally, physiological reflex syncope (vasovagal) occurs during pulmonary angiography as with many other procedures (8,43). Although rarely necessary, this can be medically treated with atropine sulfate.

Pulmonary artery pressures tend to increase after the injection of contrast material. The reasons for this increase in pressure remain unclear, although a number of theories exist. Contrast material in the pulmonary vascular system causes arterial constriction, venous constriction or both, resulting in increased arterial pressure (44,45). Hypertonic solutions tend to produce changes in red blood cells such as aggregation and crenation, which can result in capillary blockage and increased pulmonary pressure (46). Data also support the view that increased pressure may be related to contrast viscosity (47). Finally, the volume of the injection alone may be responsible for increased pressure (48). As would be expected with the above theories, the increase in pressure following the injection of high-osmolar ionic contrast material tend to be greater than those with low-osmolar non-ionic media (49,50).

Increases in pulmonary artery pressure during angiography generated much interest in early reports. Death from pulmonary angiography was attributed to the sequelae of pulmonary hypertension (2,5,26). Severe underlying pulmonary hypertension presumably places the right heart in an extremely compromised state such that any sudden increase in pulmonary pressure may result in right heart decompensation and possibly death. If the association of increased right heart pressure and cardiac failure were to hold true, the rate of mortality from pulmonary angiography should decrease with low-osmolar non-ionic agents, since they result in significantly less elevation of pulmonary pressure than high-osmolar ionic agents, as discussed above. Combining two series of studies by Hudson et al. (8) and Zuckerman et al. (10), a total of 1981 pulmonary angiograms were performed using low-osmolar non-ionic contrast material without mortality. These findings indeed lend credence to the idea that pulmonary angiography is safer with low-osmolar non-ionic agents.

A number of patients experience respiratory insufficiency and/or cardiac arrest following pulmonary angiography, which could be based on the volume of fluids given to patients during angiography. Often a relatively large amount of fluids, including contrast material, angiographic flush solutions and intravenous support fluids, are used during the procedure. As many of these patients are already severely compromised, additional intravascular volumes could be deleterious. Finally, there are unusual situations where respiratory failure can be due to other causes, again often due to the difficulty with the clinical diagnosis of PE and the need to perform angiography in compromised patients. Acute respiratory failure has been reported in patients being treated with amiodarone for arrhythmias (51,52). Obviously, care should be taken prior to pulmonary angiography in all patients and their respiratory status must be fully evaluated prior to angiography.

Cardiac arrest has been reported with pulmonary angiography (2,5,25). Many causes may result in cardiac arrest, as described above, but the exact aetiology in individual patients remains largely unclear.

MATERIALS

It is imperative that modern materials are used to decrease the chances of complications. A standard pigtail catheter, or modifications thereof, are generally used. The size of catheters may vary from 5F to 7F (Figure 10.2), depending on the manufacturer (53). Balloon catheters have been reported to be helpful, especially in patients with a large right atrium/ventricle. In our experience, these catheters do not have a place with the majority of patients, since catheterization is usually achieved without difficulty. Nevertheless, they may be beneficial in patients in whom amended contrast injections are required for fear of right ventricular overload. Balloon occlusion angiography may be able to reduce the total amount of contrast used in these patients (7).

Introducer sheaths are not required in most patients, since we are dealing with a vena puncture with a low-pressure system, which reduces the chance of pericatheter bleeding.

Guidewires may be used, but should be made of atraumatic material (9,54). When using guidewires, care must be taken not to perforate the heart (the atrial appendix is most at risk), while the pulmonary arterial tree is vulnerable for intima lesions.

As described above, low-osmolar contrast agents should be used for pulmonary angiography. It has been shown that both ionic and non-ionic agents lead to a slight increase in pulmonary arterial pressure after injection, but the increase is slight and reversible (41,49,55). A minimum concentration of 300 mg/mL of iodine is required for optimal opacification of the pulmonary arterial tree.

X-RAY EQUIPMENT

Fast film exchange systems have been nearly completely replaced by digital subtraction angiography (DSA) units. Technically, the spatial resolution of conventional cut film remains superior to

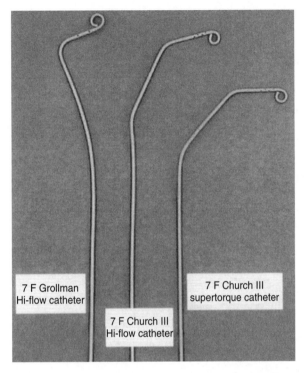

Figure 10.2 Three 7F pulmonary artery catheters. The combined use of the Grollman and Church catheter shapes is always successful even without the use of guidewires.

that of digital subtraction angiography; however, the resolution of modern DSA units is very high. In addition, the added use of cinematic review and workstation manipulation appear to be beneficial for the interpretation of pulmonary angiography. These benefits are noticeable in terms of inter-observer variation, adequacy of opacification of smaller branches and diagnostic performance (54,56,57).

A Swedish study showed that cine arteriography at frame rates of 25/s produced high diagnostic accuracy and a low number of inconclusive results in patients with suspected PE (58). In the latest digital subtraction equipment, images at 8–12 frames/s may be obtained with similar results.

TECHNIQUE

Although a brachial jugular and femoral venous approach may be applied, the latter is the entry point of choice. The right femoral vein has the additional benefit of a nearly straight approach to the vena cava and right atrium, whereas a relatively acute angle may be present where the left iliac vein enters the inferior vena cava. The femoral vein is generally located approximately 1 cm medial to the artery (sometimes the vein may actually be posterior to the artery). Following local anaesthesia using 1% lidocaine-HCl, the femoral vein is punctured. This is best achieved by asking the patient to perform a Valsalva manoeuvre, which causes the vein to distend. Subsequently, the Seldinger technique is employed and the pigtail catheter is advanced over the wire.

In case a non-guidewire passage of the heart is chosen, the Church catheter can directly pass the tricuspid valve by turning it clockwise at the level of the valve through the cusps;

then, after a 2 cm advance, a 180° anti-clockwise turn will bring it straight to the pulmonary valve, at which moment a 5 cm advance will position the catheter centrally in the pulmonary trunk.

If one decides to use a guidewire, the pigtail catheter is turned so that the end-hole faces antero-medially. The guidewire will easily pass through the tricuspid valve into the right ventricle. The next part of the manoeuvre consists of withdrawing the catheter and wire to straighten the catheter. Once this has been achieved, the catheter can be repositioned to let the end-hole face upwards and the guidewire may now be passed through the pulmonary valve into the pulmonary trunk (Figure 10.3). Once the catheter is moved forward over the guidewire, a trial injection of contrast should be administered by hand to check for large central emboli. If central emboli are seen on fluoroscopy, it is advised that a full X-ray series is obtained with contrast injection in the right ventricle. However, if the trial injection does not reveal central emboli, the wire

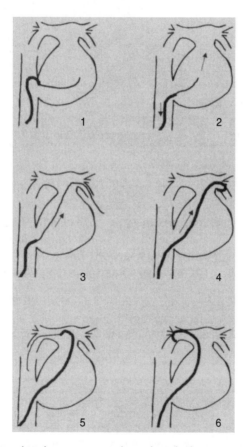

Figure 10.3 Guidewire steered catheter passage through right heart to pulmonary vessels. (1) Pigtail catheter position in right atrium; guidewire through tricuspid valve. (2) Stretching of the catheter by advancing guidewire. (3) Guidewire passing pulmonary valve through conus pulmonaris deep into left pulmonary artery. (4) Stretched catheter advanced over guidewire to left pulmonary artery; guidewire withdrawal, reshaping of catheter to pigtail configuration. Position for selective pulmonary angiography. (5) Slight catheter withdrawal into conus pulmonaris and 180° turning of pigtail position; stretching of catheter by guidewire, which is advanced deep into the right main pulmonary artery. (6) Catheter advanced over guidewire. Guidewire withdrawal and reshaping of catheter to pigtail configuration; position for selective right pulmonary angiography.

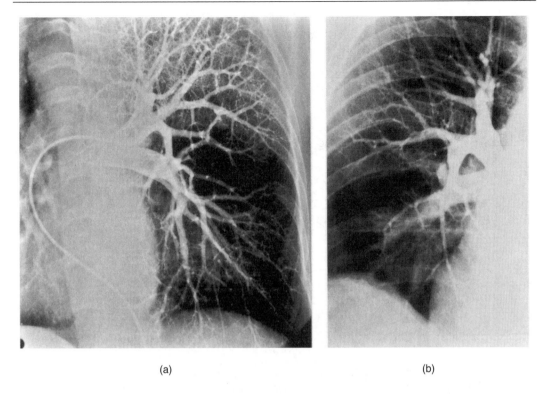

(a)   (b)

Figure 10.4   (a) Early branching of left upper lobe artery and (b) right upper lobe artery.

and catheter may be advanced into the right or left pulmonary artery. Care must be taken that early branching of the left or right upper lobe artery may occur (Figure 10.4), which could result in insufficient opacification of these lobes. Furthermore, a small bolus injection must be given prior to obtaining a full radiographic series to ascertain that the catheter tip is positioned adequately and is not wedged into a small side branch (Figure 10.5) or in a subintimal position (Figure 10.6).

Using an injection into the main pulmonary artery, adequate opacification of all segmental and subsegmental branches is usually obtained. However, in patients with atelectasis or with pain-related splinting of the diaphragm, inadequate visualization of the lower lobe branches may occur, which may even suggest the presence of large emboli (Figure 10.7a). In these patients, it is necessary to perform more selective catheterization and injection of contrast to depict these branches (Figure 10.7b). Also, an inadequate injection protocol can mimic a major pulmonary embolism (Figure 10.7c).

Contrast injection should be performed using an automated injector system. A linear rise of 0.5 s is advised to reduce catheter recoil. Thereafter, 40 mL of contrast is given at a rate of 20 mL/s at a pressure of 600 psi ($42\,kg/cm^2$). In patients with pulmonary hypertension, lesser amounts are administered more selectively to prevent acute right ventricular overload. Similarly, if contrast injections are performed into lobar or segmental arteries, the total amount of contrast is reduced to 10–15 mL/s for 2 s.

A minimum of two radiographic series are required. The standard projections used are anterior–posterior and 20–40° left and right posterior oblique for the left and right lung, respectively (59). However, in some patients additional series are required, especially if more selective angiography is needed in non-opacified segments.

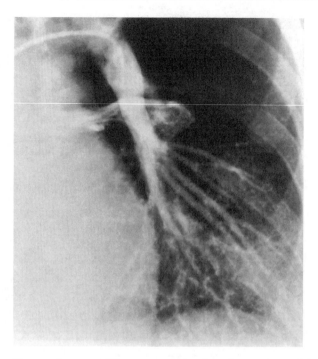

Figure 10.5 Early capillary and venous filling as a result of wedging of tip of the catheter in a small side branch of the pulmonary artery. The resultant image may suggest arteriovenous malformation if not adequately recognized.

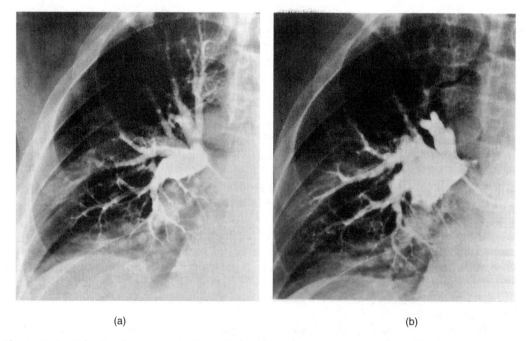

(a)   (b)

Figure 10.6 Subintimal contrast injection into the right pulmonary artery (a). Note that the proximal artery is abnormally distended, while the side-holes of the catheter give insufficient filling of peripheral branches. One second later (b), there is contrast extravasation into the perivascular space of the interstitium.

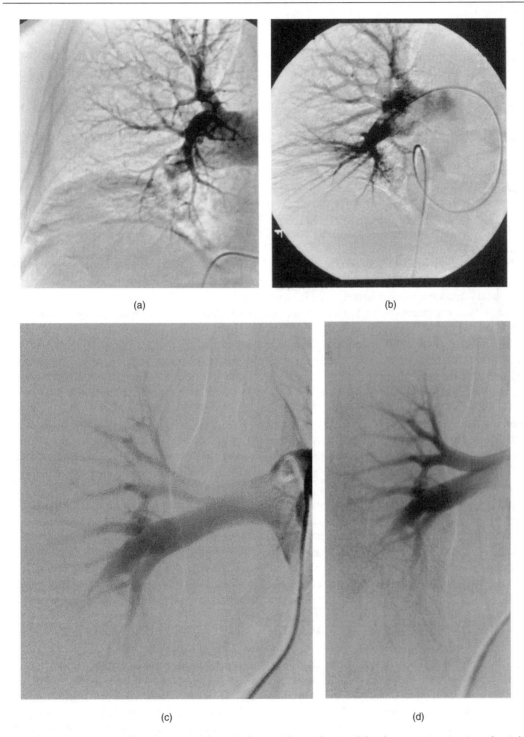

(a)

(b)

(c)

(d)

Figure 10.7 Patients with atelectasis of the right lower lobe with raised diaphragm. Injection into the right pulmonary artery shows cut-off of the right lower lobe artery (a). Subsequent more selective injection into the right lower lobe artery shows normal vasculature without evidence of PE (b). A contrast filling defect is seen in the right ascending upper lobe artery (c). This was caused by an insufficient injection protocol of 15 mL/s × 2 s. Complete filling of the artery after optimal injection of 22 mL/s × 2 s (d).

ANATOMY

The pulmonary trunk originates from the right ventricle at the level of the infundibulum. The trunk divides into a left and right pulmonary artery. The left artery runs a more or less straight upwards and then anterior oblique course, whereas the right artery is in a more caudal position and traverses underneath the aortic arch in a more horizontal plane. Subsequently, the pulmonary arteries divide into three lobar arteries. The upper lobe arteries originate first and may actually originate within the mediastinum. The middle lobe or lingular lobe arteries stem from the descending part of the main right or left pulmonary arteries, respectively. The segmental distribution is analogous to the lung segment chart as shown in Figure 10.8. Rotational views give a good insight into the different projections of the pulmonary arteries depending on the beam angle (Figure 10.9).

It is important to recognize anatomical variations, which are mainly related to left vena cava, atrial septum defects or patent foramen ovale. Even rarer anomalies are an aberrant course of vessels as in pulmonary sling or an aberrant vascular supply to lung segments as in pulmonary sequestration.

Haemodynamic measurements are an integral part of pulmonary angiography. Nevertheless, some people feel that they may be omitted since echocardiography is currently able to measure adequately pressures non-invasively (see Chapter 11). If one decides to perform pressure measurements, it is valuable to determine right atrial, right ventricular and pulmonary artery pressure. The last is most important, since it may signal pulmonary hypertension, which implies that one uses a linear rise of up to 1 s and injects less contrast agent (we prefer 30 mL at 15 mL/s). Alternatively, one could resort to super-selective catheterization of lobar or segmental arteries, where an occlusion balloon may be used to reduce further the amount of contrast injected. These measures will reduce the risks of acute right ventricular overload in patients with pulmonary hypertension (18,19).

The criteria for acute PE were defined over 40 years ago (2,60). Large studies have consistently used them and demonstrated that these criteria are valid. There are direct angiographic signs of PE, which are complete obstruction of a vessel (preferably with concave border of the contrast column) or a filling defect (2,6,61). These criteria have been shown to be reliable in various studies, which assessed intra- and inter-observer variations (6,54,62). It was also demonstrated that the same criteria may be applied in DSA with equally good observer agreement (54,56,57). However, one should be aware that the reliability of pulmonary angiography decreases with diminishing calibre of the vessels, i.e., the interpretation becomes much more difficult after the subsegmental level (62). Another factor which influences diagnostic accuracy of pulmonary angiography is related to patient selection. In 140 patients who were referred for pulmonary angiography after a non-diagnostic lung scan had been obtained, the kappa values of cut-film angiography ranged between 0.28 and 0.59, and this increased to a range of 0.66–0.89 if DSA was used (54). Nevertheless, these values were lower than those obtained in non-selected patient populations (6,62), possibly because underlying pulmonary and cardiac diseases had a negative influence on the interpretation of images.

Indirect signs of PE may be slow flow of contrast media, regional hypoperfusion and delayed or diminished pulmonary venous flow. These signs could direct one's attention to a specific region, but they cannot be used for diagnostic purposes. None of these signs have been validated and one should not diagnose PE in the absence of direct angiographic signs. Chronic pulmonary thromboembolism may be diagnosed by pulmonary angiography and is identifiable for several reasons (63). First, thrombi will be adherent to the vessel wall and will not move during the series of images. Second, signs of revascularization are usually present, such as collateral vessels and stenotic segments. In fact, it may be difficult to distinguish chronic pulmonary thromboembolism from inflammatory lesions such as Takayasu's arteritis. Finally, the results of incomplete thrombus resolution may lead to complete obstruction, webs, bands and irregularity of the vessel wall (63).

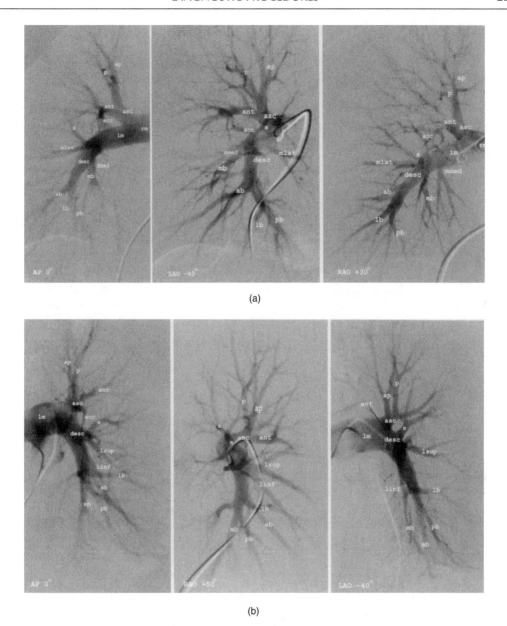

(a)

(b)

Figure 10.8 (a) Anatomy of the right arterial pulmonary tree: ab, anterior basal segmental artery lower lobe; acc, accessory upper lobe artery; ant, anterior segmental branch right upper lobe; ap, apical posterior segmental branch upper lobe; asc, ascending branch of upper lobe; desc, descending branch of lower lobe; im, interlobar; lb, lateral basal segmental artery lower lobe; mb, medial basal segmental artery lower lobe; mlat, medial lobe lateral segment; mmed, medial lobe medial segment; p, posterior segmental artery upper lobe; pb, posterior basal segmental artery lower lobe; rm, right main pulmonary artery; s, superior segmental artery lower lobe. (b) Anatomy of the left arterial pulmonary tree: ab, anterior basal segmental artery lower lobe; ant, anterior segmental branch left upper lobe; ap, apical posterior segmental branch upper lobe; asc, ascending branch of upper lobe; desc, descending branch of lower lobe; lb, lateral basal segmental artery lower lobe; linf, lingula inferior segmental branch; lm, left main pulmonary artery; lsup, lingula superior segmental branch; mb, medial basal segmental artery lower lobe; p, posterior segmental artery upper lobe; pb, posterior basal segmental artery lower lobe; s, superior segmental artery lower lobe.

PE SCORING SYSTEMS

Several attempts have been made to quantify the degree of pulmonary vascular obstruction. The main aim was to develop some form of objective scoring for the assessment of the effectiveness of fibrinolytic therapy in large clinical trials, such as those described in Chapter 24.

The Miller index, which was developed in Europe, is based on the size and number of filling defects and contrast flow (31). The presence of one or more filling defects is scored with one

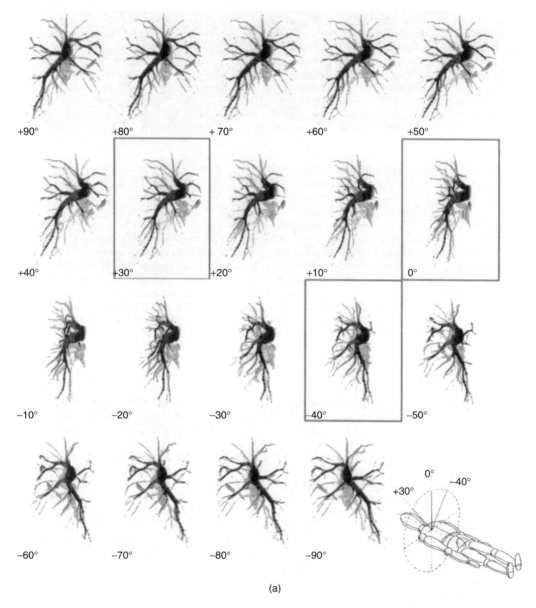

(a)

Figure 10.9 Rotational projections of the right (a) and left (b) arterial pulmonary tree over 180° from +90 lateral view to −90 lateral view; the marked projections are the standard views in arterial pulmonary angiography.

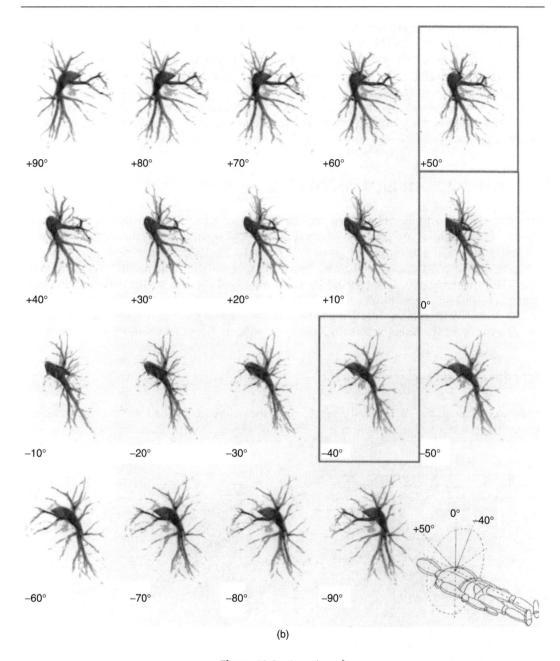

+90°   +80°   +70°   +60°   +50°

+40°   +30°   +20°   +10°   0°

−10°   −20°   −30°   −40°   −50°

−60°   −70°   −80°   −90°

(b)

Figure 10.9   (*continued*)

point, giving a maximum of 16 points (nine on the right and seven on the left). The presence of a filling defect proximal to segmental branches is scored as equal to the segmental branches arising distally. A slightly impaired flow in one-third of each lung accounts for one point, delayed flow in one-third of each lung sores one point and no contrast flow scores 3 points for each one-third of each lung. Due to the difficulty of measuring flow, most centres score only the filling defects (64).

The Walsh scoring system was developed in urokinase–streptokinase PE trials (65). This scoring system only takes central to segmental branches into consideration, and does not account for more peripheral perfusion defects. Neither the Miller index nor the Walsh system separate the elements of clot size and degree of occlusion.

The latest scoring system, which was developed by Simon *et al.*, separated clot size and degree of occlusion and yielded a true quantitative score which was a measure of severity of occlusion of the pulmonary vascular tree (66).

None of the mentioned scoring systems has gained widespread acceptance. This is partly due to the relative subjectivity of scoring, its time-consuming nature and finally its lack of clinical impact.

ANATOMICAL DISTRIBUTION OF PE

Pulmonary emboli vary greatly in size and distribution of emboli may be important for other, less-invasive modalities. An overview of pulmonary embolism at the different anatomic locations and levels in the pulmonary tree is given in Figures 10.10–10.15. In one study in 76 patients with proven pulmonary emboli, emboli were located exclusively in subsegmental arterial branches in 23 (30%) patients (67). In the PIOPED study, 6% of all patients who underwent pulmonary angiography had their emboli limited to subsegmental vessels (68). Similarly, in a selected group of 140 patients who underwent angiography following a non-diagnostic lung scan, the largest emboli were in subsegmental vessels in 3 out of 20 patients (15%) in whom PE was proven (9).

REFERENCE METHOD

Pulmonary angiography is generally regarded as the reference method for the diagnosis and (maybe more importantly) the exclusion of PE. This does not mean that pulmonary angiography

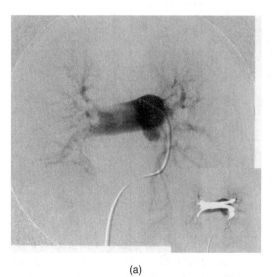
(a)

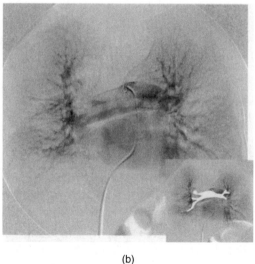
(b)

Figure 10.10   Central pulmonary emboli. The large central emboli extend to both upper and lower lobe arteries (a, b). Both patients were in deceptively good clinical condition, therefore this diagnostic outcome was totally unexpected. One patient showed almost no perfusion of the lower lobes (b) (see insets of delineation of emboli extension).

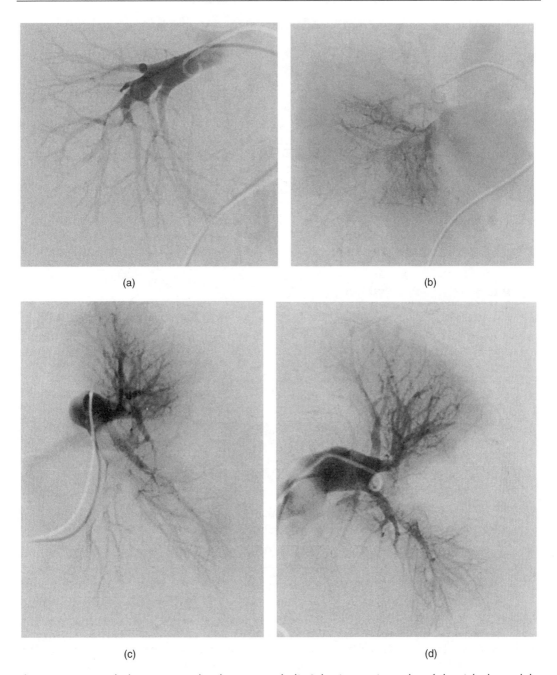

(a)

(b)

(c)

(d)

Figure 10.11 Occluding segmental pulmonary emboli. Selective angiography of the right lower lobe artery (bypassing the ascending upper lobe artery) reveals a large embolus in RAO projection. Only partial occlusion is seen of the medial basal segmental artery (a). The posterior and lateral basal segmental arteries show complete occlusion leading to a wedge-shaped perfusion defect in the corresponding segmental areas (b). Selective angiography of the left main pulmonary artery shows a cut-off of the lower lobe and inferior longula arteries in RAO projection (c); a subtle outline of contrast medium along the embolus can be noticed. Two large, wedge-shaped perfusion defects are seen corresponding with the lower lobe and inferior longula arteries except for the segment of the superior longula artery in AP projection (d).

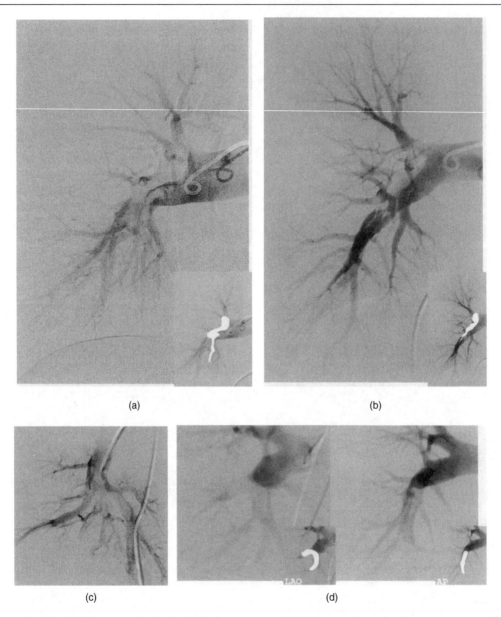

(a)

(b)

(c)

(d)

Figure 10.12   (Sub)segmental emboli of right lower and middle lobe arteries. Selective angiography of the right main pulmonary artery shows a large embolus attached to the centre wall of interlobar pulmonary artery in RAO projection (a). Although the thrombus extends along the ascending upper lobe artery and the superior segmental artery of the lower lobe, these vessels still show good filling. Only the lateral segment of the lower lobe shows complete cut-off and partial filling, respectively (see insets). Such large emboli in the same position, sliding over the right upper, medial and lower lobe segmental arterial ostia, often do not cause cut-off arteries and show normal enhancement of all segmental arteries (b). The lateral branch of the medial lobe artery and the superior segment of the lower lobe artery seem to originate on the surface of the embolus. Superselective angiography of the right lower lobe arterial segment reveals in LAO projection a casting of the emboli in all sub-segments except the anterior basal artery without any arterial cut-off (c). The shape of the embolus can differ depending on the projection angle. A saddle embolus in the right medial and descending branch of the right lower lobe pulmonary artery in horseshoe LAO projection and linear AP projection configuration (d); this causes the so called tramline configuration.

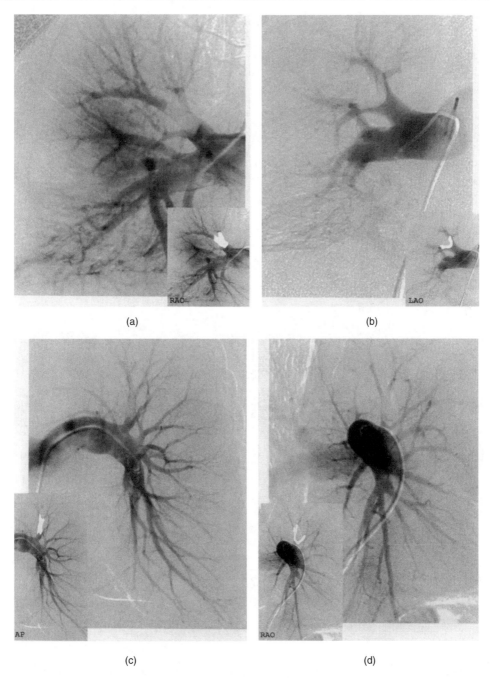

(a)

(b)

(c)

(d)

Figure 10.13 (Sub)segmental emboli of upper lobe arteries. Selective angiography of the right main pulmonary artery reveals extensive pulmonary emboli in the upper and lower lobes. The anterior segmental upper lobe artery shows a separate branching directly from the interlobar artery. The apical and posterior segmental branches show a linear-shaped embolus in RAO projection (a) but a saddle embolus in LAO projection (b): another example of separate branching of the left upper lobe segmental arterial branches. The anterior upper lobe branch originates directly from the descending left pulmonary artery. A linear filling defect is shown in the apical and posterior segmental upper lobe arteries in AP projection (c). In RAO projection a saddle embolus is seen over the crossing of these arteries (d).

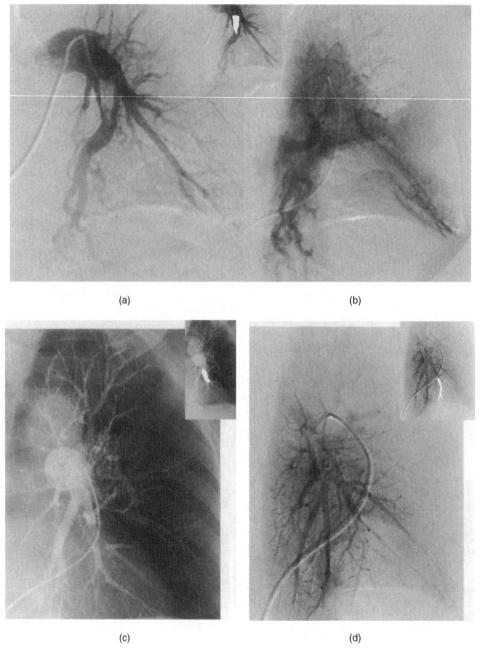

(a)

(b)

(c)

(d)

Figure 10.14 (Sub)segmental emboli of lingula and left lower lobe arteries. Selective angiography of the descending left pulmonary artery shows several vessel cut-offs in AP projection of the inferior lingula, lateral, anterior and posterior basal arteries. Only the left medial basal segmental artery is still opacified (a). Corresponding wedge-shaped perfusion defects are shown in the perfusion phase in RAO projection (b). Selective angiography in RAO projection of the left lower lobe segmental arteries show a typical 'tramline' of contrast medium attenuation along the posterior basal segmental artery (c). An orthogonal branching half-way along this vessel causes a sharp white circular contrast enhancement with a central filling defect, nicely depicted in this non-subtracted image. Filling defects with 'tramline' demarcation are seen in the anterior basal (sub)segmental artery of the left lower lobe at selective angiography in RAO projection (d).

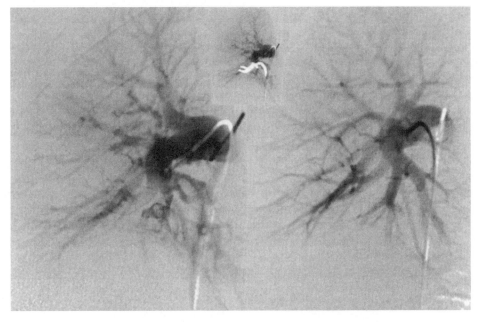

(a)

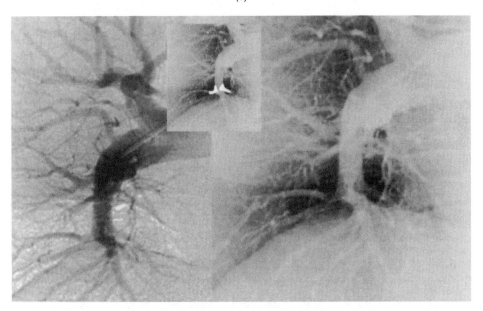

(b)

Figure 10.15 The selective angiography in LAO projection of the descending pulmonary artery shows a typical casting of emboli and/or thrombi in the lower lobe segmental arteries together with an elevated right diaphragm (a) (see inset). Repeat angiography 1 month later shows no filling defects after anticoagulant therapy (b). Circumscribed filling defects, rounded, firmly attached to the descending right pulmonary artery wall are demonstrated at selective angiography in AP projection (c). The lower lobe segmental arteries are curved by the elevated right diaphragm (d), the anterior and medial basal segments show renewed opacification after 1 cm. The round shape protruding in the lumen and the fixation to the vessel wall and restoration of peripheral flow fit the diagnosis of chronic (sub)segmental emboli. Note that the cause of abnormal vessel orientation can be missed at subtractive images.

is infallible. Since angiography is the reference method, the sensitivity and specificity of this technique cannot be formally evaluated.

The clinical validity of a normal pulmonary angiogram was assessed in five well-designed studies (9,27,60,68–70). Anticoagulants were withheld in 840 patients with clinically suspected PE in whom a normal pulmonary angiogram was obtained. All patients were followed-up for a minimum of 3 months. Recurrent thromboembolic events were demonstrated in 16 patients (1.9%; 95% CI: 1.4 to 3.2%) and three of these were fatal events (0.3%; 95% CI: 0.09 to 1.08%). Hence it is regarded safe clinical practice to withhold anticoagulants in patients with chest symptoms and a normal pulmonary arteriogram.

From these data, it may be concluded that the sensitivity of pulmonary angiography is in the region of 98%. Similarly, the specificity is thought to be between 95 and 98%. This value is slightly lower than the sensitivity due to other illnesses, which may mimic the criteria for pulmonary emboli, such as obstruction of a pulmonary artery by a mass.

In conclusion, pulmonary angiography is still a valid and valuable part of the diagnostic arsenal for the diagnosis of PE and the assessment of chronic thromboembolic pulmonary hypertension. However, given the excellent results of multidetector row CTPA, its role should be reserved for the few patients in whom non-invasive tests do not give a conclusive outcome (or where the result is totally opposite to the clinical view of the patient) and where patients are undergoing pre-surgical evaluation for thromboendarterectomy.

REFERENCES

1. Ludwig JW. Heart and coronaries – the pioneering age. In: Rosenbusch G, Oudkerk M, Amman E (eds), *Radiology in Medical Diagnostics – Evolution of X-Ray Applications 1895–1995*. Blackwell Science, Oxford, 1995, pp. 213–224.
2. Dalen JE, Brooks HL, Johnson LW, *et al*. Pulmonary angiography in acute PE: indications, techniques and results in 367 patients. *Am Heart J* 1971; **81**:175–185.
3. Sasahara AA, Hyers TM, Cole CM, *et al*. The urokinase PE trial. *Circulation* 1973; **47**:1–108.
4. Bell WR, Simon TL. A comparative analysis of pulmonary perfusion scans with pulmonary angiograms. *Am Heart J* 1976; **92**:700–706.
5. Mills SR, Jackson DC, Older RA, *et al*. The incidence, etiologies and avoidance of complications of pulmonary angiography in a large series. *Radiology* 1980; **136**:295–299.
6. Stein PD, Athanasoulis C, Alavi A, *et al*. Complications and validity of pulmonary angiography in acute PE. *Circulation* 1992; **85**:462–468.
7. Van Rooy WJJ, den Heeten GJ, Sluzewski M. PE: diagnosis in 211 patients with use of selective pulmonary digital subtraction angiography with a flow-directed catheter. *Radiology* 1995; **195**:793–797.
8. Hudson ER, Smith TP, McDermott VG, *et al*. Pulmonary angiography performed with iopamidol: complications in 1434 patients. *Radiology* 1996; **198**:61–65.
9. Van Beek EJR, Reekers JA, Batchelor D, Brandjes DPM, Peeters FLM, Büller HR. Feasibility, safety and clinical utility of angiography in patients with suspected PE and non-diagnostic lung scan findings. *Eur Radiol* 1996; **6**:415–419.
10. Zuckerman DA, Sterling KM, Oser RF. Safety of pulmonary angiography in the 1990s. *J Vasc Intervent Radiol* 1996; **7**:199–205.
11. Nilsson T, Carlsson A, Mare K. Pulmonary angiography: a safe procedure with modern contrast media and technique. *Eur Radiol* 1998; **8**:86–89
12. Kwaliteitsinstituut voor de Gezondheidszorg CBO. Richtlijn diagnostiek, preventie en behandeling van veneuze trombo-embolie en secundaire preventie arteriële trombose. www.cbo.nl
13. Van Beek EJR, Brouwers E, Song B, Stein PD, Oudkerk M. Clinical validity of a normal pulmonary angiogram in patients with suspected pulmonary embolism – a critical review. *Clin Radiol* 2001; **56**:838–842.
14. British Thoracic Society Standards of Care Committee Pulmonary Embolism Guideline Development Group. British Thoracic Society guidelines for the management of suspected acute pulmonary embolism. *Thorax* 2003; **58**:470–484.

15. Stein PD, Sostman HD, Bounameaux H, *et al.* Challenges in the diagnosis acute pulmonary embolism. *Am J Med.* 2008; **121**:565–571.
16. Schoepf UJ, Goldhaber SZ, Costello P. Spiral computed tomography for acute pulmonary embolism. *Circulation.* 2004; **109**:2160–2167.
17. Oudkerk M, van Beek EJ, Wielopolski P, *et al.* Comparison of contrast-enhanced magnetic resonance angiography and conventional pulmonary angiography for the diagnosis of pulmonary embolism: a prospective study. *Lancet* 2002; **359**:1643–1647.
18. Perlmutt LM, Braun SD, Newman GE, Oke EJ, Dunnick NR. Pulmonary arteriography in the high-risk patient. *Radiology* 1987; **162**:187–189.
19. Nicod P, Peterson K, Levine M, *et al.* Pulmonary angiography in severe chronic pulmonary hypertension. *Ann Intern Med* 1987; **107**:565–568.
20. Stein PD, Hull RD, Pineo GF. Strategy that includes serial noninvasive leg tests for diagnosis of thromboembolic disease in patients with suspected acute pulmonary embolism based on data from PIOPED. *Arch Intern Med* 1995; **155**:2101–2104.
21. Grollman KJ. Pulmonary angiography. *Cardiovasc Intervent Radiol* 1992; **15**:166–170.
22. Newman GE. Pulmonary angiography in pulmonary embolic disease. *J Thorac Imag* 1989; **4**:28–39.
23. Grollman JH, Gyepes MT, Helmer E. Transfemoral selective bilateral pulmonary arteriography with a pulmonary-artery-seeking catheter. *Radiology* 1970; **96**:202–204.
24. Mills CS, Van Aman ME. Modified technique for percutaneous pulmonary angiography. *Cardiovasc Intervent Radiol* 1986; **9**:52–53.
25. Ranniger K. Pulmonary arteriography: a simple method for demonstration of clinically significant pulmonary emboli. *AJR Am J Roentgenol* 1969; **106**:558–562.
26. Marsh JD, Glunn M, Torman HA. Pulmonary angiography: application in a new spectrum of patients. *Am J Med* 1983; **75**:763–769.
27. Cheely R, McCartney WH, Perry JR, *et al.* The role of noninvasive tests versus pulmonary angiography in the diagnosis of PE. *Am J Med* 1981; **70**:17–22.
28. Winrow D, Beckmann CF, Lacomis JM, *et al.* Entanglement of a pigtail catheter by the chordae tendineae of the tricuspid valve during pulmonary angiography. *Cardiovasc Intervent Radiol* 1996; **19**:275–277.
29. Stein PD, Athanasoulis C, Alavi A, *et al.* Complications and validity of pulmonary angiography in acute pulmonary embolism. *Circulation* 1992; **85**:462–468.
30. Moore RD, Steinberg EP, Powe NR, *et al.* Nephrotoxicity of high osmolality versus low osmolality contrast media: randomized clinical trial. *Radiology* 1992; **182**:649–655.
31. Barrett BJ, Parfrey PS, Vavasour HM, *et al.* Contrast nephropathy in patients with impaired renal function: high versus low osmolar media. *Kidney Int* 1992; **41**:1274–1279.
32. Manske CL, Sprafka JM, Strony JT, *et al.* Contrast nephropathy in azotemic diabetic patients undergoing coronary angiography. *Am J Med* 1990; **89**:615–620.
33. Rudnick MR, Goldfarb S, Wexler L, *et al.* Nephrotoxicity of ionic and nonionic contrast media in 1196 patients: a randomized trial. *Kidney Int* 1995; **47**:254–261.
34. Levy EM, Viscoli CM, Horwitz RI. The effect of acute renal failure in mortality. A cohort analysis. *JAMA* 1996; **275**:1488–1494.
35. Palmer FG. The RACR survey of intravenous contrast media reactions. *Final report. Aust. Radiol* 1988; **32**:426–428.
36. Wolf GL, Arenson RL, Cross AP. A prospective trial of ionic vs nonionic contrast agents in routine clinical practice: comparison of adverse effects. *AJR Am J Roentgenol* 1989; **152**:930–944.
37. Katayama H, Yamaguchi K, Kozuka T, *et al.* Adverse reaction to ionic and nonionic contrast media. Report from the Japanese Committee on the Safety of Contrast Media. *Radiology* 1990; **175**:621–628.
38. Grollman JH. Complications of pulmonary arteriography. *Semin Intervent Radiol* 1994; **11**:113–120.
39. Baltaoglu F, Balkanci F, Tirnaksiz B. Fatal reaction after intraarterial injection of nonionic contrast medium. *AJR Am J Roentgenol* 1994; **162**:231.
40. Smith DC, Lois JF, Gomes AS, *et al.* Pulmonary arteriography: comparison of cough stimulation effects of diatrizoate and ioxaglate. *Radiology* 1987; **162**:617–618.
41. Saeed M, Braun SD, Cohan RH, *et al.* Pulmonary angiography with iopamidol: patient comfort, image quality and hemodynamics. *Radiology* 1987; **165**:345–349.
42. Agarwal JB, Baile EM, Palmer WH, *et al.* Reflex systemic hypotension due to hypertonic solution in pulmonary circulation. *J Appl Physiol* 1969; **27**:251–255.
43. Stein MA, Winter J, Grollman JH. The value of the pulmonary-artery-seeking catheter in percutaneous selective pulmonary angiography. *Radiology* 1975; **114**:299–304.

44. Binet L, Burstein M. Sur les effets cardiovasculaires du sérum salé hypertonique. *C R Séances Soc Biol Fil* 1953; **147**:1997–2000.
45. Eliakim MD, Rosenberg SZ, Braun K. Effect of hypertonic saline on the pulmonary and systemic pressures. *Circ Res* 1958; **6**:357–362.
46. Read R, Meyer M. The role of red cell agglutination in arteriographic complications. *Surg Forum* 1959; **10**:472–475.
47. Tajima H, Kumazaki T, Ito K, *et al.* Effect of an iso-osmolar contrast medium on pulmonary arterial pressure at pulmonary angiography. *Acta Radiol* 1991; **32**:134–136.
48. Krovetz LJ, Benson RW, Neumaster T. Hemodynamic effects of isotonic 67 solutions rapidly injected into the heart and great vessels. *Am Heart J* 1967; **73**:525–533.
49. Tajima H, Kumazaki T, Tajima N, Ebata K. Effect of iohexol and diatrizoate on pulmonary arterial pressure following pulmonary angiography. *Acta Radiol Scand* 1988; Suppl 29:487–490.
50. Almen T, Aspelin P, Levin B. Effect of ionic and non-ionic contrast medium on aortic and pulmonary arterial pressure. *Invest Radiol* 1990; **25**:519–443.
51. Malden ES, Tartar VM, Gutierrez FR. Acute fatality following pulmonary angiography in a patient on an amiodarone regimen: a case report. *Angiology* 1993; **44**:152–155.
52. Wood DL, Osborn MJ, Rooke J, *et al.* Amiodarone pulmonary toxicity: report of two cases associated with rapidly progressive distress syndrome after pulmonary angiography. *Mayo Clin Proc* 1985; **60**:601–603.
53. Grollman JH, Gyepes MT, Helmer E. Transfemoral selective bilateral pulmonary arteriography with a pulmonary artery seeking catheter. *Radiology* 1970; **96**:102–104.
54. Van Beek EJR, Bakker AJ, Reekers JA. Interobserver variability of pulmonary angiography in patients with non-diagnostic lung scan results: conventional versus digital subtraction arteriography. *Radiology* 1996; **198**:721–724.
55. Smit EMT, van Beek EJR, Bakker AJ, Reekers JA. A blind, randomized trial evaluating the hemodynamic effects of contrast media during pulmonary angiography for suspected PE – ioxaglate vs iohexol. *Acad Radiol* 1995; **2**:609–613.
56. Johnson MS, Stine SB, Shah H, *et al.* Possible pulmonary embolus: evaluation with digital subtraction versus cut-film angiography – prospective study in 80 patients. *Radiology* 1998; **207**:131–138.
57. Hagspiel KD, Polak JF, Grassi CJ, Faitelson BB, Kandarpa K, Meyerovitz MF. PE: comparison of cut-film and digital pulmonary angiography. *Radiology* 1998; **207**:139–145.
58. Nilsson T, Carlsson A, Mare K, *et al.* Validity of pulmonary cine arteriography for the diagnosis of PE. *Eur Radiol* 1999; **9**:276–280.
59. Johnson BA, James AE. Oblique and selective pulmonary angiography in diagnosis of PE. *AJR Am J Roentgenol* 1973; **118**:801–808.
60. Bookstein JJ. Segmental arteriography in PE. *Radiology* 1969; **93**:1007–1012.
61. Hull RD, Hirsh J, Carter CJ, *et al.* Pulmonary angiography, ventilation lung scanning and venography for clinically suspected PE with abnormal perfusion lung scan. *Ann Intern Med* 1983; **98**:891–899.
62. Quinn MF, Lundell CJ, Klotz TA, *et al.* Reliability of selective pulmonary arteriography in the diagnosis of PE. *Am J Radiol* 1987; **149**:469–471.
63. Moser KM, Auger WR, Fedullo PF, Jamieson SW. Chronic thromboembolic pulmonary hypertension: clinical picture and surgical treatment. *Eur Respir J* 1992; **5**:334–342.
64. Görge G, Schuster S, Ge J, Meyer J, Erbel R. Intravascular ultrasound in patients with acute PE after treatment with intravenous urikinase and high-dose heparin. *Heart* 1997; **77**:73–77.
65. Walsh PN, Greenspan RH, Simon M, *et al.* An angiographic severity index for PE. *Circulation* 1973; **47** (Suppl 2):11–101.
66. Simon M, Sharma GVRK, Sasahara AA. An angiographic method for quantitating the severity of PE. *Int Angiol* 1984; **3**:389–392.
67. Oser RF, Zuckerman DA, Gutierrez FR, Brink JA. Anatomic distribution of pulmonary emboli at pulmonary angiography: implications for cross-sectional imaging. *Radiology* 1996; **199**:31–35.
68. PIOPED Investigators. Value of the ventilation-perfusion scan in acute PE: results of the Prospective Investigation of PE Diagnosis (PIOPED). *JAMA* 1990; **263**:2753–2759.
69. Novelline RA, Baltarowich OH, Athanasoulis CA, *et al.* The clinical course of patients with suspected PE and a negative pulmonary arterio-gram. *Radiology* 1978; **126**:561–567.
70. Henry JW, Relyea B, Stein PD. Continuing risk of thromboemboli among patients with normal pulmonary angiograms. *Chest* 1995; **107**:1375–1378.

CHAPTER 11

Echocardiography in Pulmonary Embolism

Günter Görge[1] and Raimund Erbel[2]

[1]Innere Medizin II, Klinikum Saarbrücken, Saarbrücken, Germany
[2]Universitätsklinikum Essen, Center for Internal Medicine,
Clinic for Cardiology, Essen, Germany

INTRODUCTION

Acute massive pulmonary embolism (PE) is an often missed but significant disease, with an estimated 2000 cases diagnosed per 1 000 000 inhabitants per year in western countries. The estimated prevalence of acute PE among 51 645 hospitalized patients was 1.0% and PE in hospitalized patients contributed or caused death in 0.2% (1). The incidence of clinically unrecognized PE has not diminished during three decades, despite advances in non-invasive diagnosis. Even fatal PE is not diagnosed in 51–70% of cases confirmed at post mortem investigation (1). In most patients suffering a fatal PE in hospital, co-morbid disease is present and many have a poor prognosis even before PE occurs (2,3). It has been estimated that most deaths occur during the first 2 hours after the initial event. Therefore, rapid identification of patients with high risk of dying and the prompt initiation of appropriate therapy are crucial for short term prognosis. Unfortunately, many proposed diagnostic strategies in patients with suspected PE are time consuming, require transportation of the patients to other wards or diagnostic facilities and often focus on 'probabilities' instead of direct visualization of thrombus or haemodynamic consequences of massive PE (2).

In the view of many clinicians, echocardiography and computed tomographic pulmonary angiography (CTPA) can both play a crucial role as rapid, reliable, first-line diagnostic tools for risk stratification and differential diagnosis of patients with clinically suspected PE (3). Echocardiography is particularly useful as a bedside non-invasive screening test for patients in unstable clinical conditions with suspected acute or chronic pulmonary hypertension, who may not be able to be moved directly to a central radiology facility to undergo CT studies (3).

Deep Vein Thrombosis and Pulmonary Embolism   Edited by Edwin J.R. van Beek, Harry R. Büller and Matthijs Oudkerk
© 2009 John Wiley & Sons, Ltd

ECHOCARDIOGRAPHY IN PULMONARY HYPERTENSION

Transthoracic echocardiography (TTE) usually enables one to determine non-invasively the pulmonary artery pressure, the right ventricular volumes and multiple functional parameters and thus the haemodynamic consequences of a pulmonary embolus (3). However, there exists no commonly accepted definition of right ventricular dysfunction (RVD) (3). Current guidelines see the role of TTE in patients with massive PE in those where CTPA is not available or practically infeasible (3).

Trans-oesophageal echocardiography (TEE) has the additional advantage of directly identifying proximal pulmonary artery embolism in a high percentage of patients with this condition and is most useful in patients with impaired transthoracic imaging (4,5)

Intravascular ultrasound (IVUS) is an invasive echo-based technique allowing imaging of the lumen and the vessel wall in patients with various forms of pulmonary hypertension (6–8). However, its limited availability, its invasiveness, the additional costs and time and mainly the lack of outcome data make IVUS in PE patients a pure research tool.

Examples of patients with PE and pulmonary hypertension as shown on various echocardiographic and IVUS studies are demonstrated in Figures 11.1–11.6.

Transthoracic Echo (TTE)

TTE has the advantage of being non-invasive. The echo-transducer (usually 2.25–5 MHz) is placed in the fourth or the fifth left intercostal space, at the apex of the heart, and positioned at the jugular notch for suprasternal images in some patients. The apical four-chamber view is the most valuable, because it allows the estimation of the size of the right and left heart chambers and the estimation

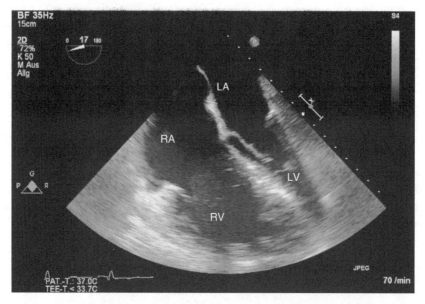

Figure 11.1 Transoesophageal echocardiography in a 75-year-old patient with acute pulmonary embolism. Right ventricular (RV) and right atrial (RA) enlargement, RV/LV ratio>1.

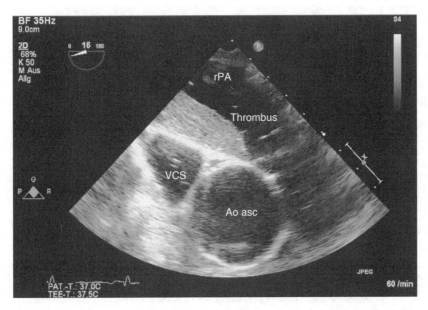

Figure 11.2   Transoesophageal imaging of the right pulmonary artery with large wall-adherent thrombus. Dilatation of pulmonary artery to 3.3 cm. Ao asc, ascending aorta; VCS, vena cava superior.

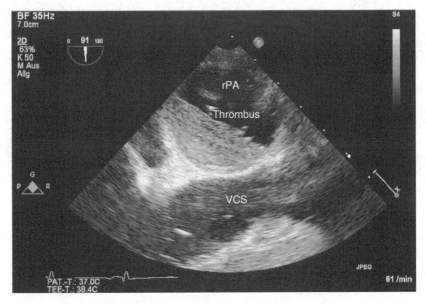

Figure 11.3   Short axis view, showing approximately 50% narrowing of the right pulmonary artery (rPA). A full colour version of this image appears in the plate section of this book.

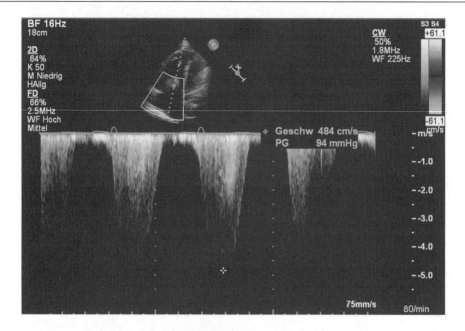

Figure 11.4 Systolic pulmonal artery pressure 94 mmHg.

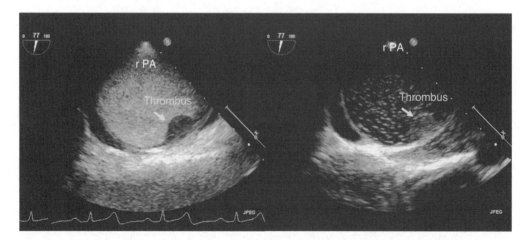

Figure 11.5 Right pulmonary artery in a patient with pulmonary embolism studied with (left) and without (right) echocontrast. Better visibility of thrombus with echocontrast.

of the gradient over the tricuspid valve by continuous Doppler examination. Pulmonary emboli can be seen either directly or indirectly.

Direct echocardiographic signs of pulmonary emboli are:

- thrombus in the pulmonary artery(ies)
- thrombus in the heart itself or thrombus 'in transit'.

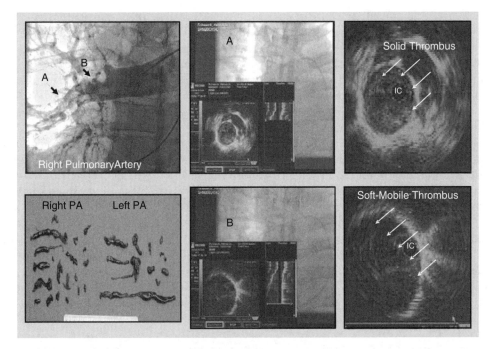

Figure 11.6 Typical example of IVUS imaging in a 61-year-old male patient with pulmonary embolism (modified from Ref. 56 with permission of the authors). Upper left: pulmonary angiogram showing complete and partial occlusion of the right pulmonary artery. Letters A and B indicate different positions of the IVUS catheter. In position A, IVUS shows solid thrombus (upper right, white arrows) as seen in angiography. In position B, soft, partly mobile thrombus is visualized by IVUS in addition to only partially visible thrombus found by angiography (white arrows). Lower left: thrombus removed during successful surgery from the left and right pulmonary circulation. IC, IVUS catheter; PA, pulmonary artery. A full colour version of this image appears in the plate section of this book.

Indirect echocardiographic signs of pulmonary hypertension are:

- dilatation of the right atrium, with or without dilatation of the right ventricle
- pulmonary artery pressure in patients with tricuspid insufficiency >30 mmHg
- RV/LV end-diastolic diameter >1
- RV end-diastolic diameter 30 mm
- RV dysfunction (RVD; mild, moderate, severe)
- compression of the left ventricle
- paradoxical motion of the septum
- increased isovolumetric relaxation time of the right ventricle
- shortening of the pulmonary artery acceleration time
- hypertrophy of the right ventricle in primary pulmonary hypertension or in recurrent embolic events.

The systolic pulmonary artery pressure is calculated as follows:

$$\text{systolic pulmonary artery pressure} = 4V_{max}^2 + \text{estimated or measured right atrial pressure}$$

TTE is available around the clock in most hospitals (3). Unlike other imaging devices in pulmonary hypertension, the echo console can be brought to the patient. TTE can directly demonstrate thrombus within the right heart chambers, the pulmonary arteries or the dynamic appearance of thrombus in transit. Acute and chronic pulmonary hypertension can be distinguished by the thickness of the right ventricular free wall (thinned in acute, hypertrophic in chronic pressure overload) and by the estimation of the pulmonary artery systolic pressure (9,10). In case of poor signal quality, the addition of echo-contrast agents injected into a peripheral vein or a central catheter will improve the Doppler signal quality in most patients.

In addition to the estimation of systolic pulmonary artery pressure by tricuspid regurgitation, the diagnostic value of the 'right ventricular isovolumetric relaxation time' and the 'acceleration time'(AcT) have been estimated in patients with PE. Table 11.1 gives an overview of the results of various groups, which compared echo parameters with invasive pressure measurements.

In the European Cooperative study, the morphological appearances of right-sided heart thrombi were described in 119 patients as either type A (long, thin, extremely mobile, snake-like thrombi) or type B (less mobile, more amorphous thrombi). PE was of type A morphology in 48 patients and these patients had higher risk of deep vein thrombosis (DVT), whereas cardiac thrombogenic disorders were more prevalent in the 57 patients with type B thrombi. Type A thrombi had a significantly worse outcome, with 89% developing significant PE with 42% mortality, whereas type B thrombi were more benign and, although 40% suffered PE, none of these were fatal. In 14 cases, a classification could not be established and these had intermediate prognosis for PE and outcome (11).

TTE is a very reliable, safe and easy to use method for both diagnosis and risk stratification in patients with PE, especially in those with massive PE or high pre-test probability. Echocardiography is the only bedside technique to allow for rapid assessment of right ventricular function, measurement of pulmonary artery pressures and direct visualization of central thrombus or thrombus in transit in selected patients. Negative aspects are the operator dependence, the requirement

Table 11.1 Example of studies comparing Doppler echocardiographic pressure measurements versus invasive measurements in patients with pulmonary hypertension. For details, see text

Study Study	Patients (n)	Technical success (%)	Pressure estimated[a]	r	Standard error (mmHg)
Tricuspid regurgitation					
Yock (43)	62	87	SPAP	0.93	8
Chan (44)	50	72	SPAP	0.87	8
Hamer (45)	51	61	SPAP	0.96	6.8
Gallet (46)	24	71	SPAP	0.91	5.4
Torbicki (47)	72	24	SPAP	0.92	7.7
Tramarin (48)	100	30	SPAP	0.66	11.9
Isovolumetric relaxation time (RV)					
Hatle (49)	48	100	SPAP	0.84	n.a.
Acceleration time					
Kitabatake (50)	48	100	MPAP	−0.88	n.a.
Matsuda (51)	67	100	MPAP	−0.75	7.9
von Bibra (52)	70	100	MPAP	−0.77	17.4
Morera (53)	68	97	SPAP	−0.98	5.2
Migueres (54)	66	91	MPAP	−0.73	n.a.
Sajkov (55)	81	84	SPAP	−0.96	3.9

[a]SPAP, systolic pulmonary artery pressure; MPAP, mean pulmonary artery pressure.

for good access and limitations in obese patients and those with chronic obstructive lung disease and emphysema. Some of the latter shortcomings can be overcome by TEE.

Trans-oesophageal Echocardiography (TEE)

The main advantage of TEE is the direct imaging of thrombi, rather than by relying on indirect signs. This is largely the result of the superior image quality of TEE as there is a much shorter distance to the structures under evaluation from the oesophageal lumen (4,5). By TEE examination, thrombus can be found in the right atrium, the right ventricle, sometimes trapped in the Chiari network or at the tricuspid or pulmonary valve. Most often, however, thrombi are found at the bifurcation of the pulmonary artery or in the main right or left pulmonary artery.

Although there is high image quality in some parts of the pulmonary circulation, imaging is limited in other parts of the pulmonary artery. Whereas the right pulmonary artery can usually be followed until the branching point into the right lobar pulmonary arteries, visualization is limited in the left pulmonary artery due to the interposition of the left main bronchus, which results in an acoustic shadow and prevents imaging of the middle segment of the left pulmonary artery.

TEE has its own limitations, which include the need for sedation in often already hypoxic patients, leading to intubation and ventilation in some, its limited availability and its operator dependence. However, TEE has an important role in patients with unexplained cardiac arrest or pulseless electrical activity, as demonstrated in a study in 1246 patients during basic life support by Kürkciyan et al., where 5% had PE diagnosed as the underlying cause (12).

DIAGNOSTIC VALUE OF ECHOCARDIOGRAPHY IN SUSPECTED PULMONARY EMBOLISM

In acute PE without previous obstruction of the pulmonary circulation, maximum pulmonary artery systolic pressures almost never exceed 35–40 mmHg. The reason for this observation is that the relatively muscle-weak right ventricle cannot achieve higher pressures acutely. However, the most recent available reference intervals for pulmonary artery pressure reported a mean value of 28 ± 5 mmHg with a wide range from 15 to 57 mmHg, mainly depending on age and body mass index (BMI) (13).

Because pulmonary artery pressures as high as 57 mmHg may be normal, the diagnosis of acute or chronic pulmonary hypertension cannot be based on pressure measurements alone. All diagnoses based on pressures alone will result in a significant number of false-positive results, especially in the growing percentage of obese patients, older patients and patients with pulmonary diseases leading to elevated pulmonary artery pressures.

Because of the limited specificity of peak pulmonary artery pressure for the diagnosis of PE, other echo markers have been defined. The two most important are as follows:

1. McConnell et al. described 'moderate' or 'severe' ventricular free-wall hypokinesia but normal contraction and 'sparing' of the right ventricular apex. This so called 'McConnell sign' seems to be most useful in distinguishing between patients with acute and persistent pulmonary hypertension (14).
2. Kurzyna et al. prospectively assessed the diagnostic value of disturbed RV ejection pattern defined as acceleration time equal or less than 60 ms in the presence of tricuspid pressure gradient lower than 60 mmHg and named it the '60/60 sign'. The sensitivity and specificity for

definitive PE in 100 patients with suspected PE were 81% and 45% for pressure overload, 25% and 94% for the '60/60 sign' and 19% and 100% for the McConnell sign, respectively. The combination of the '60/60 sign' and the McConnell sign yielded a specificity and sensitivity of 36% and 94%, respectively (15).

Casazza *et al.* analysed 161 patients with proven PE or right ventricular infarction from an echo database. The McConnell sign was found in 70% of patients with proven PE and 67% with right ventricular infarction. The McConnell sign was absent in 33% of PE and 30% of RV infarction patients, resulting in a negative predictive value of 36%. Therefore, the McConnell sign is a specific marker of PE only in patients without right ventricular infarction (16).

Other signs of pulmonary hypertension or PE have also been described and may be of some value. A tricuspid gradient >45 mmHg was shown to be a significant indicator for pulmonary hypertension in patients with scleroderma who underwent right cardiac catheterization (17). In those with proven pulmonary hypertension, dilatation of the right ventricle was present in 71%, compression of the left ventricle was seen in 38% and paradoxical movement of the septum in 42% (17). On the other hand, the possibility of false-negative Doppler echocardiographic results should be considered in cases of otherwise high clinical likelihood of massive pulmonary hypertension (17). Furthermore, in a comparative study of patients with proven PE and those where the diagnosis was excluded, a tricuspid peak regurgitant velocity >2.5 m/s was found in 84% of cases, compared with 10% in the control group. An enlarged right ventricle (>25 mm) was found in 67% of all patients with PE but only in 11% of all controls. Echocardiographic septum motion abnormalities were observed in 42% versus 9%, respectively (18).

In patients in sinus rhythm, tissue Doppler parameters are helpful in patients with signs of PE. Hsiao *et al.* calculated a right ventricular performance index in 50 patients with proven PE and compared it with that for 150 patients without pulmonary hypertension (19). The 'M-index' was defined as peak early diastolic inflow velocity divided by the right ventricular myocardial performance index (RV MPI), obtained during tissue Doppler imaging over the lateral tricuspid annulus. Peak early diastolic mitral inflow velocity was significantly less and RV MPI was greater in patients with PE than those without. An RV MPI of >0.55 identified PE with a sensitivity of 85% and a specificity of 78%. An M-index of <122 had a sensitivity of 92% and a specificity of 92%.

In summary, the absence of signs of elevated pulmonary artery pressure excludes most forms of massive PE, but not smaller PE.

RECOMMENDATIONS FOR ECHOCARDIOGRAPHY IN ACUTE PULMONARY EMBOLISM

The most recent 2008 ESC guidelines define only a limited role for echocardiography in patients with suspected PE (3). Echocardiography is not recommended in stable patients. In unstable patients with massive PE, echocardiography should be considered as first-line diagnostic tool only if CTPA is not immediately available. However, in high-risk patients with signs of RVD, the decision for thrombolysis can be based on clinical assessment and echocardiography alone. Absence of RVD excludes massive PE. The ESC guidelines define the role of echocardiography mainly to assign patients with suspected PE to the intermediate- or low-risk group in the absence of RVD.

In patients without signs of pulmonary pressure elevation, PE is not excluded, but they represent a patient group with a very favourable short-term prognosis provided that they receive full-dose anticoagulation. In this patient group, the further diagnostic work-up (D-Dimer, CTPA, venous Doppler, lung scintigraphy) can be performed over the ensuing several hours. Transportation to a radiology department for imaging studies is usually safe in this subgroup of patients. Patients with very high pulmonary artery pressures are unlikely to have an isolated acute episode of PE, but rather tend to suffer from primary pulmonary hypertension or chronic thromboembolic disease.

Echocardiography seems to have its main clinical application in patients with significant clinical impairment (2,3,20). The value of echocardiography is dependent on the pre-test probability. Echo is most useful in patients with a relatively high likelihood of PE. Roy *et al.* showed that echocardiography was inferior in ruling out PE compared with lung scans, CT and MR angiography, but was within the range of leg vein ultrasonography (20). However, in patients with a pre-test likelihood of PE of >70%, echocardiography had a high clinical usefulness for rapid confirmation PE.

PROGNOSTIC VALUE OF ECHOCARDIOGRAPHY IN PULMONARY EMBOLISM

Approximately 10–20% of patients with PE are in shock and have a poor short-term prognosis. Those without shock have a much better prognosis. However, one needs to consider that the risk for major recurrent clinical events in PE is not binary but rather a continuum. In the group without shock, 27–55% of patients show one or more signs of RVD (21–26). These patients have a better prognosis than those who are in shock, but have inferior outcomes compared with those without RVD. Therefore, the identification of this large subgroup of patients seems important during the initial diagnosis of patients with suspected PE. At present, the most rapid tool to assign patients with to PE to the high-, intermediate- or low-risk group is echocardiography.

Detection of Patent Foramen Ovale (PFO)

Echo contrast is sometimes useful to enhance the signal quality of the tricuspid regurgitation signal during TTE and to assess right to left shunting due to a PFO. Patients with a PFO have more lung perfusion deficits at a given pulmonary artery pressure. Additionally, echo contrast is useful during TEE in suspected thrombus formation in the right pulmonary artery, giving a negative contrast in wall-adherent thrombus formation (see Figure 11.6). In patients with PE, detection of a PFO identifies those at high risk for arterial thromboembolic complications and death. In a study of 139 consecutive patients with PE and presence of a PFO, Konstantinides *et al.* used multivariate analysis to demonstrate a 10-fold increase in mortality and a 5-fold increase in major adverse events (27). Therefore, every echo examination in patients with suspected PE should include assessment of potential presence of PFO.

ECHOCARDIOGRAPHY COMPARED WITH OTHER DIAGNOSTIC TOOLS

In a survey of 1001 consecutive patients with suspected PE, the role of echocardiography for decision making was compared with other techniques (28). Echocardiography was the most frequently performed diagnostic procedure (74%). Lung scan or pulmonary angiography was performed in 79% of clinically stable patients but much less frequently (32%) in those with circulatory collapse at presentation. The overall in-hospital mortality rate ranged from 8.1% in the group of stable patients to 25% in those presenting with cardiogenic shock and to 65% in patients needing cardiopulmonary resuscitation (28).

The finding or exclusion of right ventricular afterload stress by echocardiography had a high prognostic value. In a total of 317 patients with clinically suspected PE, who were prospectively evaluated by echocardiography for the presence of right ventricular afterload stress and right heart or pulmonary artery thrombi by Kasper *et al.*, objective confirmation of PE by lung scan or pulmonary angiography was obtained in 164 patients (52%) (25). The presence of DVT was established in 90 of 158 patients (57%) who underwent phlebographic or Doppler sonographic studies. Right ventricular afterload stress was diagnosed in 87 patients (27%). Objective confirmation of PE and diagnosis of DVT was more common in patients with right ventricular afterload stress than in those without (83% versus 40% and 46% versus 22%). This was also true for the detection of thrombi in the right heart and major pulmonary arteries (12 patients versus one patient; *p<* 0.001) and also for the in-hospital mortality from venous thromboembolism (13% versus 0.9%; *p<* 0.001). One year mortality from PE was 13% in patients with right ventricular afterload stress at presentation compared with only 1% in those without (25).

Table 11.2 summarizes five studies addressing the prognostic significance of RVD in acute PE. Unfortunately, the definition of RVD differed between studies. In all studies, patients with normal right ventricular function had a very low in-hospital mortality.

In a systematic review of the literature on the prognostic value of RVD detected by echocardiography and its association with adverse outcomes in patients with PE, ten Wolde *et al.* found 62 studies addressing the subject. However, only seven studies fulfilled the following criteria (29):

1. prospective cohort study or randomised controlled study in clinically suspected PE.
2. baseline echocardiography in all patients with proven PE and additional assessment of right ventricular size, right ventricular wall motion, pulmonary systolic pressure, tricuspid valve regurgitation, right ventricular wall thickness and paradoxical septal wall movement.
3. patient follow-up for a minimum of 14 days or death during 'in-hospital period'.

Table 11.2 Prognostic value of right ventricular dysfunction in acute pulmonary embolism[a]

Study	Patients (*n*)	Patient characteristics	Echo criteria	Mortality (%) RVD positive	RVD negative
Kucher (26)	1035	BP >90 mmHg	RVD	16.3	9.4 (30-day all causes)
Kasper (25)	317	Normo- and hypotensive	RV >30 mm or TI >2.8 m/s	13	0.9
Grifoni (23)	162	BP >100 mmHg	RV >30 mm or RV/LV >1 or paradox systolic septum motion or AcT<90 ms or TIPG>30 mmHg	4.6	0
Ribeiro (22)	126	Normo- and hypotensive	RVD	12.8	0
Goldhaber (21)	101	Normotensive	RV hypokinesis or dilatation	4.3	0
			Mean (of %)	10.2	2.1

[a]Mortality, in-hospital PE related except Kucher *et al.*; RVD, right ventricular dysfunction; BP, blood pressure; RV right ventricle; LV, left ventricle; TI, tricuspid insufficiency; AcT, acceleration time of right ventricular ejection; TIPG, tricuspid insufficiency peak gradient. Modified from Reference 3.

In those seven studies, 40–70% of patients had RVD. Only two studies allowed for an assessment of normotensive patients. If only these studies were analysed, RVD in haemodynamically stable patients had a predictive value for in-hospital mortality of 4% and 5%, respectively. These results found a low absolute PE-related mortality in normotensive patients with RVD, but it was still much higher than in normotensive patients without RVD. The smaller absolute difference in this patient subgroup may explain the mixed outcome of results when the indication for thrombolysis in normotensive patients was based solely on the presence of signs of RVD by echocardiography or ECG (30).

FOLLOW-UP AFTER PULMONARY EMBOLISM

Serial echocardiograms in patients with large PE studied by McConnell showed 'moderate' or 'severe' ventricular free-wall hypokinesia but normal contraction and 'sparing' of the right ventricular apex. Although the McConnell sign may be useful in distinguishing between patients with acute and persistent pulmonary hypertension, the mechanisms accounting for this observation are not fully understood (14). Additionally, a false positive McConnell sign can be found in patients with right ventricular infarction (16).

The effects of treatment can be monitored clinically, by invasive monitoring or by repeated echo examinations (14). In selected cases, the resolution of the thrombus itself can be monitored by repeated TEE (31). The estimation of the gradient over the tricuspid valve allows for the assessment of pulmonary artery pressures and the right ventricular morphology as they normalize in patients with successful treatment (31).

FUTURE PERSPECTIVE: IVUS STUDIES IN PULMONARY CIRCULATION

Intravascular ultrasound (IVUS) has developed from a research tool to an intrinsic part of invasive imaging. An echo device for use in blood vessels must combine high frequency to provide sufficient resolution with a penetration of 2–10 mm. The frequencies used at present are usually in the range 10–40 MHz (6).

Although the value of angiography in the detection of a complete obstruction is uniformly accepted, the imaging of partially occluded vessel segments has been prone to misinterpretation. As a contour method, angiography cannot be adequate in the visualization of soft, wall-adherent thrombus formation. Furthermore, cross-sectional imaging of the entire vessel wall is impossible. IVUS is, in contrast, a technique allowing imaging of the lumen and the vessel wall.

The strengths of IVUS as a tomographic method in addition to angiography and other tomographic techniques are the assessment of vessel wall motion, imaging of very small pulmonary arteries (diameter 1.5–3 mm), assessment of vessel wall changes in patients with pulmonary hypertension without thromboembolic events and visualization of thin wall-adherent or 'soft' thrombus, not visible by angiography.

Pandian's group described the role of IVUS in patients with various pulmonary artery diseases and the response of the pulmonary circulation in patients with chronic heart failure (32). Kravitz and Scharf examined a patient with pulmonary atherosclerosis, not visualized by angiography (33). A detailed description of pulmonary anatomy by IVUS has been reported by Kawano (34). In patients with different degrees of pulmonary hypertension, he found a three-layered appearance of the pulmonary vessels in comparison with the monolayer found normally. Additionally, he found evidence of a plaque-like structure in one patient. These findings were confirmed and extended by Stähr et al. in ex vivo studies: wall-adherent organized thrombi in chronic thromboembolic pulmonary hypertension could be detected by IVUS as a second inner vessel layer

(35). Therefore, IVUS may represent an additional tool for detecting chronic thromboembolic pulmonary hypertension when the results of pulmonary angiography or CT are inconclusive.

Our group reported the first IVUS findings in acute PE. It was possible to cross complete obstructions and to identify both wall-adherent and free-floating thrombus (7). Tapson *et al.* reported their initial experience with IVUS in a canine model of PE and found a higher sensitivity of IVUS for detection of residual thrombus in comparison with angiography (36,37). Scott *et al.* reported their initial experience with IVUS in three patients with acute massive PE (38). Ricou *et al.* were the first to report on a larger series of IVUS in patients with recurrent thromboembolic disease (8,39). Again, IVUS was superior to angiography in revealing wall-adherent thrombus formation. We reported on a larger series of patients with IVUS after acute massive PE (6). IVUS was superior to angiography for the identification of residual thrombus formation. Unfortunately, IVUS in the pulmonary circulation still has significant shortcomings:

- IVUS is an invasive method and the positioning of IVUS catheters is often time consuming and results in additional X-ray exposure.
- Present IVUS catheters are not steerable. Hence their position cannot be controlled easily in the pulmonary circulation.
- Because of the difficulties in steering the catheter, only a limited number of vessels in the pulmonary circulation can be examined.

The limitations in steerability could be overcome by using steerable IVUS catheters and forward-viewing catheters (40). Furthermore, the combination of pressure, Doppler, steerability, IVUS and angioscopy could allow the complete morphological and functional assessment of the pulmonary circulation. IVUS has already gained some clinical importance in bedside ultrasound-guided vena cava filter placement. Ebaugh *et al.* reported successful IVUS-guided vena cave filter placement in 24 of 26 patients without additional fluoroscopy (41). Figure fig11.6 summarizes typical IVUS findings in PE.

CONCLUSION

Echocardiography is a very important non-invasive diagnostic tool in patients with suspected pulmonary hypertension, and it may play a significant role in selected patients with suspected PE. Transthoracic echocardiography and transoesophageal echo in selected patients can distinguish patients with or without haemodynamic impairment.

Echocardiography allows for rapid risk stratification in most and guides therapy in many patients. Appropriate treatment or further diagnostic strategies can be based on the echo findings. However, better standardization in imaging is needed to compare better trials assessing the value of echocardiography and to follow up patients over time, especially those with chronic pulmonary hypertension (42).

Acknowledgements

The outstanding help and support of Drs Thomas Buck, Hagen Kälsch and Thomas Konorza is highly appreciated.

REFERENCES

1. Stein PD, Henry JW. Prevalence of acute pulmonary embolism in a general hospital. *Chest* 1995; **108**:978–981.
2. Goldhaber SZ. Pulmonary embolism. *Lancet* 2004; **363**:1295–305
3. Task Force for the Diagnosis and Management of Acute Pulmonary Embolism of the European Society of Cardiology. Guidelines on the diagnosis and management of acute pulmonary embolism: the Task Force for the Diagnosis and Management of Acute Pulmonary Embolism of the European Society of Cardiology (ESC). *Eur Heart J* 2008; **29**:2276–315.
4. Nixdorff U, Erbel R, Drexler M, Meyer J. Detection of thrombembolus of the right pulmonary artery by transesophageal two-dimensional echocardiography. *Am J Cardiol* 1988; **61**:448–9.
5. Wittlich N, Erbel R, Eichler A, *et al.* Detection of central pulmonary artery thrombemboli by transesophageal echocardiography in patients with severe pulmonary embolism. *J Am Soc Echocardiogr* 1992; **5**:515–24.
6. Görge G, Schuster S, Ge J, Meyer J, Erbel R. Intravascular ultrasound in patients with acute pulmonary embolism after treatment with intravenous urokinase and high-dose heparin. *Heart* 1997; **77**:73–7.
7. Görge G, Erbel R, Schuster S, Ge J, Meyer J. Intravascular ultrasound in diagnosis of acute pulmonary embolism [letter]. *Lancet* 1991; **337**:623–4.
8. Ricou F, Nicod PH, Moser KM, Peterson KL. Catheter-based intravascular ultrasound imaging of chronic thromboembolic pulmonary disease. *Am J Cardiol* 1991; **67**:749–52.
9. Erbel R, Drozdz J, Ge J, *et al.* Bildgebende Verfahren in der Kardiologie: akute und chronische pulmonale Hypertonie. *Internist* 1994; **35**:1039–55.
10. Kasper W, Meinertz T, Kersting F, Löllgen H, Limbourg P, Just H. Echocardiography in assessing acute pulmonary hypertension due to pulmonary embolism. *Am J Cardiol* 1980; **45**:567–72.
11. European Working Group on Echocardiography. The European Cooperative Study on the clinical significance of right heart thrombi. *Eur Heart J* 1989; **10**:1046–59.
12. Kürkciyan I, Meron G, Sterz F, *et al.* Pulmonary embolism as a cause of cardiac arrest: presentation and outcome. *Arch Intern Med* 2000; **160**:1529–35.
13. McQuillan BM, Picard MH, Leavitt M, Weyman AE. Clinical correlates and reference intervals for pulmonary artery systolic pressure among echocardiographically normal subjects. *Circulation* 2001; **104**:2797–802.
14. McConnell MV, Solomon SD, Rayan ME, Come PC, Goldhaber SZ, Lee RT. Regional right ventricular dysfunction detected by echocardiography in acute pulmonary embolism. *Am J Cardiol* 1996; **78**:469–73.
15. Kurzyna M, Torbicki A, Pruszczyk P, *et al.* Disturbed right ventricular ejection pattern as a new Doppler echocardiographic sign of acute pulmonary embolism. *Am J Cardiol.* 2002; **90**:507–11.
16. Casazza F, Bongarzoni A, Capozi A, Agostoni O. Regional right ventricular dysfunction in acute pulmonary embolism and right ventricular infarction. *Eur J Echocardiogr* 2005; **6**:11–14.
17. Mukerjee D, St George D, Knight C, *et al.* Echocardiography and pulmonary function as screening tests for pulmonary arterial hypertension in systemic sclerosis. *Rheumatology* 2004; **43**:461–6.
18. Nazeyrollas P, Metz D, Jolly D, *et al.* Use of transthoracic Doppler echocardiography combined with clinical and electrocardiographic data to predict acute pulmonary embolism. *Eur Heart J* 1996; **17**:779–86.
19. Hsiao SH, Chang SM, Lee CY, Yang SH, Lin SK, Chiou KR. Usefulness of tissue Doppler parameters for identifying pulmonary embolism in patients with signs of pulmonary hypertension. *Am J Cardiol* 2006; **98**:685–90.
20. Roy PM, Colombet I, Durieux P, Chatellier G, Sors H, Meyer G. Systematic review and meta-analysis of strategies for the iagnosis of suspected pulmonary embolism. *Br Med J* 2005; **331**:295–304.
21. Goldhaber SZ, Haire WD, Feldstein ML, *et al.* Alteplase versus heparin in acute pulmonary embolism: randomised trial assessing right-ventricular function and pulmonary perfusion. *Lancet* 1993; **341**:507–11.
22. Ribeiro A, Lindmarker P, Juhlin-Dannfelt A, Johnsson H, Jorfeldt L. Echocardiography Doppler in pulmonary embolism: right ventricular dysfunction as a predictor of mortality rate. *Am Heart J* 1997; **134**:479–87.

23. Grifoni S, Olivotto I, Cecchini P, *et al.* Short-term clinical outcome of patients with acute pulmonary embolism, normal blood pressure and echocardiographic right ventricular dysfunction. *Circulation* 2000; **101**:2817–22.
24. Kreit JW. The impact of right ventricular dysfunction on the prognosis and therapy of normotensive patients with pulmonary embolism. *Chest* 2004; **125**:1539–45.
25. Kasper W, Konstantinides S, Geibel A, Tiede N, Krause T, Just H. Prognostic significance of right ventricular afterload stress detected by echocardiography in patients with clinically suspected pulmonary embolism. *Heart* 1997; **77**:346–9.
26. Kucher N, Luder CM, Dörnhöfer T, Windecker S, Meier B, Hess OM. Novel management strategy for patients with suspected pulmonary embolism. *Eur Heart J* 2003; **24**:366–76.
27. Konstantinides S, Geibel A, Kasper W, Olschewski M, Blümel L, Just H. Patent foramen ovale is an important predictor of adverse outcome in patients with major pulmonary embolism. *Circulation* 1998; **97**:1946–51.
28. Kasper W, Konstantinides S, Geibel A, *et al.* Management strategies and determinants of outcome in acute major pulmonary embolism: results of a multicenter registry. *J Am Coll Cardiol* 1997; **30**:1165–71.
29. ten Wolde M, Söhne M, Quak E, MacGillavry MR, Büller HR. Prognostic value of echocardiographically assesd right ventricular dysfunction in patients with pulmonary hypertension. *Arch Intern Med* 2004; **164**:1685–9.
30. Konstantinides S, Geibel A, Heusel G, Heinrich F, Kasper W. Heparin plus alteplase compared with heparin alone in patients with submassive pulmonary embolism. *N Engl J Med* 2002; **347**:1143–50.
31. Bruch C, Othman T, Görge G, *et al.* Intensive medical monitoring with transesophageal echocardiography in fulminant pulmonary embolism. *Dtsch Med Wochenschr* 1996; **121**:829–33.
32. Porter TR, Taylor DO, Fields J, Cycan A, Akosah K, Mohanty PK, Pandian NG. Direct in vivo evaluation of pulmonary arterial pathology in chronic congestive heart failure with catheter-based intravascular ultrasound imaging. *Am J Cardiol* 1993; **71**:754–7.
33. Kravitz KD, Scharf GR, Chandrasekaran K. In vivo diagnosis of pulmonary atherosclerosis. Role of intravascular ultrasound. *Chest* 1994; **106**:632–4.
34. Kawano T. Wall morphology of the pulmonary artery–intravascular ultrasound imaging and pathological evaluations. *Kurume Med J* 1994; **41**:221–32.
35. Stähr P, Rupprecht HJ, Voigtländer T, *et al.* Comparison of normal and diseased pulmonary artery morphology by intravascular ultrasound and histological examination. *Int J Card Imaging* 1999: **15**:221–31.
36. Tapson VF, Davidson CJ, Gurbel PA, Sheikh KH, Kisslo KB, Stack RS. Rapid and accurate diagnosis of pulmonary emboli in a canine model using intravascular ultrasound imaging. *Chest* 1991; **100**:1410–13.
37. Tapson VF, Davidson CJ, Kisslo KB, Stack RS. Rapid visualization of massive pulmonary emboli utilizing intravascular ultrasound. *Chest* 1994; **105**: 888–90.
38. Scott PJ, Essop AR, al-Ashab W, Deaner A, Parsons J, Williams G. Imaging of pulmonary vascular disease by intravascular ultrasound. *Int J Card Imaging* 1993; **9**:179–84.
39. Ricou F, Ludomirsky A, Weintraub RG, Sahn DJ. Applications of intravascular scanning and transesophageal echocardiography in congenital heart disease: tradeoffs and the merging of technologies. *Int J Card Imaging* 1991; **6**:221–30.
40. Görge G, Ge J, Haude M, Baumgart D, Buck T, Erbel R. Initial experience with a steerable intravascular ultrasound catheter in the aorta and pulmonary artery. *Am J Card Imaging* 1995; **9**:180–4.
41. Ebaugh JL, Chiou AC, Morasch MD, Matsumura JS, Pearce WH. Bedside vena cava filter placement guided with intravascular ultrasound. *J Vasc Surg* 2001: **34**:21–6.
42. Van Beek EJR. Thromboembolic disease: can echocardiography assist management? *Chest* 2000; **118**; 888–9.
43. Yock PG, Popp RL. Noninvasive estimation of right ventricular systolic pressure by Doppler ultrasound in patients with tricuspid regurgitation. *Circulation* 1984; **70**:657–62.
44. Chan KL, Currie PJ, Seward JB, *et al.* Comparison of three Doppler ultrasound methods in the prediction of pulmonary artery pressure. *J Am Coll Cardiol* 1987; **9**:549–54.
45. Hamer HPM, Takens BL, Posma JL, Lie KL. Noninvasive measurement of right ventricular systolic pressure by combined color-coded and continuous-wave Doppler ultrasound. *Am J Cardiol* 1988; **61**:668–71.
46. Gallet B, Saudemont JP, Bourdon D, *et al.* Evaluation of pulmonary arterial hypertension by Doppler echocardiography in chronic respiratory insufficiency. *Arch Mal Coeur Vais* 1989; **82**:1575–83.
47. Torbicki A, Skwarski K, Hawrylkiewicz I, Pasierski T, Miskiewicz Z, Zielinski J. Attempts at measuring pulmonary arterial pressure by means of Doppler echocardiography in patients with chronic lung disease. *Eur Respir J* 1989; **2**:856–60.
48. Tramarin R, Torbicki A, Marchandise B, Laaban JP, Morpurgo M. Doppler echocardiographic evaluation of pulmonary artery pressure in chronic obstructive pulmonary disease. A European multicentre study.

Working Group on Noninvasive Evaluation of Pulmonary Artery Pressure. European Office of the World Health Organization, Copenhagen. *Eur Heart J* 1991; **12**:103–11.

49. Hatle L, Angelsen BAJ, Tromsdal A. Non-invasive estimation of pulmonary artery systolic pressure with Doppler ultrasound. *Br Heart J* 1981; **45**:157–65.

50. Kitabatake A, Inoue M, Asao M, *et al.* Noninvasive evaluation of pulmonary hypertension by a pulsed Doppler technique. *Circulation* 1983; **68**:302–9.

51. Matsuda M, Sekiguchi T, Sugishita Y, Kuwako K, Iida K, Ito I. Reliability of non-invasive estimates of pulmonary hypertension by pulsed Doppler echocardiography. *Br Heart J* 1986; **56**:158–64.

52. von Bibra H, Ulm K, Klein G, Sebening H, Blömer H. Die Diagnose der Pulmonalen Hypertonie mittels gepulster Dopplerechokardiographie. *Z Kardiol* 1987; **76**:149–58.

53. Morera J, Hoadley SD, Roland JM, *et al.* Estimation of the ratio of pulmonary to systemic pressures by pulsed-wave Doppler echocardiography for assessment of pulmonary arterial pressures. *Am J Cardiol* 1989; **63**:862–66.

54. Migueres M, Escamilla R, Coca F, Didier A, Krempf M. Pulsed Doppler echocardiography in the diagnosis of pulmonary hypertension in COPD. *Chest* 1990; **98**:280–5.

55. Sajkov D, Cowie RJ, Bradley JA, Mahar L, McEvoy RD. Validation of new pulsed Doppler echocardiographic techniques for assessment of pulmonary hemodynamics. *Chest* 1993; **103**:1348–53.

56. Kälsch H, Sack S, Erbel R, Jakob H. Acute massive pulmonary embolism detected with angiography and intravascular ultrasound treated by pulmonary embolectomy. *Herz* 2006; **31**:366–7.

CHAPTER 12

Ultrasonography of Deep Vein Thrombosis

Sebastian M. Schellong

Division of Internal Medicine II, Krankenhaus Dresden-Friedrichstadt Dresden, Germany

INTRODUCTION

Venous ultrasound of the leg veins has become the main tool for diagnosing patients with clinically suspected deep vein thrombosis (DVT) (1). In addition, it is increasingly being used to screen patients without symptoms in the leg in different clinical or experimental situations. Finally, authorities accept or even recommend venous ultrasound as an endpoint measure in phase II or phase III drug trials. This chapter describes the methodology of venous ultrasound, discusses the different options in performing it and reviews the data regarding its reliability and validity in different clinical situations.

ULTRASOUND ANATOMY OF THE LEG VEIN SYSTEM

Ultrasonography of DVT requires visualization of the leg veins. They are easily accessible from the groin downwards since no physical obstacles, such as bones or air-containing structures, are present between the skin surface and leg veins. The pelvic veins and the inferior vena cava may also be visualized; however, visibility is highly dependent on superimposed bowel structures and on body mass.

When followed from the groin to the ankle, there are at least four anatomical patterns which have to be identified by an appropriate ultrasound examination technique (Figure 12.1). At the groin level, the common femoral vein invariably can be found medially to the common femoral artery, and the venous bifurcation into the superficial and the deep femoral veins is situated 1–2 cm distal to the arterial bifurcation. At the thigh level, the femoral vein accompanies the femoral artery, changing its position from medial to dorsal to laterodorsal. The deep femoral vein is visible only in case of a predominant configuration. A double femoral vein or venous segment may be easily identified by ultrasound. At the popliteal level, the popliteal vein has a dorsal position to the popliteal artery, before branching in three stem veins for the three paired calf vein groups of the

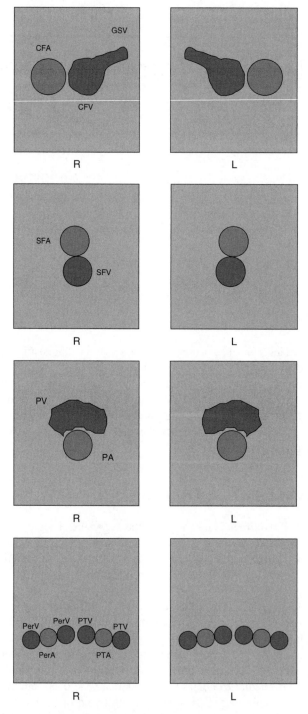

Figure 12.1 Four typical patterns of venous leg ultrasound anatomy. Cross-sections of (a) the groin, (b) the thigh, (c) the popliteal fossa and (d) the calf. CFV, common femoral vein; CFA, common femoral artery; GSV, greater saphenous vein; SFV, superficial femoral vein; SFA, superficial femoral artery; DFV, deep femoral vein; PV, popliteal vein; PA, popliteal artery; PC, peroneal confluens; PTC, posterior tibial confluens; PerV, peroneal vein; PerA, peroneal artery; PTV, posterior tibial veins; PTA, posterior tibial artery. A full colour version of this image appears in the plate section of this book.

anterior tibial veins, the posterior tibial veins and the peroneal veins. With regard to the direction of blood flow, the stems may be referred to as 'confluens segments'. The anterior confluens is usually not visible due to its steep course perforating the fascia of the anterior compartment. However, only 1–2 cm distally, the branching into the two remaining confluens segments is prominent, the posterior confluens taking a medial and the peroneal a lateral position. At the calf level, the three paired vein groups have fixed positions in relation to the bones. From a dorso-medial view, the peroneal group is located closely medial to the fibula and is normally the dominant vein group. The posterior tibial group is to be found dorsal to the tibia and will gain a greater distance to the bone as it courses down the leg. The anterior tibial group is accessible from antero-laterally close to the interosseous membrane; from proximal to distal it runs from the fibula to the tibia.

Uncertainty has risen about the distinction between proximal and distal veins as identified by ultrasound. By anatomical nomenclature it is defined that the popliteal vein is part of the proximal veins and that all veins beyond the popliteal vein are part of the distal veins. However, when examined by ultrasound, the popliteal fossa displays the transition zone between the (single) popliteal vein and the three paired calf vein groups. At this trifurcation the popliteal vein branches into the anterior, the posterior the peroneal confluens. However, as the anterior confluens is not visible, the ultrasound examination gives the appearance of a bifurcation (popliteal vein into posterior and peroneal confluens). The level of this bifurcation varies between patients (Figure 12.2). In most cases it is at the very level of the knee joint space. In a considerable number of patients, however, it is above or below this level. If it is above the knee joint, this may lead to the misconception and misnomer of a double popliteal vein; they are in fact the posterior and the peroneal confluentes. In addition, with the growing frequency of ultrasound examinations, the barrier between proximal and distal veins has been changed in the perception of sonographers and the physicians depending on their reports. All veins visible in the popliteal fossa now tend to be addressed as proximal, whereas all veins visible when examining the calf are addressed as distal. Although this is incorrect in terms of anatomical nomenclature, it is now widely accepted to name the veins of the popliteal fossa 'popliteal veins' or 'popliteal vein and trifurcation area' and to consider these as proximal. In this concept, distal veins are the paired calf veins and the calf muscle veins.

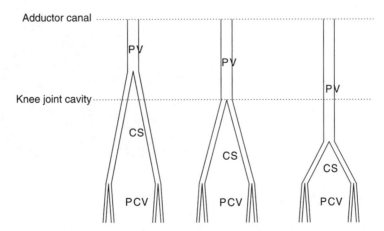

Figure 12.2 Schematic representation of the trifurcation area extending from the adductor canal to the proximal calf. (a) Branching point of popliteal vein above the knee joint cavity; (b) branching point at the very level of the knee joint level; (c) branching point below the knee joint cavity. PCV, paired calf veins; CR, confluens segments; PV, popliteal vein.

Regarding distal veins, it has been said – and often reiterated – that they have a large anatomical variability, which was one reason for the difficulties in appropriately examining them. However, variability only exists as to whether they are really paired or, by contrast, triplicate or single. It is an important aspect of sonographer education to train the fast and reliable identification of the deep distal vein groups (2).

Unlike venography, ultrasonography is easily capable of visualizing the entire calf muscle vein system (Figure 12.3). The gastrocnemius veins – mostly paired and accompanying a small artery – are drained into the popliteal vein. The soleal veins perforate the fascia underlying the soleus muscle and drain at different levels into the paired calf veins.

The greater and lesser saphenous veins are the most convenient to detect since they are in the near field of the ultrasound transducer. Once identified at any level of interest, they can be followed to their drainage point into the deep vein system with the lesser saphenous vein draining into the popliteal vein and the greater saphenous vein entering into the common femoral vein.

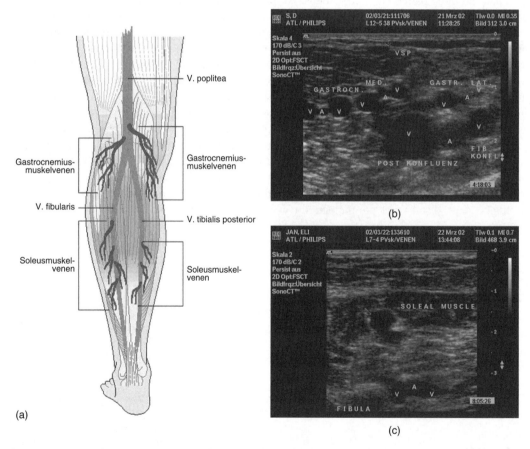

Figure 12.3 Muscle vein system of the calf. (a) Schematic representation. (b) Cross-section of the lower part of the popliteal fossa. The popliteal artery is accompanied by the two confluens segments of the paired calf veins The gastrocnemius arteries and veins are approaching from the medial and the lateral part of the calf The small saphenous vein is approaching from dorsal. (c) Cross-section of the mid-calf region. The peroneal artery is located near the fibular bone accompanied by the paired peroneal veins A segmental soleal vein is approaching from dorsal. A, artery; V, vein; VSP, small saphenous vein; arrow, soleal muscle vein. A full colour version of (a) appears in the plate section of this book.

ULTRASOUND MODALITIES

DVT may be visualized by all different ultrasound modalities such as B-mode imaging, pulse wave (PW) Doppler or colour Doppler methods. Paradoxically, the most direct ultrasound criterion, i.e., visualization of the clot itself, is the least valuable. Indirect signs establish the diagnosis more reliably. Table 12.1 gives a description of the diagnostic ultrasound criteria for DVT.

The most valid ultrasound criterion is lack of compressibility of a venous segment under investigation (Figure 12.4). Only B-mode imaging is required. When compressed, the vein collapses while the accompanying artery remains patent due to the much higher intravascular pressure. This observation is based on the presumption that if the vein does not collapse despite compression, some solid content has to be in it, i.e., a clot. Compression is carried out by exerting pressure with the ultrasound probe. A linear transducer should be used in order to transfer the pressure from the skin surface to the tissue in a predictable direction. Only cross-sections of the veins should be compressed since in the longitudinal view the vein may slip out of the field of view while moving the transducer. The manoeuvre has crucial requirements in order to yield a definitive result: The venous segment under investigation has to be identified unequivocally in terms of anatomy; no obstacle must be present preventing the pressure from being directly transferred to the vein; veins have to be distended by blood in order to allow for significant compression; the pressure has to be applied in the direction of the ultrasound beam; the pressure has to be sufficient to overcome the intravascular pressure within the vein. If all these requirements are met, compression ultrasound does not need support from other modalities. The only exception might be a very soft and/or mobile clot which moves out of the field of view under the increasing pressure of the compression manoeuvre. However, this kind of thrombus will not generate flow phenomena strong enough to be reliably established by colour Doppler or PW-Doppler methods.

The diagnostic criterion of DVT with colour Doppler is the lack of a Doppler signal at the very site of the thrombus (Figure 12.5). This directly resembles the 'filling defect' criterion of venography. However, absence of a colour Doppler signal may easily be an artefact if colour Doppler presets such as velocity scale, gain or angle are not chosen appropriately. Since visualization of intravascular flow is reliable only in longitudinal sections of the vessel, steering of the transducer for obtaining full longitudinal sections requires significantly more precision than is required for

Table 12.1 Diagnostic criteria for DVT by venous ultrasound

Modality	Direct	Indirect
B-mode	• Enlarged vein diameter • Enhanced thrombogenicity within the vessel lumen • Visible shape of the thrombus	• Lack of compressibility
PW Doppler	• Lack of Doppler signal	• Reduced spontaneous flow (velocity, modulation by respiratory movements) due to proximal obstruction • Reduced augmented flow (after tissue compression distally) due to distal obstruction
Colour Doppler	• Lack of Doppler signal	• Reduced spontaneous flow (velocity, modulation by respiratory movements) due to proximal obstruction

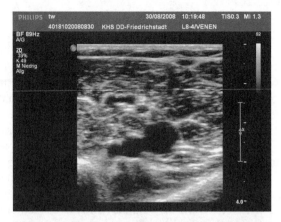

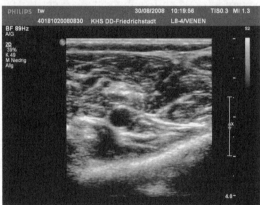

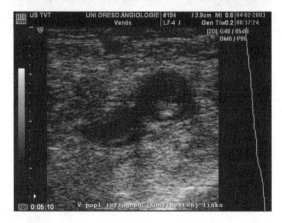

Figure 12.4   Cross-section of the popliteal fossa with popliteal artery, the two confluens segments and gastrocnemius artery and vein. (a) Without compression: veins and arteries visible. (b) Under compression: veins collapsed, arteries remain open. (c) Under compression: vein incompressible, echogenic thrombus within the venous lumen.

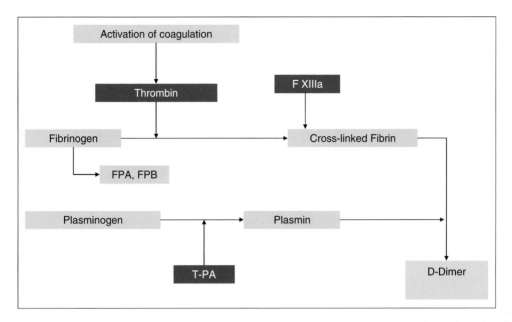

Plate 1   Schematic representation of D-dimer formation. Activated coagulation results in thrombin formation. Thrombin cleaves fibrinopeptides A and B (FPA and PPB) from the fibrinogen molecule, turning it into a fibrin monomer that polymerizes into soluble fibrin. Simultaneously, thrombin activates coagulation factor XIII (F XIII a), which then stabilizes the soluble fibrin. The activation of plasmin by the tissue-type plasminogen activator begins fibrin degradation and leads to the generation of D-dimer.

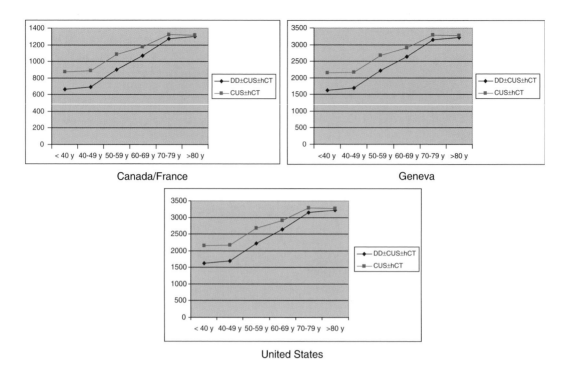

Canada/France

Geneva

United States

Plate 2 Costs in dollars of diagnostic strategies with and without ELISA D-dimer according to age and to the costs in different countries. Adapted from Righini M, Nendaz M, G LEG, *et al*. Influence of age on the cost-effectiveness of diagnostic strategies for suspected pulmonary embolism. *J Thromb Haemost* 2007; **5**:1869–77.

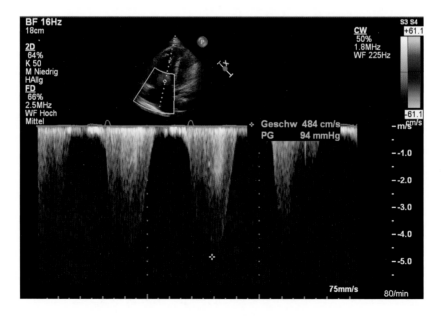

Plate 3 Systolic pulmonal artery pressure 94 mmHg.

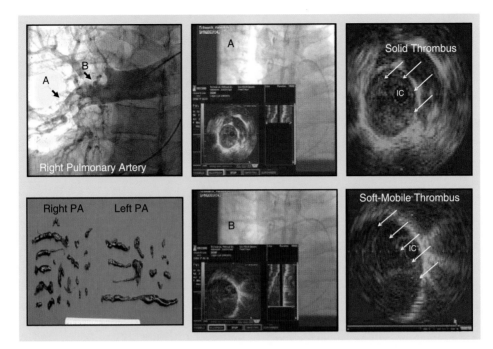

Plate 4 Typical example of IVUS imaging in a 61-year-old male patient with pulmonary embolism (modified from Ref. 56 with permission of the authors). Upper left: pulmonary angiogram showing complete and partial occlusion of the right pulmonary artery. Letters A and B indicate different positions of the IVUS catheter. In position A, IVUS shows solid thrombus (upper right, white arrows) as seen in angiography. In position B, soft, partly mobile thrombus is visualized by IVUS in addition to only partially visible thrombus found by angiography (white arrows). Lower left: thrombus removed during successful surgery from the left and right pulmonary circulation. IC, IVUS catheter; PA, pulmonary artery.

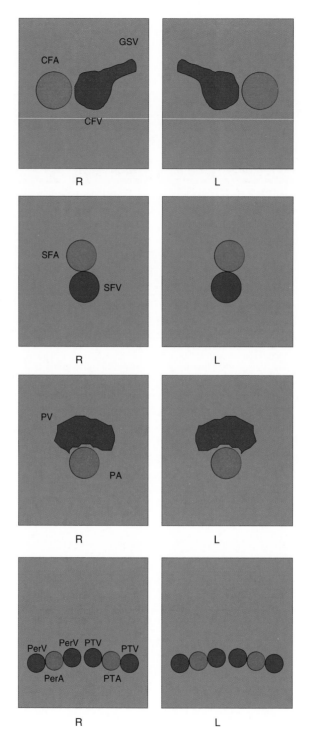

Plate 5 Four typical patterns of venous leg ultrasound anatomy. Cross-sections of (a) the groin, (b) the thigh, (c) the popliteal fossa and (d) the calf. CFV, common femoral vein; CFA, common femoral artery; GSV, greater saphenous vein; SFV, superficial femoral vein; SFA, superficial femoral artery; DFV, deep femoral vein; PV, popliteal vein; PA, popliteal artery; PC, peroneal confluens; PTC, posterior tibial confluens; PerV, peroneal vein; PerA, peroneal artery; PTV, posterior tibial veins; PTA, posterior tibial artery.

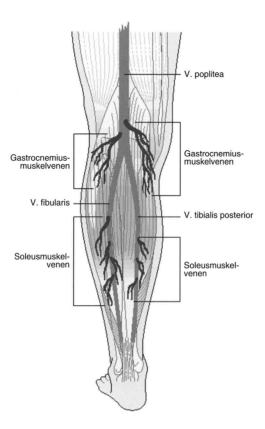

Plate 6 Muscle vein system of the calf-schematic representation.

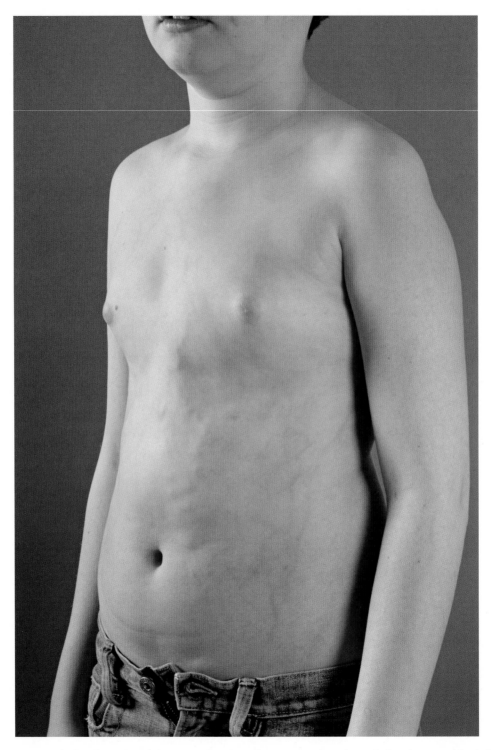

Plate 7 Extended collateral circulation in the skin after venous thromboembolic disease of both legs. Reprinted from van Ommen CH, Peters M. A new diagnosis in children: the post-thrombotic syndrome. *Progr Pediatr Cardiol* 2005; **21**:23–9, with permission of Elsevier.

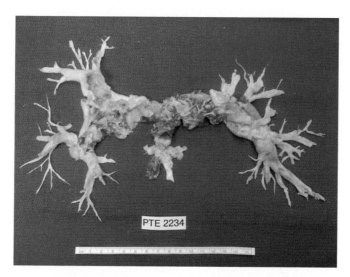

Plate 8 Surgical specimen removed from a patient with type I disease. The specimen is arrayed in anatomical position. Large amount of proximal thromboembolic material is noted in the main and both right and left pulmonary arteries. The thickened fibrous material seen in the distal vessels is characteristic of remodelled thrombus. Note that simple removal of large proximal thromboembolic material, without a complete endarterectomy, will leave a significant amount of distal disease behind and will result in the patient's demise.

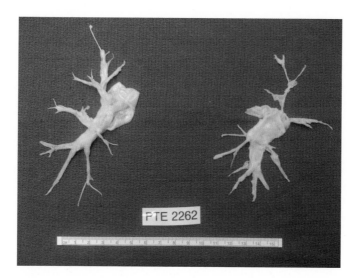

Plate 9 Surgical specimen removed from a patient with type II disease. Both pulmonary arteries have evidence of chronic thromboembolic material, but there is no evidence of fresh thromboembolic material. Note the distal tails of the specimen in each branch. Full resolution of pulmonary hypertension is dependent on complete removal of all the distal tails.

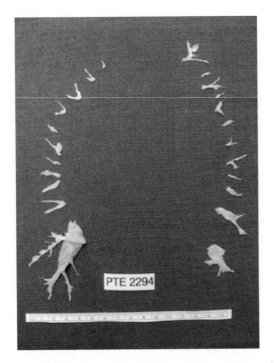

Plate 10 Surgical specimen removed from a patient with type III disease. Note that in this group of patients the disease is more distal and the plane of dissection has to be raised individually at each segmental level.

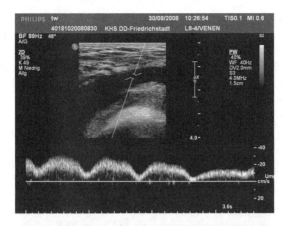

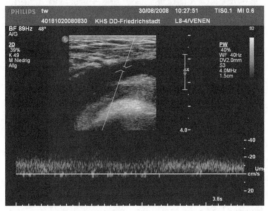

Figure 12.5 Pulsed wave Doppler signal from the common femoral vein. (a) Normal wave form with modulation by respiratory movements and by arterial pulsation from the adjacent artery, indicating patent iliac veins and inferior cava. (b) Pathological wave form without modulation, indicating venous obstruction (thrombus, compression) proximal to the common femoral vein.

cross-sectional ultrasonography. The criterion is only valid if the unaffected part of the vein displays flow and the occluded one does not, while in the same field of view. However, if this is the case, the clot would have been easily detected by compression ultrasound alone in the majority of patients. Thus, the added value of colour Doppler as compared with B-mode imaging is not so much in detecting the thrombus, but rather in helping to identify arterial signals in anatomically complex regions with reduced visibility. Once identified, the artery guides to the veins which can then be examined by compression manoeuvres.

The PW-Doppler method has the same limitation as colour Doppler and therefore does not add information to B-mode imaging as far as the leg veins are considered. However, a compromised PW flow signal in the common femoral vein with reduced velocity or respiratory changes being flattened or absent is a strong hint of an obstruction or occlusion of the iliac veins. The criterion is even more valid if there is a clear difference between the two legs. If positive, the iliac veins must be visualized directly and it may be necessary to obtain imaging of the inferior vena cava.

It is tempting to estimate thrombus age on the basis of its ultrasound appearance. However, there is no validated criterion, first because there is no gold standard to define thrombus age. On a qualitative rather than quantitative basis, the recently formed venous thrombus in a symptomatic patient enlarges the venous diameter to as much as double the size of the adjacent artery. During the natural history of DVT, the thrombus shrinks, and later recanalization occurs. The thrombus then becomes wall adherent, leaving space for a recanalized lumen; sometimes filaments crossing the lumen are visible. After some years, the thrombus is no longer present, but the vessel wall may display some degree of thickening; the total venous diameter is much smaller than that of the artery. At the thigh level, collateral veins are present in many cases, touching the artery from atypical directions, e.g., frontal or lateral. Recently formed clots have a low or even no echogenicity. The echo pattern of thrombi in organization resembles that of the surrounding tissue. Venous scars have a high thrombogenicity.

Despite the highly suggestive and plausible explanation of findings in the course of an individual disease that is offered by these qualitative descriptions, they do not allow for precisely distinguishing between residual thrombus and relapsing disease in a previously unknown patient. In the strictest sense, a relapse may only be diagnosed if there is a clear description of a previous ultrasound examination allowing for comparison. The most valid sign of relapse is a clot in a previously unaffected venous segment. Good evidence has been established for the criterion of an increase in residual thrombus diameter of 4 mm or more within the same vein segment (3). However, this requires a detailed report from the past. Even if present, sonography of relapsing DVT remains unreliable (4). Therefore, in an unknown patient with a history of DVT in the same leg, the diagnosis of relapsing disease may only be made in the context of clinical and laboratory findings. The ultrasound examination at best contributes one of the elements within the diagnostic process.

ULTRASOUND PROTOCOLS

Unlike other ultrasound procedures, for instance echocardiography, ultrasound of the leg veins has not yet been standardized. However, at least three structured approaches can be derived from the literature. All of them refer to B-mode compression ultrasound (CUS) only (Figure 12.6). Approaches including colour Doppler are less well structured. In most cases, the description of the procedure only has a list of modalities to be used without giving an order of examination steps. All these approaches may be referred to as 'unstructured' or 'intuitive'.

The elementary leg vein ultrasound procedure is the so-called 'two-point CUS' (Figure 12.6). It comprises B-mode imaging in cross-sections at two levels. The first level is the groin, where the common femoral vein and the bifurcation into the superficial and deep femoral veins can be examined. The second level is the popliteal fossa, where the popliteal vein can be examined. This protocol aims to rule in or exclude the presence of proximal DVT. The reason for skipping the entire length of the femoral vein is based on the findings in a venography study, which showed that the clot was present at least at one of these two levels in all 166 patients with proximal DVT (5). It is important to realize that this observation applied to symptomatic patients only. The advantage of this protocol is its almost universal feasibility. Several studies have demonstrated that it may be used effectively by emergency room physicians without specialized training in ultrasonography (6,7). Hence it fits well into diagnostic algorithms focusing on proximal DVT in symptomatic patients.

With increasing interest in the trifurcation area and conceptualization of the stems of the posterior tibial and the peroneal veins as proximal veins, a more elaborate protocol emerged. It may be referred to as 'extended CUS' (Figure 12.6). Again, only B-mode imaging and cross-section compression ultrasound are used. However, the entire length of the thigh veins is evaluated in addition to the popliteal vein and the entire trifurcation area. The examination stops when the respective bifurcations into the paired calf veins have been reached. This protocol also seems

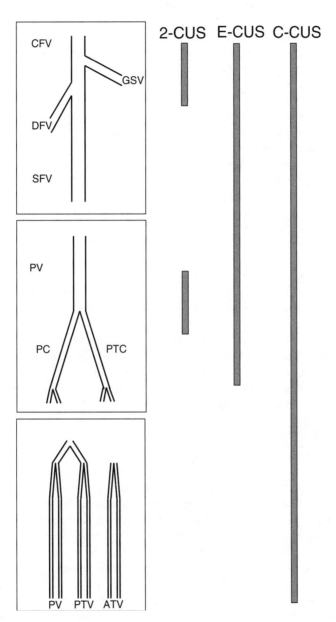

Figure 12.6 Schematic representation of the three main structured venous ultrasound protocols. 2-CUS, two-point compression ultrasound; E-CUS, extended compression ultrasound; C-CUS, complete (comprehensive) compression ultrasound; CFV, common femoral vein; GSV, greater saphenous vein; SFV, superficial femoral vein; DFV, deep femoral vein; PV, popliteal vein; PC, peroneal confluens; PTC, posterior tibial confluens; PV, peroneal veins; PTV, posterior tibial veins; ATV, anterior tibial veins.

suitable for the detection of proximal DVT in asymptomatic patients, since clots in these patients tend to be less extensive and often limited to segmental thrombi. Only one study systematically investigated the added value of the extended CUS versus two-point CUS. No additional DVT was identified. However, this was not in patients with suspected DVT, but with suspected PE. Nevertheless, with increasing popularity of venous ultrasound, most sonographers will use some type of extended CUS rather than the pure two-point CUS.

Many sonographers follow the leg veins through the calf down to the ankle level. In some countries, this is part of the education of professional ultrasound technicians. At least one well-structured protocol has been suggested which may be referred to as 'complete' or 'comprehensive' CUS (Figure 12.6) (8). Again, it relies on B-mode ultrasound and cross-sections only. The patient is examined from the popliteal fossa down to the ankle in the sitting position with the legs dangling over the edge of the examination table or placed on a stool. Pre-filling of distal veins by means of hydrostatic pressure guarantees maximum visibility; it therefore facilitates anatomic orientation and enhances the reliability of compression manoeuvres. The posterior tibial veins and the peroneal veins should be followed separately in order have the correct angle for compression. The anterior tibial veins can easily be identified and examined. However, isolated findings in these groups are exceedingly rare. Calf muscle veins are examined in both parts of the gastrocnemius muscle and in the soleal muscle. Colour Doppler may be used in cross-sections to identify the lower leg arteries if the anatomical orientation is complex, e.g., in the proximal calf. Longitudinal sections should be avoided as should colour imaging of paired veins. It is time consuming and offers no additional information.

It is an unmet need in the field of vascular ultrasound to standardize clearly the leg vein examination procedure. Strict standardization is the foundation on which education in ultrasound may be based. Accordingly it is essential for yielding and reporting meaningful scientific results. By contrast, intuitive examination procedures are cumbersome to perform and yield results which cannot be compared between investigators.

FEASIBILITY

There is a general consensus that the feasibility of ultrasound of proximal leg veins is excellent. No major validation or management study has reported consistent figures on non-evaluability for proximal veins. This is particularly true for the two-point CUS protocol. In extended CUS, the region of the adductor canal sometimes has reduced visibility due to adjacent tendineous structures. However, this can be overcome by an improved examination technique in most patients.

For distal veins, there is the suspicion that a significant proportion of patients are not evaluable for several reasons, including leg oedema, obesity or lack of accessibility due to presence of wounds, wound dressings or plaster casts. Again, it seems possible to overcome some of these difficulties by an in-depth understanding of lower leg anatomy and dedicated hands-on training. This is indicated by the reported rates of non-evaluable distal veins in the four major outcome studies dealing with comprehensive leg ultrasound in symptomatic patients, which range from 0.4 to 1.4% with an average of 0.98% (95% CI: 0.68 to 1.37%). Examination of distal veins has repeatedly been discussed as being highly time consuming. Objective data, however, are scarce. In fact, Gottlieb et al. in 1997 reported an examination time of 30 min (9), and this improved in a 2004 report by Stevens et al. to 10–15 min per leg (10). If the examination technique is strictly standardized and if only compression ultrasound without Doppler modalities is used, examination times should be much shorter. As an example, Schwarz et al. in 2002 reported 4–6 min per lower leg (11). As this measure comprised DVT-positive and -negative patients, it is obvious that a negative ultrasound study of a symptomatic leg in its entire length will not require more than

5 min to be completed. A positive finding, however, may take longer in order to identify correctly and document all affected segments. Again, these figures depend on the training status of the sonographer and also on the degree of standardization of the procedure itself.

INTERNAL VALIDITY

Inter-observer variability in terms of Cohen's kappa is considered one of the main measures of internal validity of a diagnostic test. For venous ultrasound, a few studies have assessed inter-observer variability. Most of them were done in symptomatic patients. Inter-observer variability for proximal veins was found to be excellent, with Cohen's kappa ranging from 0.9 to 1.0 (12). For distal veins, figures between 0.85 and 0.95 were reported (13,14). One study calculated separate kappa values for posterior tibial and peroneal veins, yielding figures of 0.84 and 0.77, respectively. Even muscle vein thrombosis demonstrated a reasonable kappa of 0.6 (11). These figures, of course, only apply for dedicated vascular laboratories with special interest in ultrasound of distal veins. However, they demonstrate the potential of the method if properly trained personnel are available.

For venous ultrasound in asymptomatic patients, Bressollette *et al.* investigated hospitalized medical patients and found kappa values for intra- and inter-observer variability of 0.56 and 0.88, respectively (15). In another study, Elias *et al.* investigated asymptomatic patients at least 8 days after total hip replacement and found a kappa of 0.84 (95% CI:0.66 to 1.00) (16). In both studies, isolated calf vein thromboses were included. In general, these figures compare well with inter-observer variability assessments for venography (17). However, for both diagnostic tests, inter-observer variability appears to be a function of operator training and experience rather than of the method itself.

EXTERNAL VALIDITY IN SYMPTOMATIC PATIENTS

Traditionally, the most reliable quality measure of a diagnostic test is its accuracy as validated against an objective standard. Even if venography itself has never been formally validated, it serves as an external standard for validation of newer tests for DVT. Therefore, there are many studies available that report on the accuracy of venous ultrasound as assessed by venography. Patients with leg symptoms and also asymptomatic screening patients have been studied. The patient groups need to be considered separately since the results differ considerably. The most likely reason behind this disparity is that clot morphology differs between symptomatic and asymptomatic patients, affecting its detectability for ultrasound.

The first comprehensive review of accuracy data in symptomatic patients was done by the McMaster Diagnostic Imaging Practice Guidelines Initiative and published in 1998 (18). According to strict selection criteria (ultrasound and venography evaluated independently; consecutive patients; prospective; at least 50 patients), 18 diagnostic cohorts were included. The accuracy figures are displayed in Table 12.2. It should be noted that for all result categories, i.e., all DVT, proximal DVT and distal DVT, the test for heterogeneity was statistically significant. This implies that different research groups – by using different ultrasound protocols – yield differing results. For instance, sensitivities for distal veins ranged from 100% down to 11% and even for proximal DVT figures were calculated between 100% and 77%. Very consistent, however, was the difference between proximal and distal veins, which led to the recommendation that, in order to rule out reliably the diagnosis of any DVT on the day of referral, venous ultrasound capable of excluding proximal DVT had to be combined with clinical probability assessment or D-dimer testing.

Table 12.2 Accuracy of venous ultrasound as assessed against the reference standard of venography

Study	Patient population	DVT type	Sensitivity (%) (95% CI)	Specificity (%) (95% CI)	Diagnostic odds ratio
Kearon (18)	Symptomatic	All	89 (85 to 92)	94 (90 to 98)	
		Proximal	97 (96 to 98)		
		Distal	73 (54 to 93)		
Goodacre (19)	Symptomatic	All		94 (93 to 94)	
		Proximal	94 (93 to 95)		
		Distal	64 (60 to 67)		
Kearon (18)	Asymptomatic	All	47 (37 to 57)	94 (91 to 98)	
		Proximal	62 (53 to 71)		
		Distal	53 (32 to 74)		
Kassai (24)	Asymptomatic	All			39 (12 to 121)
		Proximal			645 (170 to 2450)
		Distal			35 (12 to 105)

A more recent meta-analysis used a slightly different methodology (19). Studies were eligible if they comprised more than 10 rather than 50 patients, while prospective or consecutive recruitment was not mandatory. Interpretation of venography or ultrasound was not required to be blinded against each other. By means of this, 100 diagnostic cohorts were selected for analysis. Sensitivity figures were slightly lower than calculated previously (Table 12.2); overall sensitivity was comparable. Again, the results were subject to significant heterogeneity. Due to additional data capturing and the larger number of studies, the following predictors of heterogeneity could be identified by meta-regression. Sensitivity was influenced by the following factors: interpretation by a radiologist (lower), prevalence of DVT (higher if more prevalent), the proportion of proximal DVT (higher if more prevalent) and the date of publication (higher if more recent). Specificity was higher if patients with a previous episode of DVT were excluded. An inverse impact on sensitivity and specificity resulted from the ultrasound protocol, i.e., whether only compression ultrasound was used, only colour Doppler or Duplex and Triplex ultrasound. However, heterogeneity was still present in those subgroups of studies, the nature of which could not be identified.

Since the result of the more recent meta-analysis does not contradict the previous one, it supports the widespread perception that ultrasound is the method of choice for detecting proximal DVT in symptomatic patients. However, for distal DVT it is less accurate and cannot be regarded as a standard test. Hence, if only ultrasound of proximal veins is performed, a diagnostic gap is created which has to be filled by other tests or strategies.

Patient outcome may be considered as an alternative reference standard for external validation of a diagnostic test. This is the basis for management studies in the field of diagnosis of venous thromboembolism. Strategies which combine several tests – or repeated tests – are reported in Part IV of this book. However, for ultrasound as a single test, the external validity is reported here. For complete or comprehensive venous ultrasound comprising examination of the whole leg from the groin to the ankle as a single and definitive test, four prospective management studies have been published (10,20–22). The main outcome variable was the rate of diagnostic failures, defined as symptomatic episodes of venous thromboembolism during 3 months of follow-up after the initial work-up. The range was 0.2–0.8% with upper limits of the 95% confidence intervals between 1.2 and 2.3%. This is a very consistent result across the independent studies and demonstrates that there is no safety issue due to a lack of sensitivity if the single comprehensive ultrasound test is used. There are at least three interpretations of this contradiction between accuracy studies

Table 12.3 Diagnostic findings (%) with complete compression ultrasound

Study	All DVT	Proximal/All	Distal/All	MVT/Distal
Elias (20)	32.8	54.9	45.1	nr
Schellong (21)	16.7	44	56	49.4
stevens (10)	13.7	68.8	31.2	nr
Subramanian (22)	21.5	43.4	56.6	nr
Total		**49.6**	**50.4**	**49.4**

nr = not reported

and management studies. First, application of a reasonably sensitive test to a population with low disease prevalence results in a high negative predictive value anyway. Second, the natural history of distal DVT overlooked by a single distal ultrasound is generally benign and does not lead to clinical events during the following months. A third explanation could be that venous ultrasound performed by dedicated sonographers does not have a lower sensitivity for distal than for proximal DVT. This would fit into the observation that there is significant heterogeneity regarding accuracy within groups of ultrasound protocols with comparable gross features. Better performance within protocols can mainly be attributed to standardized training and standardized examination procedures.

If the whole leg is examined, high proportions of distal DVTs are detected. The rates within the four management studies are given in Table 12.3. A large proportion of distal DVT cases will not require treatment. So far, there are no criteria for how to identify them. Therefore, the single complete ultrasound test has the potential for overtreatment, which can only be minimized by appropriately designed treatment studies for distal DVT (23).

EXTERNAL VALIDITY IN ASYMPTOMATIC PATIENTS

The first large-scale meta-analysis of ultrasound validation studies in asymptomatic patients was also made by Kearon *et al.* (18). Applying the same selection criteria as for symptomatic patients, they identified 16 studies to be included. The result demonstrated that the sensitivity of ultrasound is low in detecting asymptomatic DVT, although slightly better for proximal DVT than for distal DVT. Specificity, however, was comparable to that observed in symptomatic patients (Table 12.2).

In 2004, Kassai *et al.* published a larger meta-analysis, differentiating level 1 from level 2 studies according to design criteria (consecutive patients, blinded interpretation of test results) (24). They included 47 studies, mostly in patients who underwent orthopaedic surgery, 31 of them having been rated as level 1. The outcome criterion was the 'diagnostic odds ratio (DOR)', not having been used before by other authors for this purpose. Therefore, the result cannot easily be compared with those of previous analyses (Table 12.2). The DOR was higher for proximal than for distal DVT. In studies with more stringent methodology, it was found to be lower than in level 2 studies. However, it was still high enough to allow for the authors' conclusion that ultrasound is an accurate method in asymptomatic patients, at least for proximal DVT and in patients after major orthopaedic surgery.

The most vigorous attempt to validate ultrasound externally against venography in the setting of a drug trial was made as a sub-study (VENUS) of two dose-finding studies within the clinical development programme of the direct oral factor Xa inhibitor rivaroxaban (25). For the first time, centrally adjudicated ultrasound of proximal and distal veins was compared with centrally adjudicated venography. The results were surprisingly disappointing, with an overall sensitivity of

31% and a specificity of 93% in the patient-based comparison. The sensitivity for proximal DVT was even lower than for distal DVT. The first-line consequence of the VENUS trial is that – at present – centrally adjudicated venous ultrasonography is not able to substitute venography for confirmatory drug trials in patients early after major orthopaedic surgery. Nevertheless, several important observations may made from the VENUS study. First, asymptomatic DVT early after major orthopaedic surgery probably is the least convenient type for ultrasound to detect and clearly document, since it is transient, non-occlusive, flaccid and – in particular in the proximal venous system – very tiny with a length of less than 2 cm in most cases. Patients 5 weeks after major orthopaedic surgery or medically ill patients mostly have the regular ascending type of DVT resembling the distribution pattern of symptomatic DVT more closely (26). Second, unlike venography, there is no uniform and worldwide examination and documentation standard for venous ultrasound in asymptomatic patients. If ultrasound is expected to play a role in future confirmatory drug trials – and regulatory authorities seemingly go into this direction – this shortcoming has to be overcome. Third, central adjudication of venous ultrasound documents has a learning curve in general and in every individual reader. As it is more time consuming than venography reading, it requires comparably large reader teams in order to deal with high patient volumes of several thousands. General and individual experience will grow only over time. Fourth, the optimal adjudication process for venous ultrasound has not yet been defined. Unlike venography, ultrasound has a substantial subjective component because the alertness of the examiner drives the focus and overall quality of the ultrasound document. At some point in the adjudication process, the local reading has to be built in formally.

DOCUMENTATION OF VENOUS ULTRASOUND

Documentation of venous ultrasound has to be adjusted to the need of the particular clinical situation in which the ultrasound examination was performed. If in a symptomatic patient the diagnosis of DVT was established, at least one affected segment should be documented in order to prove the necessity for therapeutic anticoagulation (and to avoid medico-legal issues). Separate B-mode scans should display the uncompressed and the compressed state, annotation has to be unequivocal with regard to patient identification, date and venous segment. Scans for colour Doppler or PW Doppler may be added to support the diagnostic finding.

For the symptomatic patient in whom DVT was ruled out, the requirements are different. Since most patients have a work-up following a diagnostic algorithm, the algorithm applied has to be documented step by step with the respective results. Regarding sonography, the examination protocol should be specified and the qualification of the sonographer has to be documented somewhere in the laboratory records. To document a negative ultrasound scan extensively for clinical purposes seems overdone.

In the disease course of venous thromboembolic disease, it is very helpful to document the leg vein finding after 3 or 6 months or at any time the physician deems the disease to be stable and chronic. At this point in time, the affected segments should be listed and this can serve as the new baseline situation. The key segments (common femoral, proximal femoral, popliteal) should undergo measurement of residual thrombus in the anterior–posterior extension, the measurement documented by a still image. This allows for comparison in case of a suspected relapse later on. Since an increase in residual thrombus is the only validated criterion for relapse in a formerly affected segment, this kind of documentation should be implemented into clinical practice.

An entirely different situation is ultrasound documentation of DVT in the framework of clinical trials. If symptomatic DVT is the inclusion criterion for study enrolment, this DVT will have to be documented as the qualifying event. As it is a yes/no criterion, very few images will be sufficient. If thrombus burden during treatment is an endpoint, thrombus diameter will have to be measured in key segments. No standard exists on how to document mandatory case finding ultrasound examinations in thromboprophylaxis trials in which the rate of asymptomatic DVT is the main component of the endpoint. Technically, several options exist:

- *Still images versus movies:* Still images are easy to generate and do not require much space for physical or electronic storage. Movies are much more informative and avoid misinterpretation; reading is more time consuming.
- *B-mode images only versus Doppler modalities:* Doppler modalities may offer additional information compared with pure B-mode images. On the other hand, it is cumbersome to capture them and, in the case of colour Doppler, documentation will be imperfect. The gain in information is low for DVT but is much higher in venous insufficiency.
- *Main segments versus entire length:* If the entire length of the veins is captured, the ultrasound document closely resembles a venogram and allows independent reading. However, this is technically more demanding and reading is time consuming.

Documentation in clinical trials is closely related to the issue of adjudication. For confirmation of a symptomatic event, the least elaborate documentation is sufficient for adjudication. Central adjudication of asymptomatic findings, positive or negative, may follow different pathways:

- *Confirmation only:* Positives will be centrally confirmed only if locally identified; negatives will be confirmed without central reading; only a quality check of a sample of negative segments will be adjudicated in order to confirm that the entire examination was adequate.
- *Full blinded central adjudication:* This resembles venography adjudication with two independent central readers, resolving discrepancies by consensus reading. This methodology, based on movies, was used in the PREVENT trial (27).
- *Modified central adjudication:* One blinded central adjudication is compared with the local reading. Discrepancies require central re-reading. This strategy, based on still images, was chosen in the EXCLAIM trial (28). This approach is less time consuming than full blinded adjudication.

Since authorities increasingly favour ultrasound over venographic endpoints, the scientific community needs to agree upon the most reliable and convenient adjudication procedure followed by strict standardization and widespread training. However, currently insufficient data exist that would allow a decision to be made for this process.

REFERENCES

1. Cronan JJ. History of venous ultrasound. *J Ultrasound Med* 2003; **22**:1143–1146.
2. Quinlan DJ, Alikhan R, Gishen P, Sidhu PS. Variation in lower limb venous anatomy: Implications for US diagnosis of deep vein thrombosis. *Radiology* 2003; **228**:443–448.
3. Prandoni P, Cogo A, Bernardi E, Villalta S, Polistena P, Simioni P, Noventa F, Benedetti L, Girolami A. A simple ultrasound approach for detection of recurrent proximal-vein thrombosis. *Circulation* 1993; **88**:1730–1735.
4. Linkins LA, Stretton R, Probyn L, Kearon C. Interobserver agreement on ultrasound measurements of residual vein diameter, thrombus echogenicity and Doppler venous flow in patients with previous venous thrombosis. *Thromb Res* 2006; **117**:241–247.
5. Cogo A, Lensing AWA, Prandoni P, Hirsh J. Distribution of thrombosis in patients with symptomatic deep vein thrombosis. Implications for simplifying the diagnostic process with compression ultrasound. *Arch Intern Med*, 1993; **153**:2777–780.

6. Blaivas M, Lambert MJ, Harwood RA, Wood JP, Konicki J. Lower-extremity Doppler for deep venous thrombosis – can emergency physicians be accurate and fast? *Acad Emerg Med* 2000; **7**:120–126.

7. Theodoro D, Blaivas M, Duggal S, Snyder G, Lucas M. Real-time B-mode ultrasound in the ED saves time in the diagnosis of deep vein thrombosis (DVT). *Am J Emerg Med* 2004; **22**: 197–200.

8. Schellong S. Complete compression ultrasound for the diagnosis of venous thromboembolism. *Curr Opin Pulm Med*. 2004; **10**:350–355.

9. Gottlieb RH, Voci SL, Syed L. Randomized prospective study comparing routine versus selective use of sonography of the complete calf in patients with suspected deep vein thrombosis. *Am J Roentgenol* 2003; **180**:241–245.

10. Stevens SM, Elliott CG, Chan KJ, Egger MJ, Ahmed KM. Withholding anticoagulation after a negative result on duplex ultrasonography for suspected symptomatic deep venous thrombosis. *Ann Intern Med* 2004; **140**:985–991.

11. Schwarz T, Schmidt B, Schmidt B, Schellong SM. Interobserver agreement of complete compression ultrasound for clinically suspected deep vein thrombosis. *Clin Appl Thrombosis/Hemostasis* 2002; **8**:45–49.

12. Lensing AW, Prandoni P, Brandjes D, Huisman PM, Vigo M, Tomasella G, Krekt J, Wouter ten Cate J, Huisman MV, Büller HR. Detection of deep-vein thrombosis by real-time B-mode ultrasonography. *N Engl J Med* 1989; **320**:342–345.

13. Barrellier MT, Somon T, Speckel D, Fournier L, Denizet D. Duplex ultrasonography in the diagnosis of deep vein thrombosis of the leg. Agreement between two operators. *J Mal Vasc* 1992; **17**:196–201.

14. Mantoni M, Strandberg C, Neergaard K, Sloth C, Jørgensen PS, Thamsen H, Tørholm C, Paaske BP, Rasmussen SW, Christensen SW, Wille-Jørgensen P. Triplex US in the diagnosis of asymptomatic deep venous thrombosis. *Acta Radiol* 1997; **38**:327–331.

15. Bressollette L, Nonent M, Oger E, Garcia JF, Larroche P, Guias B, Scarabin PY, Mottier D. Diagnostic accuracy of compression ultrasonography for the detection of asymptomatic deep venous thrombosis in medical patients – the TADEUS project. *Thromb Haemost* 2001; **86**:529–533.

16. Elias A, Cadène A, Elias M, Puget J, Tricoire JL, Colin C, Lefebvre D, Rousseau H, Joffre F. Extended lower limb venous ultrasound for the diagnosis of proximal and distal vein thrombosis in asymptomatic patients after total hip replacement. *Eur J Vasc Endovasc Surg* 2004; **27**:438–444.

17. Kalodiki E, Nicolaides AN, Al Kutoubi A, Cunningham DA, Mandalia S. How 'gold' is the standard? Interobservers' variation on venograms. *Int Angiol* 1998; **17**:83–88.

18. Kearon C, Julian JA, Newman TE, Ginsberg JS. Noninvasive diagnosis of deep venous thrombosis: McMaster Diagnostic Imaging Practice Guidelines Initiative. *Ann Intern Med* 1998; **128**:663–677.

19. Goodacre S, Sampson F, Thomas S, van Beek E, Sutton A. Systematic review and meta-analysis of the diagnostic accuracy of ultrasonography for deep vein thrombosis. *BMC Med Imaging* 2005; **5**:6–14.

20. Elias A, Mallard L, Elias M, Alquier FG, Gauthier B, Viard A, Mahouin P, Vinel A, Boccalon H. A single complete ultrasound investigation of the venous network for the diagnostic management of patients with a clinically suspected first episode of deep venous thrombosis of the lower limb. *Thromb Haemost* 2003; **89**:221–227.

21. Schellong SM, Schwarz T, Halbritter K, Beyer J, Siegert G, Oettler W, Schmidt B, Schroeder HE. Complete compression ultrasonography of the leg veins as a single test for the diagnosis of deep vein thrombosis. *Thromb Haemost* 2003; **89**:228–234.

22. Subramaniam RM, Heath R, Chou T, Cox K, Davis G, Swarbrick M. Deep venous thrombosis: anticoagulation therapy after negative complete lower limb US findings. *Radiology* 2005; **237**:348–352.

23. Righini M, Bounameaux H. Clinical relevance of distal deep vein thrombosis. *Curr Opin Pulm Med* 2008; **14**:408–413.

24. Kassai B, Boissel JP, Cucherat M, *et al.* A systematic review of the accuracy of ultrasound in the diagnosis of deep venous thrombosis in asymptomatic patients. *Thromb Haemost* 655–666.

25. Schellong SM, Beyer J, Kakkar AK, Halbritter K, Eriksson BI, Turpie AG, Misselwitz F, Kälebo P. Ultrasound screening for asymptomatic deep vein thrombosis after major orthopaedic surgery: the VENUS study. *J Thromb Haemost* 2007; **5**:431–437.

26. Schmidt B, Michler R, Klein M, *et al.* Ultrasound screening for distal vein thrombosis is not beneficial after major orthopaedic surgery. A randomized controlled trial. *Thromb Haemost* 2003; **90**:949–954.

27. Leizorovicz A, Cohen PH, Turpie AG, Olsson CG, Vaitkus PT, Goldhaber SZ, PREVENT Medical Thromboprophylaxis Study Group. Randomized, placebo-controlled trial of dalteparin for the prevention of venous thromboembolism in acutely ill medical patients. *Circulation* 2004; **1108**:74–79.

28. Hull RD, Schellong SM, Tapson VF, Monreal M, Samama MM, Turpie AG, Wildgoose P, Yusen RD. Extended-duration thromboprophylaxis in acutely ill medical patients with recent reduced mobility: methodology for the EXCLAIM study. *J Thromb Thrombol* 2006; **22**:31–38.

CHAPTER 13

Conventional, Computed Tomographic and Magnetic Resonance Venography

John T. Murchison[1], John H. Reid[2] and Ian N. Gillespie[1]

[1]Department of Clinical Radiology,
Royal Infirmary of Edinburgh, Edinburgh, Scotland
[2]Department of Clinical Radiology,
Borders General Hospital NHS Trust, Melrose, UK

VENOGRAPHIC DIAGNOSIS OF VENOUS THROMBOSIS

Deep venous thrombosis (DVT) is the progenitor of most cases of potentially life threatening pulmonary embolism (PE) and the cause of significant chronic venous morbidity. Consequently it remains a frequent and occasionally elusive imaging challenge. The incidence of DVT in the general population is reported to be as much as 84/100,000 per year (1) and in a non-specialist setting, between one in four and one in five investigations for DVT is positive. The vast majority of haemodynamically significant emboli arise from the deep veins of the lower extremity. The diagnostic strategy of choice depends on a number of factors including local expertise, available equipment, research interests involving clinical trials and most importantly the clinical scenario. Common clinical scenarios include:

- A symptomatic limb suggestive of de novo DVT.
- Limb symptoms and history consistent with recurrent DVT.
- Asymptomatic limb but high risk patient, particularly where PE exclusion is the aim.

When the clinical presentation is primarily that of a symptomatic lower limb, Doppler ultrasound is an excellent choice on the grounds of ready availability and high accuracy (see Chapter 12). In the context of PE investigation however, when diagnosis of culprit DVT acts as an arbiter of an indeterminate lung study (most frequently in the setting of asymptomatic lower limbs),

Deep Vein Thrombosis and Pulmonary Embolism   Edited by Edwin J.R. van Beek, Harry R. Büller and Matthijs Oudkerk
© 2009 John Wiley & Sons, Ltd

ultrasound fares less well (2). In this scenario direct thrombus imaging by an essentially angiographic technique (contrast venography (CV), computerised tomography venography (CTV) or magnetic resonance venography (MRV)) may be desirable. The presence of isolated thrombus in those areas where ultrasound is technically challenged such as the calf or iliocaval segment also favours a venographic approach. In a review of the anatomic distribution of symptomatic DVT, Cowell *et al.* demonstrated that almost a third of positive cases of lower limb DVT are isolated below knee thrombi (3). CTV and MRV, may also act as an adjunct to the primary PE imaging technique.

CONVENTIONAL CONTRAST VENOGRAPHY

Contrast venography has a venerable history. Berberich and Hirsch's first report of phlebography in 1923 (4) and the introduction of iodinated contrast materials in the 1930's by Moniz and colleagues in Portugal (5), heralded a revolution in vascular imaging that paved the way for angiographic innovation which would lead to Greitz's publication on phlebography in 1957 (6) and Rabinov and Paulin's original paper in 1972 standardising the technique for CV (7). This formed the basis of a technique which has undergone some modification to improve technical success and observer agreement in subsequent decades (8,9). CV has also formed the reference standard against which newer techniques have been measured (10).

The principal advantages of phlebography include high spatial resolution particularly of the smaller calf veins, its superior definition of anatomy including variants, and its ability to be reviewed off site by someone other than the operator.

Technique

Two basic techniques are recognised. The original publication by Rabinov and Paulin described insertion of a cannula into a superficial dorsal pedal vein with the patient in a semi-upright position while supporting his/her weight on the contralateral leg. The volume of contrast used is approximately 100 ml of 300 mg/ml non-ionic medium, hand injected with a 100 ml chaser of saline to flush the deep system.

The semi-upright position (30–45°) on a tilting fluoroscopy table directs contrast into the deep veins. Once adequate filling of the calf veins has been achieved, multiple digital spot images are taken in straight and oblique projections. As contrast progresses up the limb further spot images are taken of the knee and thigh. Finally, the image intensifier is positioned over the pelvis and the patient may be asked to perform a Valsalva manoeuvre or take their weight on the affected leg to allow muscle pumping. If this fails to produce sufficient opacification the table can be brought horizontal and the leg is lifted to produce a bolus of contrast for the pelvic image. It is of interest that Rabinov and Paulin specifically stated that the use of tourniquets could be counterproductive and introduce spurious filling defects.

The second method is the 'long leg' technique. This differs from that described above by using a greater volume of contrast per leg (approximately 150 ml), an over couch tube, the use of tourniquets and long conventional films in a Bucky film tray on a horizontal table. In a paper by Lensing *et al.*, the long-leg technique produced examinations of which only 2% were considered inadequate for interpretation compared with up to 20% for the Rabinov-Paulin technique (8).

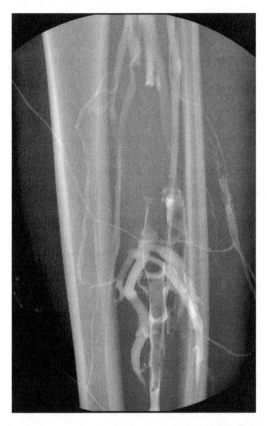

Figure 13.1 Spot film showing deep calf vein thrombi exhibiting filling defects, cut-offs, expansion of vessels and diversion of flow.

Upper limb DVT arising either as a primary phenomenon or secondarily as a result of intravascular foreign bodies such as intravenous lines requires a slightly different approach (11). A medial antecubital or more distal vein is cannulated and 30 ml of contrast injected without tourniquets. The arm is extended and slightly abducted to prevent anatomical compression of the veins at the level of the axilla.

A quartet of cardinal radiological signs signifying DVT were described by Rabinov and Paulin:

- Constant clear cut filling defects seen on more than one view. Acute thrombus often appears to expand the affected vessel.
- Abrupt cut-offs of the contrast column.
- Non-filling of the entire deep veins or part thereof.
- Diversion of flow.

It is generally accepted that the first two signs offer the greatest diagnostic confidence, although in many positive cases there is a mixture of all four (Figure 13.1). The diagnostic criteria agreed upon by the PIOPED II investigators were a complete filling defect (central filling defect which may

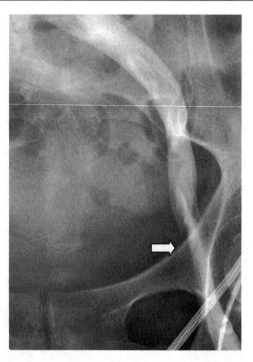

Figure 13.2   Spot film from normal contrast venogram demonstrating flow artefact commonly seen at the level of the junction of external iliac vein and femoral vein.

enlarge and completely occlude the affected deep vein) and b) a partial filling defect completely surrounded by intravenous contrast (12).

Complete non-visualisation of a deep vein can occasionally be a misleading sign and may be due to faulty technique. In common with many direct angiographic techniques a variety of interpretation errors have been reported for venography (13). Difficulties with interpretation include:

- Underfilling of the deep venous system, producing artefacts particularly in the upper thigh and pelvic veins (Figure 13.2). This can be exaggerated in the calf by weight bearing on the affected limb.
- Overlapping deep or superficial veins on a single view producing pseudo 'tramlining'.
- Contrast mixing and layering defects.
- Large varicosities with multiple incompetent perforators.
- Over projection of surgical hardware, such as used in orthopaedic surgery.

Contraindications

Contraindications to venography include previous contrast anaphylaxis, renal failure, and local foot infection. Head up tilt may have to be significantly limited in frail, elderly or hypotensive patients. Technical factors may also preclude the successful completion of the examination including poor or absent foot veins, cellulitis and gross pedal oedema. A modification of the technique, which uses the dorsal vein of the big toe as a cannulation site, may overcome some of these problems (9).

Complications

Venography has a (perhaps unfair) reputation for being a painful procedure, but it can be uncomfortable, which can lead to patient non-compliance and a failed examination.

Most complications are related to the contrast medium, including anaphylaxis, nephrotoxicity and local necrosis from extravasation, even though these complications are relatively rare. Contrast induced DVT is well recognised with figures of up to 2% being reported even with newer contrast agents (14,15). Wash out of the deep venous system after contrast injection is an attempt to minify this complication.

Accuracy

Overall technical failure rates are about 5%. Wheeler and Anderson also suggest that up to 30% of CV will fail to visualise some segment of the deep venous system (16). Kalebo *et al.* (17) indicated that the single most common reason (16%) for an incomplete examination was insufficient contrast filling of the veins, particularly in the calf. However, since other techniques (notably ultrasound) do not have the same accurate spatial and anatomic record, particularly below the knee, this is probably an overstatement. There is no doubt about venography's superior accuracy in the distal vessels and particularly in those patients with asymptomatic limbs (2,18).

Comparison of contrast venography with sonography is dependant on the clinical scenario:

1. De-novo symptomatic lower limb: It is now widely accepted that contrast venography has been supplanted by Doppler and compression ultrasonography in most modern healthcare systems recognising sonography's high accuracy in diagnosing DVT in the symptomatic lower limb. This almost certainly reflects the fact that by the time clinical symptoms of DVT appear, there is a significant volume of occlusive or near-occlusive thrombus in the deep venous system. Even early studies in the development of Doppler ultrasound methods confirmed it's near comparable accuracy to current techniques and contrast venography (Table 13.1).
   The ability of ultrasound to delineate other non-thrombotic causes of leg pain such as ruptured Baker's cyst, muscle tear and haematoma, clearly give it an advantage over venography in the symptomatic limb scenario. However, even in the best hands there is a small but measurable failure rate of ultrasonography to detect symptomatic DVT particularly in the calf veins with the attendant consequences of calf vein thrombus propagation (25). For a further detailed discussion of ultrasonography, see Chapter 12.
2. Possible recurrent DVT: A patient with previous proven DVT has a permanently elevated risk of developing a further event and up to one third of patients will re-present within a year with symptoms suggestive of recurrent thrombosis. Thrombi are less likely to resolve if the initial clot burden is large or if the patient has cancer. Previous thrombosis may damage the deep venous valves causing reflux and increased stasis leading to a higher likelihood of recurrence. Collateral venous channels may develop which can themselves be the site of future acute thrombosis. It is recognised that venous abnormalities remain detectable in approximately half of those patients who suffer a de-novo DVT one year after the event (26). Luminal obliteration, collaterals, decreased calibre and fibrotic bands are all recognised sequelae (Figure 13.3). Consequently, the ability of both venography and ultrasonography to identify fresh thrombus appears to be almost equally hampered by the presence of significant pre-existing venous disease.
   Venographic diagnosis of recurrent DVT is made considerably easier if previous examinations are available as a baseline for comparison.

Table 13.1   Studies comparing ultrasound with venography controls in patients with symptomatic lower extremities

Investigators	No. of patients	US Sensitivity (%)	US Specificity (%)
Appleman *et al.* [19]	112	89	100
Vogel *et al.* [20]	54	92	100
Dauzat *et al.* [21]	145	94	100
Foley *et al.* [22]	47	94	100
Montefusco *et al.* [23]	171	100	99
Lensing *et al.* [24]	209	100	95

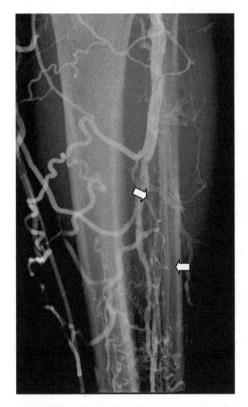

Figure 13.3   Spot film of the calf veins in a patient with chronic DVT demonstrating small calibre vessels, collaterals, luminal obliteration and fibrotic bands. Two small segments of more recent thrombus can be seen.

3. Asymptomatic limb but high risk patient (e.g., patient with an indeterminate lung study for investigation of possible PE):
    This scenario exposes the potential weakness of ultrasonographyy to detect the generally smaller residual clot burden in these cases which may often be situated in the calf and which are also frequently non-occlusive. A number of studies have highlighted this problem (Table 13.2) and led to recommendations that stress that a single negative leg ultrasound can not reliably exclude DVT in a patient with minimal leg symptoms and a possibility of PE (27). The problem has been addressed by devising investigative protocols which make use of at least two consecutive ultrasound scans if the first is negative (28).

Table 13.2 Studies comparing ultrasound with venography controls in patients with high risk but asymptomatic lower extremities

Investigators	No. of patients	Sensitivity (%)	Specificity (%)
Ginsberg *et al.* [29]	134	52	97
Davidson *et al.* [30]	385	38	92
Elliott *et al.* [31]	179	63	92
Mattos *et al.* [32]	190	67	100
Barnes *et al.* [33]	158	79	98
Agnelli *et al.* [34]	100	57	99

CT VENOGRAPHY

Direct computed tomography venography

DVT has been described using CT scanning since the late 1970's although initial reports were usually of incidental findings in patients undergoing abdominal or pelvic CT scans for other reasons (35–37). Focused imaging of peripheral veins became possible with the advent of volumetric CT. The first dedicated assessments of the lower extremity veins by CT were performed using a direct CT venography (CTV) technique, similar to conventional contrast venography as described above, followed by CT scanning of the legs and pelvis to allow visualisation of lower extremity thrombus. In a series of 52 patients direct CTV was shown to be comparable to standard venography with a sensitivity of 100% and a specificity of 96% for both femoropopliteal and calf vein thromboses (38). Opacification of the pelvic veins and IVC appeared to be better than with standard contrast venography resulting in improved diagnosis of thrombus extension into these veins (39). Another advantage of this technique was the 10 fold reduction in contrast used compared to conventional venography. The authors postulated that the dilute contrast might be expected to reduce the risk of post venography phlebitis compared with conventional venography (40). The disadvantages of direct CTV include the need of an additional contrast injection, the requirement for the additional venous puncture in a swollen lower extremity and the risk of false positive studies due to flow artefacts and layering of contrast (38,41). Inter and intra-observer variability for direct CT venography was good in the single limited study in which it was reported with kappa values ranging from 0.81 to 0.94, which was slightly better than those observed for conventional venography in the same study (range 0.71 to 0.92). Direct CTV demonstrated statically significant greater opacification than conventional venography in all regions of the thigh and pelvic veins, including the IVC and the peroneal and posterior tibial veins. It was suggested that this reduced variability in image interpretation may be due to improved venous opacification using CT (38). There was no statistical significant difference in opacification of the anterior tibial and popliteal veins when direct CTV was compared with conventional venography.

Direct computed tomography venography technique

With the patient lying supine a cannula is placed in a dorsal vein of each foot. The patient's legs are supported at the heel and upper thigh to avoid compression of the deep veins and a tourniquet placed around each ankle to limit filling of superficial veins. Using an pump injector, 40 ml of 300/mg ml non-ionic contrast medium diluted with 200 ml of saline are injected automatically via a Y adaptor into both legs simultaneously at 4 mL/sec. The automated injection protocol achieves a flow of 2 mL/sec for each leg. After a 35 second delay, a 100 cm section is imaged from the ankle to the inferior vena cava (IVC) with a volume acquisition, at 120 kV and a maximum of 250 mA. Immediately after the study, 100 ml of saline is injected into both cannulas to flush contrast material from the veins (38).

Indirect computed tomography venography

The evidence regarding direct CTV is limited. Foot vein cannulation can be time consuming and disruptive in a busy CT department and the technique was soon superseded by indirect CTV. With indirect CTV peripheral veins are imaged following blood pool venous enhancement after intra venous injection of contrast. Indirect CTV with single-slice CT was first introduced by Loud *et al.* in 1998 (42). Although there have been a couple of studies looking at indirect CTV as a primary imaging investigation for DVT, CTV is primarily advocated as an adjunct to helical CT for the detection of concurrent DVT using a single imaging technique for detection of venous thromboembolism (VTE). CT Pulmonary Angiography (CTPA) is the imaging investigation of choice for investigation of PE in most institutions. The pulmonary arteries are first evaluated to detect pulmonary embolism during the pulmonary arterial phase of the injection. The same bolus of contrast then enhances the deep lower extremity veins which are imaged with a delayed scan without injection of additional contrast for detection of DVT.

There are several rationales proposed to support adoption of this technique:

1. CTPA is recommended as the investigation of choice for most cases of suspected PE but even with multi-detector CT (MDCT) sensitivity does not reach 100% (43). Hence, diagnostic algorithms for investigation of suspected PE often advocate imaging of the leg veins in non-diagnostic or negative CTPA studies as a surrogate marker of PE (44–46) The addition of CTV to the standard CTPA examination protocol allows instant evaluation of the leg veins in these equivocal cases adding only 3 minutes to the examination time potentially obviating the need for a separate lower extremity examination that could further delay diagnosis and management (42,47). If DVT is detected then the patient is treated as if PE is present. The addition of lower limb venous imaging such as indirect CTV to CTPA imaging may improve the negative predictive value of the test (48).
2. The major risk of death with VTE is from recurrent PE, which originates from the lower limb veins in more than 90% of cases (49,50). Combined CTPA and CTV demonstrates residual clot burden in the deep veins of the lower limbs and identifies those patients most at risk of recurrent events (51). This may be another important CT finding to determine prognosis and optimize management and treatment in patients with PE. A large DVT burden in a patient who cannot receive anticoagulation may require placement of an IVC filter (52).
3. PE and DVT are part of the spectrum of the same disease process. Patients with VTE can present with either suspected PE or DVT, or both. At present this often requires two separate diagnostic tests to diagnose each condition. CTPA is now the imaging investigation of choice (53,54) for the diagnosis of PE in most cases and it has been suggested that it would be more convenient and cost-effective to provide immediate assessment of the pulmonary arteries and the deep veins of the lower limb all in one study. Because both require anticoagulation the finding of either or both confirms the diagnosis of VTE. There will be cases where the CTPA is truly negative but the patient does have leg thrombus where the addition of the CTV will result in appropriate therapy for patients who have only DVT.

Indirect CTV technique

Contrast is injected into an arm vein with imaging timed to coincide with opacification of the deep veins of the lower extremities to allow identification of thrombi within these vessels. To obtain adequate venous enhancement around 130–150 mls of IV is used. Scanning is usually started at 3–3.5 minutes after commencing the bolus injection with images obtained from iliac crest to popliteal fossa using either contiguous or non-contiguous slices.

Suggested CT venography viewing windows are: window width 250–300 HU; window level, 40–80 HU (55).

Opimizing enhancement of leg veins

- *Volume of contrast:* There is little data available concerning the optimal volume and dose of contrast to use. In an early study Garg *et al.* found no significant difference in the percentage of studies graded as good when comparing 100 versus 150 ml doses of low-osmolar contrast material (55). Most studies, however, use 135–150 ml of contrast (56,57), or standardize the amount of iodine per kilogram of body weight. For example Michel *et al.* used a standard dose of 430 mg of iodine per kilogram body weight (58). These relatively large doses of contrast are potentially nephrotoxic, particularly in critically ill patients and those with renal insufficiency (59). When this contrast dose is being used as a routine for a CTPA examination, extending the scan to include the lower limbs is not an issue. However with modern generation multidetector scanners, scan times are becoming shorter and shorter allowing the use of contrast sparing protocols for assessing the pulmonary arteries. By reducing the iodinated contrast required these protocols save cost and reduce the risk of nephrotoxic effects but also reduce the diagnostic usefulness of CTV. It is unlikely that adequate venous pool enhancement will be routinely achieved using such protocols to allow confident exclusion of DVT.
- *Osmolarity of contrast:* Isosmolar contrast material provides significant improvement in delayed opacification of the external iliac veins in comparison with conventional low-osmolar contrast media. In two studies enhancement was on average 6–7 HU (7–12.5%) greater in the isosmolar group than in the low-osmolar group (60,61) and the enhancement was rated as very good or excellent significantly more often in the isosmolar group. There was also less interobserver variability in the isosmolar group (61). Low osmolar contrast agents have an osmolarity at least twice the osmolarity of blood and it is postulated that the influx of water into the intravascular space when these agents are used prevents optimal venous opacification on delayed images accounting for the better enhancement with the isosmolar group. The diagnostic importance of this small increase in venous attenuation is uncertain and in view of its increased cost it is not clear if this modest increase justifies its routine use. Where it may have a place is in the imaging of patients with suspected VTE who have marginal renal function as isosmolar contrast has been shown to produce significantly less renal function impairment than low osmolar contrast (62).
- *Scan Timing:* The veins should ideally opacify to 80–110 HU to allow differentiation from thrombus. (47,57). Time density curves have shown that maximal venous enhancement occurs about 2 minutes after contrast injection. (47). The time density curves of venous enhancement in a group of 50 patients without clinical suspicion of DVT or PE showed mean peak enhancement values of the inferior vena cava and the iliac, femoral, popiteal, anterior tibial, posterior tibial, and peroneal veins were, respectively, 112+/−16, 103+/−17, 93+/−23, 98+/−30, 112+/−28, 137+/−28, and 124+/-29HU. These were reached at 93+/−9.5, 129+/−15, 135+/−20, 147+/−57, 124+/−32, 123+/−17, and 123+/-18 seconds (63). However, early scanning can

result in false positive findings due to flow artefact. As important as degree of enhancement is homogeneity of enhancement. In the same study homogenous opacification of lower limb veins was obtained after 210 seconds. Homogeneous opacification was found in all the iliac, femoral, and popliteal veins; in 30% of the calf veins; and in 60% of the inferior caval veins (63). At three minutes, 85% of patients were within 90% of peak enhancement. The delay in obtaining homogeneous opacification in veins is due to the low flow dynamics in capacious vessels. According to the results of Szapiro et al., (63) the optimal window for sequential CTV was between 210 and 240 seconds for the below knee veins and 180–300 seconds for the above knee veins. Because endoluminal homogeneity is present for a shorter time at the calf level, the triggering of the scan for below-knee veins investigation should be timed to optimise this. On the basis of this the authors advised a delayed caudocranial acquisition starting 210 seconds after a bolus injection to allow optimal contrast enhancement for maximal clot detection when using a single slice scanner covering all deep veins from calf to diaphragm (63). With faster scanning techniques using MDCT scanners and covering shorter areas the choice of acquisition direction is irrelevant. This timing protocol starting 210 seconds after contrast injection has also been advocated by authors who have shown that CT venography of the abdomen, pelvis and lower extremities begun 3 minutes after the start of contrast injection routinely produces high mean levels of contrast enhancement with average attenuation of the iliac, femoral, and popliteal veins is in the range of 85–110 HU (56,57,61,64).

- *Non-homogeneous opacifaction:* Flow artifact due to non-homogeneous opacification of veins can be confused with non-occlusive clot (65) and lead to false positive studies (55). Flow artifact is due to non-homogenous mixing of contrast-enhanced and unenhanced blood and is especially seen in the IVC at the level of the renal veins. Flow artifacts are more commonly seen in patients with pulmonary arterial hypertension, cardiomyopathy, peripheral arterial disease and congestive heart failure. A longer delay of 4–5 minutes post injection has been advocated for these patients with suspected slow flow or abnormal hemodynamic status (55,66).
- *Insufficient Venous Opacification:* Although mean levels of enhancement appear good, insufficient venous opacification can occur in as many as 15% of patients. This is a particular problem at the sural veins level despite optimal timing (67). Suboptimal enhancement of veins may result in false negative diagnosis (60). Lower levels of venous enhancement may occur in patients with reduced blood flow to the legs. This may be caused by severe arterial disease, extrinsic compression of abdominal or pelvic veins, or extensive bilateral DVT (68).
- *Compressive stockings:* Contrast enhancement of deep leg veins can be significantly improved by the use of compressive stockings during imaging. The use of venous stockings was shown to result in a mean increase of venous density of 30–34% compared with that of patients without stockings with average HU levels increasing from around 85 HU in the group without stocking to around 112 HU in the extremity veins of the patients with stockings (69). The use of venous stockings adds time and expense to the study and despite the reported benefits does not appear to have been widely adopted in clinical practice.

Scan Interpretation (Table 13.3)

- *Acute Deep Venous Thrombus:* The most reliable CT signs of thrombus are a complete (Figure 13.4) or partial intravascular filling defect surrounded by contrast material that presents the 'polo-mint sign' (Figure 13.5) in sections which were perpendicular to the long axis of the vessel. The presence of thrombus produces the "railway or tramtrack sign" in reconstructed

Table 13.3 DVT findings on CTV

Acute DVT findings	Chronic DVT findings
Partial filling defect with polo mint appearance	Irregular margins
Tramline appearance in longitudinal reformats	Calcifications
Homogeneous hyper-attenuating attenuation 50–70 HU	Thick walled
Additional findings:	Small vessel
- venous expansion	Multiple collateral vessels
- wall enhancement	Lower attenuation than
- peri-venous edema	acute thrombus
	May be heterogeneous
	with small areas of high
	attenuation

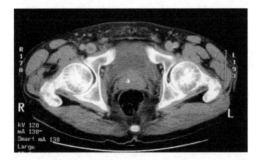

Figure 13.4 CT scan post contrast at level of groins demonstrates filling defect in the right common femoral vein indicating proximal thrombosis.

long axis coronal or sagital sections parallel to the long axis of the leg. The involved vein is frequently dilated compared with similar vessels on the contra-lateral side and is often twice the size of the accompanying artery (65), although this may be more difficult in bilateral DVT (Figure 13.6). Other indirect signs of DVT include perivenous soft-tissue infiltration suggestive of edema, most visible in the thigh and popliteal regions where fat surrounds the vein. A dense rim may be seen around the thrombosed vein with enhancement to a level equal to or greater than the adjacent muscle due to contrast staining in the vasa vasorum or contrast accumulation around the intraluminal clot. Mean attenuation of all thrombus was measured as 51 HU (57) Attenuation of thrombi however varies with time. Thrombus in clots judged clinically to be present fewer than 8 days were predominantly hyper-attenuating (compared with that of muscle) and homogeneous with an average attenuation of (66+/- 7 HU) and an attenuation greater than 60 HU in 74% of the patients (38).

- *Chronic Deep Venous Thrombus:* The age of the thrombus affects its attenuation. Clots present for more than 8 days were more inhomogeneous than the acute thrombi and contained small areas of high attenuation. Their average attenuation was lower than acute thrombi at (55+/- 11 HU) (38) The most specific features of chronic thrombus include an irregular margin and the presence of calcifications (67). Veins with chronic thrombosis tend to be smaller than normal veins but the differences are usually slight. The involved vein may look thick walled and poorly enhancing, often with multiple deep or superficial collaterals. Partial clot recanalisation may

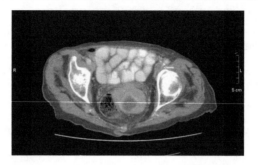

Figure 13.5 Left common iliac thrombus in patient with uterine malignancy.

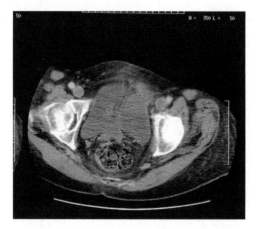

Figure 13.6 Bilateral common femoral DVT.

result in a heterogeneously enhancing lumen. Other features include eccentric thrombus with a large portion adherent to the vein wall. Chronic thrombus can result in a small retracted vein or replacement of the vein with a fibrous cord (65,70). By identifying thrombus as chronic rather than acute or recurrent is important in defining management and may prevent inappropriate thrombolytic therapy (70).

Additional findings

CTV frequently shows additional non-venous finding in the pelvis and lower limbs. This includes pathologies causing leg symptoms mimicking DVT such as Baker's cyst, intramuscular haematoma, acute compartment syndrome, ileopectineal bursitis and bone metastasis (65,67,71), Venous anatomical variants can also be identified (65). The most common lower limbs venous anatomical variant is a duplicated venous segment. The superficial femoral vein is duplicated over at least a short segment in 15–20% of patients and the popliteal vein is duplicated in up to 35% of patients (72). Variable venous pathways and congenital absence of a vein can also occur and are more readily demonstrated at CTV than on sonography or ascending venography. (67). DVT is more common in patients with venous duplication. Iliac vein compression syndrome (May-Thurner Syndrome) is associated with pelvic DVT and is better demonstrated by CTV than by US (71). Additional incidental abdominal and pelvic findings affecting patient management can also be identified, such as thrombus in an inferior cava filter (Figure 13.7). This is more likely to occur when a large field is covered. In a series of 300 patients Katz *et al.* (73), who scanned from the diaphragm to ankles during their venous phase, reported a subcapsular fluid collection, a psoas haematoma and three renal call carcinomas (Figure 13.8) as well as less significant additional findings.

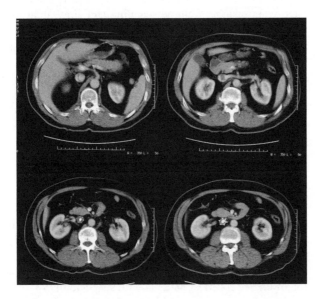

Figure 13.7   Thrombosed IVC filter with thrombus extending cranially.

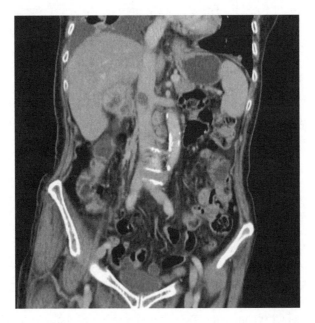

Figure 13.8   IVC thrombus due to renal carcinoma demonstrated on coronal reformatted images.

Pitfalls in interpretation of CTV

Non-venous normal and abnormal structures can mimic DVT. Examples include thrombosed native arteries. These should be readily differentiated from a venous thrombosis by the presence of calcification in the vessel wall and by knowledge of normal anatomy (65). Other potential mimics of DVT include inguinal lymph nodes with fatty or necrotic centres, muscular hematoma or abcess, popliteal cyst, normal or tumoral sciatic nerve and normal aponeurosis and tendon (67). These are more readily differentiated when using a volume scanning technique than interrupted scanning as the structure in question can then be followed on serial images. CTV can demonstrate extra-luminal anatomical structures causing extrinsic venous compression and allow the visualization of not only the lumen but also the wall of the vein.

Beam hardening artefacts result in hypodense or hyperdense streaking generated by high attenuation material such as orthopaedic material, dense contrast in the urinary bladder, arterial calcification and bone. They can mimic thrombus but are usually readily distinguished from DVT because they extend through the perivascular tissue and are straight in contrast to clot which is rounded and can be seen on consecutive images (57,67,70).

Sensitivity and specificity

CT imaging appears to have an excellent sensitivity and specificity for proximal DVT when compared with ultrasound (74). A meta-analysis (75,76) of published data demonstrated a pooled estimate of sensitivity of 95% (95% CI 91-97%; Figure 13.9) and the pooled estimate of specificity of 97% (95% CI 95 to 98%; Figure 13.10). These findings are close to that of ultrasound which is the imaging investigation of choice for most patients with suspected DVT (64). However estimates of both sensitivity and specificity were subject to significant heterogeneity. Reported sensitivity ranged from 71 to 100% in the individual studies, while specificity ranged from 93 to 100% (47, 55, 57, 64, 68, 77–9).There are various technical aspects of image acquisition which varied between studies which may account for this. These include the variety of CT scanners used, the scanning

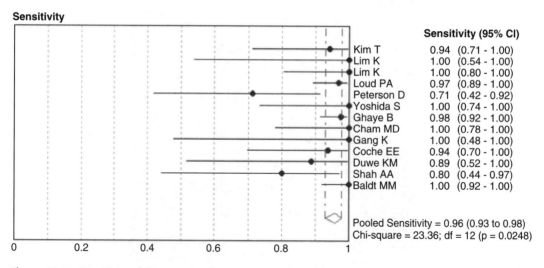

Figure 13.9 Sensitivity of CT scanning for DVT. Reproduced from Thomas *et al.*, (2008) *Clinical Radiology*; **63**: 299–304 [76].

Specificity

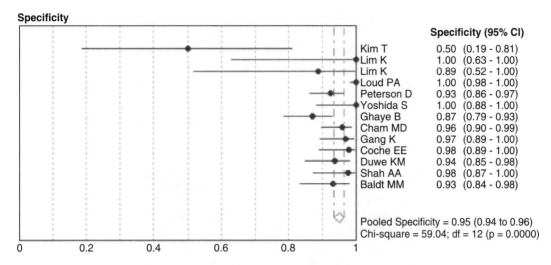

	Specificity (95% CI)
Kim T	0.50 (0.19 - 0.81)
Lim K	1.00 (0.63 - 1.00)
Lim K	0.89 (0.52 - 1.00)
Loud PA	1.00 (0.98 - 1.00)
Peterson D	0.93 (0.86 - 0.97)
Yoshida S	1.00 (0.88 - 1.00)
Ghaye B	0.87 (0.79 - 0.93)
Cham MD	0.96 (0.90 - 0.99)
Gang K	0.97 (0.89 - 1.00)
Coche EE	0.98 (0.89 - 1.00)
Duwe KM	0.94 (0.85 - 0.98)
Shah AA	0.98 (0.87 - 1.00)
Baldt MM	0.93 (0.84 - 0.98)

Pooled Specificity = 0.95 (0.94 to 0.96)
Chi-square = 59.04; df = 12 (p = 0.0000)

0   0.2   0.4   0.6   0.8   1

Figure 13.10 Specificity of CT scanning for DVT. Reproduced from Thomas *et al.*, (2008) *Clinical Radiology*; **63**: 299–304 [76].

parameters employed and anatomical areas covered (76). It might be hoped that as multi-row CT scanners become more common that diagnostic accuracy will improve across the board. There are several other factors which need to be borne in mind when assessing these figures. Firstly most of these studies of indirect CTV limited analysis to popliteal and more proximal DVT so these results can only be applied to proximal DVT and not calf DVT (39). In a series of 42 patients who underwent indirect CTV for primary investigation of leg swelling (71), 12 patients had DVT and sensitivity and specificity were both 100% compared with ultrasound. However the data looking at distal DVT is too limited to allow accurate estimate of sensitivity of indirect CTV for diagnosis of distal DVT. Secondly the reference standard for all of these indirect CTV studies was ultrasonography which has limitations itself. Sensitivity of ultrasound in detection of DVT is particularly reduced in asymptomatic DVT, pelvic DVT and below knee DVT. As ultrasound does not have perfect sensitivity and specificity this may lead to overestimation or underestimation of the diagnostic accuracy of CTV (76). Thirdly most studies are in patients with suspected PE and many of the papers reported high rates of PE detection. This suggests a selection bias as patients with PE might be expected to have a higher incidence of proximal DVT and thus inflate estimates of sensitivity. On this basis it may be safe to conclude that CT has a similar sensitivity and specificity to US in patients with suspected PE where investigation of suspected DVT is required. It is not clear whether these figures would still apply when ruling out DVT in lower-risk patients (75) and the diagnostic accuracy of CT in patients with suspected DVT alone is limited. (76).

False positive studies are more common with CTV than false negative studies (57,66) This raises the concern that some patients with a negative CTPA and isolated evidence of DVT on CTV may be falsely labelled positive and treated for thromboembolism. It has been suggested on this basis that patients with isolated DVT on a CTA-CTV imaging protocol may benefit from confirmatory ultrasound of the lower extremity. When reviewing the PIOPED II data in patients with suspected PE, Goodman and colleagues found that CTV was positive more often (60%) in patients with signs and symptoms of DVT than in those without (8%). CTV was also positive more often (26%) in patients with a history of DVT than in those without (13%). Patients without a history of DVT and asymptomatic patients have a relatively low incidence of DVT and derive less benefit from CTV than symptomatic patients (74). In the PIOPED II population only 10% of patients had signs or symptoms of DVT and 5% history of DVT.

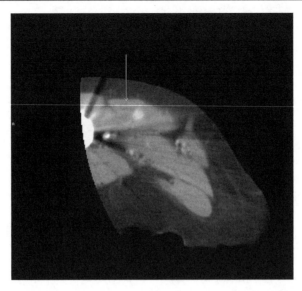

Figure 13.11   Acute common femoral vein thrombus visible as "polo-mint" filling defect (arrow) despite presence of streak artefact from hip prosthesis.

Study quality

Non-diagnostic studies

Non-diagnostic indirect CTV examinations occur in 4–16% of patients (55, 57, 67, 80,) and are even more common in the population of critically ill patients (24%). Insufficient venous opacification is identified as the cause of the indeterminate study in 66–80% of cases (55,81). This is a particular problem at the sural vein level and occurs despite apparent optimal scan timing (55). The presence of peripheral vascular disease can result in poor delivery of contrast bolus to the peripheral veins. Suboptimal enhancement of veins may result in false negative diagnosis (55). The next most common cause of a non-diagnostic study is beam hardening artifacts 12–25% (81,55) due to orthopedic hardware or dense arterial calcification (Figure 13.11). These factors partially account for the increase in non-diagnostic studies in the ICU/ITU population (82). Patient related factors including motion and image noise also produced non-diagnostic studies. (80). The mid superficial femoral vein is relatively poorly visualised in some patients. This may be due to inherent physiological compression of the superficial femoral vein in the mid to distal thigh caused by adjacent muscles (adductor or Hunter's canal) and the position of the legs on the CT table. The common femoral vein and popliteal vein which are better seen are generally surrounded by fat (60). Obese patients (BMI > 35) were twice as likely to have suboptimal studies compared with other patients. This can be accounted for by a decreased signal to noise ratio (SNR) caused by radiation scatter. Furthermore, these patients often receive less IV contrast per kilogram of body weight than non-obese patients (74).

Interobserver variation

Inter observer agreement in interpretation of indirect CTV is moderately good with published figures of kappa around 0.65 (range 0.59–0.88) in the general patient population. (66, 83,). Results were less good in an ICU/ITU population where, with 3 readers the average kappa value was lower at 0.49. This was attributed to altered cardiovascular function and frequency of orthopaedic hardware in this population (81). Inter-observer variation is more common in the interpretation of pelvic veins. The course of the pelvic veins, which in some segments is not perpendicular to the imaging plane, may result in volume averaging, which could potentially result in pseudo-filling defects and account for the increased inter-observer variation in this region (38,83). False positive studies are more likely to happen when the scan is read by a less experienced radiologist (66).

Incremental effect with CTPA

The addition of indirect CT venography to CT pulmonary angiography incrementally increases the detection rate of thrombo-embolic disease by 15–38% (57,64,83,84). The incremental effect measures the number of additional patients in whom VTE is identified by indirect CTV, who did not have PE demonstrated at CTPA. This increase in VTE diagnosis which was first reported with single slice scanners is also seen with multi-detector row CT where the addition of indirect CT venography increased the diagnosis of VTE in 17–27% of patients (85,86). However, with the advance of multi-detector row CT into the 16-slice and higher domain, the additional diagnostic value is expected to be less as PE diagnosis becomes more sensitive.

Positive indirect CTV rates

The positive rates of indirect CTV are relatively low ranging from 7–13% in most studies (57,66,77,79,80). Occasionally higher rates have been reported up to 18.8% (85). These variations are likely to be related to differences in patient populations involved with resulting differences in the pretest probability of disease (80).

Another way of looking at the incremental effect is to look at the absolute increase in number of patients diagnosed with venous thromboembolism (VTE) in the whole populations studied rather than in the increase in percentage of positive case. In most series this varies between 1–4% (676, 77). Looking at it this way only one to four patients in every hundred will have their management changed by undergoing a CTV at the same time as their CTPA. The reported incremental effect of indirect CTV after CTPA appears high but the actual absolute percentage of cases with additional positive findings are much less impressive. The results are therefore variably described as significantly improving the diagnosis of VTE (80), or too high a cost and radiation burden to make it worthwhile.

Radiation dose

The addition of CTV substantially increases the overall patient radiation dose. The main issue is the amount of pelvic irradiation. Estimates of pelvic radiation vary considerably according to the specific CT venography protocol used (87). Rademaker *et al.* using a single-slice spiral CT scanning mode, calculated a radiation dose of approximately 2.2.mSv chest and 2.5 mSv to the pelvis (88). Issue of dose is particularly pertinent to radiosensitive tissues such as ovaries and testis. The ovarian dose increased by a factor of 500 to 4.7 mSv if a CTPA study was followed by a CTV. The testicular dose increased even more by a factor of 2000 to 6.7 mSv using the same protocol (87). In PIOPED II patients were scanned continuously from the iliac crest to the tibial plateau in 7.5 mm intervals. The patient radiation exposure varied with scanner manufacturer and scanner generation but average calculated radiation dose to the chest, pelvis and thighs were 3.8, 6.0 and 3.2 mSv respectively (87). Begeman *et al.* using a 4 row scanner calculated an effective dose including pelvis of 8.26 mSv with a gonadal dose of 3.87 mSv (78). These authors concluded that due to the dose the indications have to be considered very carefully and suggested that the procedure should be limited or withheld in younger patients and women of childbearing age.

Dose reduction

- *Pelvic scanning:* Frequency of isolated pelvic DVT is low being identified in 1%–4% of all cases positive for DVT (56, 64, 89). In PIOPED II IVC or iliac clot was only detected in 3% of patients and in all these cases thrombus was also detected in the pulmonary arteries at CTPA. Since the pelvic component contributes significantly to the overall dose but does not significantly improve the detection of VTE it has been suggested that scans should cover the area from the accetabulum rather than from the iliac crest (90). The PIOPED II investigators also recommended that scanning should start at the accetabulum in female patients of reproductive age to reduce gonadal irradiation.
- *Contiguous versus non-contiguous slices:* Protocols using spaced sections rather than spiral acquisition help reduce radiation but risk missing smaller thrombi. Opinion varies about whether contiguous imaging or discrete 5 mm transverse images every 2–5 cm should be employed. Some investigators advocate the use of inter- slice gaps of 2 – 5 cm rather than contiguous sections (55,56,42,64).

Using 16 slice MDCT scanner and a continuous spiral scanning CT protocol from iliac crest to popliteal fossa, Das *et al.* recorded doses of 8.5 mSv for men and 8.8 mSv for women (91). With 10/20 protocol effective estimated dose was reduced to 5.6 mSv for men and 5.5 mSv for women. The effective radiation dose was further reduced with a 10/50 sequential protocol to 4.1 mSv for men was and 4.0 mSv for women. Using a discontinuous strategy starting at the acetabulum can reduce radiation by approximately 75–80% (89).

A negative aspect of this technique is that it may reduce the specificity of the study. It can produce interpretive errors (65,67,92). As with PE detection it is useful to identify thrombus on two or more consecutive images before making a definite diagnosis. This is particularly useful in assessing the leg veins, where contrast enhancement is relatively low and where differences in attenuation within the veins can be subtle. As the consecutive image may not be available using interrupted protocols, the diagnosis of DVT may have to be made on less certain evidence. Partial volume artefacts which mimic clot can be produced when vessels such as the iliac and popliteal veins run oblique to the transverse plane of scanning. Without adjacent CT slices to assess, diagnosis of thrombus in these circumstances can again be tentative. Smaller clots are more likely to be missed with interrupted protocols. It has been shown that 6% clots measure 2 cm or less in size, 18% clots measure 3 – 4 cm length and 76% clots are more than 4 cm in length. The 6% of clots that are smaller than 2 cm may be missed with discontinuous scanning every 2 cm and many of the 24% of clots less that 4 cm in length could be missed when a 10/50 protocol is used. Because interrupted protocol indirect CT venography can lead to false negative diagnosis and consequent mistreatment some clinicians prefer the spiral scanning mode with contiguous sections despite the increased radiation dose involved (91).

Modern MDCT scanners are equipped with dose reducing algorithms that automatically modulate the tube current according to the patient's body habitus. The use of such technology can further reduce the patient dose. However, this tends to increase the image noise which may have implications for image quality (89).

Given the high costs, the radiation burden and the low yield, researchers argued that indirect CTV should not be performed routinely in all patients evaluated for PE. Patient groups which might particularly benefit include those with a high pre-test probability of VTE including those with a history of VTE and possible malignancy (93). Patients who are clinically unstable and need an immediate diagnosis and treatment (78) and patients who are required to have a second CTPA due to a technically unsatisfactory or equivocal initial study (52).

Although concerns about radiation exposure should not preclude clinically indicated examinations, physicians should be aware of the deleterious effects, particularly in younger patients, and remember that CT imaging contributes to the bulk of medical radiation exposure (59).

Upper extremity DVT

Upper extremity DVT is a rare thrombotic disorder (1–4% of all DVT) which has the potential for considerable morbidity. Ultrasound can be limited in the assessment of these patients and it has been suggested that CT venography may have a role (94). Sabharwal *et al.* reported demonstration of sub-clavian DVT using a direct upper limb CTV technique. The method that they employed was to inject 100 ml of 50% diluted (with normal saline) non-ionic contrast material 300 mg iodine per ml injected with an automated injector at a flow rate of 2 ml/s into a cannula placed in a dorsal vein of the affected hand with the arm placed along the patient's side. The patient was scanned from the level of the neck down to the wrist, with scanning commenced following visualisation of contrast in the SVC.

CT Venography summary

Indirect CTV has been refined as an investigation but its role in imaging of DVT remains contradictory (Table 13.4). If it has a place in routine imaging it is as an adjunct to CTPA as a one-stop shop (88) where it has been shown to increase the rate of VTE diseases detection compared with CTPA alone. Whether it should replace ultrasound, be used routinely or just in selected patient groups remains to be determined. Because of its ease of scheduling, its short examination time, its ability to evaluate the iliac veins and the reassurance of the negative study it has proved popular and was recommended as routine practice by 70% of PIOPED II investigators. What is also not certain is whether the additional radiation dose, time and expense (95) it entails justifies the additional diagnostic yield the test produces. Data on the usefulness of CTV as a primary test in patients with suspected DVT is very limited and further research is required in patients with suspected DVT, but without suspected PE is required before it can be recommended as an alternative definite test for DVT in patients in whom US is not feasible (76).

Table 13.4 Advantages and disadvantages of combined CTPA and CTV imaging in patients with suspected PE

Advantages	Disadvantages
One stop shop	Radiation dose
Incremental effect	Requires iodinated contrast-risk of
Diagnostic accuracy similar to US	contrast nephropathy
Detects other pathologies	Cannot be performed at bedside
Lack of operator depenance	Inability to study venous valve function
Out of hours availability	Higher cost
Ability to assess pelvic veins	Inaccuracy of detection of below knee
	thrombus

MAGNETIC RESONANCE VENOGRAPHY

A variety of diagnostic tests have been investigated, ranging from ultrasonography to CTV, radionuclide imaging techniques and magnetic resonance venography (MRV) (96). Of these, ultra-sonography and CTV have been most readily accepted for clinical practice thus far.

A variety of magnetic resonance techniques have been developed over the last two decades to enable visualisation of the veins of leg, pelvis, upper extremity and central veins. These techniques have the advantage over conventional and CT venography that they avoid exposure to ionising radiation and use less nephrotoxic contrast media. They can therefore be used in patients in whom iodinated contrast or radiation may be contraindicated, such as patients with pre-existing renal impairment (albeit with caution), history of contrast allergy, and pregnant women. It must be noted however that there are a number of contraindications to the use of MRI especially in relation to the presence of metallic implants and there are a significant number of claustrophobic patients who cannot tolerate the examination. MRI techniques may be categorised into those which do not use contrast agents and those dependent on using well tolerated paramagnetic contrast agents.

Initial developments in magnetic resonance of the venous system utilised flowing blood to generate signal which differentiates blood vessels from surrounding stationary tissue without administration of an intravascular contrast agent. Both spin-echo (SE) and gradient-echo (GRE) pulse sequences were investigated in early reports. Erdman et al. used spin-echo imaging to assess DVT of upper and lower limbs and found that it was both reliable and demonstrated more central disease than conventional venography with a sensitivity of 90% and specificity of 100% (97). Pope et al. looked at both techniques and reported that GRE imaging was optimal for detecting DVT and commented that SE images were less suitable due to signal arising within vessels containing both flowing and non flowing blood (98). SE techniques have the advantages of decreased sensitivity to field inhomogeneity and metallic artefacts and better evaluation of surrounding tissues. However GRE images are acquired more rapidly allowing shorter examination times and are less susceptible to motion artefact which is important in pelvic vein imaging.

Time-of-flight (TOF) and phase-contrast (PC) techniques are both dependent on flowing blood to generate signal against suppressed background (99,100). Other non-contrast techniques are independent of flow and exploit the longer T2 of blood in comparison with surrounding tissues by using heavily T2-weighted fast spin echo (FSE) sequences to demonstrate venous anatomy (101–104).

Direct thrombus imaging does not depend on blood flow or intravenous contrast administration but instead uses the paramagnetic properties of methaemoglobin formed from oxidation of haemoglobin in thrombus to generate a signal. Methaemoglobin reduces T1 and results in high signal intensity in fresh clot against a suppressed dark background (105,106).

Contrast enhanced (ce) 3D MRV is an extension of widely accepted arteriography techniques which require administration of paramagnetic contrast agents into a peripheral vein or directly into pedal veins. These agents, of which chelates of Gadolinium are most commonly used, shorten the T1 relaxation time of spins in the vicinity of the paramagnetic particles in proportion to their concentration in blood. Image contrast is dependent on differences in T1 relaxation times between blood and surrounding tissues and not on velocity dependent inflow or phase shift effects. Acquisition timing can be adjusted to capture passage of contrast in veins rather than arteries and images acquired during the phase of venous filling may be subtracted from arterial phase or background images to reveal only veins. The resulting raw data can then be interrogated axially on a workstation or subjected to volumetric post processing techniques which usually present maximum intensity projection (MIP) images of venous anatomy similar to those obtained by conventional venography. Contrast enhanced 3D MRV enjoys the advantages of faster acquisition times, better SNR, and greater specificity in slow flow states and in tortuous venous anatomy when compared with non-contrast enhanced techniques (107).

MRV techniques and their relative accuracy as defined in the published literature will now be discussed in more detail in the following sections. Useful reviews of these techniques and literature are provided in articles by Butty and colleagues (110) and Vogt and colleagues (104).

A. Flow dependent techniques

1. Time- of- flight (TOF): TOF venography is based on gradient recall echo (GRE) sequences using a short repetition time (TR). TR is set well below the T1 relaxation time of stationary tissues and there is therefore insufficient time for T1 recovery and thus signal from stationary tissue is effectively saturated by the application of multiple radiofrequency (RF) pulses resulting in low signal intensity. As blood enters the imaging slice its longitudinal magnetisation is tipped into the transverse plane by an excitation pulse producing high signal intensity – "inflow enhancement". Spins in flowing blood are constantly refreshed and therefore appear bright and this enhancement phenomenon is maximised when blood receives only one RF pulse before leaving the imaging plane. At lower velocities blood protons remain within the imaging volume longer reducing signal intensity and this may lead to difficulties in demonstrating patency of low flow veins (109–111).

   Similarly when longer vessel segments lie within the image plane such as when the vessel is aligned parallel to that plane flowing spins receive multiple excitations (spin saturation within flowing blood) which may reduce signal intensity to that of surrounding stationary tissue and thus lead to loss of vessel contrast differentiation (105). Use of a short echo time (TE) reduces signal from stationary fat and a low flip angle minimises in-plane flow saturation. The flip angle is also selected according to whether the slice orientation is longitudinal to direction of flow (in-plane) or through-flow. Venous signal is maximised by acquiring slices perpendicular to the direction of flow.

   Both arteries and veins are displayed. Arterial enhancement which would otherwise also appear bright is removed by the application of a presaturation band in the upstream direction of arterial flow. This saturates protons in arteries outside the volume of acquisition and effectively eliminates arterial inflowing spins which therefore do not contribute to the bright signal in the resulting images.

   For venous imaging most published series utilise the 2D acquisition technique where thin sequential slices are acquired which affords coverage of a large area and the ability to detect small vessels with low flow. However 2D TOF does suffer the disadvantages of in-plane flow saturation (which may lead to incorrect determination of absent flow especially in tortuous vessel segments where acquisition is inevitably not always orthogonal to direction of flow) and respiratory artefact (so-called venetian-blind appearance). Turbulent flow at venous confluences may yield focal low signal which can be misinterpreted as thrombi. 3D acquisition excites a whole volume of tissue that is subsequently divided into thin contiguous sections but the prolonged imaging times are not usually achievable within a single breath-hold and it is therefore not generally applicable to venous imaging. The progressive saturation of blood as it passes through the volume also reduces in-plane spatial resolution (111). Very slow flow such as is found in small vessels may saturate the vascular signal which results in low signal intensity and limits the application of this technique below the knee (112).

   Spritzer *et al.* have reported their results using GRE magnetic resonance imaging for DVT extensively and in those cases with correlative imaging (mostly by venography) achieved sensitivity of 97% and specificity of 95% in 79 cases (113–115). Similarly, Carpenter *et al.* reported sensitivity against venography of 100% and specificity of 96% in 85 patients (100). Sensitivity of 100% and specificity of 96% was also determined when comparing duplex sonography against venography in a subset of 33 of these patients. Evans *et al.* conducted a prospective blinded study comparing MRV with contrast venography in 61 cases of suspected DVT and used additional techniques in equivocal cases (femoral vein puncture, PC, SE, cine MR imaging) (99). Sensitivity and specificity for detection of DVT in the pelvis, thigh and calf was 100% and 95%, 100% and 100%, and 87% and 97%, respectively.

In a study comparing MRV with contrast venography to diagnose proximal thrombosis after joint surgery Larcom *et al.* produced a sensitivity of only 45% when MRV examinations were reported by staff radiologists but this increased to 91% when reviewed by a dedicated MR angiographer (116). When comparing 2D TOF MRV and colour Doppler sonography against contrast venography from popliteal veins upwards Laissy *et al.* showed sensitivity and specificity of MRV to be 100% and 100%, whilst that for sonography was 87% and 83%. (117). MRV was 95% sensitive and 99% specific in determining the extent of DVT compared to sensitivity of 46% and specificity of 100% for sonography. Catalano *et al.* evaluated the role of TOF MRV in the detection of pelvic DVT and in selected cases of uncertainty also undertook cine-PC acquisitions to differentiate flow disturbance artefact signal loss on TOF from true thrombus (118), The authors reported sensitivity of 100% and specificity of 94% when compared to contrast venography and commented that MRV is particularly useful in the pelvis where other imaging modalities (venography and ultrasound) experience significant limitations. Spritzer a *et al.* identified a higher rate of isolated pelvic DVT in 20% of 769 TOF MR venograms performed on patients with suspected DVT than has been reported previously in studies using ultrasound or venography (119). Although it is possible that this could in part represent a high false positive rate, several authors feel that pelvic DVT is underreported in studies based on venography or ultrasound.

In a prospective study by Evans *et al.*, comparing MRV (GRE sequential axial imaging) with sonography, the sensitivity and specificity of MRV for detecting femoropopliteal thrombus was 100% (120). The sensitivity of sonography was 77% and specificity was 98%. No other direct comparison between MRV and sonography has been found in the literature.

Montgomery and colleagues undertook preoperative screening of patients with acetabular fractures by MRV (2D TOF) and identified asymptomatic thrombi in 34% of popliteal veins and above (121). A large proportion of these patients underwent preoperative IVC filter insertion and only 1 of 101 patients screened suffered a non fatal pulmonary embolus. A high rate of pelvic vein DVT (46%) was reported in a study utilising TOF MRV in moderate to high risk women following caesarean section performed by Rodger *et al.* (122).

2. Phase contrast: Phase contrast (PC) techniques depend on the observation that transverse magnetisation within a voxel containing flowing blood has a different phase position than that within adjacent stationary tissue. Thus, moving spins in a magnetic field gradient have different phases when compared to stationary spins and the phase difference between 2 successively acquired images represents the phase shift from moving spins only. As the measured phase difference is directly related to flow velocity in the flow encoded direction the resulting image represents a velocity map. Flow sensitivity can be adjusted so that it is set slightly higher than the fastest velocity in the target vessel. Velocity encoding values of 20 cm/sec are used for venography and determine the highest measurable velocity (123).

There are few reports in the literature applying PC MR to the investigation of DVT although some authors mentioned in the preceding section used PC techniques selectively to clarify equivocal appearances on TOF examinations. Phase contrast imaging is time consuming, susceptible to motion artefacts, and sensitive to turbulence and pulsatility and is not normally utilised for lower limb venography (104).

B. Flow independent non-enhanced MRV

Blood has a relatively long T2 value which varies according to oxygen saturation and this observation may be exploited by using heavily T2-weighted fast spin echo (FSE) sequences to produce high intravascular signal compared to other tissues. In addition to oxygen saturation the T2 of blood varies with tau180 (time between 180 degrees refocusing pulses and presence of signal is in the transverse plane). The T2 of venous blood measures 150–100 ms for FSE sequences with tau180 at 14–17 ms, which is significantly longer than other extremity tissues. In comparison with TOF where small low flow veins (eg calf) result in low signal intensity and PC which when made sensitive to low flow results in greater motion artefact FSE sequences may be used to demonstrate small peripheral veins such as those below the knee because of the lack of flow dependence and increased resolution. FSE techniques may therefore be of value in demonstrating extremity veins especially in the calf and forearm with relatively high resolution and in addition to DVT may also be helpful in evaluating conditions such as vascular malformations. However the high sensitivity to small vessels may yield complex MIPs, which may be difficult to interpret (112).

More recently described flow-independent techniques utilise true fast imaging with steady state precession (FISP) (124,125). These are gradient echo sequences with short TR and TE and a large flip angle to maintain high signal contrast between vessels and muscle due to the high T2/T1 ratio of blood. Because true FISP images are inherently T2 weighted they may demonstrate oedema in soft tissues surrounding an acutely thrombosed vein. Cantwell *et al.* demonstrated high sensitivity and specificity (100%) in the pelvis and thigh but low sensitivity (68%) below the popliteal vein (125). Superior visualisation of all pelvic veins including internal iliac veins and IVC was achieved when compared with contrast venography. Pedrosa *et al.* compared true FISP images with those obtained from 3D contrast enhanced MRV in a small group of patients and found that true FISP was much less sensitive in diagnosing DVT of central veins of the chest, abdomen, and pelvis (sensitivity 66% and specificity 70%) (126). A disadvantage of true FISP images is that they are susceptible to pulsation artefact which may be mistaken for thrombus, particularly in veins that are adjacent larger arteries.

C. Contrast – enhanced MRV

Gadolinium is a metal which exerts a strong paramagnetic effect (due to its 6 unpaired electrons) and shortens T1 relaxation times of protons in its immediate vicinity, thus producing a transient increase in signal intensity from blood vessels following intravascular injection. When protons and neutrons exist in pairs in nuclei their magnetic moments orientate in opposite directions and cancel out. Nuclei with odd numbers of protons and neutrons have a net nuclear magnetic moment which precesses at the Larmor frequency when placed in an external magnetic field. The surrounding electrons also respond to the external magnetic field and the resulting dipole moments are larger than the nuclear magnetic moments. The large magnetic dipole moments of paramagnetic molecules will interact with adjacent protons to shorten their relaxation time. Tissue T1 relaxation is inherently slow compared to T2 so the predominant effect is on T1 (111).

The shortening of T1 relaxation time is proportional to the concentration of Gadolinium in the blood and image contrast is based on differences in T1 relaxation between arterial blood, venous blood and surrounding tissues. Thrombus is demonstrated as a dark intraluminal defect within the bright signal of blood vessels. Unlike conventional TOF and PC techniques, which depend on motion of inflowing blood all vessels containing contrast are demonstrated regardless of flow characteristics. Contrast enhanced imaging eliminates motion and flow artefacts and enables in-plane imaging of blood vessels thus reducing the number of image sections required to demonstrate large vascular territories. Image acquisition times are thereby greatly reduced (107).

As free Gadolinium is toxic it is delivered in the form of tightly bound chelates with a safety profile which compares favourably with iodinated contrast. Osmolality differs between different proprietory agents but total osmolar load is very small due to the low doses administered. Gd chelates diffuse rapidly into interstitial tissues after a short intravascular phase because of their low molecular weight and are excreted by the kidneys with a plasma half-life of about 90 minutes (this is prolonged in patients with renal impairment). The rapid diffusion of Gd into extravascular tissue means that venous signal intensity decreases rapidly and timing must be set to capture k-space acquisition to coincide with the venous phase of the contrast bolus passage.

Although the safety profile of MR contrast agents compares very favourably with iodinated contrast in terms of allergic and idiosyncratic reactions (107) in recent years an association between nephrogenic systemic fibrosis and administration of gadolinium chelates to patients with severely impaired renal function has been observed. The risk appears to affect patients whose GFR is <30 ml/min./1.73m (most patients are already on renal replacement therapy) and this systemic condition for which there is no effective treatment carries a mortality of 5% (94,95). As a result of this the FDA in the USA have issued a black box warning for Gd containing contrast agents. The risk may be dose dependent (129) and cumulative (130). Other risk factors have also been implicated and include recent inflammatory events such as surgery or thrombotic events (130), high dose erythropoietin (131), and peritoneal dialysis (128).

Newer "blood-pool" contrast agents, which either bind to albumen or possess a macromolecular structure which prevents their leakage into extravascular tissues are under evaluation. These agents also possess markedly increased relaxivity compared to conventional extracellular agents and may therefore be used in much lower doses than conventional agents. The longer half-life of these agents ensures constant high intravascular concentration during the steady state phase and facilitates the acquisition of higher spatial resolution images. Prince has commented that improving both arterial and equilibrium phase images should result in a superior final pure venogram (132) Sharafuddin et al. demonstrated much improved visualisation of ilio-caval venous opacification in a clinical trial using one such agent compared to a conventional gadolinium product (133).

Ultrasmall superparamagnetic iron oxide (USPIO) substances are also under investigation as positive contrast agents in T1 weighted imaging. Aschauer et al. investigated the use of a new superparamagnetic blood-pool agent (iron oxide) and found advantages in the depiction of pelvic veins and IVC in comparison to conventional venography (134). Overall sensitivity and specificity compared to conventional venography was 93% and 96%. Larsson et al. confirmed the safety and tolerability of another iron oxide contrast agent when used in MRV, though only intermediate agreement was achieved for veins above the knee when compared with conventional venography (135). USPIO particles accumulate in thrombus and may therefore be of value in determining the age of thrombus (136).

Spoiled gradient echo sequences are obtained to achieve maximum T1 weighting and the images are collected in the plane of the vessels of interest enabling large vessel territories to be imaged in the coronal plane with short acquisition times. The volumetric data may be viewed on a work station in any plane and images are usually presented in MIP format thus simulating those obtained by conventional venography.

The Fourier nature of 3D MR data acquisition collects the entire data set prior to any reconstruction unlike the rapid acquisition of multiple 2D CT slices which are then reconstructed in 3D format. Motion artifacts can be averaged away as they are spread across the whole dataset. The SNR of vessel-to–background contrast is improved and is not flow dependent. Prospective coronal acquisitions have better in-plane spatial resolution than coronal reformations from data acquired axially.

Contrast may be injected either indirectly into a non-target vein (usually the antecubital vein) or directly into the target venous territory (e.g., pedal vein for lower limb venous examinations). With the **indirect** method contrast dose may be large as it is diluted on passage through the lungs and arterial system before reaching the veins. Imaging of the venous bed must be performed during the first pass before significant interstitial tissue redistribution of contrast occurs. Timing is therefore crucial but the use of very short TR and TE enables consecutive 3D dataset acquisitions in short timeframes. Venous phase images can be subtracted from arterial phase images to improve the contrast to noise ratio and subtraction techniques are ideal for the lower limbs as spatial misregistration artefacts caused by respiratory motion do not occur.

Subtraction techniques are now routinely used in MR arteriography and have been applied to MRV. Lebowitz *et al.* described using contrast enhanced 3D FISP sequence venography acquiring two to four identical volume acquisitions after contrast injection (137). The image set with most intense venous signal was then used as the template from which the earlier arterial dataset was subtracted to generate venous MIP images.

Fraser *et al.* described a variant of standard ce 3D MRV utilising a double subtraction algorithm (138). A single 500 mm field of view enabled inclusion of lower IVC, iliac and femoral veins. 8 successive image acquisitions were obtained each lasting 30 s. 20 mg of contrast was injected into the antecubital vein at 1 ml/s after 15 s of the first acquisition had elapsed. A double subtraction algorithm, which in most cases involved subtraction of the sum of the first two and last two measurements, yielded images retaining summated venous signal whilst removing arterial and background signal. A single AP MIP was produced and compared with results of conventional venography. This technique was called VESPA (venous enhanced subtracted peak arterial) MRV and was shown to be diagnostic in 95% of 55 cases. Sensitivity and specificity at femoral vein level was 100% and 97%, and 100% and 100% for iliac veins respectively in this group of symptomatic patients. More extensive proximal thrombus in iliac veins or cava was seen than in conventional venography and this may be of clinical relevance when insertion of a caval filter or thrombolysis is under consideration. Contrast enhancement of the vessel wall was also noted in cases of acute but not chronic thrombosis as described in previous studies (139). They concluded that this rapid technique is ideally suited to assessing proximal extent of above-knee thrombus and represents an advance over TOF imaging. It can be performed quickly using standard angiography sequences and post-processing software and does not require timing studies. The value of VESPA MRV was further demonstrated in a study by Fraser *et al.*, which confirmed persistent occlusion of left iliac vein in association with right common iliac artery/left common iliac vein compression syndrome when compared with recanalisation rates of other iliofemoral deep vein thrombosis of the legs (140).

Conversely Baarslag *et al.* produced disappointing results for MRV (both TOF and 3D CE MRV) in detecting thrombosis of upper limb veins when compared with conventional venography (141). However a high number of patients were unable to undergo MRV and other technical factors identified by the authors may have contributed to the poor results.

Time-resolved MRA has the potential benefit of clear demonstration of both arterial and venous circulation in the periphery, Du *et al.* used a time-resolved sequence that combined under sampled projection reconstruction in-plane and Cartesian slice encoding through-plane to depict both high temporal-resolution and high-spatial resolution images of the arterial and venous systems (142). An automated segmentation algorithm based on a contrast arrival time threshold can be applied to separate the contrast dynamics in the venous system from those in the arterial system and may produce high resolution images of calf veins.

Kluge *et al.* performed MR pulmonary angiography (true FISP and CE 3D FLASH (fast low angle shot combined thoracic)) with indirect MRV (also 3D FLASH) using the contrast administered for the thoracic MR sequences in an attempt to provide a "one-stop shopping" approach for diagnosis of both pulmonary embolism and deep venous thrombosis (143). The lower leg, upper leg, and pelvis were imaged using a stepping table and evaluated by viewing raw data and multi planar reconstructions rather than utilising subtraction techniques and producing MIP images. MRV detected more DVT than duplex sonography, especially in the pelvis, and the addition of MRV to thoracic MRI revealed 17% more patients with thromboembolic disease. This corresponds well with previous studies where CT venography has been added to thoracic CTA (64,77,83).

A number of techniques have been developed in recent years which employ ultra fast sequences to provide time resolved vessel information. An example is to use parallel imaging techniques such as SENSE (sensitivity encoding). It is accepted that application of SENSE will reduce acquisition time, but that this will be at the expense of SNR. Reiderer *et al.* investigated the relative SNR provided by 2D SENSE applied to 3D CE MRA (144). When an elliptical centric (EC) phase encoding order is used to map the waning magnetisation of the contrast bolus to k-space the application of SENSE provides a signal amplification over corresponding non accelerated acquisitions which improves SNR and spatial resolution and hence clinical acceptability of highly accelerated CE MRA or MRV acquisitions.

The **direct** technique involves injection of contrast into a vein proximal to the area of interest and the contrast is diluted ratio1:20 to avoid T2 shortening effects thus reducing contrast dose significantly. Repeated acquisitions may be obtained of the draining venous territory upstream of the injection site and superior contrast-to-noise ratios are achieved though the examination is limited to the veins draining the injection site(110).

Ruehm *et al.* utilised direct contrast injection into pedal veins, a peripheral vascular coil and 3D spoiled GRE sequences obtained of the upper and lower veins with and without tourniquets to demonstrate initially the deep and then superficial venous system of the legs (145,146). Although not performed in patients with suspected DVT, the results of MRV were comparable to those of conventional venography for depiction of venous anatomy. Depiction of veins on MRV not seen on contrast venography likely reflects the limitations of the conventional technique rather than false positives for MRV. They reported similar results in the upper limb venous territory and conclude that direct MRV not only reduces the dose of administered contrast significantly but also obviates the need for arterial subtraction and may be completed in under 10 minutes examination time (146).

D. Direct thrombus imaging

Magnetic resonance direct thrombus imaging (MRDTI) visualises acute thrombus directly against a suppressed background utilising a T1 weighted magnetisation-prepared 3D GRE sequence. As such it is distinct from other MR techniques which demonstrate thrombus as filling defect in high signal venous blood. When blood clots methaemoblobin is generated in the thrombus and this reduces the T1 time of clot which is seen as bright signal against a suppressed dark background (Figure 13.12). This high signal intensity is seen initially at the edges of thrombus on T1 weighted images and extends towards the centre as the clot matures (106). Macrophages invade the margins of thrombus and consume haemoglobin degradation products as thrombus becomes organised and this is seen as a loss of signal intensity in the periphery of clot on T2 weighted images. These changes in clot signal may therefore be utilised to estimate age of thrombus. An inversion recovery pulse may be used to nullify signal from unclotted blood and in addition to the signal generated by fresh thrombus further enhances contrast between clot and blood. Fat signal can be suppressed by selective radiofrequency excitation of water molecules thus reducing background signal in the T1 weighted image.

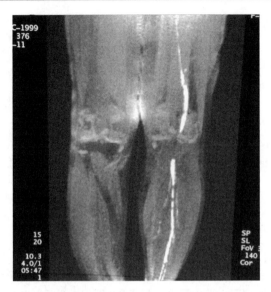

Figure 13.12 DTMRI image demonstrating extensive left lower limb DVT and normal contralateral leg. Courtesy of Dr Alan Moody, Toronto, Canada.

The 3D acquisition which enables multiplanar reconstruction provides improved SNR and resolution and this technique is not subject to the artefacts such as in-plane flow saturation which bedevil flow-dependent techniques TOF and PC. There are specific advantages to this technique as dressings and plaster casts do not interfere and nor does the effect of the pregnant uterus on surrounding pelvic veins. There may be an important contribution in research into the natural history of thromboembolic disease and in screening high-risk patients as well as monitoring response to therapy (106).

Fraser *et al.* undertook a prospective blinded study of MRDTI for the diagnosis of lower limb DVT (105). The scan time in this study was 12 minutes and no special patient preparation or contrast was required. Overall sensitivities of 96% and 94% and specificities of 90% and 92% for two readers was achieved when compared to conventional venography. Sensitivities ranged were 92% and 83% for isolated calf DVT and 100% and 100% for ileofemoral DVT, respectively. Specificities ranged from 94% and 96% in the calf to 100% and 100% for femoropopliteal and ileofemoral DVT. Interobserver variability measured by weighted kappa ranged from 0.89 to 0.98. These figures were affected by using contrast venography as the gold standard for comparison in spite of its well recognised imperfections. These include inaccuracies caused by incomplete filling of veins, overlying vessels, difficulties in differentiating acute from chronic thrombus, and dilution effects in the pelvis. The authors stated that as the errors of MRDTI and venography are independent the figures quoted above are likely to underestimate the accuracy of MRDTI. As signal generation does not depend on flow or filling of vessels with contrast, flow artefacts, low flow in small veins, and venous occlusion due to extrinsic compression and chronic thrombus do not affect this technique. One patient in this series whose MRDTI was falsely negative for popliteal thrombus had had previous femoropopliteal thrombosis six months earlier and on this occasion had a low d-dimer suggesting that the clot seen on venography was probably old.

It has been shown that high signal in fresh clot is visible within eight hours of the onset of symptoms (106). High signal lasts for up to several months. At six months 43 patients with initially positive MRDTI examinations were rescanned and none was positive although some had persistent deep venous occlusion on ultrasound. Thus it may be possible to exclude fresh thrombus in patients with recurrent DVT.

A further study looked at MRDTI using a high field system magnet (3T) and found that thrombi were clearly visible as high signal against a suppressed anatomical background in a small group of patients and healthy volunteers (147). The use of a high field strength system leads to a gain in SNR which in turn improves spatial resolution, but such magnets are mostly available in research rather than hospital practice at present.

MR Venography Summary

Most of the published literature on MRV relates to TOF and more recently CE MRV techniques. TOF has been shown to be accurate for identification of iliofemoral DVT and thrombus extending into the IVC but suffers the disadvantages of long acquisition times and susceptibility to flow and in-plane saturation artifacts. These may result in false positive examinations particularly in the pelvis in relation to venous junctions. Slices may be acquired with gaps between sections in order to maximise in-plane spatial resolution but keep imaging times to acceptable levels and 3D reconstruction cannot then be employed. Where contiguous sections are used the imaging times increase significantly and may restrict access to MRI scanners which are heavily utilised in other clinical applications. Contrast enhanced 3D MRV reduces image acquisition times substantially and examinations may be completed in a few minutes following an injection of contrast into the antecubital vein. The application of subtraction algorithms and post processing multiplanar reconstruction tehniques produce venous images analogous to those produced by conventional venography where thrombus is demonstrated as a filling defect or non-visualisation of a venous segment. Direct pedal injection of contrast may further improve signal to noise ratios and substantially reduce the contrast load but only allows examination of the veins above the injection site and requires venous cannulation of a foot vein which may not always be possible. There are only a few reports in the literature looking at direct thrombus imaging or fast imaging sequences at present.

The accompanying Table 13.5 shows results of the accuracy of MRV techniques in the literature taken from series which clearly apply a reference standard (usually contrast venography) (148,75).

Table 13.5 Summary of studies using MR venography for the diagnosis of DVT and respective sensitivity and specificity compared to contrast venography and/or ultrasonography

First Author	Year	n	Technique	Reference standard	Sensitivity	Specificity
Erdman 97	1990	36	T1 SE	Venography	90%	100%
Pope 98	1991	17	GRE, SE	Venography	100%	100%
Spritzer 115	1993	79	GRE some SE	Venography54 Ultrasound 16 CT 9	97%	95%
Evans 99	1993	61	GRE some SE,PC,cine		100% 100% 87%	95% pelvis 100%thigh 97% calf
Carpenter100	1993	101	2D TOF, SE	Venography	100%	96%
Evans 120	1996	75	GRE some SE,PC,cine	Sonography	100%	100%
Larcom 116	1996	203	2D TOF	Venography	91%	99%
Laissy 117	1996	21	2D TOF	Venography	100%	100%
Catalano 120	1997	43	2D TOF, cine PC	Venography	100%	94%
Fraser 105	2002	101	MRDTI	Venography	94%	92%
Fraser 138	2003	55	VESPA 3DCEMRV	Venography	100%	97%

Sampson *et al.* undertook a systematic review and meta-analysis of the accuracy of MRI in diagnosis of suspected DVT (148). Only 14 articles met the inclusion criteria and pooled sensitivity of 91.5% and specificity of 94.8% was estimated. There were 3 articles (not included in the table above) with markedly lower sensitivities than the rest, probably due to failure to detect distal thrombi and in the case of one article due to the inexperience of the radiologist performing the initial image review and these will have affected the pooled data. Of note, the sensitivity for proximal DVT was 93.9% compared to a sensitivity of only 62.1% for distal (below knee) DVT. This compares with sensitivity of ultrasound for proximal thrombus of 94% and for distal thrombus of 64% (149).

There are no reports of direct comparison of CTV with MRV in the literature, though early reports of CTV are encouraging when used in patients undergoing CTPA for suspected pulmonary embolus. It is not known how CT will perform as the primary investigation of suspected DVT alone. The results of a recent study by Kluge suggest comparable results may be obtained from "one-stop-shopping" addition of peripheral MRV to MR pulmonary angiography (143). CT suffers from the major disadvantages of a substantial radiation dose and the risks of iodinated contrast media and it therefore unlikely to replace ultrasound as the first investigation of choice for DVT. Conventional venography has been supplanted by ultrasound in everyday practice as it also involves significant irradiation and the use of intravascular contrast administered via pedal injection. This is not always possible and may be contraindicated in pregnant patients or those with a history of contrast allergy. It is an imperfect reference standard for assessment of other imaging modalities as patent veins are not always demonstrated and dilutional effects may impair demonstration of pelvic veins.

The results outlined above demonstrate similar performance for MRV and ultrasound in the detection of lower limb DVT and in both cases sensitivity is much greater for proximal rather than below-knee thrombus. However MRV has an advantage over ultrasound in detection of pelvic DVT and it is not operator dependent (although dedicated training is required). It may also be used in patients who cannot be examined adequately by ultrasound due to body habitus, the presence of plaster casts or surgical wounds, etc. Diagnosis of new thrombosis in a post thrombotic limb may also be possible with MRI (39). Disadvantages of MRV include costs, availability, requirement for experienced specialist interpretation, and the fact that not all patients can undergo MR examinations due to the presence of metallic implants or claustrophobia. Ultrasound has the advantage that it is cheaper and much more readily available and is therefore unlikely to lose its role as first choice imaging modality for investigation of DVT to MRI. MRV does have a role in the further assessment of patients in whom ultrasound has produced equivocal results or when isolated pelvic DVT is suspected such as in pregnant patients.

The literature base on MRV techniques is small and heterogeneous both in study populations and techniques utilised and it is a field which is constantly evolving. The present state of knowledge suggests that MRV and ultrasound share similar accuracy in detecting DVT in symptomatic patients and both perform rather poorly below the knee. Given the cost and difficulty in obtaining access to MRI scanners there is currently insufficient evidence to justify using MRI as an alternative to venography or ultrasound in routine clinical practice except where other techniques are contraindicated, or results are equivocal (148). Future developments in both software and hardware may extend the role of MRI in the investigation of venous disease in the future.

REFERENCES

1. Anderson FA Jr, Wheeler HB, Goldberg RJ *et al.* A population-based perspective of the hospital incidence and case-fatality rates of deep vein thrombosis and pulmonary embolism. The Worcester DVT study. *Arch Intern Med* 1991; **151**:933–938.

2. Burke B, Sostman HD, Carroll BA, Witty, LA. The diagnostic approach to deep venous thrombosis.. *Clin Chest Med* 1995; **16**:253–268.

3. Cowell GW, Reid JH, Simpson AJ, Murchison, JT. A profile of lower limb deep-vein thrombosis: the hidden menace of below knee DVT. *Clinical Radiology*; 2007: **62**:858–863.

4. Berberich J, Hirsch S. Die rontgenologische Darstellung der Arterien und Venen im lebenden Menschen. *Klin Wschr* 1923; **49**:2226.

5. Moniz E. Diagnostic des tumours cerebrales et epreuve de l'encephalographie arterielle, Paris 1931.

6. Greitz T. The technique of ascending phlebography of the lower extremity. *Acta Radiologica* 1954; **42**:421–441.

7. Rabinov K, Paulin S. Roentgen diagnosis of venous thrombosis in the leg. *Arch Surg* 1972; **104**:134–144.

8. Lensing AWA, Buller HR, Prandoni P, *et al*. Contrast venography the gold standard for the diagnosis of deep-vein thrombosis: improvement in observer agreement. *Thromb Haemost* 1992; **67**:8–12.

9. Sidhu PS, Alikhan R, Ammar T, Quinlan DJ. Lower limb contrast venography: a modified technique for use in thromboprophylaxis clinical trials for the accurate evaluation of deep vein thrombosis. *British Journal of Radiology* 2007; **80**:859–865.

10. Redman HC. Deep venous thrombosis: is contrast venography still the diagnostic 'gold standard'? *Radiology* 1988; **168**:277–278.

11. Baarslag HJ, van Beek EJR, Tijssen JGP, van Delden OM, Bakker AJ, Reekers JA. Deep venous thrombosis of the upper extremity. Intra- and interobserver study of digital subtraction venography. *Eur Radiol* 2003; **13**:251–255.

12. Gottschalk A, Stein PD, Goodman LR, Sostman HD. Overview of Prospective Investigation of Pulmonary Embolism II. *Seminars in Nuclear Medicine* 2002; **32**:173–182.

13. McLachlan MSF, Thomson JG, Taylor DW, Kelly ME, Sackett DL. Observer variation in the interpretation of lower limb venograms. *Am J Radiol* 1979; **132**:227.

14. Lensing AWA, Prandoni P, Buller HR, Casara D, Cogo A, ten Cate WJ. Lower extremity venography with Iohexol: results and complications. *Radiology* 1990; **177**:503–505.

15. Lea TM, Keeling FP, Piaggio RB, Treweeke PS. Contrast agent induced thrombophlebitis following leg phlebography: iopamidal versus meglumine iothalamate. *British Journal of Radiology* 1984; **57**:205–207.

16. Wheeler HB, Anderson FA Jr. Diagnostic methods for deep vein thrombosis. *Haemostasis* 1995; **25**:6–26.

17. Kalebo P, Eriksson BI, Zachrisson BE. Central assessment of bilateral phlebograms in a major multicentre thromboprophylactic trial. Reasons for inadequate results. *Acta Radiologica* 1999; **40**:29–32.

18. Rose S, Zwiebel W, Murdock L *et al*. Insensitivity of color Doppler flow imaging for detection of acute calf deep venous thrombosis in asymptomatic postoperative patients. *J Vasc Interv Radiol* 1993; **4**:111–117.

19. Appleman PT, DeJong TE, Lampmann LE Deep venous thrombosis of the leg: US findings. *Radiology* 1987; **163**:743–746.

20. Vogel P, Laing FC, Jeffrey RB, *et al*. Deep venous thrombosis of the lower extremity: US evaluation. *Radiology* 1987; **163**:747–751.

21. Dauzat MM,: Laroche JP, Charras C, *et al*. Real-time B-mode ultrasonography for better specificity in the non-invasive diagnosis of deep venous thrombosis. *J Ultrasound Med* 1986; **5**:625–631.

22. Foley WD, Middleton WD, Lawson TL, *et al*. Colour Doppler ultrasound imaging of lower-extremity venous disease. *Am J Roentgol* 1989; **152**:371–376.

23. Montefusco-von Kleist CM, Bakal C, Sprayregen S, *et al*. Comparison of duplex ultrasonography and ascending contrast venography in the diagnosis of venous thrombosis. *Angiology* 1993; **44**:169–175.

24. Lensing AW, Prandoni P, Brandjes D, *et al*: Detection of deep vein thrombosis by real-time B-mode ultrasonography. *N Engl J Med* 1989; **320**:342–345.

25. Theodorou SJ, Theodorou DJ, Kakitsubata Y. Sonography and venography of the lower extremities for diagnosing deep vein thrombosis in symptomatic patients. *Clinical Imaging* 2003; **3**:180–183.

26. Kearon C. The natural history of venous thromboembolism. *Circulation* 2003; **107**:1–22.

27. British Thoracic Society guidelines for the management of suspected acute pulmonary embolism. British Thoracic Society Standards of Care Committee Pulmonary Embolism Guideline Development Group. *Thorax* 2003; **58**:470–484.

28. Cogo A, Lensing AWA, Koopman MMW, Piovella F *et al*. Compression ultrasonography for diagnostic management of patients with clinically suspected deep vein thrombosis: prospective cohort study. *British Medical Journal* 1998; **316**:17–20.

29. Ginsberg JS, Caco CC, Brill-Edwards PA, *et al*: Venous thrombosis in patients who have undergone major hip or knee surgery: Detection with compression US and impedance plethysmography. *Radiology* 1991; **181**:651–654.

30. Davidson BL, Elliott CG, Lensing AW: Low accuracy of colour Doppler ultrasound in the detection of proximal leg vein thrombosis in asymptomatic high-risk patients. *Ann Intern Med* 1992; **117**:735–738.

31. Elliott CG, Suchyta M, Rose SC, *et al*: Duplex ultrasonography for the detection of deep-vein thrombi after total hip or knee arthroplasty. *Angiology* 1993; **44**:26–33.

32. Mattos MA, Londrey GL, Leutz DW, *et al*: Color-flow duplex scanning for the surveillance and diagnosis of acute deep venous thrombosis. *J Vasc Surg* 1992; **15**:366–375.

33. Barnes CL, Nelson CL, Nix ML, *et al*: Duplex scanning versus venography as a screening examination in total hip arthroplasty patients. *Clin Orthop* 1991; **271**:180–189.

34. Agnelli G, Volpato R, Radicchia S, *et al*: Detection of asymptomatic deep vein thrombosis by real-time B-mode untrasonography in hip surgery patients. *Thromb Haemost* 1992; **68**:257–260.

35. Steele JR, Sones PJ, Haeffner LT. The detection of inferior vena cava thrombosis with computed tomography. *Radiology* 1978; **128**:385–386.

36. Zerhouni EA, Barth KH, Siegelman SS. Demonstration of venous thrombosis by computed tomography. *AJR.* 1980; **134**:753–758.

37. Shah AA, Buchshee N, Yankelevitz DF, Henschke CI. Assessment of Deep Venous Thrombosis using routine pelvic CT. *AJR.* 1999; **173**:659–63.

38. Baldt MM, Zontsich T, Stumpflen A, Fleischmann D, Schneider B, Minar E, Mostbeck GH Deep Venous Thrombosis of the Lower Extremity: Efficacy of Spiral CT venography Compared with Conventional Venography in Diagnosis. *Radiology* 1996; **200**:423–8.

39. Orbell JH, Smith A, Burnand KG, Waltham M. Imaging of deep vein thrombosis. *British Journal of Surgery* 2008; **95**:137–46.

40. Bettman MA, Paulin S, leg phlebography: the incidence, nature and modification of undesirable side effects. *Radiology.* 1977; **122**:101–104.

41. Stehling MK, Rosen MP, Weintraub J, Kim D, Raptopoulos V. Spiral CT of the lower extremity. *AJR* 1994; **163**:451–453.

42. Loud PA, Grossman ZD, Klippenstein DL, Ray CE. Combined CT venography and pulmonary angiography: a new diagnostic technique for suspected thromboembolic disease. *AJR* 1998; **170**:951–954.

43. Winer-Muram HT, Rydberg J, Johnson MS *et al* Suspepected acute pulmonary embolism: evaluation with multi-detector row CT versus subtraction pulmonary arteriography. *Radiology* 2004; **233**:806–815.

44. Goodman LR, Lipchik RJ, Kuzo RS. Acute pulmonary embolism: the role of computed tomographic imaging. *J Thorac Imaging.* 1997; **12**:83–86.

45. Stein PD, Hull RD, Saltzman HA, Pineo G,. strategy for diagnosis of patients with suspected acute pulmonary embolism. *Chest* 1993; **103**:1553–1559.

46. Wildberger JE, Mahnken AH, Das M, Kuttner A, Lell M, Gunter RW. CT imaging in acute pulmonary embolism: diagnostic strategies. *European Radiology.* 2005; **15**:919–929.

47. Yankelevitz DF, Gamsu G, Shah A *et al.* Optimization of combined pulmonary CT angiography with lower extremity CT venography. *AJR* 2000; **174**:67–69.

48. Quiroz R, Kucher N, Zou KH, Kipfmueller F, Costello P, Goldhaber SZ, Schoepf UJ. Clinical validity of a negative computed tomography scan in patients with suspected pulmonary embolism. *JAMA.* 2005; **239**:2012–2017.

49. Moser KM. Venous thromboembolism. *Am Rev Respir Dir* 1990; **141**:235–249.

50. Ghaye B, Ghuysen A, Bruyere P-J, D'Orio V, Donderlinger RF. Can CT Pulmonary Angiography Allow Assessment of Severity and Prognosis in Patients Presenting with Pulmonary Embolism? What the Radiologist Needs to Know. (2006) *Radiographics*; **26**:24–40.

51. Dalen JE, Alpert JS. Natural history of pulmonary embolism. *Prog Cardiovasc Dis* 1975; **17**:259–270.

52. Reid JH. Multisclice CT pulmonary angiography and CT venography. *British Journal of Radiology.* 2004; **77**:S39–S45.

53. Remy-Jardin M, Remy J. Spiral CT angiography of the pulmonary circulation. *Radiology* 1999; **212**:615–636.

54. Stein PD, Hull RD, Multidetector computed tomography for the diagnosis of acute pulmonary embolism. *Current Opinions in Pulmonary Medicine.* 2007; **13**:384–388.

55. Garg K, Kemp JL, Wojcik D *et al* Thromboembolic disease: comparison of combined CT pulmonary angiography and venography with bilateral leg sonography in 70 patients. *AJR* 2000; **175**:997–1001.

56. Bruce D, Loud PA, Klippenstein DL, Grossman ZD, Katz DS. Combined CT venography and pulmonary angiography: how much venous enhancement is routinely obtained? *AJR* 2001; **176**:1281–1285.

57. Cham MD, Yankelevitz DF and Shaham D, *et al*, Deep venous thrombosis detection by using indirect CT venography, The Pulmonary Angiography-Indirect CT Venography Cooperative Group. *Radiology* **216** (2000) 744–751.

58. Michel SJ, Friel AM, Sinha S, Wilson J, Bensadoun E, Arnold S, Buck JL. Comparison of Iodixanol with Iohexol for delayed pelvic venous opacification: A preliminary study of potential use for CT venography. *AJR.* 2004; **183**:123–126.

59. Kanne JP, Lalani T. Role of computed tomography and magnetic resonance imaging for deep venous thrombosis and pulmonary embolism. *Circulation*. 2004; **109** supplement: I–15- I-21.

60. Garg K, Kemp JL, Russ PD, Baron AE. Thromboembolic disease variability of interobserver agreement in the interpretation of CT angiography. *AJR*, **176** (2001) 1043–1047.

61. Goodman LR, Gulsum M, Nagy P, Washington L. CT of the deep venous thrombosis and pulmonary embolus: Does iso-osmolar contrast agent improve vascular opacification? *Radiology.* 2005; **234**:923–928.

62. Asplin P, Aubry P, Fransson SG, Strasser R, Willenbrock R, Berg KJ. Nephrotoxic effects in high risk patients undergoing angiography. *N Engl J Med*. 2003; **348**:491–499.

63. Szapiro D, Ghaye B, Willems V, Zhang L, Albert A, Dondelinger RF. Evaluation of CT time-density curves of lower-limb veins. *Investigative Radiology* 2001; **36**:164–169.

64. Loud PA, Katz DS, Bruce DA, Klippenstein DL, Grossman ZD. Deep Venous thrombosis with suspected pulmonary embolism: detection with combined CT venography and pulmonary angiography. *Radiology* 2001; **219**:498–502.

65. Ciccotosto C, Goodman LR, Washington L, Quiroz F. Indirect CT venography following CT pulmonary angiography: spectrum of CT findings. *J Thorac Imaging* 2002; **17**:18–27.

66. Richman PB, Dominguez S, Kasper D, Chen F, *et al*. Interobserver agreement for the diagnosis of venous thromboembolism on computed tomography chest angiography and indirect venography of the lower extremities in emergency department patients. *Academic Emergency Medicine* 2006; **13**:295–301.

67. Ghaye B, Szapiro D, Willems V and Donderlinger RF. Pitfalls in CT Venography of Lower Limbs and Abdominal Veins. 2002 *American Journal of Radiology:* **178**:1465–1471.

68. Duwe KM, Shiau M, Budorick NE, *et al*. Evaluation of the lower extremity veins in patients with suspected pulmonary embolism: a retrospective comparison of helical CT venography and sonography. *AJR* 2000; **175**:1525–1531.

69. Abdelmoumene Y, Chevallier P, Barghouth G, Portier F, Qanadli SD, Doenz F, Schnyder P, Denys A. Optimisation of multidetector CT venography performed with elastic stockings on patients' lower extremities: a preliminary study of non-thrombosed veins. *AJR.* 2003; **180**:1093–1094.

70. Park, E-A, Lee W, Min W, Choi S-I, Jae HJ, Chung JW, Park JH. Chronic-stage deep venous thrombosis of the lower extremities: Indirect CT venographic findings. *Journal of Computer Assisted Tomography*. 2007; **31**:649–656.

71. Yoshida S, Akiba H, Tamakawa M, Yama N, Takeda M, Hareyama M. Spiral CT venography of the lower extremities by injection via an arm vein in patients with leg swelling. *British Journal of Radiology* 2001; **74**:1013–1016.

72. Chung JK, Yoon CJ, Jung SI, Kim H-C, Lee W, Young I, Jae HJ, Park JH. Acute Ileofemoral Deep Vein Thrombosis: Evaluation of underlying Anatomical Abnormalities by Spiral CT Venography. *Journal of Vascular and Interventional Radiology.* 2004; **15**:249–256.

73. Katz DS, Loud PA, Klippenstein DL, Shah RA, Grossman ZD. Extra-thoracic findings on the venous phase of combined CT venography and pulmonary angiography. *Clin Radiol* 2000; **55**:177–181.

74. Goodman LR, Stein PD, Matta F, Sostman HD, Wakefield TW, Woodard PK, Hull R, Yankelevitz DF, Beemath A. CT Venography and compression sonography are diagnostically equivalent: Data from PIOPED II *AJR.* 2007; **189**:1071–1076.

75. Goodacre S, Sampson F, Stevenson M, Wailoo A, Sutton A, Thomas S. *et al*. Measurement of the clinical and cost-effectiveness of non-invasive diagnostic testing strategies for deep vein thrombosis. *Health Technology Assessment* 2006; **10**:1–168.

76. Thomas SM, Goodachre SW, Sampson FC, van Beek EJR. Diagnostic value of CT for deep vein thrombosis: results of a systemic review and meta-analysis. *Clinical Radiology* 2008; **63**:299–304.

77. Cham MD, Yankelevitz DF, Henschke CI. Thromboembolic Disease Detection at Indirect CT Venography versus CT Pulmonary Angiography (2005) *Radiology*; **234**:591–594.

78. Begemann PG, Bonacker M. Kemper J, Guthoff AE, Hahn KE, Steiner P, Adam G. Evaluation of the deep venous system in patients with suspected pulmonary embolism with MDCT: a prospective study in comparison to doppler sonography. *J Comput Assist Tomogr.* 2003; **27**:399–409.

79. Stein PD, Fowler SE, Goodman LR *et al* Multidetector computed tomography for acute pulmonary embolism. *N Engl J Med.* 2006; **354**:2317–27.

80. Rhee KH, Iyer RS, Cha S, Naidich DP, Rusinek H, Jacobowitz GR, Ko JP. Benefits of CT venography for the diagnosis of thromboembolic disease. *Clinical Imaging* 2007; **31**:253–258.

81. Kelly AM, Patel S, Carlos RC, Cronin P, Kazerooni EA. Multidetector Row CT Pulmonary Angiography and Indirect Venography for the diagnosis of Venous Thromboembolic Disease in Intensive Care Unit Patients. *Academic Radiology* 2006; **13**:486–495.

82. Taffoni MJ, Ravenel JG, Ackerman SJ. Prospective comparison of indirect CT venography versus sonography in ICU patients. *AJR*. 2005; **185**:457–462.

83. Coche EE, Hamoir XL, Hammer FD, Hainaut P, Goffette PP. Using dual-detector helical CT angiography to detect deep venous thrombosis in patients with suspicion of pulmonary embolism diagnostic value and additional findings *AJR* **176** (2001) 1035–1039.

84. Cham MD, Yankelevitz DF and Henschke CI, Thromboembolic disease detection at indirect CT venography versus CT pulmonary angiography, *Radiology* **234** (2005) 591–594.

85. Ghaye B, Nchimi A, Noukoua CT, Dondelinger RF. Does Multi-detector row CT pulmonary angiography reduce the incremental value of indirect CT venography compared with single-detector row CT pulmonary angiography? *Radiology* 2006; **240**:256–262.

86. Nchimi A, Ghaye B, Noukoua CT, Dondelinger RF, Incidence and distribution of lower extremity deep venous thrombosi at indirect computed tomography venography in patients suspected of pulmonary embolism. *Thrombosis and Haemostasis*. 2007; **97**:566–572.

87. Rademaker J, Griesshaber V, Hidajat N, Oestmann JW, Felix R. Combined CT pulmonary angiography and venography for the diagnosis of pulmonary embolism and deep vein thrombosis: radiation dose. *Journal of Thoracic Imaging*. 2001; **16**:297–299.

88. Remy-Jardin M, Pistolesi M, Goodman LR *et al* Management of suspected acute pulmonary embolism in the era of CT angiography: A statement from the Fleischner Society. 2007; **245**:315–329.

89. Goodman LR, Venousthromboembolic disease: CT evaluation. *Q J Nuc Med* 2001; **45**:302–310.

90. Kalva SP, Jagannathan JP, Hahn PF, Wicky ST. Venous Thromboembolism: Indirect CT Venography during CT Pulmonary Angiography- Should the pelvis be imaged? *Radiology* 2008; **246**:605–611.

91. Das M, Muhlenbruch G, Mahnken AH, Weis C, Schoepf UJ, Leidecker C, Gunther RW, Wildberger JE, Optimized image reconstruction for detection of deep venous thrombosis at multidetector-row CT venography. *European Radiology*. 2006. **16**:269–275.

92. Ghaye B, Dondelinger RF. Non-traumatic thoracic emergencies: CT venography in the integrated diagnostic strategy for pulmonary embolism and venous thrombosis. *Eur Radiology* 2002; **12**:1906–1921.

93. Hunsaker AR, Zou, KH, Angeline CP, Trotman-Dickenson B, Jacobson FL, Gill RR, Goldhaber SZ. Routine Pelvic and Lower Extremity CT Venography in Patients Undergoing Pulmonary CT Angiography. *AJR* 2008; **190**:322–326.

94. Sabharwal R, Boshell D, Vladica P Multidetector spiral CT venography in the diagnosis of upper extremity deep venous thrombosis. *Australasian radiology* 2007; **51** Suppl: B253–6.

95. Peterson DA, Kazerooni EA, Wakefield TW, Knipp BS, Forauer AR, Bailey BJ, Sullivan VV, Proctor MC, Henke PK, Greenfield LJ, Stanley JC, Upchurch GR. Computed tomographic venography is specific but not sensitive for diagnosis of acute lower-extremity deep venous thrombosis in patients with suspected pulmonary embolus. *Journal of Vascular Surgery*. 2001; **34**:798–803.

96. Wells PS, Forgie MA. Diagnosis of deep vein thrombosis. *Biomed Pharmacother* 1996; **50**:235–42.

97. Erdman WA, Jayson HT, Redman HC, Miller GL, Parkey RW, Peshock RW. Deep venous thrombosis of extremities: role of MR imaging in the diagnosis. *Radiology* 1990; **174**:425–31.

98. Pope CF, Dietz MJ, Ezekowitz MD, Gore JC. Technical variables influencing the detection of acute deep vein thrombosis by magnetic resonance imaging. *Magn Reson Imaging* 1991; **9**:379–88.

99. Evans AJ, Sostman HD, Knelson MH, Spritzer CE, Newman GE, Paine SS *et al*. 1992 ARRS Executive Council Award. Detection of deep venous thrombosis: prospective comparison of MR imaging with contrast venography. *AJR* 1993; **161**:131–9.

100. Carpenter JP, Holland GA, Baum RA, Owen RS, Carpenter JT, Cope C. Magnetic resonance venography for the detection of deep venous thrombosis: comparison with contrast venography and duplex doppler ultrasonography. *J Vasc Surg* 1993; **18**:734–41.

101. Wright GA, Nishimura DG, Macovski A. Flow-independent magnetic resonance projection angiography. *Magn Reson Med*. 1991; **17**:126–40.

102. Brittain JH, Olcott EW, Szuba A *et al*. Three-dimensional flow-independent peripheral angiography. *Magn Reson Med*. 1997; **38**:343–54.

103. Gronas R, Kalman PG, Kucey DS *et al*. Flow-independent angiography for peripheral vascular disease: initial in-vivo results. *J Magn Reson Imaging*. 1997; **7**:637–43.

104. Vogt FM, Herbon CU, Goyen M. MR venography. *Mag Res Imaging Clinic of N Amer*. 2005; **13**:113–29.

105. Fraser DG, Moody AR, Morgan PS, Martel AL, Davidson I. Diagnosis of lower limb deep venous thrombosis: a prospective blinded study of magnetic resonance direct thrombus imaging. *Ann Intern Med.* 2002; **136**:89–98.
106. Moody AR, Pollock JG, O'Connor AR, Bagnall M. Lower limb deep venous thrombosis: direct MR imaging of the thrombus. *Radiology.* 1998; **209**:349–55.
107. Prince MR, Grist TM, Debatin JF. *3D Contrast MR Angiography*. 1999 Springer *
108. Bradley WG, Waluch V. Blood flow: magnetic resonance imaging. *Radiology.* 1985; **154**:443–450.
109. Dumoulin CL, Hart HR. Magnetic resonance angiography. *Radiology.* 1986; **161**:717–20.
110. Butty S, Hagspiel KD, Leung DA, Angle JF, Spinosa DJ, Matsumoto AH. Body MR venography. *Radiol Clin N Amer.* 2002; **40**:899–919.
111. Nitz W. In *Clinical MR imaging: a practical approach*. Eds Riemer P, Parizel PM, Stichnoth FA. Chapter1 pages 1–35. Principles of magnetic resonance imaging and magnetic resonance angiography Springer. 1999.*
112. Bluemke DA, Wolf RL, Tani I, Tachiki S, McVeigh ER, Zerhouni EA. Extremity veins: evaluation with fast-spin echo MR venography. *Radiology* 1997; **204**:562–65.
113. Spritzer CE, Sussman SK, Blinder RA, Saeed M, Herfkens RJ. Deep venous thrombosis evaluation with limited flip-angle, gradient refocused MR imaging: preliminary experience. *Radiology.* 1988; **166**:371–75.
114. Spritzer CE, Sostman HD, Wilkes DC, Coleman RE. Deep venous thrombosis: experience with gradient-echo MR imaging in 66 patients. *Radiology* 1990; **177**:235–241.
115. Spritzer CE, Norconk JJ, Sostman HD, Coleman RE. Detection of deep venous thrombosis by magnetic resonance imaging. *Chest* 1993; **104**:54–60.
116. Larcom PG, Lotke PA, Steinberg ME, Holland G, Foster S. Magnetic resonance venography versus contrast venography to diagnose thrombosis after joint surgery. *Clin Orthop* 1996; **331**:209–215.
117. Laissy J-P, Cinqualbre A, Loshkajian A, Henry-Feugeas M-C, Crestani B, Riquelme C, Schouman-Claeys E. Assessment of deep venous thrombosis in the lower limbs and pelvis: MR venography versus duplex Doppler sonography. *AJR* 1996; **167**:971–975.
118. Catalano C, Pavone P, Laghi A, Scipioni A, Fanelli F, Assael FG *et al.* Role of MR venography in the evaluation of deep vein thrombosis. *Acta Radiologica* 1997; **38**:907–912.
119. Spritzer CE, Arata MA, Freed KS. Isolated pelvic deep venous thrombosis: relative frequency as detected with MR imaging. *Radiology* 2001; **219**:521–525.
120. Evans AJ, Sostman HD, Witty LA, Paulson EK, Spritzer CE, Hertzberg BS, *et al.* Detection of deep venous thrombosis: prospective comparison of MR imaging and sonography. *J Magn Reson Imaging* 1996; **6**:44–51.
121. Montgomery KD, Potter HG, Helfet DL. The detection and management of proximal deep venous thrombosis in patients with acute acetabular fractures: a follow-up report. *J of Orthop* 1997; **11**:330–33.
122. Rodger MA, Avruch LI, Howley HE, Olivier A, Walker MC. Pelvic magnetic resonance venography reveals high rate of pelvic vein thrombosis after caesarean section. *American Journal of Obstetrics and Gynecology* 2006; **194**:436–7.
123. Constantinesco A, Mallett JJ, Bonmartin A. Spatial or flow velocity phase encoding gradients in NMR imaging. *Magn Reson Imaging.* 1984; **2**:335–340.
124. Spuentrup E, Buecker A, Stuber M *et al.* MR venography using high resolution True-FISP. *Rofo* 2001; **173**:686–690.
125. Cantwell CP, Cradock A, Bruzzi J, Fitzpatrick P, Eustace S, Murray J. MR venography with true fast imaging with steady-state precession for suspected lower limb deep vein thrombosis. *Journal of Vascular and Interventional Radiology* 2006; **17**:1763–69.
126. Pedrosa I, Morrin M, Oleaga L, Baptista J, Rofsky NM. Is true FISP imaging reliable in the evaluation of venous thrombosis? *AJR* 2004; **185**:1632–40.
127. Michaely HJ, Thomsen HS, Reiser MF, Schoenberg SO. Nephrogenic systemic fibrosis – implications for radiology. *Radiologe* 2007; **47**(9):785–93.
128. Saab G, Cheng S. Nephrogenic systemic fibrosis: a nephrologist's perspective. *Haemodialysis International* 2007; **11**:S2–S6.
129. Broome DR, Girguis MS, Baron PW, Cottrell AC, Kjellin I, Kirk GA. Gadodiamide-associated nephrogenic systemic fibrosis: why radiologists should be concerned. *AJR* 2007; **188**:586–92.
130. Sadowski EA, Bennett LK, Chan MR *et al.* Nephrogenic systemic fibrosis: risk factors and incidence estimation. *Radiology* 2007; **243**:148–57.
131. Swaminathan S, Ahmed I, McCarthy JT *et al.* Nephrogenic fibrosisng dermopathy and high dose erythropoietin therapy. *Ann Intern Med* 2006; **145**:234–5.
132. Prince MR, Sostman HD. MR venography: unsung and underutilised. *Radiology* 2003; **226**:630–32.

133. Sharafuddin MJ, Stolpen AH, Dang YM, Andresen KJ, Roh B-S. Comparison of MS 325 and gado-diamide MR venography of iliocaval veins. *Journal of Vascular and Interventional Radiology* 2002; **13**:1021–27.

134. Aschauer M, Deutschmann HA, Stollberger R, Hausegger KA, Obernosterer A, Schollnast H, Ebner F. Value of a blood pool contrast agent in MR venography of the lower extremities and pelvis: preliminary results in 12 patients. *Magn Reson in Med* 2003; **50**:993–1002.

135. Larsson E-M, Sunden P, Olsson C-G, Debatin J, Duerinckx AJ, Baum R, Hahn D, Ebner F. MR venography using an intravascular contrast agent: results from a multicenter phase 2 study of dosage. *AJR* 2003; **180**:227–232.

136. Schmitz SA, Winterhalter S, Schiffler S *et al*. USPIO- enhanced direct thrombus MRI. *Acad Radiol.* 2002; **9**:S339–40.

137. Lebowitz JA, Rofsky NM, Krisky GA, Weinreb JC. Gadolinium-enhanced body MR venography with subtraction technique. *AJR* 1997; **169**:755–58.

138. Fraser DGW, Moody AR, Davidson IR, Martel AL, Morgan PS. Deep venous thrombosis: diagnosis by using venous enhanced subtracted peak arterial MR venography versus conventional venography. *Radiology* 2003; **226**:812–20.

139. Froehlich JB, Prince MR, Greenfield LJ, Downing LJ, Shah NL, Wakefield TW. " Bulls-eye" sign on gadolinium enhanced venography determines thrombus presence and age: a preliminary study. *J Vasc Surg* 1997; **26**:809–16.

140. Fraser DGW, Moody AR, Morgan PS, Martel A. Iliac compression syndrome and recanalisation of femoropopliteal and iliac venous thrombosis: a prospective study with magnetic resonance venography. *J Vasc Surg* 2004; **40**:612–19.

141. Baarslag HJ, Van Beek EJR, Reekers JA. Magnetic resonance venography in consecutive patients with suspected deep vein thrombosis of the upper extremity: initial experience. *Acta Radiologica* 2004; **45**:38–43.

142. Du J, Thornton FJ, Mistretta CA, Grist TM. Dynamic MR venography: an intrinsic benefit of time-resolved MR angiography. *J Magn Reson Imaging* 2006; **24**:922–27

143. Kluge A, Mueller C, Strunk J, Lange U, Bacmann G. Experience in 207 combined MRI examinations for acute pulmonary embolism and deep vein thrombosis. *AJR* 2006; **186**:1686–96.

144. Riederer SJ, Hu HH, Kruger DG, Haider CR, Campeau NG, Huston III J. Intrinsic signal amplification in the application of 2D SENSE parallel imaging to 3D contrast-enhanced elliptical centric MRA and MRV. *Magn Reson Med.* 2007; **58**:855–64.

145. Ruehm SG, Weisner W, Debatin J. Pelvic and lower extremity veins: contrast-enhanced three-dimensional MR venography with a dedicated vascular coil – initial experience. *Radiology* 200; **215**:421–427.

146. Ruehm SG, Zimny K, Debatin J. Direct contrast-enhanced 3D MR venography. *Eur Radiol* 2001; **11**:102–12.

147. Schmitz SA, O'Regan DP, Gibson D, Cunningham C, Allsop J, Larkman DJ, Hajnal JV. Magnetic resonance direct thrombus imaging at 3T field strength in patients with lower limb deep vein thrombosis: a feasibility study. *Cin Rad* 2006; **61**:282–86.

148. Sampson FC, Goodacre SW, Thomas SM, van BEEK EJR. The accuracy of MRI in diagnosis of suspected deep vein thrombosis: systematic review and meta-analysis. *Eur Radiol* 2007; **17**:175–81.

149. Goodacre S, Sampson F, Thomas S, van Beek EJ, Sutton AJ. Systematic review and meta-analysis of the diagnostic accuracy of ultrasonography for deep vein thrombosis. *BMC Med Imaging* 2005 vol **5**:6. pages 1–13

PART IV

Diagnostic Management Strategies

Diagnostic Management Strategies in Patients with Suspected Deep Vein Thrombosis

Philip S. Wells

Division of Hematology, Canada Research Chair,
University of Ottawa, Department of Medicine and the
Ottawa Health Research Institute, Ontario, Canada

INTRODUCTION

Venous thromboembolism (VTE), manifesting as deep vein thrombosis (DVT) or pulmonary embolism (PE), is one of the most common cardiovascular disorders in industrialized countries, affecting about 5% of people in their lifetime (1). PE is highly fatal and in 22% of cases is not diagnosed before causing death (2,3). The signs and symptoms of both DVT and PE are largely non-specific and, as a consequence, many patients presenting with leg pain or swelling or chest pain or dyspnea are investigated but ultimately do not have DVT or PE. Mismanagement of PE has been a frequent problem (4), at least in part due to the limitations of diagnostic tests. Although imaging tests still have some limitations, these can be better managed since the diagnostic work-up for suspected PE has now evolved to an integrated approach that includes clinical pre-test probability assessment and D-dimer testing in combination with imaging.

Detailed evaluation of the clinical presentation of DVT is described in Chapter 3 (DVT), while individual diagnostic tests for DVT are described in Chapters 5 (Clinical Prediction Rules), 6 (Plasma D-dimer), 12 (Ultrasonography of DVT) and 13 (Venography). In this chapter, the literature on imaging tests, clinical probability assessment and D-dimer assays for the diagnostic management of DVT will be briefly summarized with a focus on integration of these diagnostic modalities. Integrated strategies permit the application of Bayes' theorem, i.e., pre-test odds times the likelihood ratio (especially pertinent is the negative likelihood ratio of 1 minus sensitivity divided by specificity) = post-test odds (5,6).

Deep Vein Thrombosis and Pulmonary Embolism   Edited by Edwin J.R. van Beek, Harry R. Büller and Matthijs Oudkerk
© 2009 John Wiley & Sons, Ltd

DIAGNOSIS OF DVT

Imaging tests for DVT

The test of choice for clinically suspected DVT is venous compression ultrasonography, which is highly specific; a positive result is sufficiently predictive in most patients so that treatment can be initiated (7–10). The exceptions to this approach are patients with a previous history of DVT and low pre-test probability in which the positive predictive value carries less diagnostic value (11).

In many centres, ultrasonographic testing is limited to the proximal veins (from the level of the femoral veins to the level of the trifurcation of the calf veins into the popliteal vein just below the knee), since the sensitivity for proximal DVT has been reported as 97%, whereas it is considerably less (in the 70–75%) for calf DVT (12). In these centres, it has been suggested that a negative ultrasound test (where compression of the veins is normal) should be repeated 1 week later (serial testing) to detect extending calf DVT (8). However, in symptomatic patients only 10–20% of thrombi detected are isolated to the calf and only 20–30% of these extend, rendering routine serial testing both inefficient and inconvenient. Indeed studies suggest very few patients (1–2% in two recent studies) who have a negative initial ultrasound test will be confirmed to have proximal DVT upon serial testing (12,13). As a result, serial testing is not cost-effective (14,15). Three recent studies have suggested that imaging of the entire deep vein system, excluding DVT with a single negative result, is a safe strategy (16–18). These studies suggest that calf vein imaging by experienced sonographers, and as described by Schellong et al. (17), has a sensitivity much higher than 73%. Inexperienced sonographers are likely to miss DVT (19). Since it is unlikely that further studies comparing whole-leg ultrasound with venography will be performed, the true sensitivity for calf vein DVT is unclear, but the litmus test of a management study is a reasonable surrogate that suggests higher sensitivity. However, no prospective randomized trials have compared the safety of this approach with strategies that only evaluate the proximal venous system. It is unknown if the single whole-leg vein assessment can be widely applied with the accuracy described in these studies, it is more laborious and it would still result in many needless tests. In Schellong et al.'s study only 0.2% of patients with low clinical probability had DVT. As will be discussed below, a strategy that employs a combination of D-dimer, clinical probability and ultrasound imaging appears to be the ideal combination to improve efficiency and cost-effectiveness in the diagnosis of DVT.

Computed tomographic venography (CTV) using intravenous iodinated contrast agents may be a reasonable alternative diagnostic tool, but experience in patients with suspected DVT is limited (20,21). Very few studies have been performed, which clearly enrolled selected patients given the very high rates of DVT. Pooling of data is not possible since most studies evaluated CTV as a tool for diagnosis of DVT in patients with suspected PE. On the basis of the sensitivity and specificity for proximal DVT in patients with suspected PE, 96% and 95%, respectively, it is likely to be a reasonably accurate test for suspected DVT (21). Magnetic resonance imaging (MRI) may have an accuracy close to that of ultrasound, but the techniques are not well standardized, relatively few studies have been published and it is clearly more expensive and less widely available (22). The ideal place for MRI may be for diagnosis of recurrent DVT when ultrasound is equivocal (23,24).

Clinical diagnosis of DVT

Although the clinical diagnosis of DVT is non-specific, it has now been well established that a clinical prediction rule incorporating signs, symptoms and risk factors can be accurately applied

Table 14.1 Simplified clinical model for assessment of DVT[a]

Clinical variable	Score
Active cancer (treatment ongoing or within previous 6 months or palliative)	1
Paralysis, paresis or recent plaster immobilization of the lower extremities	1
Recently bedridden for 3 days or more or major surgery within the previous 12 weeks requiring general or regional anaesthesia	1
Localized tenderness along the distribution of the deep venous system	1
Entire leg swelling	1
Calf swelling at least 3 cm larger than that on the asymptomatic leg (measured 10 cm below the tibial tuberosity)	1
Pitting oedema confined to the symptomatic leg	1
Collateral superficial veins (non-varicose)	1
Previously documented DVT	1
Alternative diagnosis at least as likely as DVT	−2

[a]≥ 2 probability of DVT is 'likely' ≤ 1 probability for DVT is 'unlikely'. Alternatively, <1 is low probability, moderate is 1 or 2 and high is >2.

to categorize patients as low, moderate or high probability for DVT (Table 14.1). Alternatively, the same rule can be used to categorize patients as 'DVT likely' or 'DVT unlikely' (25). A recent systematic review (all studies included used the same clinical prediction rule) demonstrated that the prevalence of DVT in the low, moderate and high clinical probability groups was 5.0% (95% CI: 4.0 to 8.0%), 17% (95% CI: 13 to 23%) and 53% (95% CI: 44 to 61%), respectively (26). Inter-observer reliability has not been widely evaluated, but the reported studies involved many different physicians with a wide range of clinical experience, including junior residents. One study specifically demonstrated the model's reproducibility by resident physicians (27).

Determination of pre-test probability allows for several potential diagnostic strategies. Used in combination with ultrasound imaging, it has been demonstrated that patients at low pre-test probability can have DVT safely excluded on the basis of a single negative ultrasound test without serial testing (11). However, the pre-test probability determination may be best used in algorithms with the subsequent use of D-dimer. Constans *et al.* demonstrated the usefulness of the Wells rule in hospitalized patients and derived a new rule (St André score) that enabled more patients to be classified as low probability (28). In a validation study in outpatients, the Wells score proved superior to the St André score (29). A new ambulatory score derived in that study has not been validated. Finally, a New Zealand group proposed a Hamilton score for patients presenting to the emergency department and compared it with the Wells rule (30). This rule provided no advantage over the Wells rule and is yet to be validated.

Oudega *et al.* developed a rule specifically for use in primary care (31). This rule also incorporates specific patient demographics, signs, symptoms and risk factors. It differs from the Wells rule in that the D-dimer result (based on a highly sensitive D-dimer assay) is incorporated into the score and indeed is the most heavily weighted factor. Their data suggests this strategy may be able to exclude DVT in 21% of patients but it has yet to be validated in practice (32). This strategy would require verification with other D-dimer assays before widespread application can be advised.

D-dimer for the diagnosis of DVT

D-dimer, a degradation product of a cross-linked fibrin, is typically elevated with acute VTE. D-dimer levels may also be increased by a variety of non-thrombotic disorders including recent major surgery, haemorrhage, trauma, malignancy or sepsis and D-dimer levels increase with age and through pregnancy (33–36). Thus, D-dimer assays are sensitive but non-specific markers for VTE and positive D-dimer results are *not* useful to 'rule in' the diagnosis; rather, the potential value is for a negative test result to 'rule out' the diagnosis. Although the negative predictive value of the D-dimer test increases proportionately as the sensitivity increases, as with all tests the negative predictive value of the D-dimer is inversely related to the prevalence of VTE in the population under study. Specificity is important since use of a very non-specific assay or the testing of very ill hospitalized patients would be of limited value due to the expected high number of positive results, many in patients without VTE (i.e., false positives). Data suggest that most D-dimer assays lie on the same receiver operating characteristic (ROC) curve (37–40), although one meta-analysis suggests three tests had significantly worse diagnostic odds ratios then the reference D-dimer assay used in the analysis (the Vidas assay) (41). The most comprehensive analysis of D-dimer assay accuracy found a trade-off between sensitivity and specificity without obvious evidence of any method being inferior to others with regard to both sensitivity and specificity (40). Enzyme-linked immunofluorescence assays, microplate ELISA and latex quantitative assays were found to have comparably high sensitivity but lower specificity than whole-blood D-dimer and latex semiquantitative and latex qualitative assays. No randomized comparative studies have been performed. It is probably best to consider D-dimer assays as those with moderate sensitivity and moderate specificity or those with high sensitivity and poor specificity. The former consist of latex agglutination assays (semiquantitative and qualitative) and the whole-blood assays. The sensitivities and specificities for these assays were in that ranges 85–90% and 50–80%, respectively. Qualitative D-dimer assays have the advantages that they are simple, have a rapid turnaround time and are inexpensive, but since they are interpreted by visual inspection, it is advisable that only trained observers perform and interpret them (42). The rapid, automated enzyme-linked immunofluorescence assay (Vidas D-dimer test; bioMérieux, Marcy l'Etoile, France), has demonstrated the highest sensitivity at an average of 93–98% but with a specificity of 36–52%.

DIAGNOSTIC STRATEGIES

Recommended approach to patients for the diagnosis of a first episode of DVT

Patients with leg symptoms compatible with DVT should initially have a determination of pre-test probability of DVT using an established prediction model/rule such as the one which was previously validated (Table 14.1). It is important that a history and physical examination be done first and only if DVT remains a diagnostic possibility should the model be applied. If it is obvious that the symptoms are due to an alternative problem (e.g., muscle strain or infection), DVT does not need to be a diagnostic possibility. If doubt remains or if DVT risk factors exist, the physician can apply the model. After the pre-test probability has been determined, a D-dimer test should be performed. Performing the D-dimer test prior to clinical assessment should be avoided since positive results are likely to influence the physician's clinical impression incorrectly. If moderate-sensitivity D-dimer assays are used, the pre-test clinical probability should be <10% to enable a negative D-dimer to exclude the diagnosis without the need for ultrasonography. A score of ≤ 1 (unlikely DVT) by the modified Wells model is sufficient to use with a qualitative D-dimer such as the IL-test or the SimpliRED (Figure 14.1). However, most studies have employed the

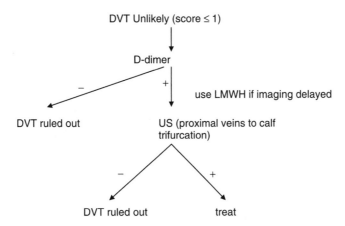

Figure 14.1 Diagnostic algorithm using clinical probability, D-dimer and ultrasound in patients with suspected DVT. DVT, deep vein thrombosis; US, ultrasound; LMWH, low molecular weight heparin.

earlier Wells scoring system and as such use a score of zero or less to allow exclusion of DVT with a negative moderate-sensitivity D-dimer test (26,27). The use of the unlikely category should enable up to 40% of outpatients referred with suspected DVT to have the diagnosis excluded without imaging tests. It should be kept in mind that ultrasonography may provide information helpful to establish an alternative diagnosis but ultrasound imaging for DVT is not required to rule out DVT with low/unlikely probability in combination with a negative D-dimer test result. Due to its better negative likelihood ratio of 0.08 (vs 0.20 for moderate-sensitivity assays), a negative Vidas D-dimer test (and other high-sensitivity assays) may be used to exclude the diagnosis of VTE when the pre-test probability is less than 20%, corresponding to a score ≤ 2 (43). There is widespread consensus that a D-dimer assay is *unable* to exclude DVT in patients who are in the high pre-test probability category.

Clinical assessment and D-dimer testing have the further advantage of allowing management at times when imaging is not available. Patients with moderate/high clinical probability may receive an injection of low molecular weight heparin (treatment dose) and imaging can subsequently be arranged the following day (Figures 14.1 and 14.2) (44,45). Patients at low risk (by clinical models or negative sensitive D-dimer) may have diagnostic imaging delayed for a 12–24 hour period without the need for anticoagulants. When imaging is indicated ultrasound is performed, limited to the proximal veins from the groin proceeding distally to the trifurcation region. If the test is positive (lack of complete vein compressibility), the diagnosis is confirmed. If the veins are completely compressible, a repeat ultrasound no more then 1 week later has generally been recommended. At least four studies reported sufficient data to determine that a negative D-dimer result with a clinical probability estimate of moderate/high and normal initial ultrasound permits exclusion of DVT without a serial ultrasound test (25,44–47). Serial testing after an initially normal ultrasound result can be confined to high-probability patients with positive D-dimer results (Figure 14.2). Note that false-negative D-dimer results may occur in patients with prolonged symptoms of DVT or after prolonged heparin therapy (more than 24 hours) (48).

Finally, it is important that the D-dimer test should only be employed if the physician is convinced that DVT is a diagnostic possibility and is not suitable as a screening test. Indiscriminate use of D-dimer as a screening test will result in many unnecessary ultrasound tests. Two retrospective analyses in emergency departments have confirmed the effectiveness of the approach outlined in Figures 14.1 and 14.2 in a real-life setting (49,50).

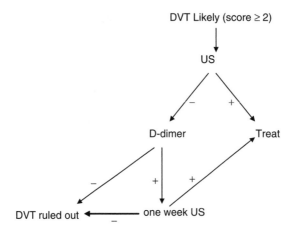

Figure 14.2 Diagnostic algorithm using clinical probability of DVT likely, D-dimer and ultrasound in patients with suspected DVT. DVT, deep vein thrombosis; US, ultrasound; LMWH, low molecular weight heparin.

Other approaches

In at least one study, it has been demonstrated that a negative ultrasound result combined with a negative D-dimer test can be used to exclude the need for a serial test. This strategy obviates the need for clinical pre-test probability assessment but there are no further data to support this approach (51). As described above, full leg ultrasound without use of D-dimer or clinical assessment results in safe management of patients but the strategy is likely to be more expensive and less convenient given that many patients could have been excluded from imaging with clinical assessment and D-dimer testing (17). Furthermore, the clinical relevance of the inevitably detected calf vein and muscular vein thrombi are unclear and may lead to unnecessary treatment (52).

A remarkably extensive review published by the UK Health Technology Assessment group concluded that the most cost-effective approach for the diagnosis of DVT includes a combination of clinical assessment, D-dimer and ultrasound imaging (53).

SPECIAL SITUATIONS

Cancer

The derivation, validation and randomized trial using the Wells model and the strategy advocated above included patients with cancer. De Nisio *et al.* demonstrated that the model for the determination of pre-test clinical probability works in cancer patients since the prevalence of DVT was 9.5, 25 and 68% in the low-, moderate- and high-probability categories, respectively (54). In this study, the SimpliRED D-dimer had a negative predictive value of 100% in low- and moderate-probability patients but negative D-dimer results occurred less frequently. However, it is clear that cancer patients are more likely to have elevated D-dimer levels. In one report in patients with suspected PE, only 11% of cancer patients had a negative D-dimer result (55). Pooled data from three studies demonstrated that 42% of a cohort of 200 patients with cancer had DVT. The D-dimer had a 100% negative predictive value but only 6% of patients with a low pre-test probability and 12% of patients with an 'unlikely' pre-test probability had a negative D-dimer (56). As such, the strategy is still effective but may not be cost-effective in patients with cancer.

Critical care unit patients

Critical care patients are unique in that they are at high risk, but in many cases they are unable to communicate due to mechanical ventilation, sedation or other conditions. Crowther *et al.* evaluated the Wells clinical model in these patients and determined that the DVT rates were 9% in patients deemed unlikely and 20% in those considered DVT likely (57). However, no patient had a negative D-dimer result and therefore the integrated strategy described above cannot be applied in this patient population. There may be value in the clinical determination in that it should suggest the possibility of a false-positive or clinically irrelevant thrombosis that does not require treatment in patients deemed unlikely to have DVT, but prospective management trials are required to evaluate this possibility.

Recurrent DVT and patients on oral anticoagulant therapy

A randomized trial demonstrated the safety of combining clinical probability, D-dimer and ultrasound testing for the diagnosis of recurrent DVT (25). This has been confirmed in at least one other study (58). The greatest concern is the occurrence of false-positive ultrasound results. It is helpful to recognize that if the ultrasound reveals thrombosis, which is echogenic, non-occlusive or discontinuous, then chronic DVT should be considered. Serial testing or venography can help clarify the issue. If previous ultrasound results are available, an increase in clot diameter by at least 4 mm is suggestive of recurrence (59). A recent study suggested that a negative sensitive D-dimer test result can exclude recurrence without ultrasound, but Bayes' theorem demonstrates the danger of this strategy since high pre-test probability patients may have over a 20% probability of DVT after a negative highly sensitive D-dimer test (60).

There are very few data on the utility of D-dimer in patients with suspected DVT who are on therapeutic doses of oral anticoagulants. One small study provides preliminary evidence that D-dimer may have insufficient sensitivity in this setting (61). In the 26 patients with an unlikely pre-test probability and a negative D-dimer result, two (7.7%) had DVT during follow-up. In addition, two of the 10 patients with a negative D-dimer who had a 'likely' pre-test probability had DVT on the initial ultrasound. Clearly, further study is required.

Pregnancy

Most diagnostic and treatment studies of DVT have excluded pregnant women, hence it is difficult to formulate evidence-based recommendations for this population. Serial impedance plethysmography has been demonstrated to rule out DVT safely, but it is no longer widely employed (62). D-dimer is often positive in the later stages of pregnancy, lowering the utility of this test to rule out DVT (63,64). However, a recent prospective cohort study in 149 pregnant patients with suspected DVT suggests the SimpliRED D-dimer may be useful in this population (65). In this management study, 13 women were diagnosed with DVT. The sensitivity and the negative predictive values of the SimpliRED D-dimer were both 100%. Importantly, 81 patients had a negative D-dimer result and almost 60% of patients in the study were in the third trimester. This study used serial ultrasound testing on days 3 and 7. Further research is needed to evaluate the role of pre-test probability assessment and to determine the safety of withholding serial testing given no patient converted upon serial testing.

CONCLUSION

Recent advances in the management of patients with suspected DVT have both improved diagnostic accuracy and made management algorithms safer and more accessible. Ongoing clinical trials are evaluating whether these diagnostic processes can be made even easier and less expensive. Patients at low risk (as determined by a validated clinical assessment score) with a negative D-dimer can avoid imaging tests and those at moderate risk with a negative high-sensitivity D-dimer can have VTE excluded without the need for imaging. Diagnostic strategies should include pre-test clinical probability, D-dimer assays and non-invasive imaging tests. Future research should be directed at refining the diagnostic process in pregnant patients and those with suspected recurrent DVT.

REFERENCES

1. Spencer FA, Emery C, Lessard D, Anderson F, Emani S, Aragam J, et al. The Worcester Venous Thromboembolism Study. A population-based study of the clinical epidemiology of venous thromboembolism. *J Gen Intern Med* 2006; **21**:722–7.
2. Heit JA, Silverstein MD, Mohr DN, Petterson TM, O'Fallon WM, Melton LJ III. Risk factors for deep vein thrombosis and pulmonary embolism: a population-based case–control study. *Arch Intern Med* 2000; **160**:809–15.
3. Heit, JA, O'Fallon WM, Petterson TM, Lohse CM, Silverstein MD, Mohr DN, et al. Relative impact of risk factors for deep vein thrombosis and pulmonary embolism: a population-based study. *Arch Intern Med* 2002; **162**:1245–8.
4. Schluger N, Henschke C, King T, Russo R, Binkert B, Rackson M, et al. Diagnosis of pulmonary embolism at a large teaching hospital. *J Thorac Imaging* 1994; **9**:180–4.
5. Bayes, T. An essay towards solving a problem in the doctrine of chances. *Philos Trans R Soc London* 1763; **53**:370–418.
6. Heller I, Topilsky M, Shapira I, Isakov A. Graphic representation of sequential Bayesian analysis. *Methods Inf Med* 1999; **38**:182–6.
7. Anand SS, Wells PS, Hunt D, Brill-Edwards P, Cook D, Ginsberg JS. Does this patient have deep vein thrombosis? *JAMA* 1998; **279**:1094–9.
8. Cogo A, Lensing AWA, Koopman MMW, Piovella F, Siragusa S, Wells PS, et al. Compression ultrasonography for diagnostic management of patients with clinically suspected deep vein thrombosis: prospective cohort study. *Br Med J* 1998; **316**:17–20.
9. Heijboer H, Buller HR, Lensing AWA, Turpie AGG, Colly LP, ten Cate JW. A comparison of real-time compression ultrasonography with impedance plethysmography for the diagnosis of deep-vein thrombosis in symptomatic outpatients. *N Engl J Med* 1993; **329**:1365–9.
10. Lensing AW, Prandoni P, Brandjes DPM, Huisman PM, Vigo M, Tomacella G, et al. Detection of deep-vein thrombosis by real-time B-mode ultrasonography. *N Engl J Med.* 1989: **320**:342–5.
11. Wells PS, Anderson DR, Bormanis J, Guy F; Mitchell M, Gray L, et al. Value of assessment of pre-test probability of deep-vein thrombosis in clinical management. *Lancet* 1997; **350**:1795–8.
12. Kearon C, Julian JA, Newman TE, Ginsberg JS. Noninvasive diagnosis of deep vein thrombosis. *Ann Intern Med* 1998; **128**:663–77.
13. Wells PS, Lensing AWA, Davidson BL, Prins MH, Hirsh J. Accuracy of ultrasound for the diagnosis of deep venous thrombosis in asymptomatic patients after orthopedic surgery. A meta-analysis. *Ann Intern Med* 1995; **122**:47–53.
14. Perone N, Bounameaux H, Perrier A. Comparison of four strategies for diagnosing deep vein thrombosis: a cost-effectiveness analysis. *Am J Med* 2000; **110**:33–40.

15. Hillner BE, Philbrick JT, Becker DM. Optimal management of suspected lower-extremity deep vein thrombosis.An evaluation with cost assessment of 24 management strategies. *Arch Intern Med* 1992; **152**:165–75.

16. Elias A, Mallard L, Elias M, Alquier C, Guidolin F, Gauthier B, *et al.* A single complete ultrasound investigation of the venous network for the diagnostic management of patients with a clinically suspected first episode of deep venous thrombosis of the lower limbs. *Thromb Haemost* 2003; **89**:221–7.

17. Schellong, SM, Schwarz T, Halbritter K, Beyer J, Siegert G, Oettler W, *et al.* Complete compression ultrasonography of the leg veins as a single test for the diagnosis of deep vein thrombosis. *Thromb Haemost* 2003; **89**:228–34.

18. Stevens SM, Elliot CG, Chan KJ, Egger MJ, Ahmed KM. Withholding anticoagulation after a negative result on duplex ultrasonography for suspected symptomatic deep venous thrombosis. *Ann Intern Med* 2004; **140**:985–91.

19. Jacoby J, Cesta M, Axelband J, Melanson S, Heller M, Reed J. Can emergency medicine residents detect acute deep venous thrombosis with a limited, two-site ultrasound examination? *J Emerg Med* 2007; **32**:197–200.

20. Baldt MM, Zontisch T, Stumpflen A, Fleischmann D, Schneider B, Minar E, *et al.* Deep venous thrombosis of the lower extremity: efficacy of spiral CT venography compared with conventional venography in diagnosis. *Radiology* 1996; **200**:423–8.

21. Thomas SM, Goodacre SW, Sampson FC, van Beek EJ. Diagnostic value of CT for deep vein thrombosis: results of a systematic review and meta-analysis, *Clin Radiol* 2008; **63**:299–304.

22. Sampson FC, Goodacre, SW, Thomas SM, van Beek EJ. The accuracy of MRI in diagnosis of suspected deep vein thrombosis: systematic review and meta-analysis. *Eur Radiol* 2007; **17**:175–81.

23. Sirol M, Fuster V, Badimon JJ, Fallon JT, Moreno PR, Toussaint JF, *et al.* Chronic thrombus detection with in vivo magnetic resonance imaging and a fibrin-targeted contrast agent. *Circulation* 2005; **112**:1594–600.

24. Moody AR. Magnetic resonance direct thrombus imaging. *J Thromb Haemost* 2003; **1**:1403–9.

25. Wells PS, Anderson DR, Rodger M, Forgie MA, Kearon C, Dreyer JF, *et al.* Evaluation of D-dimer in the diagnosis of suspected deep-vein thrombosis. *N Engl J Med* 2003; **349**:1227–35.

26. Wells PS, Owen C, Doucette S, Fergusson D, Tran H. Does this patient have deep vein thrombosis? *JAMA* 2006; **295**:199–207.

27. Penaloza A, Laureys M, Wautrecht JC, L'Heureux Ph, Motte S. Accuracy and safety of pre-test probability assessment of deep vein thrombosis by physicians in training using the explicit Wells clinical model. *J Thromb Haemost* 2006; **4**:278–81.

28. Constans J, Nelzy ML, Salmi LR, Skopinski S, Saby JC, Le Metayer P, *et al.* Clinical prediction of lower limb deep vein thrombosis in symptomatic hospitalized patients. *Thromb Haemost* 2001; **86**:985–90.

29. Constans J, Boutinet C, Salmi LR, Saby JC, Nelzy ML, Baudouin P, *et al.* Comparison of four clinical prediction scores for the diagnosis of lower limb deep venous thrombosis in outpatients. *Am J Med* 2003; **115**:436–40.

30. Subramaniam RM, Snyder B, Heath R, Tawse F, Sleigh J. Diagnosis of lower limb deep venous thrombosis in emergency department patients: performance of Hamilton and modified Wells scores, *Ann Emerg Med* 2006; **48**:678–85.

31. Oudega R, Moons KG, Hoes AW. Ruling out deep venous thrombosis in primary care. A simple diagnostic algorithm including D-dimer testing. *Thromb Haemost* 2005; **94**:200–5.

32. Toll DB, Oudega R, Bulten RJ, Hoes AW, Moons KG. Excluding deep vein thrombosis safely in primary care. *J Fam Pract* 2006; **55**:613–8.

33. Bombeli T, Raddatz MP, Fehr J. Evaluation of an optimal dose of low-molecular-weight heparin for thromboprophylaxis in pregnant women at risk of thrombosis using coagulation activation markers. *Haemostasis* 2001; **31**:90–8.

34. Bosson JL, Labarere J, Sevestre MA, Belmin J, Beyssier L, Elias A, *et al.* Deep vein thrombosis in elderly patients hospitalized in subacute care facilities. A multicenter cross-sectional study of risk factors, prophylaxis and prevalence. *Arch Intern Med* 2003; **163**:2613–8.

35. Righini M, Goehring C, Bounameaux H, Perrier A. Effect of age on the performance of common diagnostic tests for pulmonary embolism. *Am J Med* 2000; **109**:357–61.

36. Freyburger G, Trillaud H, Labrouche S, Gauthier P, Javorschi S, Bernard P, *et al.* D-dimer strategy in thrombosis exclusion. A gold standard study in 100 patients suspected of deep vein thrombosis or pulmonary embolism: 8 DD methods compared. *Thromb Haemost* 1998; **79**:32–7.

37. Kraaijenhagen RA, Lijmer JG, Bossuyt PMM, Prins MH, Heisterkamp SH, Buller HR. The accuracy of D-dimer in the diagnosis of venous thromboembolism: a meta-analysis. In Kraaijenhagen RA (ed), *The Etiology, Diagnosis and Treatment of Venous Thromboembolism*, Academic Medical Centre, Amsterdam, The Netherlands, 2000, pp.159–83.

38. Philbrick JT, Heim SW. The D-dimer test for deep venous thrombosis: gold standards and bias in negative predictive value. *Clin Chem* 2003; **49**:570–4.

39. Stein PD, Hull RD, Patel KC, Olson RE, Ghali WA, Brant RF, *et al.* D-dimer for the exclusion of acute venous thrombosis and pulmonary embolism. A systematic review. *Ann Intern Med* 2004; **140**:589–602.

40. Di Nisio M, Squizzato A, Rutjes AW, Buller HR, Zwinderman AH, Bossuyt PM. Diagnostic accuracy of D-dimer test for exclusion of venous thromboembolism: a systematic review. *J Thromb Haemost* 2007; **5**:296–304.

41. Heim SW, Schectman JM, Siadaty M. S, Philbrick JT. D-dimer testing for deep venous thrombosis: a metaanalysis. *Clin Chem* 2004; **50**:1136–47.

42. Turkstra F, van Beek EJR, Buller HR. Observer and biological variation of a rapid whole blood D-dimer test. *Thromb Haemost* 1998; **79**:91–3.

43. Keeling DM; Mackie IJ, Moody A, Watson HG. The diagnosis of deep vein thrombosis in symptomatic outpatients and the potential for clinical assessment and D-dimer assays to reduce the need for diagnostic imaging. *Br J Haematol* 2004; **124**:15–25.

44. Anderson DR, Kovacs MJ, Kovacs G, Stiell I, Mitchell M, Khoury V, *et al.* Combined use of clinical assessment and D-dimer to improve the management of patients presenting to the emergency department with suspected deep-vein thrombosis (the EDITED Study). *J Thromb Haemost* 2003; **1**: 645–51.

45. Bauld DL, Kovacs MJ. Dalteparin in emergency patients to prevent admission prior to investigation for venous thromboembolism. *Am J Emerg Med* 1999; **17**:11–4.

46. Bates SM, Kearon C, Crowther MA, Linkins L, O'Donnell M, Douketis JD, *et al.* A diagnostic strategy involving a quantitative latex D-dimer assay reliably excludes deep venous thrombosis. *Ann Intern Med* 2003; **138**:787–94.

47. Schutgens REG, Ackermark P, Haas FJ, Nieuwenhuis HK, Peltenburg HG, Pijlman AH, *et al.* Combination of a normal D-dimer concentration and a non-high pre-test clinical probability score is a safe strategy to exclude deep venous thrombosis. *Circulation* 2003; **107**:593–7.

48. Stricker H, Marchetti O, Haeberli A, Mombelli G. Hemostatic activation under anticoagulant treatment: a comparison of unfractionated heparin vs. nadroparin in the treatment of proximal deep vein thrombosis. *Thromb Haemost* 1999; **82**:1227–31.

49. Arnason T, Wells PS, Forster AJ. Appropriateness of diagnostic strategies for evaluating suspected venous thromboembolism. *Thromb Haemost* 2007; **97**:195–201.

50. de Bastos MM, Bastos MR, Pessoa PC, Bogutchi T, Carneiro-Proietti AB, Rezende SM. Managing suspected venous thromboembolism in a mixed primary and secondary care setting using standard clinical assessment and D-dimer in a noninvasive diagnostic strategy. *Blood Coagul Fibrinol* 2008; **19**:48–54.

51. Bernardi E, Prandoni P, Lensing AW, Agnelli G, Guazzaloca G. D-dimer testing as an adjunct to ultrasonography in patients with clinically suspected deep vein thrombosis: prospective cohort study. The Multicentre Italian D-dimer Ultrasound Study Investigators Group., *BMJ* 1998; **317**:1037–40.

52. Palareti G, Agnelli G, Imberti D, Moia M, Ageno W, Pistelli R, *et al.* A commentary: to screen for calf DVT or not to screen? The highly variable practice among Italian centers highlights this important and still unresolved clinical option. Results from the Italian MASTER registry. *Thromb Haemost* 2008; **99**:241–4.

53. Goodacre S, Sampson F, Stevenson, M, Wailoo A, Sutton A, Thomas S, *et al.* Measurement of the clinical and cost-effectiveness of non-invasive diagnostic testing strategies for deep vein thrombosis. *Health Technol Assess* 2006; **10**(15):1–151.

54. Di Nisio M, Rutjes AW, Buller HR. Combined use of clinical pre-test probability and D-dimer test in cancer patients with clinically suspected deep venous thrombosis. *J Thromb Haemost* 2006; **4**:52–7.

55. Righini M, Le Gal G, De Lucia S, Roy P-M, Meyer G, Aujesky D, *et al.* Clinical usefulness of D-dimer testing in cancer patients with suspected pulmonary embolism. *Thromb Haemost* 2006; **95**:715–9.

56. Carrier M, Lee A, Bates SM, Anderson DR, Wells PS. Accuracy and usefulness of a clinical prediction rule and D-dimer testing in excluding deep vein thrombosis (DVT) in cancer patients. *J Thromb Haemost* 2007; **5**(Suppl 2): Abstract P–S-555.

57. Crowther MA, Cook DJ, Griffith LE, Devereaux PJ, Rabbat CC, Clarke FJ, *et al.* Deep venous thrombosis: clinically silent in the intensive care unit. *J Crit Care* 2005; **20**:334–40.

58. Aguilar C, Del Villar V. Combined D-dimer and clinical probability are useful for exclusion of recurrent deep venous thrombosis. *Am J Hematol* 2007; **82**:41–4.

59. Heijboer H, Jongbloets LMM, Buller HR, Lensing AWA, ten Cate JW. Clinical utility of real-time compression ultrasonography for diagnostic management of patients with recurrent venous thrombosis. *Acta Radiol* 1992; **33**:297–300.
60. Rathbun SW, Whitsett TL, Raskob, GE. Negative D-dimer result to exclude recurrent deep venous thrombosis: a management trial. *Ann Intern Med* 2004; **141**:839–45.
61. Aguilar C, Del Villar V. Diagnostic value of D-dimer in outpatients with suspected deep venous thrombosis receiving oral anticoagulation. *Blood Coagul Fibrinol* 2007; **18**:253–7.
62. Hull RD, Raskob GE, Carter CJ. Serial impedance plethysmography in pregnant patients with clinically suspected deep-vein thrombosis. Clinical validity of negative findings. *Ann Intern Med* 1990; **112**:663–7.
63. Epiney M, Boehlen F, Boulvain M, Reber G, Antonelli E, Morales M, *et al.* D-dimer levels during delivery and the postpartum. *J Thromb Haemost* 2005; **3**:268–71.
64. Eichinger S. D-dimer testing in pregnancy. *Semin Vasc Med* 2005; **5**:375–8.
65. Chan WS, Chunilal S, Lee A, Crowther M, Rodger M, Ginsberg JS. A red blood cell agglutination D-dimer test to exclude deep venous thrombosis in pregnancy. *Ann Intern Med* 2007; **147**:165–70.

CHAPTER 15

Diagnostic Management Strategies in Patients with Suspected Pulmonary Embolism

Renée A. Douma[1], Pieter W. Kamphuisen[1], Edwin J.R. van Beek[2], Matthijs Oudkerk[3] and Harry R. Büller[1]

[1]Department of Vascular Medicine, Academic Medical Center, Amsterdam, The Netherlands
[2]Department of Radiology, Carver College of Medicine, University of Iowa, USA
[3]Department of Radiology, Academic Medical Centre, Groningen, The Netherlands

INTRODUCTION

Venous thromboembolism (VTE), consisting of pulmonary embolism (PE) and deep vein thrombosis (DVT) is a frequently occurring disease. A large and growing number of patients suspected with PE are evaluated at hospital emergency departments each year. The disease can be fatal in 25% of patients if left untreated (1), but this rate lowers to 1.5% in patients treated with anticoagulant therapy (2). However, treatment with anticoagulants has its own risks, most notably an annual bleeding incidence of 2–7% (3,4).

Prevalence and diagnosis of PE

The prevalence of confirmed PE in patients suspected of having the disease has decreased in recent decades. Whereas the diagnosis was confirmed in 30–35% of patients 20 years ago (5), this number has decreased to 20–25% in recent management studies (6,7) and even lower in some other reports (8). This decrease in prevalence most likely reflects an increase in patients in whom PE is suspected, since there is no evidence that the absolute number of detected cases of PE has increased simultaneously (9). It may therefore point towards an increase in the awareness of PE and also a decreased threshold for testing as diagnostic protocols have been increasingly simplified and made available around the clock. Adequate diagnosis is essential to prevent PE-related mortality and morbidity on the one hand and unnecessary treatment on the other. Preferably, excluding the diagnosis is performed using safe, efficient and non-invasive diagnostic methods.

Where do we come from?

Until the introduction of pulmonary angiography and ventilation/perfusion scintigraphy (10,11), the tests available for physicians to diagnose or exclude PE mainly existed of an arterial blood gas, the chest X-ray and an electrocardiogram. With the advent of imaging tests, it became possible to directly or indirectly visualize the presence of clots in the lungs and to exclude or diagnose PE with more certainty (12). The V/Q scan is a non-invasive imaging test with relatively low radiation exposure. It is well established that a normal perfusion lung scan rules out PE and that anticoagulant therapy can be safely withheld (5,13–16). On the other hand, a high-probability V/Q scan, defined as at least one segmental perfusion defect with locally normal ventilation, confirms the presence of the disease with a positive predictive value of 85–90% in a patient population with a PE prevalence of approximately 30% (5,17). However, a significant number of investigated patients (40–60%) have a non-diagnostic test result and further investigation is necessary. Another drawback of this diagnostic method is the need for expensive ventilation materials, which are not always available. Pulmonary angiography was long regarded as the diagnostic gold standard. By direct opacification of the pulmonary arteries with contrast media after catheterization, the diagnostic yield is high and non-diagnostic test results are obtained in approximately 4% of patients (18). However, because of the risk of major complications with this invasive test (fatal complications in 0.5% and non-fatal in 1%) (18), physicians remain reluctant to perform angiography. Moreover, it is an expensive test which requires expertise that is not available in all hospitals. Because of the drawbacks of these techniques, other tests and diagnostic strategies were developed.

The need for integrated strategies

Over the last two decades, many new diagnostic methods and strategies have been introduced for the diagnostic work-up of patients with suspected PE. Individual signs and symptoms have low sensitivity and specificity, meaning that there is no single risk factor or clinical sign that can be used to confirm or exclude the diagnosis (19). The available diagnostic tests also have several limitations: they can be invasive, non-specific and/or costly. These limitations may contribute to over or undertreatment of PE, an occurrence that is not uncommon (20–22). To enforce an accurate diagnosis, concurrently reducing costs and invasiveness, diagnostic tests have now been integrated in diagnostic algorithms consisting of clinical pre-test probability and D-dimer testing followed by imaging.

This chapter focuses on different integrated diagnostic strategies that have been evaluated in proper management studies. First, however, the individual diagnostic tests will be discussed briefly in so far they have not been mentioned already (for detailed information, the reader is referred to the previous chapters).

DIAGNOSTIC TESTS

Clinical probability

The first step in the approach to patients with suspected PE is a thorough clinical history and physical examination, in order to determine the clinical probability of the presence of PE. Although not sensitive or specific when used alone, specific information regarding clinical signs and symptoms can be used to categorize the patients in probability categories, by using either implicit judgement or validated clinical decision rules. Several rules are available and have been validated (23–27) and recent guidelines recommend the assessment of clinical probability in each patient with suspected PE before any further objective testing is ordered (28–32).

Determining clinical probability

The simplest way is by using the physician's implicit clinical judgement. The Prospective Investigation Of Pulmonary Embolism Diagnosis (PIOPED) investigators and others were able show the potential of using the clinician's overall diagnostic impression in further diagnostic management (5,24,33–36). However, it has been criticized that this unstandardized probability assessment is dependent on the physician's expertise and training (37,38), has a high inter-physician variability (39) and probability estimates tend to follow the middle road (with fewer patients categorized as 'low' or 'high' probability) (40).

The best known clinical decision scores for explicit clinical judgment are the Geneva score (25), the Revised Geneva score (27) and the Wells rule (26,41) (Table 15.1). The Wells rule, currently the most widely applied, is composed of seven variables obtained from medical history and physical examination. Both the trichotomous (with three probability categories: low, intermediate and high) and the dichotomous version (with two categories: unlikely and likely) have been extensively evaluated in outcome studies. Despite the subjective character of one of the variables ('alternative diagnosis less likely'), it has a moderate inter-rater variability and is independent of the physician's level of training (42–44). The more recently introduced Revised Geneva score (27) is composed of eight solely objective clinical variables.

The different methods of determining pre-test probability show similar accuracy. The level of experience of the treating physician seems to be of less influence with the use of an objective score compared with empirical judgment (38,39,43,45).

Advantages of clinical stratification

Because the prevalence of PE is unacceptably high in the low or unlikely probability categories (ranging from 1 to 28%) (39,46), clinical probability scores alone are insufficiently reliable to exclude PE and additional diagnostic tests are always indicated. They are, however, useful to guide the further diagnostic work-up. According to Bayes' theorem, the post-test probability is a function not only of the sensitivity and specificity of the test, but also of the pre-test probability (47). Stratifying patients into different levels of pre-test probability therefore affects the diagnostic yield of subsequent tests. Also, the cost-effectiveness of clinical stratification has been demonstrated, as the requirement for invasive tests is reduced (48).

D-dimer testing

The measurement of the specific breakdown products of cross-linked fibrin in plasma, known as D-dimers, is widely applied in patients with suspected VTE. It is a fast, easy and inexpensive method, with high sensitivity for PE, although the diagnostic accuracy of D-dimer tests for the exclusion of PE varies. D-dimer assays with a high sensitivity and high negative predictive value, such as the standard or rapid enzyme-linked immunosorbent assay (ELISA) and immuno-turbidimetric D-dimer test, may be used to rule out PE in low or intermediate clinical probability patients. There is, however, a trade-off between sensitivity and specificity, especially in specific

Table 15.1   Clinical decision scores

Wells score (26)		Geneva score (25)		Revised Geneva score (27)	
Characteristics	Points	Characteristics	Points	Characteristics	Points
Previous PE or DVT	+1.5	Previous PE or DVT	+2	Age >65 years	+1
Heart rate	+1.5	Heart rate	+1	Previous DVT or PE	+3
Recent surgery or immobilization	+1.5	Recent surgery	+1	Surgery or fracture within 1 month	+2
Clinical signs of DVT	+3	Age (years)		Active malignancy	+2
Alternative diagnosis less likely than PE	+3	60–79	+1	Unilateral lower limb pain	+3
Haemoptysis	+1	≥80	+2	Haemoptysis	+2
Cancer	+1	Arterial blood gas		Heart rate	
		CO_2 (kPa)		75–94	+3
		<4.8	+2	≥95	+5
		4.8–5.19	+1	Pain on lower limb deep vein palpation and unilateral 0edema	+4
		O_2 (kPa)			
		<6.5	+4		
		6.5–7.99	+3		
		8–9.49	+2		
		9.5–10.99	+1		
		Chest X-ray			
		Atelectasis	+1		
		Elevated hemidiaphragm	+1		
Clinical probability		*Clinical probability*		*Clinical probability*	
Low	<2	Low	0–4	Low	0–3
Intermediate	2–6	Intermediate	5–8	Intermediate	4–10
High	>6	High	≥9	High	≥11
Dichotomous (6)					
Unlikely	≤4				
Likely	>4				

patient groups such as the elderly and hospitalized patients. This results in a confident exclusion of the disease at the expense of more additional imaging testing. In a recent meta-analysis, it was found that compared with other D-dimer assays, the enzyme-linked immunofluorescence assay (ELFA), microplate ELISA and latex quantitative assay had a comparably high sensitivity, but a lower specificity than whole-blood D-dimer latex semiquantitative and latex qualitative assays (49). Whole-blood agglutination assays, such as the SimpliRED test, are less sensitive and therefore used for the exclusion of PE in patients with low clinical probability only (50,51).

CT angiography

In the diagnosis of PE, computed tomographic pulmonary angiography (CT or CTPA) has gained a position of increasing importance. Introduced in 1992, it has evolved to become the main imaging test for the diagnosis of PE. Initially, physicians were sceptical about the accuracy of detecting emboli in segmental and subsegmental arteries with early single-slice detector CT. Studies reported a sensitivity between 53% and 100% and a specificity between 81% and 100% in comparison with pulmonary angiography (52). In a meta-analysis, the pooled sensitivity and specificity of the single slice CT were 86% and 94%, respectively (53). However, with the introduction of multi-detector row CT (MDCT), the sensitivity has greatly improved and even small subsegmental emboli can now be visualized (7,54).

Contrast-enhanced CT angiography has several advantages over other imaging techniques, such as the speed with which patients can be investigated and the characterization of non-vascular structures – and therefore the possibility of finding alternative or additional diagnoses (55). Similarly to pulmonary angiography, it provides a clear result (either positive or negative), with a low number of non-diagnostic test results (<2%) (55). An important disadvantage, however, is the radiation exposure (56,57).

Ultrasonography

Ultrasonography of the lower limb veins is used as an indirect method to detect PE. In approximately 50–80% of patients with proven PE, concomitant DVT can be detected (58). This does not mean that these patients all have symptomatic DVT. In patients with clinically suspected DVT, compression ultrasonography (CUS) of the proximal deep lower limb veins has a sensitivity and specificity above 95% for the diagnosis of DVT. Although the specificity of a positive proximal CUS is also high for PE, the sensitivity is only approximately 40–50%.

INTEGRATED STRATEGIES IN PATIENTS WITH SUSPECTED PULMONARY EMBOLISM

Integrated diagnostic strategies

The success of an integrated diagnostic strategy is primarily defined by the rate of VTE eventually detected during follow-up in the patients in whom the disease was excluded (i.e., the false-negative rate) (40). In outcome studies, an observed failure rate of 1–2% is targeted, with an upper 95% confidence interval (CI) limit below 3%. This rate is comparable to the false-negative rate of VTE found for pulmonary angiography (59) or a normal V/Q scan (13,14). There are several other arguments supporting these target rates and threshold. No VTE at all (failure rate 0% over a 3–6 month period of follow-up) is very unlikely, considering that PE is a prevalent disease even in asymptomatic patients having a CT scan of the chest for other reasons (60–62). Furthermore, a threshold with an upper 95% CI level below 3% still balances favourably with the expected bleeding rate from anticoagulant therapy. Lowering the upper boundary could lead to an increase in diagnostic tests and a higher risk of false-positive results (40). A number of management studies have evaluated diagnostic algorithms with integrated approaches; they all found VTE rates below the targeted threshold (6,7,15,41,63–69) (see also Table 15.2). Prudence is in order when the overall prevalence of PE in a population is low: the negative predictive value may be misleadingly high (i.e., the false-negative result is low), while sensitivity could be low (9).

Clinical probability and D-dimer in diagnostic strategies

The advantage of using pre-test probability in the exclusion of PE is mainly achieved in combination with a D-dimer test result. The scores are therefore usually implemented at the beginning of the diagnostic algorithm, to be used in combination with D-dimer testing (see Table 15.2 and Figures 15.1–15.4). Several management studies have demonstrated that PE can safely be ruled out without imaging techniques in patients with a low, low/intermediate or unlikely clinical probability (70). This applies to 15–47% (41,63,65,66,71), 30–32% (7,72) and 32% (6) of the study population for low, low/intermediate and unlikely clinical probability, respectively (see Table 15.3). The failure rates of VTE in outcome studies is below 0.5%, indicating that the D-dimer test is a good first objective test to be used after clinical assessment to determine which patients require diagnostic imaging. The clinical usefulness is high, considering that PE can safely be excluded without imaging tests in approximately one third of the study population (Table 15.3). The straightforwardness of variables available at the bedside and a laboratory test renders high clinical utility. Because the sensitivity may vary between different D-dimer assays, it depends on the D-dimer assay whether further testing is not necessary in patients with a low, low/intermediate or unlikely probability.

Unless the D-dimer test is also used further on in the diagnostic strategy, patients who have a high or likely pre-test probability for PE should not necessarily undergo D-dimer testing: the post-test probability for PE remains too high for safely ruling out the disease (6,7,28,32,50,71). Although the negative predictive value of some D-dimer assays is very high, it is advocated that the D-dimer test should not be used as a stand-alone test (32). Further diagnostic testing is recommended in patients who have a normal D-dimer test result but a high or likely clinical probability – especially in combination with a less sensitive D-dimer test (28,49,73–76).

In some strategies, the clinical pre-test probability is combined with the result of imaging tests such as V/Q or CT scan to guide additional testing in apprehension of false-positive or false-negative results, i.e., to verify the diagnosis in patients in whom the clinical pre-test probability is discordant with the V/Q scan (15,77) or patients with a negative CT scan and a high clinical pre-test probability (64).

CTPA in diagnostic strategies

In patients with a high or likely pre-test clinical probability or patients with an abnormal D-dimer test, additional imaging is required. CTPA as the subsequent test has been studied extensively, in both accuracy and outcome studies (see Figures 15.2–15.4). In a recent randomized controlled diagnostic management study, CTPA was found to be equally capable as V/Q scanning in ruling out PE (15) (for flowcharts of the study algorithms, see Figures 15.1 and 15.2).

Table 15.2 Recent management outcome studies using clinical pre-test probability, D-dimer testing and imaging[a]

Study	Setting	No. of patients, n	Design	Prevalence of PE (%)	Failure rate[b] (%, 95% CI)
Kruip et al., 2002 (71)	In- and outpatients	234	CDR, DD, CUS, PA	22	1/182 (0.5%, 0.1 to 3.0%)
Perrier et al., 2004 (64)	Outpatients	965	CDR, DD, CUS, CT, PA	23	7/685 (1.1%, 0.5 to 2.2%)
Elias et al., 2005 (88)	Outpatients	274	CDR, DD, CUS, CT	40	1/164 (0.6%, 0.1 to 3.4%)
Wells et al., 2001 (41)	Outpatients	930	CDR, DD, V/Q (serial) CUS	910	3/492 (0.6%, 0.2 to 1.8%)
Leclercq et al., 2003 (72)	In- and outpatients	202	CDR, DD, X/Q, CUS, PA	29	0/133 (0.0%, 0.0 to 2.8%)
ten Wolde et al., 2004 (63)	In- and outpatients	631	PTP, DD, V/Q, CUS	20	6/466 (1.3%, 0.6 to 2.8%)
Anderson et al., 2007 (15)[c]	In- and outpatients	712	CDR, DD, V/Q (serial) CUS	14	6/611 (1.0%, 0.5 to 2.1%)
	In- and outpatients	694	CDR, DD, CT, (serial) CUS	19	2/561 (0.4%, 0.1 to 1.3%)
Anderson et al., 2005 (65)	Outpatients	858	CDR, DD, CT, CUS, PA	10	2/858 (0.2%, 0.1 to 0.8%)
Perrier et al., 2005 (7)	Outpatients	756	CDR, DD, CT, CUS, PA	26	5/523 (1.0%, 0.4 to 2.2%)
Righini et al., 2008 (69)	Outpatients	855	CDR, DD, CUS, CT	21	2/649 (0.3%, 0.1 to 1.1%)
	Outpatients	838	CDR, DD, CT	21	2/627 (0.3%, 0.1 to 1.2%)
Ghanima et al., 2005 (66)	Outpatients	432	DD, CDR, CT	24	2/324 (0.6%, 0.2 to 2.2%)
Christopher study, 2006 (6)	In- and outpatients	3306	CDR, DD, CT	20	23/2464 (0.9%, 0.6 to 1.4%)

[a]PE, pulmonary embolism; CDR, clinical decision rule; DD, D-dimer; CUS, compression ultrasonography; PA, pulmonary angiography; CT, computed tomography; V/Q, ventilation–perfusion scintigraphy; X/Q, perfusion scintigraphy combined with chest X-ray; PTP, pre-test probability.
[b]3 month rate of venous thromboembolism of the entire strategy.
[c]No data available on patients with unlikely CDR combined with normal DD (not included in the analysis).

Table 15.3 Clinical decision rule combined with D-dimer testing in management studies[a]

Study	Setting	Clinical decision rule	CDR cut-off	D-dimer test	Prevalence of PE (%)	n (% of patients)[b]	Failure rate n (%, 95% CI)
Wells et al., 2001 (41)	Outpatients	Wells (26)	Low	SimpliRED	10	437/930 (47%)	0/437 (0.2%, 0.0 to 1.3%)
Kruip et al., 2002 (71)	In- and outpatients	Wells '98 (77)	Low	Vidas	22	60/234 (26%)	0/60 (0.0%, 0.0 to 6.0%)
Leclercq et al., 2003 (72)	In- and outpatients	Wells '98 (77)	Low/intermediate	Tinaquant	29	64/202 (32%)	0/64 (0.0%, 0.0 to 5.6%)
ten Wolde et al., 2004 (63)	In- and outpatients	Clinical judgement	Low	Tinaquant	20	95/631 (15%)	0/95 (0.0%, 0.0 to 3.8%)
Perrier et al., 2004 (64)	Outpatients	Geneva (25) + clinical judgement	All	Vidas	23	280/965 (29%)	0/280 (0.0%, 0.0 to 1.1%)
Anderson et al., 2005 (65)	Outpatients	Wells (26)	Low	SimpliRED/IL-test	10	369/858 (43%)	0/369 (0.0%, 0.0 to 1.0%)
Ghanima et al. 2005 (66)	Outpatients	Hyers (105)	Low	STA-Liatest	24	103/432 (24%)	0/103 (0.0%, 0.0 to 3.7%)
Perrier et al., 2005 (7)	Outpatients	Geneva (25)	Low/intermediate	Vidas	26	232/756 (30%)	0/232 (0.0%, 0.0 to 2.7%)
Christopher study, 2006 (6)	In- and outpatients	Wells (26) – dichotomous	Unlikely	Vidas/Tinaquant	20	1057/3306 (32%)	5/1057 (0.5%, 0.2 to 1.1%)
Goekoop et al., 2007 (68)	Outpatients	Wells (26) – dichotomous	Unlikely	Vidas	12	450/879 (51%)	2/450 (1.8%, 0.6 to 3.0%)
Righini et al., 2008 (69)[d]	Outpatients	Revised Geneva score (27)	Low/intermediate	Vidas	21	561/1693 (33%)	0/561 (0.0%, 0.0 to 1.3%)

[a]PE, pulmonary embolism; CDR, clinical decision rule; DD, D-dimer.
[b]Proportion of patients in whom PE was excluded based on the CDR and DD result.
[c]month rate of venous thromboembolism.
[d]Per protocol analysis, patients from both study arms combined.

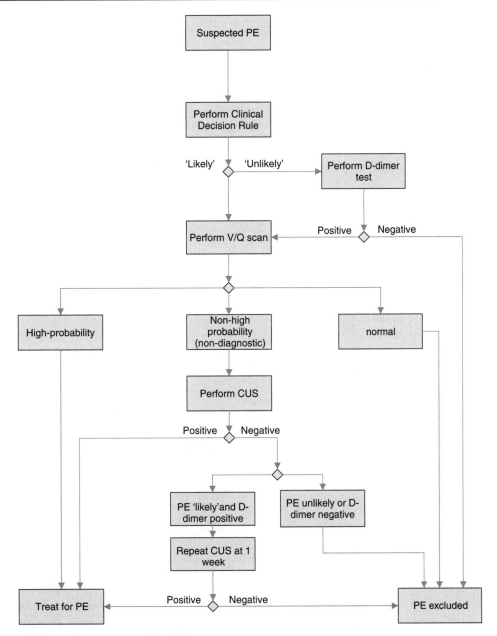

Figure 15.1 Clinical decision rule, D-dimer testing, V/Q scan and ultrasonography – algorithm used in the V/Q arm of the study by Anderson *et al.* (15). PE, pulmonary embolism; V/Q scan, ventilation–perfusion scan; CUS, compression ultrasonography.

Single-slice CT is known to be less sensitive in detecting PE, especially in the more peripheral arteries of the lungs. Studies that investigated strategies with single-slice CTPA usually demanded a compression ultrasonography or other tests after a negative CTPA (15,36,55,65), sometimes depending on the pre-test clinical probability (64). In two studies, the incidence of a positive finding with CUS after a negative CTPA was relatively high at 3.0 and 7.3%, with both studies

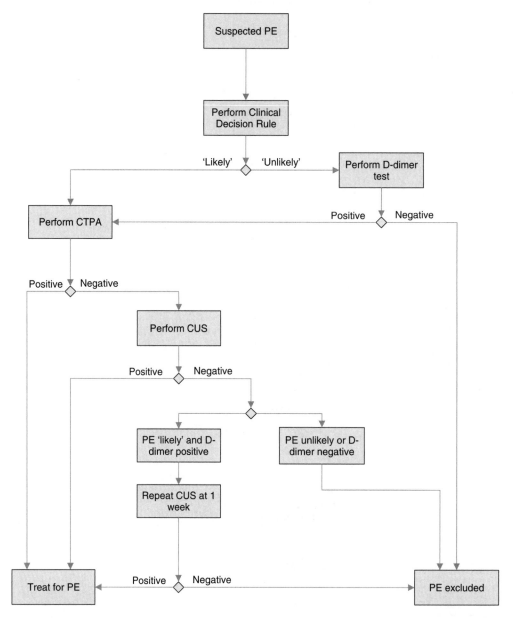

Figure 15.2 Clinical decision rule, D-dimer testing, CT scanning and ultrasonography – algorithm used in the CT arm of the study by Anderson *et al.* (15). PE, pulmonary embolism; CTPA, computed tomography of the pulmonary arteries; CUS, compression ultrasonography.

using single-slice CT (36,65). Conversely, other studies observed rates of DVT after a negative CTPA, ranging from 0.8 to 1.3% using either MDCT, single-slice CT or both (7,15,55). The total false-negative rate of CTPA in outcome studies ranged from 0.6% using MDCT to as high as 9.1% using single-slice CT (6,7,15,36,55,65,66,69) (Table 15.4). In the Christopher study, a large outcome study in which both single-slice CT and MDCT were used, comparable incidences of VTE were observed in untreated patients who underwent MDCT (14/1266, 1.1%) versus single-detector

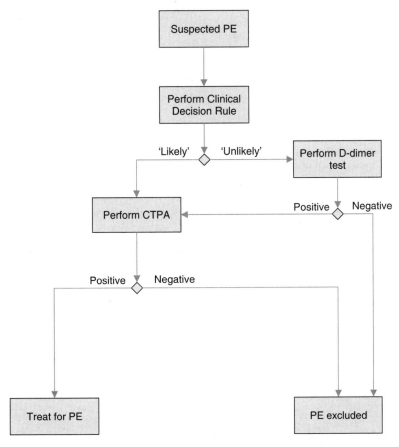

Figure 15.3 Clinical decision rule, D-dimer testing and CT – algorithm used in the Christopher study (6). PE, pulmonary embolism; CTPA, computed tomography of the pulmonary arteries.

row CT (4/170, 2.4%), but there was a trend for more false-negative results with the single-detector row CT (6).

Multiple detector row CTPA

The rate of false-negative CTPA results appears be lower when MDCT is used (Table 15.4) and a negative result on MDCT is generally accepted as excluding PE. Whether negative MDCT can be used to exclude PE in patients with a high pre-test probability remains debatable. In an accuracy study comparing MDCT with a reference diagnostic work-up composed of high-probability V/Q, abnormal findings on pulmonary angiography or abnormal findings on CUS and non-diagnostic V/Q, the negative predictive value of CTPA was 60% in patients with a high pre-test probability for PE (78). However, in two large outcome studies, the additional yield of CUS after negative MDCT was very small (Figures 15.2 and 15.4) (7,15). Furthermore, the combination of clinical probability assessment, D-dimer testing and CTPA without CUS proved safe in two large outcome studies, with a 3 month VTE rate of 0.6 and 0.9% (6,66) (for flow chart, see Figure 15.3). Finally, in a recent outcome study, MDCT alone was compared with MDCT preceded by CUS (69). Among 855 patients in the D-dimer–CUS–CT strategy, 53 (9%) showed a proximal DVT, obviating the need for MDCT. The 3 month VTE rates were 0.3% (95% CI: 0.1 to 1.1%) and 0.3% (95% CI: 0.1

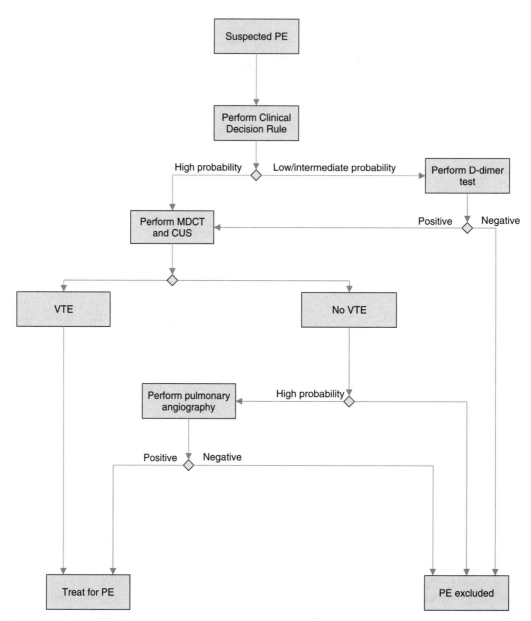

Figure 15.4   Clinical decision rule, D-dimer testing, ultrasonography, MDCT and additional testing in case of a high clinical probability – algorithm used in a study by Perrier *et al.* (7) and in one of the arms (DD–CUS–CT arm) of a study by Righini *et al.* (69). PE, pulmonary embolism; MDCT, multidetector-row computed tomography; CUS, compression ultrasonography; V/Q scan, ventilation–perfusion scan,; VTE, venous thromboembolism.

Table 15.4 Performance of CT in management outcome studies including clinical pre-test probability and D-dimer testing[a]

Study	Patients, n	CT type	False to negative (FN) CT scan results		Failure rate of the complete strategy if CUS had not been included in the diagnostic work-up[b] N (%, 95% CI)
			CUS + after CT – N (%, 95% CI)	VTE in 3 month FU N (%, 95% CI)	
Anderson et al., 2005 (65)	489	Single	13/422 (3.0%, 1.8 to 5.2%)	2/409 (0.5%, 0.1 to 1.8%)	15/791 (1.9%, 1.2 to 3.1%)
Perrier et al., 2005 (7)	524	MDCT	3/324 (0.9%, 0.3 to 2.7%)	5/292 (1.7%, 0.7 to 3.9%)	8/523 (1.5%, 0.8 to 3.0%)
Ghanima et al., 2005 (66)	329	MDCT	NA	2/221 (0.9%, 0.1 to 3.2%)	2/330 (0.6%, 0 to 2.2%)
Christopher study, 2006 (6)	2249	Both (90% MDCT)	NA	18/1436 (1.3%, 0.7 to 2.0%)	23/2464 (0.9%, 0.6 to 1.4%)
Anderson et al., 2007 (15)	694	Both (72% MDCT)	7/531 (1.3%, 0.6 to 2.7%)	2/524 (0.4%, 0.1 to 1.4%)	NDA
Righini et al., 2008 (69)	521	MDCT[c]	53 DVT before CT (9%, 7 to 12%)	2/383 (0.5%, 0.1 to 1.9%)	NDA[e]
	558	MDCT[d]	NA	2/364 (0.5%, 0.2 to 2.0%)	2/658 (0.3%, 0.1 to 1.1%)

[a]PE, pulmonary embolism; FN, false negative; CT, computed tomography; CUS, compression ultrasonography; DVT, deep vein thrombosis; MDCT, multidetector-row computed tomography; NA, not applicable; NDA, no data available; VTE, venous thromboembolism.
[b]From the total study population: proportion of patients without anticoagulants in whom PE was excluded that had VTE during follow-up or after negative CT scan.
[c]CDR–DD–CUS–CT strategy.
[d]CDR–DD–CT strategy.
[e]CUS performed before CT, therefore patients in whom DVT was detected on CUS did not undergo CT and no data are available on whether CUS had not been included in the strategy.

to 1.2%) for the D-dimer–CUS–CT strategy and the D-dimer–CT strategy, respectively. In this study, totalling 1819 patients, a strategy with MDCT alone yielded equal results to a strategy with MDCT combined with CUS. None of the patients with a high clinical probability and a negative MDCT had PE on additional testing or during follow-up. Hence adding CUS makes the strategy more complicated and more expensive.

CT venography

CT venography (CTV) is an imaging technique to detect lower extremity venous thrombi, by scanning the pelvis and leg veins 3–3.5 min after intravenous injection of contrast material for CT pulmonary angiography (30). As an alternative to venous ultrasonography, it is used as an adjuvant test after negative CTPA to increase the sensitivity for detecting VTE. There is high concordance between ultrasound and CT venography (78), while CT surpasses US in the diagnosis of pelvic DVT. The evidence remains contradictory as to what the role of CTV should be in the diagnostic algorithm for PE: whether it should be performed routinely and whether the additional diagnostic yield justifies the additional time, costs and radiation exposure. In the PIOPED II study, the sensitivity of VTE detection increased from 83 to 90% without affecting the specificity (78); this increase was not statistically significant. There was a small gain in negative predictive value, from 95 to 97%. In a recent prospective study investigating 829 patients who underwent MDCTA–CTV, isolated DVT was found in 28 (3.4%) of patients, giving an incremental value of CTV of 3.4% for the total population (79). This risk was 2.6% in patients classified as 'high risk': those with a high probability of PE, including those with a history of VTE and possible malignancy (79). The authors concluded that CTV should not be performed routinely in all patients, but may be useful in 'high-risk' patients. Nevertheless, because the necessity for lower limb vein investigation seems limited, CTV does not appear to improve the diagnostic yield of CTPA enough to justify the additional radiation.

False-positive results

After considering false-negative results and the sensitivity of CTPA, the question of whether verification tests should be performed in case of positive CTPA results should be addressed. Bayes' theorem predicts that using an assumed sensitivity of 92% and a specificity of 94% for CTPA, patients who have a low pre-test probability for PE (5%) will have a false-positive rate of approximately 55%, whereas this rate is 20% for those with a moderate pre-test probability (20%) (80). In the PIOPED II study, in patients who had a positive CTPA despite a low pre-test probability, the reference diagnosis was positive for PE in only 58% (78). Furthermore, in an accuracy study comparing MDCT with pulmonary angiography, eight of 26 positive CTPA results were not confirmed by pulmonary angiography (81), with the incorrectly identified thrombi on CT mostly detected in isolated segmental or subsegmental vessels. This was also a finding in the PIOPED II study (78). With the advent of 16-slice and even 64-slice or higher MDCT, the sensitivity of CTPA in the more distal arteries may well increase, but solely due to the higher number of clinically insignificant thrombi or false-positive results. So far, it remains unclear what the further testing in patients with such findings should be (82,83).

Strategies including V/Q scintigraphy

Large studies have shown that V/Q scanning is non-diagnostic, i.e., unable to exclude or confirm PE in the majority of patients (5), which means that these patients need additional diagnostic tests. In patients with a normal chest X-ray, the diagnostic yield of the V/Q scan is markedly increased, leading to a diagnostic outcome in up to 92% of patients (84,85). If V/Q scanning is combined with clinical probability and D-dimer testing, the proportion of patients who require additional testing remains high. After exclusion of patients with a low, low/intermediate or unlikely clinical probability and a normal D-dimer test, 48–54% of patients have a non-diagnostic V/Q scan (15,34,41,63). In a recent large diagnostic management study including patients with a likely clinical probability or an abnormal D-dimer test, 35% (247/712) of patients had normal scan results (of whom 0.8% had proximal DVT on US) and 54% (368/712) had non-diagnostic V/Q scans (of whom 7.0% were found to have VTE upon initial testing and 1% had VTE during the follow-up period) (15) (Figure 15.1).

Non-diagnostic V/Q scan

The prevalence of PE in patients with a non-diagnostic V/Q scan varies, but it is acknowledged that these patients require additional tests such as ultrasound, pulmonary angiography or CT (32). In patients with a low or moderate pre-test probability, it is assumed that a normal CUS in combination with a non-diagnostic V/Q scan excludes PE sufficiently (3 month VTE failure rate: 1.2–2.4%) (15,33,34,41,67,86). Patients with high pre-test probability and a non-diagnostic V/Q scan should undergo pulmonary angiography, CT or serial CUS. In a recent study, the CT scan was positive for PE in six out of 23 patients with a non-diagnostic V/Q scan and normal ultrasound and three out of six pulmonary angiograms were positive for PE (15). Wells *et al.* (41) used the D-dimer to guide further management after a negative CUS and non-diagnostic V/Q scan in patients with moderate or high clinical probability. If the D-dimer was positive, serial CUS or pulmonary angiography was the next step in the algorithm. This was not performed, however, in 47% of the patients in whom it was indicated (41). Kearon *et al.* also used the D-dimer test to guide further management; PE was diagnosed with additional testing in four of 140 patients with a high pre-test probability, non-diagnostic V/Q scan, normal CUS and abnormal D-dimer (2.9%) (67).

Strategies including chest X-ray–perfusion scintigraphy (X/Q scan)

Although ventilation–perfusion scintigraphy is an established diagnostic test, ventilation scintigraphy is expensive and not available daily in all hospitals. Therefore, elimination of ventilation scintigraphy will reduce costs and radiation (30). The PISA-PED study was performed to assess the value of a perfusion lung scan alone (without a ventilation imaging) in combination with clinical assessment, with pulmonary angiography as the reference standard (87). Depending on the presence of wedge-shaped defects on the lung scan, it was possible to accurately diagnose or exclude PE (sensitivity and specificity 86% and 93%, respectively) (87). To date, there has been only one modest prospective management outcome study, including 200 patients, that has investigated a strategy with clinical pre-test probability, D-dimer testing and perfusion scintigraphy (72). The chest X-ray was added in case the observed perfusion defects could result in a high-probability chest X-ray–perfusion (X/Q) scan, i.e., if there were at least two segmental perfusion defects. Ultrasonography and if necessary: pulmonary angiography were performed in case the scan was non-diagnostic. Although none of the 31 patients with a normal lung scan developed VTE during follow-up (72), caution is required in interpreting high-probability X/Q scans, since the positive predictive value of this strategy is still unclear.

Although CTPA has now largely taken over the place of pulmonary scintigraphy as the main imaging test in the diagnostic management of patients with suspected PE, it still has a role in selected patients, such as those with an iodinated contrast material allergy or renal impairment or women of reproductive age.

Strategies including ultrasonography

The role of ultrasonography as adjuvant diagnostic test after normal single-slice CTPA or non-diagnostic V/Q scan has been described earlier. The interpretation of the test outcome is dependent also on the pre-test clinical probability. Instead of functioning as a safety net after these imaging tests, some advocate that performing ultrasonography as the first imaging technique after clinical probability assessment and D-dimer testing may have advantages (34,36,64,69,71,86,88). Although due to the low sensitivity for PE a negative proximal CUS result should always be followed by additional testing, a positive ultrasound is specific for PE. A positive CUS result therefore diagnoses PE and no further testing is necessary. Ultrasonography is a safe and non-invasive imaging technique; performing CUS before (single-slice) CTPA or V/Q scanning might reduce costs and radiation exposure for a proportion of patients. However, many patients will have to be screened and the diagnostic yield is low, thereby jeopardizing the cost-effectiveness. In addition, when multi-detector row CTPA is used, the role of CUS remains debatable.

DIAGNOSTIC STRATEGIES IN SELECTED PATIENTS

Allergy to iodinated contrast material or impaired renal function

CTPA is contraindicated in patients with a moderate or severe iodine allergy or renal impairment because of the use of contrast material. These patients were usually excluded from studies and therefore the available data are limited. However, clinical assessment and D-dimer testing can still be performed. If this fails to exclude PE, then patients with mild to moderate iodine allergies may be pre-treated (with hydrocortisone and diphenhydramine) and then imaged with CT. Alternatively, V/Q scanning can be done. A normal V/Q scan excludes the diagnosis, while a high-probability V/Q scan in combination with a high clinical pre-test probability showed PE in 96% (5). In case of a non-diagnostic V/Q results (PE prevalence: 16–88%) (5), further evaluation with, for instance, ultrasonography is necessary. Gadolinium-enhanced MRA could be a welcome alternative; a large-scale study to evaluate its role in diagnostic management is currently under way.

Young women

Another group of patients for whom pulmonary scintigraphy could be the imaging test of first choice is women of reproductive age (younger than 50 years). Recently, concerns have been raised regarding the risk of cancer following radiation exposure with (repeated) CT scanning and the increased risk of breast cancer, especially in young women (56,57). In an average woman weighing 60 kg, breast irradiation with CT angiography is 10–20 mGy per breast (89,90) and up to 190 mGy with CT angiography in a woman with large breasts (91). For comparison, breast irradiation with a ventilation-perfusion scan is approximately 0.28 mGy (89). It can be expected that in these young and often otherwise healthy individuals a perfusion scan would suffice, possibly in combination with a chest X-ray (84). This strategy would reduce both costs and radiation exposure. Time and cost permitting, women of reproductive age could be another subgroup of patients who could benefit from MRA in the future. Because of the debatable additional yield in diagnosing VTE and the high (additional) radiation dose, CTV is not recommended in this group of patients (30).

In- or outpatients

Most diagnostic management studies are based on outpatients or a combination of in- and outpatients, but rarely on inpatients alone. The stratification of patients in different pre-test probability categories is effective, also in inpatients (92,93) The clinical usefulness of the D-dimer test in inpatients is limited because of the low prevalence of a normal D-dimer (7–19%) and the low specificity (92,94,95). The proportion of patients with a low/unlikely clinical probability in combination with a normal D-dimer test is therefore also smaller (10%) (93), which means that relatively more hospitalized patients need imaging testing compared with outpatients. In a recent analysis of 605 hospitalized patients, the largest cohort of hospitalized patients to date, a strategy including clinical decision rule, D-dimer and CTPA was evaluated. In this study, there were no observed VTE events during follow-up (failure rate 0%; 95% CI: 0 to 6.7%). Even so, with this number of patients the upper limit of the 95% CI was 6.7%, which may be considered too high (93). The study also showed that it was safe to withhold anticoagulant therapy in hospitalized patients with a normal CTPA as the sole imaging technique (VTE rate 1.3%; 95% CI: 2 to 4.7%) (93). Alternatively, a V/Q scan could be performed, although the diagnostic yield is expected to be much lower compared with outpatients because of the frequent co-morbidity.

The elderly

With increasing age the clinical utility of the D-dimer test decreases (96,97). This results in a lower proportion of elderly patients in whom PE can be excluded by clinical assessment and D-dimer testing (10%) (98). In a sub-study of 47 patients older than 75 years with this combination, the incidence of VTE events during the follow-up period did not differ from the total population (0%; 95% CI: 0 to 7.9%) (98). The clinical utility of the V/Q scan is also dependent on age. The diagnostic yield is almost twice as low in patients older than 70 years than in patients younger than 40 years (58% and 32% non-diagnostic test results, respectively) (99). Although the sensitivity is lower in higher age groups, subgroup analysis of patients older than 75 years showed that it was safe to withhold anticoagulant therapy in patients with a normal CTPA (failure rate 0.3%; 95% CI: 0.01 to 1.9%). A negative result on single-slice CT is not sufficient to exclude the diagnosis and further evaluation, e.g., with CUS, is necessary (99).

Patient with suspected recurrent PE

Despite the fact that 10–20% of patients with PE will have a recurrence during the first 2 years after the initial event, the data on the diagnostic management in suspected recurrent PE are very limited. Currently, there is only one study that evaluated the safety of excluding the diagnosis in patients with suspected recurrent PE on the basis of an unlikely clinical decision rule, a normal D-dimer test or a negative CTPA (100). In this sub-analysis of 259 patients with suspected recurrent PE, withholding anticoagulant therapy in patients with an unlikely clinical pre-test probability and a normal D-dimer was safe (failure rate 0%; 95% CI: 0 to 6.9%). With 16% of patients meeting these criteria, the clinical utility was lower compared with patients with a suspected first episode of PE. In the remaining patients in whom the diagnosis could not be excluded by clinical probability and D-dimer testing, anticoagulant therapy could safely be withheld based on a normal CTPA (failure rate 0.8; 95% CI: 0.02 to 4.3%) (100). To date, this is the only prospective study assessing the value of a standardized diagnostic strategy in patients with suspected recurrent PE.

COST-EFFECTIVENESS OF DIAGNOSTIC STRATEGIES

Several cost-effectiveness analyses comparing various diagnostic strategies have been published (48,101–104). Decision analysis models were used to compare the strategies, based on mortality/morbidity data or accuracy of excluding/diagnosing PE, combined with the associated costs for testing, the treatment and the extra costs for missed diagnoses. Strategies including clinical stratification according to pre-test probability assessment reduce the requirement for invasive tests and have been shown to be cost-effective (5,41,48,77). Whatever the diagnostic strategy and for patients up to the age of 80 years, D-dimer testing was highly cost saving (101). In older patients, the cost-effectiveness of D-dimer was remarkably lower; the costs were similar for strategies including or not including D-dimer testing. Of note, D-dimer testing in patients older than 80 years did not increase the costs of diagnostic strategies (101) and although the clinical usefulness may be lower, additional imaging tests can be avoided in 10% of patients when D-dimer testing is used (98). Sensitivity analyses showed that the sensitivity of CTPA was important in selecting the appropriate strategy (48). CTPA sensitivity above 85% was necessary in order to reduce mortality and to improve cost-effectiveness. Whereas MDCT-based strategies were very cost-effective, strategies including single-slice CTPA were not and were even less cost-effective than strategies including V/Q scanning (48).

In a recent cost-effectiveness analysis focusing on diagnostic strategies as a function of age, the four different strategies that were evaluated were equally safe: variations in the 3 month survival did not exceed 0.5% as compared with the most effective strategy (101) (Figure 15.5). The same group also investigated the cost-effectiveness of CTPA alone, an imaging technique that has never

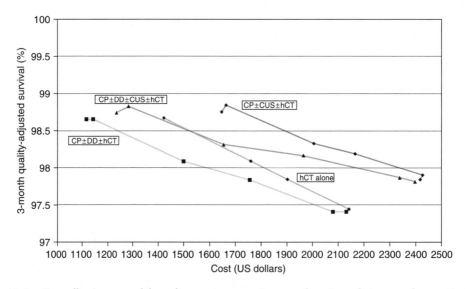

Figure 15.5 Cost-effectiveness of four diagnostic strategies as a function of six age classes. Each box represents the cost-effectiveness for increasing age class: from left to right: <40, 40–49, 50–59, 60–69, 70–79,>80 years. The 3 month quality-adjusted expected survival was selected as the main outcome measure for effectiveness. CP, clinical probability; DD, D-dimer measurement; CUS, compression ultrasonography; HCT, (multi-slice) helical computed tomography. Righini M, Nendaz M, Le Gal G, Bounameaux H and Perrier A. Influence of age on the cost-effectiveness of diagnostic strategies for suspected pulmonary embolism. J Thromb Haemost 2007; 5:1869–77. Reproduced by permission of Blackwell Publishing.

been prospectively evaluated as a single diagnostic test in management studies. Its effectiveness was only slightly lower than that of other validated diagnostic strategies. The authors speculated that it could be a less expensive strategy in hospitalized elderly patients, where the diagnostic yield from clinical probability assessment and D-dimer testing is low. This, however, has not been prospectively evaluated. The secondary advantage of finding alternative diagnoses on CTPA was not included in the cost-effectiveness analyses. According to the most recent cost-effectiveness analysis, the least expensive diagnostic strategy is composed of clinical probability and D-dimer testing, if necessary followed by MDCT (101). This is the same strategy that was proposed and studied in three large and recent outcome studies (6,7,66).

CONCLUSION

Following diagnostic algorithms improves patient care (21). To date, several diagnostic strategies have been validated. It is important to adhere to these algorithms, as inappropriate use can increase the recurrence of VTE (21). The first step in the diagnostic work-up of patients with suspected PE is to assess the clinical probability. In combination with D-dimer testing, the diagnosis can be safely excluded in a substantial proportion of patients, who will not have to undergo further testing. In patients who need additional testing, several options are possible. If the clinical status of the patient permits, the next recommended step is MDCT or V/Q scan, followed by additional testing in case of non-diagnostic test results. Further research should determine if additional testing is also necessary in case of discordance with the outcome of the pre-test probability and the imaging test. Although our current knowledge is based on large outcome studies including several thousand patients and covering a wide range of presentations and patient characteristics, in the end, the clinical status and the experience with and availability of diagnostic tools should decide what strategy is chosen.

REFERENCES

1. White RH. The epidemiology of venous thromboembolism. *Circulation* 2003; **107**(23 Suppl 1):I4–I8.
2. Douketis JD, Kearon C, Bates S, Duku EK, Ginsberg JS. Risk of fatal pulmonary embolism in patients with treated venous thromboembolism. *JAMA* 1998; **279**(6):458–62.
3. Levine MN, Raskob G, Beyth RJ, Kearon C, Schulman S. Hemorrhagic complications of anticoagulant treatment: the Seventh ACCP Conference on Antithrombotic and Thrombolytic Therapy. *Chest* 2004; **126**(3 Suppl):287S–310S.
4. Linkins LA, Choi PT, Douketis JD. Clinical impact of bleeding in patients taking oral anticoagulant therapy for venous thromboembolism: a meta-analysis. *Ann Intern Med* 2003; **139**(11):893–900.
5. Value of the ventilation/perfusion scan in acute pulmonary embolism. Results of the prospective investigation of pulmonary embolism diagnosis (PIOPED). The PIOPED Investigators. *JAMA* 1990; **263**(20):2753–9.
6. van Belle A, Büller HR, Huisman MV, *et al*. Effectiveness of managing suspected pulmonary embolism using an algorithm combining clinical probability, D-dimer testing and computed tomography. *JAMA* 2006; **295**(2):172–9.
7. Perrier A, Roy PM, Sanchez O, *et al*. Multidetector-row computed tomography in suspected pulmonary embolism. *N Engl J Med* 2005; **352**(17):1760–8.
8. Prologo JD, Gilkeson RC, Diaz M, Asaad J. CT pulmonary angiography: a comparative analysis of the utilization patterns in emergency department and hospitalized patients between 1998 and 2003. *AJR Am J Roentgenol* 2004; **183**(4):1093–6.
9. Le Gal G, Bounameaux H. Diagnosing pulmonary embolism: running after the decreasing prevalence of cases among suspected patients. *J Thromb Haemost* 2004; **2**(8):1244–6.
10. Williams JR, Wilcox C, Andrews GJ, Burns RR. Angiography in pulmonary embolism. *JAMA* 1963; **184**:473–6.

11. Wagner HN, Jr, Sabiston DC, Jr, McAfee JG, Tow D, Stern HS. Diagnosis of massive pulmonary embolism in man by radioisotope scanning. *N Engl J Med* 1964; **271**:377–84.

12. Dalen JE. Pulmonary embolism: what have we learned since Virchow? Natural history, pathophysiology and diagnosis. *Chest* 2002; **122**(4):1440–56.

13. Hull RD, Raskob GE, Coates G, Panju AA. Clinical validity of a normal perfusion lung scan in patients with suspected pulmonary embolism. *Chest* 1990; **97**(1):23–6.

14. van Beek EJ, Kuyer PM, Schenk BE, Brandjes DP, ten Cate JW, Büller HR. A normal perfusion lung scan in patients with clinically suspected pulmonary embolism. Frequency and clinical validity. *Chest* 1995; **108**(1):170–3.

15. Anderson DR, Kahn SR, Rodger MA, *et al.* Computed tomographic pulmonary angiography vs ventilation–perfusion lung scanning in patients with suspected pulmonary embolism: a randomized controlled trial. *JAMA* 2007; **298**(23):2743–53.

16. Kruip MJ, Leclercq MG, van der Heul C, Prins MH, Büller HR. Diagnostic strategies for excluding pulmonary embolism in clinical outcome studies. A systematic review. *Ann Intern Med* 2003; **138**(12):941–51.

17. Goldhaber SZ. Pulmonary embolism. *Lancet* 2004; **363**(9417):1295–305.

18. Stein PD, Athanasoulis C, Alavi A, *et al.* Complications and validity of pulmonary angiography in acute pulmonary embolism. *Circulation* 1992; **85**(2):462–8.

19. Le Gal G, Righini M, Roy PM, *et al.* Differential value of risk factors and clinical signs for diagnosing pulmonary embolism according to age. *J Thromb Haemost* 2005; **3**(11):2457–64.

20. Schluger N, Henschke C, King T, *et al.* Diagnosis of pulmonary embolism at a large teaching hospital. *J Thorac Imaging* 1994; **9**(3):180–4.

21. Roy PM, Meyer G, Vielle B, *et al.* Appropriateness of diagnostic management and outcomes of suspected pulmonary embolism. *Ann Intern Med* 2006; **144**(3):157–64.

22. Berghout A, Oudkerk M, Hicks SG, Teng TH, Pillay M, Büller HR. Active implementation of a consensus strategy improves diagnosis and management in suspected pulmonary embolism. *QJM* 2000; **93**(6):335–40.

23. Kline JA, Nelson RD, Jackson RE, Courtney DM. Criteria for the safe use of D-dimer testing in emergency department patients with suspected pulmonary embolism: a multicenter US study. *Ann Emerg Med* 2002; **39**(2):144–52.

24. Miniati M, Prediletto R, Formichi B, *et al.* Accuracy of clinical assessment in the diagnosis of pulmonary embolism. *Am J Respir Crit Care Med* 1999; **159**(3):864–71.

25. Wicki J, Perneger TV, Junod AF, Bounameaux H, Perrier A. Assessing clinical probability of pulmonary embolism in the emergency ward: a simple score. *Arch Intern Med* 2001; **161**(1):92–7.

26. Wells PS, Anderson DR, Rodger M, *et al.* Derivation of a simple clinical model to categorize patients probability of pulmonary embolism: increasing the models utility with the SimpliRED D-dimer. *Thromb Haemost* 2000; **83**(3):416–20.

27. Le Gal G, Righini M, Roy PM, *et al.* Prediction of pulmonary embolism in the emergency department: the Revised Geneva score. *Ann Intern Med* 2006; **144**(3):165–71.

28. Stein PD, Woodard PK, Weg JG, *et al.* Diagnostic pathways in acute pulmonary embolism: recommendations of the PIOPED II investigators. *Am J Med* 2006; **119**(12):1048–55.

29. Qaseem A, Snow V, Barry P, *et al.* Current diagnosis of venous thromboembolism in primary care: a clinical practice guideline from the American Academy of Family Physicians and the American College of Physicians. *Ann Fam Med* 2007; **5**(1):57–62.

30. Remy-Jardin M, Pistolesi M, Goodman LR, *et al.* Management of suspected acute pulmonary embolism in the era of CT angiography: a statement from the Fleischner Society. *Radiology* 2007; **245**(2):315–29.

31. Kamphuisen PW, Oudkerk M. Diagnosis of deep-vein thrombosis and pulmonary embolism: the new guideline of the Dutch Institute for Health Care Improvement. *Imaging Decisions MRI* 2007; **11**(3):3–7.

32. British Thoracic Society Standards of Care Committee Pulmonary Embolism Guideline Development Group. British Thoracic Society guidelines for the management of suspected acute pulmonary embolism. *Thorax* 2003; **58**(6):470–83.

33. Perrier A, Bounameaux H, Morabia A, *et al.* Diagnosis of pulmonary embolism by a decision analysis-based strategy including clinical probability, D-dimer levels and ultrasonography: a management study. *Arch Intern Med* 1996; **156**(5):531–6.

34. Perrier A, Desmarais S, Miron MJ, *et al.* Non-invasive diagnosis of venous thromboembolism in outpatients. *Lancet* 1999; **353**(9148):190–5.

35. Sanson BJ, Lijmer JG, Mac Gillavry MR, Turkstra F, Prins MH, Büller HR. Comparison of a clinical probability estimate and two clinical models in patients with suspected pulmonary embolism. ANTELOPE Study Group. *Thromb Haemost* 2000; **83**(2):199–203.

36. Musset D, Parent F, Meyer G, *et al*. Diagnostic strategy for patients with suspected pulmonary embolism: a prospective multicentre outcome study. *Lancet* 2002; **360**(9349):1914–20.

37. Kabrhel C, Camargo CA, Jr, Goldhaber SZ. Clinical gestalt and the diagnosis of pulmonary embolism: does experience matter? *Chest* 2005; **127**(5):1627–30.

38. Rosen MP, Sands DZ, Morris J, Drake W, Davis RB. Does a physician's ability to accurately assess the likelihood of pulmonary embolism increase with training? *Acad Med* 2000; **75**(12):1199–205.

39. Chunilal SD, Eikelboom JW, Attia J, *et al*. Does this patient have pulmonary embolism? *JAMA* 2003; **290**(21):2849–58.

40. Wells PS. Integrated strategies for the diagnosis of venous thromboembolism. *J Thromb Haemost* 2007; 5(Suppl 1): 41–50.

41. Wells PS, Anderson DR, Rodger M, *et al*. Excluding pulmonary embolism at the bedside without diagnostic imaging: management of patients with suspected pulmonary embolism presenting to the emergency department by using a simple clinical model and D-dimer. *Ann Intern Med* 2001; **135**(2):98–107.

42. Wolf SJ, McCubbin TR, Feldhaus KM, Faragher JP, Adcock DM. Prospective validation of Wells criteria in the evaluation of patients with suspected pulmonary embolism. *Ann Emerg Med* 2004; **44**(5):503–10.

43. Rodger MA, Maser E, Stiell I, Howley HE, Wells PS. The interobserver reliability of pretest probability assessment in patients with suspected pulmonary embolism. *Thromb Res* 2005; **116**(2):101–7.

44. Penaloza A, Melot C, Dochy E, *et al*. Assessment of pretest probability of pulmonary embolism in the emergency department by physicians in training using the Wells model. *Thromb Res* 2007; **120**(2):173–9.

45. Iles S, Hodges AM, Darley JR, *et al*. Clinical experience and pre-test probability scores in the diagnosis of pulmonary embolism. *QJM* 2003; **96**(3):211–5.

46. Tamariz LJ, Eng J, Segal JB, *et al*. Usefulness of clinical prediction rules for the diagnosis of venous thromboembolism: a systematic review. *Am J Med* 2004; **117**(9):676–84.

47. Sackett DL, Haynes RB, Guyatt GH, Tugwell P. *Clinical Epidemiology: a Basic Science for Clinical Medicine*, 2nd edn. Little, Brown, Boston, 1991.

48. Perrier A, Nendaz MR, Sarasin FP, Howarth N, Bounameaux H. Cost-effectiveness analysis of diagnostic strategies for suspected pulmonary embolism including helical computed tomography. *Am J Respir Crit Care Med* 2003; **167**(1):39–44.

49. Di Nisio M, Squizzato A, Rutjes AW, Büller HR, Zwinderman AH, Bossuyt PM. Diagnostic accuracy of D-dimer test for exclusion of venous thromboembolism: a systematic review. *J Thromb Haemost* 2007; **5**(2):296–304.

50. Stein PD, Hull RD, Patel KC, *et al*. D-dimer for the exclusion of acute venous thrombosis and pulmonary embolism: a systematic review. *Ann Intern Med* 2004; **140**(8):589–602.

51. Ghaye B, Dondelinger RF. When to perform CTA in patients suspected of PE? *Eur Radiol* 2008; **18**(3):500–9.

52. Rathbun SW, Raskob GE, Whitsett TL. Sensitivity and specificity of helical computed tomography in the diagnosis of pulmonary embolism: a systematic review. *Ann Intern Med* 2000; **132**(3):227–32.

53. Hayashino Y, Goto M, Noguchi Y, Fukui T. Ventilation-perfusion scanning and helical CT in suspected pulmonary embolism: meta-analysis of diagnostic performance. *Radiology* 2005; **234**(3):740–8.

54. Patel S, Kazerooni EA, Cascade PN. Pulmonary embolism: optimization of small pulmonary artery visualization at multi-detector row CT. *Radiology* 2003; **227**(2):455–60.

55. Van Strijen MJ, de Monye W, Schiereck J, *et al*. Single-detector helical computed tomography as the primary diagnostic test in suspected pulmonary embolism: a multicenter clinical management study of 510 patients. *Ann Intern Med* 2003; **138**(4):307–14.

56. Brenner DJ, Hall EJ. Computed tomography–an increasing source of radiation exposure. *N Engl J Med* 2007; **357**(22):2277–84.

57. Einstein AJ, Henzlova MJ, Rajagopalan S. Estimating risk of cancer associated with radiation exposure from 64-slice computed tomography coronary angiography. *JAMA* 2007; **298**(3):317–23.

58. Girard P, Musset D, Parent F, Maitre S, Phlippoteau C, Simonneau G. High prevalence of detectable deep venous thrombosis in patients with acute pulmonary embolism. *Chest* 1999; **116**(4):903–8.

59. Henry JW, Relyea B, Stein PD. Continuing risk of thromboemboli among patients with normal pulmonary angiograms. *Chest* 1995; **107**(5):1375–8.

60. Gosselin MV, Rubin GD, Leung AN, Huang J, Rizk NW. Unsuspected pulmonary embolism: prospective detection on routine helical CT scans. *Radiology* 1998; **208**(1):209–15.

61. Storto ML, Di Credico A, Guido F, Larici AR, Bonomo L. Incidental detection of pulmonary emboli on routine MDCT of the chest. *AJR Am J Roentgenol* 2005; **184**(1):264–7.

62. Cronin CG, Lohan DG, Keane M, Roche C, Murphy JM. Prevalence and significance of asymptomatic venous thromboembolic disease found on oncologic staging CT. *AJR Am J Roentgenol* 2007; **189**(1):162–70.

63. ten Wolde M, Hagen PJ, MacGillavry MR, *et al*. Non-invasive diagnostic work-up of patients with clinically suspected pulmonary embolism; results of a management study. *J Thromb Haemost* 2004; **2**(7):1110–7.

64. Perrier A, Roy PM, Aujesky D, *et al*. Diagnosing pulmonary embolism in outpatients with clinical assessment, D-dimer measurement, venous ultrasound and helical computed tomography: a multicenter management study. *Am J Med* 2004; **116**(5):291–9.

65. Anderson DR, Kovacs MJ, Dennie C, *et al*. Use of spiral computed tomography contrast angiography and ultrasonography to exclude the diagnosis of pulmonary embolism in the emergency department. *J Emerg Med* 2005; **29**(4):399–404.

66. Ghanima W, Almaas V, Aballi S, *et al*. Management of suspected pulmonary embolism (PE) by D-dimer and multi-slice computed tomography in outpatients: an outcome study. *J Thromb Haemost* 2005; **3**(9):1926–32.

67. Kearon C, Ginsberg JS, Douketis J, *et al*. An evaluation of D-dimer in the diagnosis of pulmonary embolism: a randomized trial. *Ann Intern Med* 2006; **144**(11):812–21.

68. Goekoop RJ, Steeghs N, Niessen RW, *et al*. Simple and safe exclusion of pulmonary embolism in outpatients using quantitative D-dimer and Wells' simplified decision rule. *Thromb Haemost* 2007; **97**(1):146–50.

69. Righini M, Le Gal G, Aujesky D, *et al*. Diagnosis of pulmonary embolism by multidetector CT alone or combined with venous ultrasonography of the leg: a randomised non-inferiority trial. *Lancet* 2008; **371**(9621):1343–52.

70. ten Cate-Hoek AJ, Prins MH. Management studies using a combination of D-dimer test result and clinical probability to rule out venous thromboembolism: a systematic review. *J Thromb Haemost* 2005; **3**(11):2465–70.

71. Kruip MJ, Slob MJ, Schijen JH, van der Heul C, Büller HR. Use of a clinical decision rule in combination with D-dimer concentration in diagnostic work-up of patients with suspected pulmonary embolism: a prospective management study. *Arch Intern Med* 2002; **162**(14):1631–5.

72. Leclercq MG, Lutisan JG, van Marwijk KM, *et al*. Ruling out clinically suspected pulmonary embolism by assessment of clinical probability and D-dimer levels: a management study. *Thromb Haemost* 2003; **89**(1):97–103.

73. Kelly J, Hunt BJ. A clinical probability assessment and D-dimer measurement should be the initial step in the investigation of suspected venous thromboembolism. *Chest* 2003; **124**(3):1116–9.

74. Ginsberg JS, Wells PS, Kearon C, *et al*. Sensitivity and specificity of a rapid whole-blood assay for D-dimer in the diagnosis of pulmonary embolism. *Ann Intern Med* 1998; **129**(12):1006–11.

75. Agnelli G, Becattini C, Kirschstein T. Thrombolysis vs heparin in the treatment of pulmonary embolism: a clinical outcome-based meta-analysis. *Arch Intern Med* 2002; **162**(22):2537–41.

76. Gibson NS, Sohne M, Gerdes VE, Nijkeuter M, Büller HR. The importance of clinical probability assessment in interpreting a normal D-dimer in patients with suspected pulmonary embolism. *Chest* 2008; **134**(4):789–93.

77. Wells PS, Ginsberg JS, Anderson DR, *et al*. Use of a clinical model for safe management of patients with suspected pulmonary embolism. *Ann Intern Med* 1998; **129**(12):997–1005.

78. Stein PD, Fowler SE, Goodman LR, *et al*. Multidetector computed tomography for acute pulmonary embolism. *N Engl J Med* 2006; **354**(22):2317–27.

79. Hunsaker AR, Zou KH, Poh AC, *et al*. Routine pelvic and lower extremity CT venography in patients undergoing pulmonary CT angiography. *AJR Am J Roentgenol* 2008; **190**(2):322–6.

80. Ranji SR, Shojania KG, Trowbridge RL, Auerbach AD. Impact of reliance on CT pulmonary angiography on diagnosis of pulmonary embolism: a Bayesian analysis. *J Hosp Med* 2006; **1**(2):81–7.

81. Winer-Muram HT, Rydberg J, Johnson MS, *et al*. Suspected acute pulmonary embolism: evaluation with multi-detector row CT versus digital subtraction pulmonary arteriography. *Radiology* 2004; **233**(3):806–15.

82. Le Gal G, Righini M, Parent F, van Strijen M, Couturaud F. Diagnosis and management of subsegmental pulmonary embolism. *J Thromb Haemost* 2006; **4**(4):724–31.

83. Goodman LR. Small pulmonary emboli: what do we know? *Radiology* 2005; **234**(3):654–8.

84. Forbes KP, Reid JH, Murchison JT. Do preliminary chest X-ray findings define the optimum role of pulmonary scintigraphy in suspected pulmonary embolism? *Clin Radiol* 2001; **56**(5):397–400.

85. Stein PD, Alavi A, Gottschalk A, *et al*. Usefulness of noninvasive diagnostic tools for diagnosis of acute pulmonary embolism in patients with a normal chest radiograph. *Am J Cardiol* 1991; **67**(13):1117–20.

86. Bosson JL, Barro C, Satger B, Carpentier PH, Polack B, Pernod G. Quantitative high D-dimer value is predictive of pulmonary embolism occurrence independently of clinical score in a well-defined low risk factor population. *J Thromb Haemost* 2005; **3**(1):93–9.

87. Miniati M, Pistolesi M, Marini C, *et al.* Value of perfusion lung scan in the diagnosis of pulmonary embolism: results of the Prospective Investigative Study of Acute Pulmonary Embolism Diagnosis (PISA-PED). *Am J Respir Crit Care Med* 1996; **154**(5):1387–93.

88. Elias A, Cazanave A, Elias M, *et al.* Diagnostic management of pulmonary embolism using clinical assessment, plasma D-dimer assay, complete lower limb venous ultrasound and helical computed tomography of pulmonary arteries. A multicentre clinical outcome study. *Thromb Haemost* 2005; **93**(5):982–8.

89. Cook JV, Kyriou J. Radiation from CT and perfusion scanning in pregnancy. *BMJ* 2005; **331**(7512):350.

90. Parker MS, Hui FK, Camacho MA, Chung JK, Broga DW, Sethi NN. Female breast radiation exposure during CT pulmonary angiography. *AJR Am J Roentgenol* 2005; **185**(5):1228–33.

91. Milne EN. Female breast radiation exposure. *AJR Am J Roentgenol* 2006; **186**(6):E24–.

92. Miron MJ, Perrier A, Bounameaux H, *et al.* Contribution of noninvasive evaluation to the diagnosis of pulmonary embolism in hospitalized patients. *Eur Respir J* 1999; **13**(6):1365–70.

93. Kruip MJ, Sohne M, Nijkeuter M, *et al.* A simple diagnostic strategy in hospitalized patients with clinically suspected pulmonary embolism. *J Intern Med* 2006; **260**(5):459–66.

94. Brotman DJ, Segal JB, Jani JT, Petty BG, Kickler TS. Limitations of D-dimer testing in unselected inpatients with suspected venous thromboembolism. *Am J Med* 2003; **114**(4):276–82.

95. Schrecengost JE, LeGallo RD, Boyd JC, *et al.* Comparison of diagnostic accuracies in outpatients and hospitalized patients of D-dimer testing for the evaluation of suspected pulmonary embolism. *Clin Chem* 2003; **49**(9):1483–90.

96. Sohne M, Kamphuisen PW, van Mierlo PJ, Büller HR. Diagnostic strategy using a modified clinical decision rule and D-dimer test to rule out pulmonary embolism in elderly in- and outpatients. *Thromb Haemost* 2005; **94**(1):206–10.

97. Righini M, Le Gal G, Perrier A, Bounameaux H. The challenge of diagnosing pulmonary embolism in elderly patients: influence of age on commonly used diagnostic tests and strategies. *J Am Geriatr Soc* 2005; **53**(6):1039–45.

98. Sohne M, Kruip MJ, Nijkeuter M, *et al.* Accuracy of clinical decision rule, D-dimer and spiral computed tomography in patients with malignancy, previous venous thromboembolism, COPD or heart failure and in older patients with suspected pulmonary embolism. *J Thromb Haemost* 2006; **4**(5):1042–6.

99. Righini M, Goehring C, Bounameaux H, Perrier A. Effects of age on the performance of common diagnostic tests for pulmonary embolism. *Am J Med* 2000; **109**(5):357–61.

100. Nijkeuter M, van Kwakkel EH, Sohne M, *et al.* Clinically suspected acute recurrent pulmonary embolism: a diagnostic challenge. *Thromb Haemost* 2007; **97**(6):944–8.

101. Righini M, Nendaz M, Le Gal G, Bounameaux H, Perrier A. Influence of age on the cost-effectiveness of diagnostic strategies for suspected pulmonary embolism. *J Thromb Haemost* 2007; **5**(9):1869–77.

102. Paterson DI, Schwartzman K. Strategies incorporating spiral CT for the diagnosis of acute pulmonary embolism: a cost-effectiveness analysis. *Chest* 2001; **119**(6):1791–800.

103. Hull RD, Feldstein W, Stein PD, Pineo GF. Cost-effectiveness of pulmonary embolism diagnosis. *Arch Intern Med* 1996; **156**(1):68–72.

104. Oudkerk M, van Beek EJ, van Putten WL, Büller HR. Cost-effectiveness analysis of various strategies in the diagnostic management of pulmonary embolism. *Arch Intern Med* 1993; **153**(8):947–54.

105. Hyers TM. Venous thromboembolism. *Am J Respir Crit Care Med* 1999; **159**(1):1–14.

CHAPTER 16

Management of Venous Thromboembolism in Pregnancy

Wee Shian Chan[1] and Jeffrey S. Ginsberg[2]

[1]Department of Medicine, University of Toronto Women's College Hospital,
Ontario, Canada
[2]Department of Medicine, Thromboembolism Unit, McMaster Medical Centre,
Ontario, Canada

EPIDEMIOLOGY

The risk of venous thromboembolism (VTE), which includes both deep vein thrombosis (DVT) and pulmonary embolism (PE), is increased 10-fold during pregnancy compared with age-matched non-pregnant women (1). The absolute overall risk of DVT or PE in pregnancy is nevertheless low, at 0.5–1 in 1000 pregnancies (2–4). The risk of VTE is increased in the postpartum period compared with the antepartum period (5–8) and is dependent on the mode of delivery. Results from four large population-based studies estimate that the risk of VTE is 0.9–7.5 per 10 000 patients for vaginal deliveries compared with 7.8–59 per 10 000 patients for Caesarean sections (5–8).

Despite the low incidence of VTE, it remains the major cause of maternal mortality in developed countries (8–10); an awareness, early diagnosis and appropriate management by clinicians of this condition in pregnant patients remain critical in reducing maternal mortality and morbidity.

PATHOPHYSIOLOGY OF VENOUS THROMBOEMBOLISM

The increased risk of VTE during pregnancy might partly result from changes in the haemostatic and fibrinolytic systems (11,12). Increased levels of coagulation factors, such as fibrinogen and factor VIII, and decreased levels of coagulation inhibitors, such as protein S (11,12), could serve to promote a 'prothrombotic state'. In addition to changes in the coagulation system, physiological alterations during pregnancy cause venous stasis in the lower extremities that could predispose patients to venous thrombosis (13–15). There is increased lower extremity venous diameter and decreased flow, probably as a result of hormonal influences on vascular tone and the compressive effects on the veins by the enlarging uterus (13–15). This latter physiological change, which is

Deep Vein Thrombosis and Pulmonary Embolism Edited by Edwin J.R. van Beek, Harry R. Büller and Matthijs Oudkerk
© 2009 John Wiley & Sons, Ltd

exaggerated for the left lower extremity venous system, could explain the resultant preponderance of left leg DVT observed and an overall increased risk of VTE during pregnancy (16).

The importance of accurate VTE diagnosis and appropriate management of VTE in pregnant patients, as with non-pregnant patients, is indisputable. Unfortunately, there are few well-designed clinical trials of VTE diagnosis and management in pregnant patients (17). Current recommendations in this chapter surrounding appropriate diagnosis and management of VTE during pregnancy are still mostly extrapolated from studies in non-pregnant patients and from observational data in pregnant patients.

During the last two decades, a plethora of observational studies have also been published linking adverse pregnancy events to thrombophilic disorders (18–23), and clinical trials are currently in progress to evaluate the effectiveness of anticoagulation therapy in improving pregnancy outcomes. Many of these patients, especially those with thrombophilic disorders, are referred to haematologists or thrombosis specialists for initiation of antithrombotic therapy, even in the absence of a history of VTE. In this chapter, we review the evidence for this association and present recommendations with respect to the management of these patients.

DIAGNOSIS OF VENOUS THROMBOEMBOLISM IN PREGNANCY

Deep vein thrombosis

The key diagnostic test for pregnant women with symptoms suspicious of DVT is compression ultrasound (CUS). Although prospective studies validating the accuracy of CUS in pregnant women have yet to be performed, CUS has been extensively evaluated in non-pregnant patients (24). A pooled analysis of studies (24) investigating the test characteristics of CUS in the general population showed that it is highly sensitive (97%) and specific (94%) for symptomatic proximal DVTs. CUS is probably less accurate for DVTs isolated to the calf or pelvis (i.e., iliac vein thrombosis) (24). Calf vein thromboses are significant because they comprise about 20% of DVT in symptomatic non-pregnant patients and 20% of them propagate proximally into the popliteal veins and have the potential to embolize (25). Isolated iliac DVT has also been reported to occur frequently in pregnancy (26,27), but the exact incidence is unknown. These thrombi are very important to detect because they have a high potential to cause PE.

Although CUS has some limitations in the diagnosis of DVT, these can be overcome by performing serial testing over 7 days if the initial test is normal (28,29). D-dimer testing and estimation of pre-test probability (PTP) can be used as adjuncts to CUS. The use of clinicians' PTP based on structured prediction rules and D-dimer testing in combination with CUS to aid in the diagnosis of DVT has been investigated prospectively in many studies of non-pregnant subjects (29–31). Structured prediction rules (32) for assessing PTP have not been evaluated in pregnant women. Some of the presenting signs used to develop prediction rules (e.g., leg oedema) may be too non-specific to be useful in pregnant women. In addition, risk factors for VTE associated with the general population (e.g., trauma, malignancy), which are important parts of clinical prediction rules, are rare in pregnant women. Therefore, the generalizability of available prediction rules to pregnant women is uncertain.

D-dimer levels are known to increase as normal pregnancy progresses and with pregnancy-associated conditions such as preterm labour and hypertensive disorders (33–35). Studies investigating the utility of D-dimer assays for VTE diagnosis in non-pregnant patients excluded pregnant patients. Several small observational studies have reported that most D-dimer assays have very poor specificity, severely limiting their utility in pregnant patients (36,37). However, in a recently published prospective study, the whole-blood red cell agglutination assay

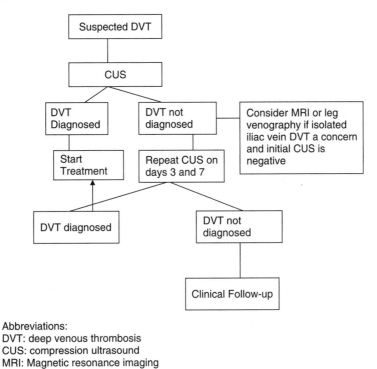

Abbreviations:
DVT: deep venous thrombosis
CUS: compression ultrasound
MRI: Magnetic resonance imaging

Figure 16.1 Diagnostic algorithm for the diagnosis of deep vein thrombosis in pregnant patients. DVT, deep vein thrombosis; CUS, compression ultrasound; MRI, magnetic resonance imaging.

appeared to show sufficient specificity to be useful in pregnant patients [81/135 (60%; 95% CI: 52 to 68%)] (38); moreover, a negative result for this test in pregnant patients with suspected DVT appeared to exclude the diagnosis of DVT [negative predictive value of 81/81 (100%; 95% CI: 95 to 100%)].

Based on the above data, investigation of pregnant patients with suspected DVT should probably begin with CUS. CUS should be repeated on days 3 and 7, if initial testing is negative, because of the uncertain ability of CUS in diagnosing calf and isolated iliac DVTs in pregnant patients (Figure 16.1). In pregnant women with an estimated high PTP, e.g., asymmetrically swollen and discoloured leg, or if recurrent DVT is suspected, clinicians should consider further testing following an initial negative CUS, with magnetic resonance imaging (MRI) (39) or venography. The risk and benefits of these imaging techniques should be weighed and discussed with the patient.

Pulmonary embolism

As with the diagnosis of DVT, there are no prospective clinical studies evaluating the objective diagnosis of PE in pregnant patients. Current recommendations regarding PE diagnosis in pregnant patients are usually derived by extrapolating results from those studies of non-pregnant patients. Pregnant women often complain of non-thrombotic symptoms such as dyspnea and chest pain, mimicking those seen in PE (40). Diagnostic imaging remains the only means objectively to exclude PE in these patients.

The diagnostic imaging tests used to diagnose PE in non-pregnant patients include pulmonary angiography (PA) (42), ventilation–perfusion (V/Q) lung scanning (43) and spiral computed tomography (CT) (44). As with the diagnosis of DVT, CUS, structured prediction rules and D-dimer testing also play integral roles in PE diagnosis (46–48). Pulmonary angiography, the 'reference standard' for the diagnosis of PE, is invasive; many diagnostic strategies for PE, circumventing the need for PA and using less invasive testing with V/Q scanning combined with CUS, structured prediction rules and D-dimer testing, have been validated in non-pregnant patients (46,47). However, as with DVT diagnosis, none of these latter ancillary tests have separately been studied for pregnant patients (46,47).

In the last decade, spiral CT has been investigated as a primary diagnostic modality for PE, in place of V/Q scanning. Spiral CT scanning is sensitive and specific for PE (48,49). In addition, many studies utilizing spiral CT scanning as the primary imaging modality have reported that this test can be safely used to diagnose and exclude PE as part of a management strategy (50,51). The additional advantage of a spiral CT scan over a V/Q scan is that other non-thrombotic causes of respiratory illness can be diagnosed (e.g., lung cancer). There are, however, many concerns with the safety of the spiral CT scan in pregnancy. Although the calculated radiation risk to the fetus is low (52) and below the threshold recommended for pregnancy (53) (Table 16.1), there remain two major concerns with this test. (a) The iodinated contrast agent can cross the placenta and could affect fetal thyroid tissue (54,55). Although neonatal hypothyroidism has not been reported to result directly from *in utero* exposure to maternal radiographic imaging (55), the safety of contrast agents has not been demonstrated. (b) The calculated minimum radiation dose to each breast of an average 60 kg woman is 20–35 mGy (56). This dose is equivalent to that received from 7–10 mammograms and is much greater than that received from V/Q scanning (<10 mGy) (56). Increasingly, there are data linking an increased risk of breast cancer to diagnostic imaging procedures (57,58). For all these reasons, the consideration to use spiral CT scanning over V/Q scanning during pregnancy should be carefully weighed.

Unlike spiral CT scanning, there are a few published reports on the performance of V/Q scanning in pregnant patients. In a retrospective study of pregnant patients, Chan *et al.* (40) reported on experience with PE diagnosis in 120 pregnant women who received V/Q scanning. Most of the V/Q

Table 16.1 Fetal radiation risks associated with diagnostic imaging for women presenting with suspected pulmonary embolism

Diagnostic test	Estimated fetal radiation exposure (mGy)
Perfusion scan with [99m]TcMAA	
3 mCi	0.18
1–2 mCi	0.6–0.12
Ventilation scan	
[99m]TcDTPA	0.07–0.35
[99m]TcSC	0.01–0.05
CT scan of chest[a]	
1st trimester	0.003–0.020
2nd trimester	0.008–0.077
3rd trimester	0.051–0.131
Chest X-ray	<0.01

[a]Source: Hurwitz LM, Yoshizumi T, Reiman RE, Goodman PC, Paulson EK, Frush DP, Toncheva G, Nguyen G, Barnes L. Radiation dose to the fetus from body MDCT during early gestation. AJR Am J Roentgenol 2006;186(3):871–876.

scans were normal (74%) or non-diagnostic (24%); high-probability scans were reported in only 2% of the patients. The low prevalence of abnormal scans in pregnant patients was further confirmed in another retrospective review at another centre (59), where 92% of the scans were normal and 1% were high probability. The prevalence of high-probability scans in pregnant women who present with suspicious symptoms is low compared with those reported in the general population [1–2% versus 10% (46,47)]. This probably reflects the fact that pregnant women are younger and tend to have fewer co-morbid conditions than the general population and that non-thrombotic symptoms which mimic those of PE are frequent during pregnancy.

The estimated fetal radiation from spiral CT and V/Q scanning is low (Table 16.1) and it is several orders of magnitude less than the fetal exposure threshold of 50–100 mGy [above this threshold of exposure, the risk of childhood malignancies may be increased (53)]. In addition, data from the study by Chan *et al.* suggesting that no adverse pregnancy outcomes (e.g., pregnancy losses) or childhood outcomes were reported is reassuring (40). The fetal radiation dose associated with V/Q scanning can further be minimized (by at least one-third) if a perfusion-only scan is performed; in most of these pregnant women presenting with suspected PE (74–91%), a normal perfusion scan is obtained and PE is effectively excluded (40,59).

Our current approach to PE diagnosis in pregnant women is shown in Figure 16.2. When PE is suspected, initial testing with bilateral CUS should be considered. Although the likelihood of asymptomatic DVT is low, if DVT is diagnosed, the presence of PE can be assumed and V/Q scanning can be obviated. If CUS is negative, a V/Q scan or perfusion-only scan should be performed. Based on the results of the V/Q scan, no further testing is needed (if normal) or anticoagulation should be initiated (if high probability). When a scan is non-diagnostic, clinicians may elect to proceed with either a spiral CT scan or with serial CUS testing alone, based on clinical suspicion and presence of risk factors. The risks and benefits of each of these procedures should always be carefully discussed with the patient.

TREATMENT

Acute VTE

Unfractionated heparin

Unfractionated heparin (UH) consists of a heterogeneous mixture of branched glycosaminoglycans and exerts its anticoagulant effect mostly via binding to and potentiating the action of antithrombin (also known as antithrombin III), which inactivates thrombin (factor IIa) and factors Xa, IXa, XIa and XIIa (60). UH is administered intravenously or subcutaneously. Initial dosing of heparin for therapeutic purposes is usually based on the patient's weight and subsequent dose adjustment is usually made based upon the results of the activated partial thromboplastin time (aPTT) and occasionally using heparin levels (target = 0.3–0.7 anti-factor Xa units/mL) (60).

UH was used extensively in pregnant patients in past decades and has been shown in a large review to be safe for the fetus (61). Because low molecular weight heparin (LMWH) has similar efficacy as UH, and it has fewer side-effects such as osteoporosis (with long-term use) and heparin-induced thrombocytopenia (67), LMWH has replaced UH for many VTE indications in non-pregnant patients.

Although UH use has also largely been supplanted by LMWH in pregnant patients, there are still several situations in which UH should be considered, for example, a patient who has had a diagnosis of acute VTE within 2–4 weeks of the expected date of delivery. The use of intravenous UH could be considered for 'bridging' therapy around the time of labour and delivery. Intravenous

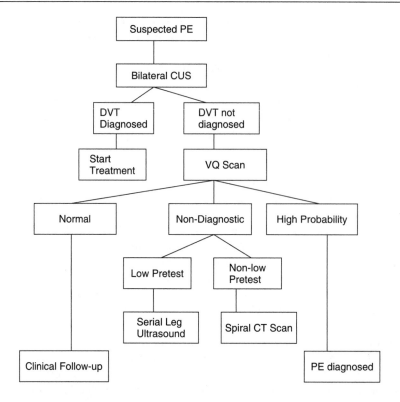

Figure 16.2 Diagnostic algorithm for the diagnosis of pulmonary embolism in pregnant patients. PE, pulmonary embolism; DVT, deep vein thrombosis; CUS, compression ultrasound; V/Q, ventilation–perfusion scan; CT, computed tomography.

UH has a short half-life (45–60 min) and levels can be monitored with aPTT measurements. In addition, UH can be readily reversed with protamine sulfate if bleeding ensues (60); 1 mg of protamine neutralizes approximately 100 U of UFH (60).

LMWH

LMWH is derived from UH by chemical or enzymatic depolymerization. The lower molecular weight of LMWH and shorter chains result in reduced anti-factor IIa activity relative to anti-factor Xa activity (less bleeding) and superior pharmacokinetic properties, while still exerting its anticoagulation effect via antithrombin-mediated inhibition of activated factor Xa (60). LMWH is less protein bound than UFH and has predictable bioavailability. Peak anti-factor Xa activity occurs 3–5 h after subcutaneous administration of LMWH and the elimination half-life of LMWHs is 3–6 h after injection, mostly via the renal route. Because of these properties, LMWH can be dosed based on body weight alone in patients with VTE, without the need to 'monitor' levels.

As stated above, LMWH has supplanted UH as the anticoagulant of choice for the treatment of VTE in pregnant patients as it has in non-pregnant patients. LMWH, like UH, does not cross the placenta and is not teratogenic (68–70). The safety of LMWH use in pregnant women has been confirmed in several large reviews of pregnant patients who were treated with LMWH (71–73). The relative efficacy and safety of one LMWH preparation compared with another, however, cannot be determined from these observational studies.

There are several advantages of LMWH over UH use in pregnant women. LMWH is associated with a low risk of heparin-induced thrombocytopenia [0% in over 2000 pregnancies (73)], low risk of osteoporosis [0.04%; 95% CI: 0 to 0.2% (73)] and of bleeding [2.0%; 95%CI 1.5 to 2.5% (73)]. However, like UH, LMWH use can result in erythematous cutaneous plaques at injection sites [1.8%; 95% CI 1.3 to 2.4% (73–75)]. When this condition arises, heparin-induced thrombocytopenia should similarly be excluded before a careful switch is made to another preparation of LMWH.

LMWH is effective for the treatment of VTE in non-pregnant patients (71–73) and is administered at a dose that is based on a patient's weight (as recommended by the respective manufacturers) (76). Unlike UH, the need for anti-factor Xa level monitoring as a measure of 'therapeutic' drug activity is largely unnecessary for LMWH. Monitoring of anti-factor Xa levels is generally recommended in patients with renal failure or morbid obesity (76).

During pregnancy, two physiological changes occur that can affect the bioavailability of LMWH: (a) progressive weight gain and (b) increased glomerular filtration rate (77). How these two factors affect LMWH dosing in pregnant patients is unclear. Several small longitudinal studies which followed peak anti-factor Xa levels (3–4 h post-injection) of therapeutic doses of LMWH for treatment of acute VTE have yielded inconsistent results: Rodie et al. (78) reported that 10% of women on therapeutic LMWH required dose reduction based on peak anti-factor Xa levels (>1.0 U/mL), while 90% did not; Barbour et al. (79) and Jacobsen et al. (80) reported that 85 and 69% of pregnancies, respectively, required upward dose adjustments. From other pharmacokinetic studies of LMWH in pregnant women, the rate of LMWH elimination is shown to increase (81–83). Taken together, these studies suggest that if a 'specific' drug level is desired, monitoring of anti-factor Xa activity may be required and twice daily dosing might be preferable to once daily dosing for VTE treatment in pregnancy.

Our recommendation for the treatment of acute VTE in pregnant patients, based largely on available evidence in non-pregnant patients, is the use of LMWH, once or twice daily, based on the patient's weight (as recommended by the manufacturers). Dose adjustments or changes may not be necessary; however, in specific situations where the risk of obstetric bleeding or risk of recurrent VTE is of concern, anti-factor Xa levels can be drawn 3–4 h post injection, to target anti-Xa levels between 0.5 and 1.0 U/mL for twice daily dosing and 1.0–1.5 U/mL for once daily dosing. These target values are empirical.

Vitamin K antagonists (VKAs)

VKAs, such as warfarin, depress synthesis of vitamin K-dependent clotting factors (factors II, VII, IX and X) by blocking reduction of the epoxide form of vitamin K (84). Because of their low molecular weight, VKAs cross the placenta, achieving clinically significant levels in the fetus (85,86). A specific pattern of congenital anomalies known as warfarin embryopathy is recognized in children exposed *in utero* to warfarin between 6 and 12 weeks of pregnancy (85–88); these anomalies, which are estimated to occur at a rate of 6.4% (95% CI: 4.6 to 8.9%), consist of nasal hypoplasia and chondrodysplasia punctata (epiphyseal and vertebral stippling) (87), and might be a result of fetal anticoagulation. Warfarin exposure after the first trimester has also been associated with central nervous system (CNS) abnormalities, such as intraventricular haemorrhages, microcephaly, hydrocephalus, cerebellar and cerebral atrophy, eye and vision abnormalities (optic atrophy, cataracts, blindness, microphthalmia), seizures and growth and mental retardation

(85–88). Beyond these *in utero* CNS side-effects, prospective studies evaluating neurodevelopmental outcomes in children exposed to warfarin *in utero* have revealed the presence of mild neurodevelopmental abnormalities in these children (89).

Despite their adverse effects on the fetus and pregnancy, VKAs are undoubtedly effective thromboprophylactic agents in pregnant women, especially those women with prosthetic mechanical heart valves, in whom UH and LMWH might be relatively less effective (87). However, for the purpose of VTE treatment and thromboprophylaxis during pregnancy, VKAs are generally avoided during pregnancy in favour of heparin and its related compounds.

Other anticoagulants

In pregnant patients who have, or develop, heparin-induced thrombocytopenia, both danapanoid and hirudin have been used successfully (90,91). The number of cases reported is small, however, and therefore adverse fetal effects cannot be completely excluded.

In recent years, fondaparinux, a synthetic pentasaccharide, has been shown to be as least as effective as UH or LMWH for thromboprophylaxis and treatment of VTE in non-pregnant patients (92,93). In a small placental *in vitro* study, fondaparinux did not appear to cross the placenta (94). In addition, it has also been successfully used to treat pregnant women who had heparin intolerance (95). The reported experience with fondaparinux is currently too limited to recommend its routine use in pregnancy for VTE treatment or thromboprophylaxis.

Thrombolytic therapy and vena cava filters

The experience with early-generation thrombolytic therapy (streptokinase, urokinase, tissue plasminogen activator) in pregnancy was summarized in a review by Turrentine *et al*. (96). In 172 patients with VTE given thrombolysis, a maternal mortality rate of 1.2% was observed; haemorrhagic complications occurred in 8.1% of cases, with 5.8% resulting in pregnancy loss. In a more recent review, Leonhardt *et al*. (97) reported on the use of recombinant tissue plasminogen activator in 28 pregnant patients for either arterial complications (stroke, myocardial infarction, prosthetic valve thrombosis) or venous complications (DVT and PE). Significant maternal mortality (23%), probably a result of these underlying diseases, was reported with 8% fetal loss. None of the livebirths, however, suffered perceptible deficits.

Based on the reported experience with thrombolytic therapy use in pregnancy, rT-PA, streptokinase and urokinase appear to have no direct placental transfer (96,97). Although the reported use of thrombolytic therapy has increased over the last decade, the indications for using thrombolytic therapy in pregnant patients who develop VTE would be similar to those in non-pregnant patients. Currently, the only clear indication for thrombolytic therapy (systemic or catheter-guided) in pregnant women is for those patients with uncontrolled haemodynamic instability from PE. Thrombolytic therapy can also be considered in pregnant women who develop limb-threatening DVT or PE with considerable haemodynamic instability (98).

The additional benefit of vena cava filter insertion in patients with VTE who were on therapeutic anticoagulation was examined in non-pregnant patients (99) in a single randomized controlled trial. Although patients with filter placement experienced a lower risk of recurrent PE compared with anticoagulation alone, the risk of DVT was also increased (20.8% in the filter group compared with 11.6% in the group with anticoagulation alone). Currently, the role of vena cava insertion remains uncertain in the management of patients with VTE who are already on adequate anticoagulation.

There is experience of vena cava filters used in pregnant patients (100,101). In the majority of pregnant patients with VTE, management with therapeutic anticoagulation alone is adequate. In the uncommon situation where patients present with extensive VTE shortly before the need for delivery (within 2 weeks) or if anticoagulation therapy has to be interrupted in the acute period because of bleeding concerns, placement of a vena cava filter should be considered. Although complications with vena cava filter insertion appear to be uncommon, careful consideration should be given to the imaging modality used for cava insertion and minimizing the amount of fetal radiation absorbed.

Duration of therapy for acute VTE

The appropriate duration of therapy for acute VTE during pregnancy is unclear. For non-pregnant patients who have an initial episode of VTE (in the presence of a secondary provoking factor such as surgery or trauma), the recommended duration of therapy in non-pregnant patients is 3 months; however, in the setting of an unprovoked VTE, recommended duration of therapy ranges from 6 months to indefinite (76).

Since pregnancy is perceived by most experts to be a 'transient' provoking factor, lasting at least 4–6 weeks after delivery, the treatment of acute VTE diagnosed during pregnancy should be continued for at least 3 months. However, ongoing anticoagulation, at either therapeutic or prophylactic doses, should be considered beyond 3 months until the end of pregnancy and for 4–6 weeks postpartum (76). Based on the results of studies in non-pregnant patients with underlying malignancy (102) or with contraindications to anticoagulation (103), reducing the intensity of anticoagulation after a period of therapeutic anticoagulation is a reasonable option (102,103).

Management of anticoagulation around labour and delivery

It is our practice to have pregnant patients who are on anticoagulation therapy seen and counselled by an anaesthetist prior to delivery so that anaesthetic options are discussed. For patients on therapeutic LMWH, planned induction of labour at approximately 38 weeks of gestation with discontinuation of LMWH approximately 24 h prior can help to ensure that neuraxial anaesthesia remains an option and bleeding risks are kept to a minimum.

For patients on therapeutic anticoagulation therapy, the last administered dose of LMWH should occur no later than 12–24 h prior to the planned induction (76). If spontaneous labour occurs within 12 h after LMWH administration or if emergent Caesarean section is required within 12 h after LMWH administration, neuraxial procedures are avoided and alternate analgesia and anaesthesia considered. In cases where excessive intrapartum bleeding results from the recent use of LMWH, protamine sulfate should be considered as it at least partly neutralizes the anticoagulant effects (60).

In certain situations where the risk of recurrence or progression of VTE is high, (e.g., acute VTE <4 weeks), 'bridging' anticoagulation with intravenous unfractionated heparin should be considered during the hours of induction and prior to delivery. The intravenous UH can be discontinued after the onset of active labour and restarted after delivery with close monitoring of aPTT activity.

For women in whom ongoing anticoagulant therapy is required in the postpartum period, i.e., those who develop acute antepartum VTE, resumption of LMWH administration should be considered 4 h or more after removal of any catheter used for neuraxial analgesia (104). Provided that haemostasis is secure, we usually restart anticoagulation therapy 12–24 h after delivery, and, when relevant, at least 4 hours after an epidural catheter is removed.

If desired, VKAs, which are compatible with breastfeeding, can be used for ongoing treatment or thromboprophylaxis of VTE in the postpartum period (105).

Management of long-term anticoagulation prior to pregnancy

Patients who are on long-term anticoagulation with a VKA for previous thromboembolic disease and who are planning conception should be carefully counselled. As stated above, VKAs exert fetopathic effects mostly between 6 and 12 weeks of gestational age (87). In addition, spontaneous loss associated with VKAs in early pregnancy cannot be totally excluded (87). Patients could opt to switch from VKAs to therapeutic LMWH prior to conception or make the switch in early pregnancy once a positive serum pregnancy test is obtained (corresponding to about 4 weeks gestational age) (76).

THROMBOPROPHYLAXIS

Previous VTE

Women with a previous episode of VTE are at an increased risk of recurrence during pregnancy. The risk of recurrent VTE events has been reported to be between 0 and 13% from early observational studies (76). More recently, two studies have provided more accurate data regarding the risk of recurrent VTE (106,107). In a retrospective cohort study (106), the risk of recurrent VTE in women who had a previous episode of VTE was reported to be 6.2% (95% CI: 1.6 to 10.9%) in women who did not receive thromboprophylaxis during pregnancy compared with no recurrences in women who did; the risk of VTE was also higher in the former cohort of patients: 5.2% in the postpartum period compared with women who received thromboprophylaxis. In a prospective study, Brill-Edwards *et al.* (107) reported that no antepartum thromboprophylaxis combined with postpartum thromboprophylaxis for 4–6 weeks after delivery resulted in an overall recurrence rate of 2.4% (95% CI: 0.2 to 6.9%). Most of the recurrences in the study occurred in women with thrombophilia and/or who had a previous unprovoked VTE (5.5%; 95% CI: 1.2 to 16%). In contrast, no women (0%; 95% CI: 0 to 8%) who had no thrombophilic disorders and a previously provoked VTE developed recurrence.

The results of these two studies suggest that withholding *antepartum* thromboprophylaxis can be considered in all pregnant patients with previous VTE, particularly in those women whose initial VTE was secondary to a transient risk factor. Women who choose this option should be counselled about symptoms suggestive of VTE and instructed to present on an emergent basis for investigation should symptoms arise. Antepartum prophylaxis should be offered, particularly in women with previous unprovoked VTE and those with a thrombophilic disorder. The choice of antepartum thromboprophylaxis regimens in the antepartum period includes 'low-dose' LMWH or UH (Table 16.2). In the postpartum period, however, thromboprophylaxis is recommended in all women with previous VTE for 4–6 weeks after delivery.

Asymptomatic thrombophilia

Because of increased screening of asymptomatic first-degree relatives of patients with VTE and hereditary thrombophilia, many women of child-bearing age who have inherited thrombophilia are being identified. In the majority of these women (with no previous history of VTE), the absolute risk of VTE is likely to be low, but increased compared with 'normal' women. For the inherited thrombophilias, estimates of the risks are one in 500 for heterozygous factor V Leiden, one in 200 for heterozygous prothrombin G20210A mutation, one in 113 for protein C deficiency, one in three for Type I AT def and one in 42 for Type II AT deficiency. Protein S deficiency could be

Table 16.2 Summary of recommendations regarding the use of thromboprophylaxis during pregnancy

Condition	Antepartum management	Peripartum management	Postpartum management
Acute VTE during pregnancy	(a) LMWH at a therapeutic dose of 200 IU/kg/day (or equivalent) in one or two divided doses	Administer the last dose of LMWH at least 24 h prior to planned induction.	LMWH is restarted 12–24 h after delivery provided adequate haemostasis is achieved. It should not be restarted within 4 h of epidural catheter removal. A switch to VKAs for ongoing anticoagulation could be made postpartum
	(b) Intravenous heparin could be considered for 5–7 days prior to a switch to subcutaneous LMWH or unfractionated heparin (6 h aPTT at 1.5–2.0 times control)	Consider 'bridging' anticoagulation with intravenous heparin if risk of recurrence is high (i.e., VTE <2–4 weeks)	
One previous episode of venous thromboembolism: (a) Unprovoked (including birth control pill use, pregnancy)	(a) LMWH at prophylactic dosing of 100 IU/kg/day or 5000 U/day	Consider withholding therapy for 24 h prior to scheduled induction	Restart prophylactic doses of LMWH or coumadin (INR 2.0–3.0) for 4–6 weeks after delivery
(b)Provoked	Or (b) Clinical surveillance or prophylaxis with LMWH (both options would be reasonable for both situations)		

(continued oveleaf)

Table 16.2 (continued)

Condition	Antepartum management	Peripartum management	Postpartum management
More than one episode of VTE, on long-term anticoagulation	Switch to LMWH at therapeutic dosing prior to conception or once pregnancy is diagnosed (≤ 4 weeks gestational age)	Administer the last dose of LMWH at least 24 h prior to planned induction.	Restart VKAs
Asymptomatic thrombophilia	Clinical surveillance or prophylaxis with LMWH	Discontinue LMWH, if administered, at term	Consider short-term anticoagulation (4–6 weeks), especially if Caesarean section is performed
Pregnancy complications: (a) Recurrent losses and APLA	(a) LMWH and low-dose ASA	Discontinue LMWH and ASA if administered, near term	Consider short-term anticoagulation (4–6 weeks), especially if Caesarean section is performed
(b) Adverse pregnancy outcomes with thrombophilia	(b) Consider LMWH in prophylactic doses or clinical surveillance		

associated with similar risks to protein C deficiency (108). The risk of VTE in pregnant women with homozygosity for factor V Leiden has been reported to be 9–16% (108,109), whereas double heterozygosity for factor V Leiden and prothrombin G20210A mutation has been reported to be associated with an risk of VTE of 4% (95% CI: 1.4–16.9%). The validity of these estimates is limited by the small numbers and the retrospective design of the relevant studies. Further, recommendations for appropriate management of these women during pregnancy are severely limited by a lack of published prospective studies. However, at a minimum, we counsel these individuals to be vigilant for symptoms of VTE and, for the higher risk thrombophilias, will discuss the possibility of antepartum and postpartum prophylaxis. However, until further high-quality information becomes available, any management recommendation must be considered empirical.

Thrombophilia and adverse pregnancy outcomes

In some patients, the presence of antiphospholipid antibodies is associated with recurrent miscarriages (110,111). In these patients, thromboprophylaxis with LMWH or UH can reduce the risk of miscarriages in subsequent pregnancies (110–112). In these small studies (110–112), the addition of low-dose UH or LMWH to low-dose aspirin improved pregnancy success. Therefore, consensus panels continue to recommend (76) the use of both low-dose aspirin (81 mg) with LMWH or UH in the management of these patients

The management of women with other inherited thrombophilic disorders and history of adverse pregnancy outcomes, however, is more uncertain. In the last few years, several systematic reviews of mostly observational studies are consistent: with associations between inherited thrombophilias and adverse pregnancy events such as early pregnancy losses [odds ratios (ORs) 1.40–6.25], late pregnancy losses (ORs 1.31–20.09), pre-eclampsia (ORs 1.37–3.49), intrauterine growth restriction (ORs 1.24–2.92) and placental abruption (ORs 1.42–7.71) (113–120).

Despite a lack of clinical trials defining the role of thromboprophylaxis in pregnant patients with inherited thrombophilias, many clinicians prescribe LMWH routinely to such women if they have a history of previous adverse pregnancy outcomes (121–123). There are currently at least two randomized controlled studies under way defining the effectiveness of LMWH for the prevention of adverse pregnancy outcomes. It is hoped that the results from these studies will clarify the utility of LMWH in pregnant thrombophilic women.

CONCLUSION

VTE continues to be a major cause of maternal morbidity and mortality during pregnancy and there is increasing evidence that inherited thrombophilias are associated with VTE and also other adverse pregnancy outcomes. Appropriate diagnosis, treatment and prevention of VTE in pregnancy are complex because of the unique problems that pregnancy poses and the lack of high-quality evidence from large clinical trials.

REFERENCES

1. Lindqvist P, Dahlback B, Marsal K. Thrombotic risk during pregnancy: a population study. *Obstet Gynecol* 1999; **94**:595–599.
2. Simpson EL, Lawrenson RA, Nightingale AL, Farmer RD. Venous thromboembolism in pregnancy and the puerperium: incidence and additional risk factors from a London perinatal database. *Br J Obstet Gynaecol* 2001; **108**:56–60.

3. Macklon NS, Greer IA. Venous thromboembolic disease in obstetrics and gynaecology: the Scottish experience. *Scott Med J* 1996; **41**:83–86.
4. Gherman RB, Goodwin TM, Leung B, Bryne JD, Hethumumi R, Montoro M. Incidence, clinical characteristics and timing of objectively diagnosed venous thromboembolism during pregnancy. *Obstet Gynecol* 1999; **94**:730–734.
5. Hauth J, for the NICHD MFMU Network. MFMU Cesarean Registry: thromboembolism – occurrence and risk factors in 39,285 Cesarean births. *Am J Obstet Gynecol* 2003; **189**:S120–.
6. Chan LY, Tam WH, Lau TK. Venous thromboembolism in pregnant Chinese women. *Obstet Gynecol* 2001; **98**:471–475.
7. Chisaka H, Utsunomiya H, Okamura K, Yaegaki N. Pulmonary thromboembolism following gynecologic surgery and Cesarean section. *Int J Gynaecol Obstet* 2004: **84**:47–53.
8. Jacobsen AF, Anders D, Klow NE, Dahl GF, Qvigstad E, Sandset PM. Deep vein thrombosis after elective Cesarean section. *Thromb Res* 2004; **113**:283–288.
9. Sachs BP, Brown DA, Driscoll ST, *et al*. Maternal mortality in Massachusetts. Trends and Prevention. *N Engl J Med* 1987; **316**:607–672.
10. Report on Confidential Enquiries into Maternal Deaths for England and Wales 1979–1981. HM Stationery Office, London, 1986.
11. Bonnar J. The blood coagulation and fibrinolytic system in the new born and mother at birth. *Br J Obstet Gynaecol* 1971; **78**:355–360.
12. Comp PC, Thurnau GR, Welsh J, Esmon CT. Functional and immunologic protein S levels are decreased during pregnancy. *Blood* 1986; **68**:881–885.
13. Cordts PR, Gawley TS. Anatomic and physiologic changes in lower extremity venous hemodynamics associated with pregnancy. *J Vasc Surg* 1996; **24**:763–767.
14. Palmgren J, Kirkinen P. Venous circulation in the maternal lower limb: a Doppler study with the Valsalva maneuver. *Ultrasound Obstet Gynecol* 1996; **8**:93–97.
15. Macklon NC, Greer IA, Bowman AW. An ultrasound study of gestational and postural changes in the deep venous system of the leg in pregnancy. *Br J Obstet Gynaecol* 1997; **104**:191–197.
16. Ray J, WS Chan. Deep vein thrombosis during pregnancy and puerperium: a meta-analysis of the period of risk and leg of presentation. *Obstet Gynecol Surv* 1999; **54**:265–271.
17. Nijkeuter M, Ginsberg JS, Huisman MV. Diagnosis of deep vein thrombosis and pulmonary embolism in pregnancy: a systematic review. *J Thromb Haemost* 2006; **4**(3):496–500.
18. Howley HE, Walker M, Rodger MA A systematic review of the association between factor V Leiden or prothrombin gene variant and intrauterine growth restriction. *Am J Obstet Gynecol* 2005; **192**(3):694–708.
19. Lin J, August P. Genetic thrombophilias and preeclampsia: a meta-analysis. *Obstet Gynecol* 2005; **105**(1):182–192.
20. Kovalevsky G, Gracia CR, Berlin JA, Sammel MD, Barnhart KT. Evaluation of the association between hereditary thrombophilias and recurrent pregnancy loss: a meta-analysis. *Arch Intern Med* 2004; **164**(5):558–563.
21. Krabbendam I, Franx A, Bots ML, Fijnheer R, Bruinse HW. Thrombophilias and recurrent pregnancy loss: a critical appraisal of the literature. *Eur J Obstet Gynecol Reprod Biol* 2005; **118**(2):143–153.
22. Rey E, Kahn SR, David M, Shrier I. Thrombophilic disorders and fetal loss: a meta-analysis. *Lancet* 2003; **361**(9361):901–908; Di Nisio M, Peters L, Middeldorp S. Anticoagulants for the treatment of recurrent pregnancy loss in women without antiphospholipid syndrome. *Cochrane Database Syst Rev* 2005; (2): CD004734–.
23. Robertson L, Wu O, Langhorne P, *et al*. The Thrombosis: Risk and Economic Assessment of Thrombophilia Screening (TREATS) Study. Thrombophilia in pregnancy: a systematic review. *Br J Haematol* 2006; **132**(2):171–196.
24. Kearon C, Julian JA, Ginsberg JS, *et al*. Noninvasive diagnosis of deep venous thrombosis. *Ann Intern Med* 1998; **128**:663–677.
25. Lohr JM, Kerr TM, Lutter KS, *et al*. Lower extremity calf thrombosis: to treat or not to treat? *J Vasc Surg* 1991; **14**:618–623.
26. Frede TE, Ruthberg BN. Sonographic demonstration of iliac venous thrombosis in the maternity patient. *J Ultrasound Med* 1988; **7**:33–37.
27. Polak JF, O'Leary DH. Deep venous thrombosis in pregnancy: noninvasive diagnosis. *Radiologu* 1988; **166**:377–379.
28. Cogo A, Lensing AW, Koopman MM, *et al*. Compression ultrasound for diagnostic management of patients with clinically suspected deep-vein thrombosis: prospective cohort study. *BMJ* 1998; **316**:17–20.

29. Perrier A, Desmaris S, Miron M-J, *et al*. Non-invasive diagnosis of venous thromboembolism in outpatients. *Lancet* 1999; **353**:190–195.

30. Bernardi E, Prandoni P, Lensing AW, *et al*. D-dimer testing as an adjunct to ultrasonography in patients with clinically suspected deep vein thrombosis: prospective cohort study. The Multicentre Italian D-dimer Ultrasound Study Investigators Group. *BMJ* 1998; **317**(7165):1037–1040.

31. Bates SM, Kearon C, Crowther M, *et al*. A diagnostic strategy involving a quantitative latex D-dimer assay reliably excludes deep venous thrombosis.Ann Intern Med 2003; **138**(10):787–794.

32. Wells PS, Anderson DR, Bormanis J, *et al*. Value of assessment of pre-test probability of deep-vein thrombosis in clinical management. *Lancet* 1997; **350**:1795–1798.

33. Nolan TE, Smith RP, Devoe LD. Maternal plasma D-dimer levels in normal and complicated pregnancies. *Obstet Gynecol* 1993; **81**:235–238.

34. Proietti AB, Johnson MJ, Proietti FA, *et al*. Assessment of fibrin (nogen) degradation products in preeclampsia using immunoblot enzyme-linked immunosorbent assay and latex-bead agglutination. *Obstet Gynecol* 1991; **77**:696–700.

35. Francalanci I, Comeglio P, Alessandrello A, *et al*. D-dimer concentrations during normal pregnancy, as measured by ELISA. *Thromb Res* 1995; **78**:399–405.

36. Kline JA, Williams GW, Hernandez-Nino J. D-dimer concentrations in normal pregnancy: new diagnostic thresholds are needed. *Clin Chem*. 2005; **51**(5):825–829.

37. Morse M. Establishing a normal range for D-dimer levels through pregnancy to aid in the diagnosis of pulmonary embolism and deep vein thrombosis. *J Thromb Haemost* 2004; **2**(7):1202–1204.

38. Chan WS, SD Chunilal, Lee A, Crowther M, Rodger M. A red blood cell agglutination D-dimer test to exclude deep venous thrombosis in pregnancy. *Ann Intern Med* 2007; **147**(3):165–170.

39. Kluge A, Mueller C, Strunk J, Lange U, Bachmann G. Experience in 207 combined MRI examinations for acute pulmonary embolism and deep vein thrombosis. *AJR Am J Roentgenol* 2006; **186**(6):1686–1596.

40. Chan WS, Ray J, Coady G, Murray S, Ginsberg JS. Clinical presentation of suspected pulmonary embolism during pregnancy, VQ lung scan: results and subsequent maternal and pediatric outcomes. *Arch Intern Med* 2002; **162**(10):1170–1175.

41. van Beek EJ, Brouwerst EM, Song B, Stein PD, Oudkerk M. Clinical validity of a normal pulmonary angiogram in patients with suspected pulmonary embolism–a critical review. *Clin Radiol* 2001; **56**:838–842.

42. Anonymous. Value of the ventilation/perfusion scan in acute pulmonary embolism. Results of the prospective investigation of pulmonary embolism diagnosis (PIOPED). *JAMA* 1990; **263**:2753–2759.

43. Stein PD, Fowler SE, Goodman LR, *et al*., PIOPED II Investigators. Multidetector computed tomography for acute pulmonary embolism. *N Engl J Med* 2006; **354**(22):2317–2327.

44. Hull RD, Raskob GE, Coates G, Panju AA, Gill GJ. A new noninvasive management strategy for patients with suspected pulmonary embolism. *Arch Intern Med* 1989; **149**:2549–5255.

45. Wells PS, Ginsberg JS, Anderson DR, Kearon C, Gent M, Turpie AG, *et al*. Use of a clinical model for safe management of patients with suspected pulmonary embolism. *Ann Intern Med* 1998; **129**:997–1005.

46. Kearon C, Ginsberg JS, Douketis J, *et al*., Canadian Pulmonary Embolism Diagnosis Study (CANPEDS) Group. An evaluation of D-dimer in the diagnosis of pulmonary embolism: a randomized trial. *Ann Intern Med* 2006; **144**(11):812–821.

47. Stein PD, Hull RD, Pineo G. Strategy that includes serial noninvasive leg tests for diagnosis of thromboembolic disease in patients with suspected acute pulmonary embolism based on data from PIOPED. Prospective investigation of pulmonary embolism Diagnosis. *Arch Intern Med* 1995; **155**(19):2101–2104.

48. Rathbun SW, Raskob GE, Whitsett TL. Sensitivity and specificity of helical computed tomography in the diagnosis of pulmonary embolism: a systematic review. *Ann Intern Med* 2000; **132**(3):227–232.

49. Stein PD, Fowler SE, Goodman LR, *et al*., PIOPED II Investigators. Multidetector computed tomography for acute pulmonary embolism. *N Engl J Med* 2006; **354**(22):2317–2327.

50. van Belle A, Büller HR, Huisman MV, *et al*., Christopher Study Investigators. Effectiveness of managing suspected pulmonary embolism using an algorithm combining clinical probability, D-dimer testing and computed tomography spiral CT. *JAMA* 2006; **295**:172–179.

51. Ghanima W, Almaas V, Aballi S, *et al*. Management of suspected pulmonary embolism (PE) by D-dimer and multi-slice computed tomography in outpatients: an outcome study. *J Thromb Haemost* 2005; **3**(9):1926–1932.

52. Hurwitz LM, Yoshizumi T, Reiman RE, *et al*. Radiation dose to the fetus from body MDCT during early gestation. *AJR Am J Roentgenol*. 2006; **186**(3):871–876.

53. Doll R, Wakefield R. Risk of childhood cancer from fetal radiation. *Br J Radiol* 1997; (70): 130–139.

54. Hill BJ, Saigal G, Patel S, Abdenour GE Jr. Transplacental passage of non-ionic contrast agents resulting in fetal bowel opacification: a mimic of pneumoperitoneum in the newborn. *Pediatr Radiol* 2007; **37**(4):396–398.

55. Weber G, Vigone MC, Rapa A, Bona G, Chiumello G. Neonatal transient hypothyroidism: aetiological study. Italian Collaborative Study on Transient Hypothyroidism. *Arch Dis Child Fetal Neonatal Ed* 1998; **79**(1):F70–F72.

56. Parker MS, Hui FK, Camacho MA, Chung JK, Broga DW, Sethi NN. Female breast radiation exposure during CT pulmonary angiography. *AJR Am J Roentgenol* 2005; **185**:1228–1233.

57. Berrington de Gonzalez A, Darby S. Risk of cancer from diagnostic X-rays: estimates for the UK and 14 other countries. *Lancet* 2004; **363**:345–351.

58. Preston DL, Mattsson A, Holmberg E, Shore R, Hildreth NG, Boice JD Jr. Radiation effects on breast cancer risk: a pooled analysis of eight cohorts. *Radiat Res* 2002; **158**(2): 220–235. Erratum:Radiat Res 2002; **158**(5):666.

59. Scarsbrook AF, Bradley KM, Gleeson FV. Perfusion scintigraphy: diagnostic utility in pregnant women with suspected pulmonary embolic disease. *Eur Radiol* 2007; **17**(10):2554–2560.

60. Hirsh J, Raschke R. Heparin and low-molecular-weight heparin. The Seventh ACCP Conference on Antithrombotic and Thrombolytic Therapy. *Chest* 2004; **126**:188S–203S.

61. Ginsberg JS, Hirsh J. Anticoagulants during pregnancy. *Annu Rev Med* 1989; **40**:79–86.

62. Koopman MM, Prandoni P, Piovella F, *et al*. Treatment of venous thrombosis with intravenous unfractionated hepari administered in the hospital as compared with subcutaneous low-molecular-weight heparin administered at home. The Tasman Study Group. *N Engl J Med* 1996; **334**:682–687.

63. Dolovich LR, Ginsberg JS, Douketis JD, Holbrook AM, Cheah G. A meta-analysis comparing low-molecular-weight heparins with unfractionated heparin in the treatment of venous thromboembolism: examining some unanswered questions regarding location of treatment, product type and dosing frequency. *Arch Intern Med* 2000; **160**:181–188.

64. Gould MK, Dembitzer AD, Doyle RL, Hastie TJ, Garber AM. Low-molecular-weight heparins compared with unfractionated heparin for treatment of acute deep venous thrombosis. A meta-analysis of randomized, controlled trials. *Ann Intern Med* 1999; **130**:800–809.

65. Monreal M, Lafoz E, Olive A, del Rio L, Vedia C. Comparison of subcutaneous unfractionated heparin with a low molecular heparin (Fragmin) in patients with venous thromboembolism and contraindications to coumarin. *Thromb Haemost* 1994; **71**:7–11.

66. Dahlman TC. Osteoporotic fractures and recurrence of thromboembolism during pregnancy and the puerperium in 184 women undergoing thromboprophylaxis with heparin. *Am J Obstet Gynecol* 1993; **168**:1265–1270.

67. Warkentin TE, Levine MN, Hirsh J, Horsewood P, Roberts RS, Gent M, Kelton JG. Heparin-induced thrombocytopenia in patients treated with low-molecular-weight heparin or unfractionated heparin. *N Engl J Med* 1995; **332**:1330–1335.

68. Forestier F, Daffos F, Capella-Pavlovsky M. Low molecular weight heparin (PK 10169) does not cross the placenta during the second trimester of pregnancy study by direct fetal blood sampling under ultrasound. *Thromb Res* 1984; **34**(6):557–560.

69. Dimitrakakis C, Papageorgiou P, Papageorgiou I, Antzaklis A, Sakarelou N, Michalas S. Absence of transplacental passage of the low molecular weight heparin enoxaparin. *Haemostasis* 2000; **30**(5):243–248.

70. Omri A, Delaloye JF, Andersen H, Bachmann F. Low molecular weight heparin Novo (LHN-1) does not cross the placenta during the second trimester of pregnancy. *Thromb Haemost* 1989; **61**(1):55–56.

71. Chan WS, Ray J. Low molecular weight heparin use in pregnancy: issues of safety and practicality. *Obstet Gynecol Surv* 1999: **54**(10):649–654.

72. Sanson BJ, Lensing AWA, Prins MH, *et al*. Safety of low-molecular-weight heparin in pregnancy: a systematic review. *Thromb Haemost* 1999; **81**:668–672.

73. Greer IA, Nelson-Piercy C. Low-molecular-weight heparins for thromboprophylaxis and treatment of venous thromboembolism in pregnancy: a systematic review of safety and efficacy. *Blood* 2005; **106**(2):401–407.

74. Verdonkschot AE, Vasmel WL, Middeldorp S, van der Schoot JT. Skin reactions due to low molecular weight heparin in pregnancy: a strategic dilemma. *Arch Gynecol Obstet*. 2005; **271**(2):163–165.

75. Kim J, Smith KJ, Toner C, Skelton H. Delayed cutaneous reactions to heparin in antiphospholipid syndrome during pregnancy. *Int J Dermatol*. 2004; **43**(4):252–260.

76. Bates SM, Greer IA, Hirsh J, Ginsberg JS. Use of antithrombotic agents during pregnancy: the Seventh ACCP Conference on Antithrombotic and Thrombolytic Therapy. *Chest* 2004; **126**(3 Suppl):627S–644S.

77. Lindheimer MD, Katz AI. Renal physiology and disease in pregnancy, in Sedin DW, Giebisch G (eds), *The Kidney: Physiology and Pathophysiolgy*, Raven Press, New York, 1992, pp. 3371–3431.

78. Rodie VA, Thomson AJ, Stewart FM, Quinn AJ, Walker ID, Greer IA. Low molecular weight heparin for the treatment of venous thromboembolism in pregnancy: a case series. *Br J Obstet Gynaecol* 2002; **109**(9):1020–1024.

79. Barbour LA, Oja JL, Schultz LK. A prospective trial that demonstrates that dalteparin requirements increase in pregnancy to maintain therapeutic levels of anticoagulation. *Am J Obstet Gynecol* 2004; **191**(3):1024–1029.

80. Jacobsen AF, Qvigstad E, Sandset PM. Low molecular weight heparin (dalteparin) for the treatment of venous thromboembolism in pregnancy. *Br J Obstet Gynaecol* 2003; **110**(2):139–144.

81. Casele HL, Laifer SA, Woelkers DA, Venkataramanan R. Changes in the pharmacokinetics of the low-molecular weight heparin enoxaparin sodium during pregnancy. *Am J Obstet Gynecol* 1999; **181**:1113–1117.

82. Norris LA, Bonnar J, Smith MP, Steer PJ, Savidge G. Low molecular weight heparin (tinzaparin) therapy for moderate risk thromboprophylaxis during pregnancy. A pharmacokinetic study. *Thromb Haemost* 2004; **92**(4):791–796.

83. Ensom MH, Stephenson MD. Pharmacokinetics of low molecular weight heparin and unfractionated heparin in pregnancy. *J Soc Gynecol Invest* 2004; **11**(6):377–383.

84. Ansell J, Hirsh J, Poller L, Bussey H, Jacobson A, Hylek E The pharmacology and management of the vitamin K antagonists: the Seventh ACCP Conference on Antithrombotic and Thrombolytic Therapy. *Chest* 2004; **126**(3 Suppl):204S–233S.

85. Hall JG, Pauli RM, Wilson KM. Maternal and fetal sequelae of anticoagulation during pregnancy. *Am J Med* 1980; **68**:122–140.

86. Shaul WL, Hall JG. Multiple congenital anomalies associated with oral anticoagulants. *Am J Obstet Gynecol* 1977; **127**:191–198.

87. Chan WS, Anand S, Ginsberg JS. Anticoagulation of pregnant women with mechanical heart valves. A systemic review of the literature. *Arch Intern Med* 2000; **160**:191–196.

88. Wong V, Cheng CH, Chan KC. Fetal and neonatal outcome of exposure to anticoagulants during pregnancy. *Am J Med Genet* 1993; **45**:17–21.

89. Wesseling J, Van Driel D, Heymans HS, *et al*. Coumarins during pregnancy: long-term effects on growth and development of school-age children. *Thromb Haemost* 2001; **85**(4):609–613.

90. Lindhoff-Last E, Kreutzenbeck HJ, Magnani HN. Treatment of 51 pregnancies with danaparoid because of heparin intolerance. *Thromb Haemost* 2005; **93**(1):63–69.

91. Aijaz A, Nelson J, Naseer N. Management of heparin allergy in pregnancy. *Am J Hematol*. 2001; **67**(4):268–269.

92. Eriksson BI, Bauer KA, Lassen MR, Turpie AG, Steering Committee of the Pentasaccharide in Hip-Fracture Surgery Study. Fondaparinux compared with enoxaparin for the prevention of venous thromboembolism after hip-fracture surgery. *N Engl J Med* 2001; **345**(18):1298–1304.

93. Büller HR, Davidson BL, Decousus H, *et al*., Matisse Investigators. Fondaparinux or enoxaparin for the initial treatment of symptomatic deep venous thrombosis: a randomized trial. *Ann Intern Med* 2004; **140**(11):867–873.

94. Lagrange F, Vergnes C, Brun JL, *et al*. Absence of placental transfer of pentasaccharide (Fonda-parinux, Arixtra) in the dually perfused human cotyledon in vitro. *Thromb Haemost* 2002; **87**(5): 831–5.

95. Mazzolai L, Hohlfeld P, Spertini F, Hayoz D, Schapira M, Duchosal MA. Fondaparinux is a safe alternative in case of heparin intolerance during pregnancy. *Blood* 2006; **108**(5):1569–1570.

96. Turrentine MA, Braema G, Ramirez MM. Use of thrombolytics for te treatment of thromboembolic disease during pregnanacy. *Obstet Gynecol Surv* 1995; **50**(7):534–541.

97. Leonhardt G, Gaul C, Nietsch HH, Buerke M, Schleussner E. Thrombolytic therapy in pregnancy. *J Thromb Thrombol* 2006; **21**(3):271–276.

98. Büller HR, Agnelli G, Hull RD, Hyers TM, Prins MH, Raskob G. Antithrombotic therapy for venous thromboembolic disease. The Seventh ACCP Conference on Antithrombotic and Thrombolytic Therapy. *Chest* 2004; **126**:401S–428S.

99. Decousus H, Leizorovicz A, Parent F, *et al*. A clinical trial of vena caval filters in the prevention of pulmonary embolism in patients with proximal deep-vein thrombosis. Prévention du Risque d'Embolie Pulmonaire par Interruption Cave Study Group. *N Engl J Med* 1998; **338**(7):409–415.

100. Aburahma AF, Mullins DA. Endovascular caval interruption in pregnant patients with deep vein thrombosis of the lower extremity. *J Vasc Surg* 2001; **33**(2):375–378.

101. Kawamata K, Chiba Y, Tanaka R, Higashi M, Nishigami K. Experience of temporary inferior vena cava filters inserted in the perinatal period to prevent pulmonary embolism in pregnant women with deep vein thrombosis. *J Vasc Surg* 2005; **41**(4):652–656.

102. Lee AY, Levine MN, Baker RI, *et al*., Randomized Comparison of Low-Molecular-Weight Heparin versus Oral Anticoagulant Therapy for the Prevention of Recurrent Venous Thromboembolism in Patients with Cancer (CLOT) Investigators. Low-molecular-weight heparin versus a coumarin for the prevention of recurrent venous thromboembolism in patients with cancer. *N Engl J Med* 2003; **349**(2):146–153.

103. Monreal M, Lafoz E, Olive A, del Rio L, Vedia C. Comparison of subcutaneous unfractionated heparin with a low molecular weight heparin (Fragmin) in patients with venous thromboembolism and contraindications to coumarin. *Thromb Haemost* 1994; **71**(1):7–11.

104. Horlocker TT, Heit JA. Low molecular weight heparin: biochemistry, pharmacology, perioperative prophylaxis regimens and guidelines for regional anesthetic mangement. *Anesth Analg* 1997; **85**:874–885.

105. Clark SL, Porter TF, West FG. Coumarin derivatives and breast-feeding. *Obstet Gynecol* 2000; **95**(6 Pt 1):938–940.

106. Pabinger I, Grafenhofer H, Kaider A, Kyrle PA, Quehenberger P, Mannhalter C, Lechner K. Risk of pregnancy-associated recurrent venous thromboembolism in women with a history of venous thrombosis. *J Thromb Haemost* 2005; **3**(5):949–954.

107. Brill-Edwards P, Ginsberg JS, Gent M, *et al*., Recurrence of Clot in This Pregnancy Study Group. Safety of withholding heparin in pregnant women with a history of venous thromboembolism. Recurrence of Clot in This Pregnancy Study Group. *N Engl J Med* 2000; **343**(20):1439–1444.

108. Martinelli I, Mannucci PM, De Stefano V, *et al*. Different risks of thrombosis in four coagulation defects associated with inherited thrombophilia: a study of 150 families. *Blood* 1998; **92**(7):2353–2358.

109. Grandone E, Margaglione M, Colaizzo D, D'Andrea G, Cappucci G, Brancaccio V, Di Minno G. Genetic susceptibility to pregnancy-related venous thromboembolism: roles of factor V Leiden, prothrombin G20210A and methylenetetrahydrofolate reductase C677T mutations. *Am J Obstet Gynecol* 1998; **179**(5):1324–1328.

110. Rai R Cohen H, Dave M, Regan L. Randomised controlled trial of aspirin and aspirin plus heparin in pregnant women with recurrent miscarriage associated with phospholipid antibodies (or antiposphpholipid antibodies). *BMJ* 1997; **314**: 253–257.

111. Kutteh WH. Antiphospholipid antibody-associated recurrent pregnancy loss: treatment with heparin and low-dose aspirin is superior to low-dose aspirin alone. *Am J Obstet Gynecol* 1996; **174**:1584–1589.

112. Brenner B, Hoffman R, Blumenfeld Z, Weiner Z, Younis JS. Gestational outcome in thrombophilic women with recurrent pregnancy loss treated by enoxaparin. *Thromb Haemost* 2000; **83**:693–7.

113. Howley HE, Walker M, Rodger MA A systematic review of the association between factor V Leiden or prothrombin gene variant and intrauterine growth restriction. *Am J Obstet Gynecol* 2005; **192**(3):694–708.

114. Lin J, August P. Genetic thrombophilias and preeclampsia: a meta-analysis. *Obstet Gynecol* 2005; **105**(1):182–92.

115. Kovalevsky G, Gracia CR, Berlin JA, Sammel MD, Barnhart KT. Evaluation of the association between hereditary thrombophilias and recurrent pregnancy loss: a meta-analysis. *Arch Intern Med* 2004; **164**(5):558–63.

116. Krabbendam I, Franx A, Bots ML, Fijnheer R, Bruinse HW. Thrombophilias and recurrent pregnancy loss: a critical appraisal of the literature. *Eur J Obstet Gynecol Reprod Biol*. 2005; **118**(2): 143–53.

117. Rey E, Kahn SR, David M, Shrier I. Thrombophilic disorders and fetal loss: a meta-analysis. *Lancet* 2003; **361**(9361):901–8; Di Nisio M, Peters L, Middeldorp S. Anticoagulants for the treatment of recurrent pregnancy loss in women without antiphospholipid syndrome. *Cochrane Database Syst Rev* 2005; (2):CD004734–.

118. Robertson L, Wu O, Langhorne P, *et al*. The Thrombosis: Risk and Economic Assessment of Thrombophilia Screening (TREATS) Study. Thrombophilia in pregnancy: a systematic review. *Br J Haematol* 2006; **132**(2):171–96.

119. Coulam CB, Jeyendran RS, Fishel LA, Roussev R. Multiple thrombophilic gene mutations rather than specific gene mutations are risk factors for recurrent miscarriage. *Am J Reprod Immunol* 2006; **55**(5):360–8.

120. Gerhardt A, Scharf RE, Beckmann MW, *et al*. Prothrombin and factor V mutations in women with a history of thrombosis during pregnancy and the puerperium. *N Engl J Med* 2000; **342**(6):374–80.
121. De Carolis S, Ferrazzani S, De Stefano V, *et al*. Inherited thrombophilia: treatment during pregnancy. *Fetal Diagn Ther* 2006; **21**(3):281–6.
122. Kalk JJ, Huisjes AJ, de Groot CJ, *et al*. Recurrence rate of pre-eclampsia in women with thrombophilia influenced by low-molecular-weight heparin treatment? *Neth J Med* 2004; **62**(3):83–7.
123. Nurk E, Tell GS, Refsum H, Ueland PM, Vollset SE. Factor V Leiden, pregnancy complications and adverse outcomes: the Hordaland Homocysteine Study. *QJM* 2006; **99**(5):289–98.

CHAPTER 17

Management Of Venous Thromboembolic Disease In Childhood

C. Heleen van Ommen, Harriët Heijboer and Marjolein Peters

Department of Paediatric Hematology,
Emma Children's Hospital/Academic Medical Centre, Amsterdam,
The Netherlands

INTRODUCTION

Over recent decades, medical progress in surgical interventions, treatment and supportive care of critically ill children has led to an impressive increase in the survival of these children with previously fatal diseases. However, this improved survival is associated with the development of new, secondary complications hitherto uncommon in children. One of these complications is venous thromboembolic disease. For example, the introduction of central venous catheters has permitted the administration of fluids, nutrition and medication to critically ill patients. However, insertion of such catheters causes damage to the vessel wall and disruption of blood flow and as a result these catheters have become the most important risk factor for venous thrombosis in both neonates and children.

Since the first registry of paediatric patients with venous thrombosis by Andrew et al. in 1994 (1), much progress has been made towards a better understanding of the underlying conditions leading to paediatric thrombosis. Thrombosis in childhood is almost always multifactorial, involving both genetic and environmental factors. Unfortunately, there have been only a few clinical trials of diagnostic methods for and treatment and prevention of paediatric thrombosis. Guidelines concerning the management of paediatric thrombosis are chiefly based on data from adult studies and uncontrolled paediatric studies.

This chapter outlines the epidemiology, aetiology, clinical presentation and management of venous thromboembolic disease in paediatric patients. Potential new anticoagulant agents are discussed. The field of paediatric thrombosis is promisingly advancing, with new studies being planned. However, to include a sufficient number of patients, these studies have to be performed in a multicentre setting. Hence collaboration is essential in order to initiate these studies. The results of multicentre, randomized trials will contribute to an evidence-based management of paediatric patients with venous thromboembolic disease in the future.

INCIDENCE

Venous thromboembolic disease (VTE) occurs less frequently in childhood than in adults. Whereas the annual incidence in adults is about 10 per 10 000 persons, various paediatric thrombosis registries estimated it to be 0.07–0.14 per 10 000 children or 5.3 per 10 000 paediatric hospital admissions and 24 per 10 000 admissions to neonatal intensive care units (1–5). Incidence rates of pulmonary embolism were 0.014 per 10 000 children or 0.86 per 10 000 paediatric hospital admissions (1–4).

Incidences of pulmonary embolism (PE) are probably underestimated. PE is frequently clinically silent or presents with symptoms that can be explained by underlying diseases. Buck *et al.* showed that in children with clinically significant PE, 50% had documented typical signs and symptoms (6). The clinical diagnosis was considered in only 15% of these children. The causes of the lower incidences of VTE in childhood compared with adults are not entirely clear; apart from decreased clinical suspicion, the lower capacity of thrombin generation, elevated levels of α-2-macroglobulin (an inhibitor of thrombin) and enhanced antithrombotic potential of the vessel wall may all contribute to the decreased incidence in childhood (7).

Age is an important modifying factor of thrombotic incidence, both in adults and in childhood. In adults, the incidence of first-time VTE rises exponentially with age, from about 30 per 100 000 per year among persons aged 25–30 years to about 300–500 per 100 000 per year among persons aged 70–79 years (8). In childhood there are two age-related frequency peaks: the first peak is during the neonatal period, followed by another peak in adolescence, with a higher frequency in females, probably as a result of the use of oral contraceptives (9) (Figure 17.1). The relatively high incidence of thrombosis in neonates compared with older children may be the result of small vessel size as most neonatal thrombi are catheter related. In adolescents, the incidence is the same as that in young adults.

RISK FACTORS

In 1856, Virchow postulated three main causes of thrombosis: damage to the vessel wall, stasis of the blood and increase in blood coagulability ('Virchow's triad') (10). Nowadays, risk factors for VTE are usually classified into acquired and congenital risk factors. The acquired risk factors may be transient or persistent over time. True idiopathic thrombosis is rare in children, in contrast to adults. Whereas in adults 25–50% of all venous thrombi are idiopathic (see Chapter 1), in more than 95% of paediatric patients at least one risk factor can be found (1,11–13) (Table 17.1).

Acquired risk factors

Central venous catheters

Currently, the presence of a central venous catheter is the most important acquired trigger for the development of VTE in paediatric patients, contributing to more than 90% of all neonatal thrombi and half of all thrombi in the older children (1,14,15). Several mechanisms play a role in the development of catheter-related thrombosis, including vessel wall injury by the catheter or the infused

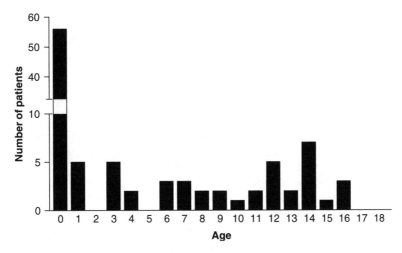

Figure 17.1   Age distribution of paediatric patients with venous thrombosis in a prospective two-year registry in The Netherlands. Reprinted from van Ommen CH, Heijboer H, Büller HR, Hirasing RA, Heijmans HS, Peters M. Venous thromboembolism in childhood: a prospective two-year registry in The Netherlands. J Pediatr 2001; 139:676–81, with permission of Elsevier.

Table 17.1   Risk Factors for the Development of Venous Thromboembolic Disease in Childhood(13)

Acquired risk factors

Disease related:	*Medication related:*	*Iatrogenic risks:*
Shock	Oral contraceptives	Central venous catheters
Septicaemia	Corticosteroids	Surgery
Malignancy	Asparaginase	Parenteral nutrition
Immobilization		Cardiac surgery (i.e., Fontan procedures)
Trauma		
Kidney disease		
Cardiac disease		
Systemic lupus erythematosus		
Inflammatory bowel disease		
Diabetes		
Sickle cell anaemia		
Prematurity		
Asphyxia		
Polycythaemia		
Hyperhomocysteinaemia		
Carbohydrate-deficient glycoprotein syndrome		
Varicella infection		

Genetic risk factors

Factor V mutation
Factor II mutation
Antithrombin deficiency
Protein C deficiency
Protein S deficiency
Hyperhomocysteinaemia

substances (especially parenteral nutrition), compromised blood flow and thrombogenic effects of the catheter material (16). Catheter-related thrombi develop both in children with long-term venous access devices for diseases such as malignancy, intestinal failure, renal insufficiency and cystic fibrosis and in children with short-term catheters in the intensive care unit or for cardiac catheterization (17–19).

Large-bore (triple lumen or pheresis) catheters placed in the relatively small vessels of infants increase the risk of thrombosis. Furthermore, the risk of thrombosis is higher with the use of external catheters compared with implantable ports (20). Finally, Male et al. showed that the risk of thrombosis is significantly greater when the catheter is placed on the left side of the body [odds ratio (OR) 2.5; 95% confidence interval (CI): 1.0 to 6.4] and in the subclavian vein (OR 3.1; 95% CI: 1.2 to 8.5) than on the right side and in the jugular vein (21).

The reported incidences of catheter-related thrombi are highly variable, from 0 to 67%, depending on the patient group, the study design and the diagnostic method (17,22–25). Many of the catheter-related thrombi are asymptomatic or diagnosed solely by radiographic tests (22). Catheter-related thrombi are mostly located in the upper central venous system where obstruction may not result in acute clinical symptoms. The development of catheter-related thrombosis is usually a gradual process, permitting collaterals to form, which minimizes the acute symptoms of arm, neck or facial swelling. These asymptomatic thrombi may be clinically noteworthy, as catheter-related thrombosis is associated with catheter-related infection and PE (19,26). Furthermore, in some children loss of venous access will jeopardize adequate management of their disease.

Cardiac disease

During the last three decades, improvements in diagnostic methods, medical treatment and surgical procedures for congenital heart disease (CHD) have increased the survival rates of affected children. Children with CHD are surviving into adulthood and are faced with the secondary complications of diagnostic and/or therapeutic interventions, such as VTE (27). Thrombotic events are well-known complications of cardiac diseases, attributed mainly to altered haemodynamics, increased blood viscosity, prosthetic materials, surgically damaged blood vessels, cardiopulmonary bypass and central venous catheters. The reported incidence of catheter-related thrombosis in children with CHD varies between 1.1% in a retrospective study and 43% in a prospective study (28). The frequency of thromboembolic events after Fontan and modified Fontan procedures is probably up to 20% (29). In children with CHD, thrombotic events have a major impact on mortality. Two retrospective studies showed that about half of the patients with CHD who developed VTE postoperatively died (28,30). In addition, in children with Fontan procedures, mortality after thrombosis has been reported to be as high as 25% (31). Multiple coagulation factor abnormalities following Fontan procedures involving both pro- and anticoagulant factors have been described (32,33). These abnormalities might contribute to the increased risk of venous thrombosis. Most of these abnormalities, however, are qualitatively and quantitatively similar to those found in patients prior to the Fontan operation, with the exception of factor VIII (34). Odegard et al. reported an increased level of factor VIII after Fontan procedure; in six of the 20 children (35%), the level was significantly above the normal range, two of whom had a thrombotic event (35).

The Antiphospholipid syndrome

The antiphospholipid syndrome is characterized by the clinical manifestations of venous or arterial thrombosis and in women it can be associated with recurrent fetal loss (36). It can occur in isolation or in the setting of autoimmune diseases, such as systemic lupus erythematosus (SLE). The diagnosis is made after the detection of persistently elevated levels of antiphospholipid antibodies. Antiphospholipid antibodies are a heterogeneous group of antibodies directed against protein antigens that bind to anionic phospholipids, such as β-2-glycoprotein 1 and prothrombin, or directed against phospholipids, such as cardiolipin. Lupus anticoagulant (LA) is detected by prolongation of in *vitro* clotting tests and is caused by the presence of anti β-2-glycoprotein 1 and/or antiprothrombin antibodies. LA is the strongest predictor of the risk of thrombotic events in patients with SLE (37). If testing for LA is not possible, anticardiolipin IgM and anti-β-2-glycoprotein 1 IgG have the highest predictive value. Levy *et al.* showed that at 33.6 months after diagnosis of SLE, 50% of 24 paediatric patients with LA-positive SLE developed thrombotic events (38). Recurrent thrombosis occurred in about one-third of the antiphospholipid syndrome paediatric patients (39,40).

Malignancy

In prospective cohort studies the general prevalence of thrombosis of all paediatric patients with cancer varied between 1 and 50%, particularly depending on the choice of the diagnostic method (22,41–45). When thrombosis was diagnosed from clinical symptoms, the prevalence was about 5-10% (41,42). In contrast, when thrombosis was diagnosed with venography, the prevalence was 37–50% (22,43). The biology of the underlying malignancy seems to be an important determinant of thrombosis. Acute lymphoblastic leukaemia (ALL) has been the most common cancer reported in association with thrombosis in children. In a meta-analysis of 17 prospective studies, the incidence rate of symptomatic thrombosis was 5.2% (95% CI: 4.2–6.4%) in children with ALL (46). Thrombotic events mainly occurred in the central venous system and in the upper limbs. Most of the thrombi developed in the induction phase of therapy. In this initial phase, the disease is still active and treatment is intense, including asparaginase and steroids (47). Both asparaginase and steroids induce a prothrombotic state by suppression of anticoagulant proteins, particularly antithrombin and plasminogen, and by elevation of factor VIII/von Willebrand factor complex, respectively. Furthermore, steroids increase plasminogen activator inhibitor, causing hypofibrinolysis. Central venous catheters are an important risk factor for site-specific venous thrombosis in children with ALL. The role of congenital prothrombotic disorders remains uncertain (46). More prospective studies are needed to provide guidelines for routine screening and prophylactic strategies.

Other conditions with acquired prothrombotic disorders

Many of the acquired risk factors are known to be associated with acquired prothrombotic disorders, such as Fontan procedures, asparaginase therapy (both discussed above), use of estrogen, varicella infection and carbohydrate-deficient glycoprotein (CDG) syndrome. Tall girls using very high-dose estrogen for reduction of growth develop protein S deficiency, which might contribute to thrombus formation in certain circumstances (48,49). After cessation of estrogen administration, plasma protein S levels return to normal values in about 4 weeks (50). A severe acquired protein S deficiency as a result of auto-antibodies may develop after varicella infection, causing thromboemboli and/or purpura fulminans (51–53). In children with CDG syndrome, blood coagulation disorders are a common finding (54–56). The characteristic biochemical feature of this disease consists of hypoglycosylation of glycoproteins, such as coagulation factors and inhibitors. The most common findings are reduced activities of antithrombin, protein C, protein S and factor XI. The imbalance between procoagulant and anticoagulant proteins leads to a prothrombotic state, which may cause venous thrombosis, especially when additional risk factors for thrombosis are present (57).

Congenital risk factors

Egeberg was the first to use the term thrombophilia, in 1965, when he described a Norwegian family that had a tendency to VTE, based on a deficiency of antithrombin (58). Various laboratory abnormalities have been discovered since then that increase the risk of venous thrombosis. In adults, the prevalence of the five established congenital defects, namely factor V G1691A mutation, factor II G20210A mutation and deficiencies of natural anticoagulants antithrombin, protein C and protein S, is estimated to be about 30% in unselected Caucasian patients with confirmed venous thrombosis (59). In paediatric patients with venous thromboembolic disease, published frequencies of single congenital prothrombotic disorders vary from 10 to 59% (60–68) and combined congenital prothrombotic disorders from 3 to 21% (60,62,65,66), depending on the age and size of the study population, the type of prothrombotic disorders studied and study design.

In addition to the five established congenital risk factors several other prothrombotic risk factors were identified in adults, such as hyperhomocysteinaemia and increased levels of factor VIII, IX, XI, fibrinogen and thrombin-activatable fibrinolysis inhibitor (69–74). Very recently, seven single-nucleotide polymorphisms were identified that were associated with DVT in two large adult population-based case–control studies in The Netherlands (75).The increased thrombotic risk is usually mild. In children, the role of these factors in the aetiology of thrombosis has yet to be established.

The usefulness and cost-effectiveness of testing for thrombophilia in paediatric patients with VTE is a matter of debate. Testing for thrombophilia may have some advantages. First, an important reason to test for thrombophilia would be the possibility of adjusting therapeutic regimes in children with VTE to prevent recurrent thrombosis. One study showed that in paediatric patients with a first spontaneous thrombotic event, the risk of recurrent thrombosis was significantly higher in patients carrying a single or combined congenital prothrombotic disorder compared with those who did not (66). These patients could be candidates for prolongation of anticoagulant treatment. Whether prolongation of treatment will improve the clinical outcome of children with VTE and thrombophilia still needs to be determined. Second, testing may improve the understanding of the causes of VTE. Especially in children, parents and their doctors would like to know the cause as thrombosis is a rare disease in children. However, most of the children with VTE have several additional acquired risk factors, which also contribute to a prothrombotic state. One study showed that thrombophilia testing is probably worthwhile in adolescents with spontaneous VTE (76), as in this group of patients a higher incidence of congenital defects was present. Finally, testing for thrombophilia can be used to identify asymptomatic family members. These adult family members have a 2–10-fold increased risk of VTE compared with non-carriers (77–79). The overall absolute risk remains low, however. One prospective study has been performed assessing spontaneous rates of VTE in children aged 1–14 years who had at least one family member known to be a carrier for a single prothrombotic disorder. This study showed that none of the 143 children developed VTE during follow-up for a mean of 5 years, despite exposure to acquired risk factors, including surgery, trauma and immobilization (80). About 60% of these children were carriers of a congenital prothrombotic disorder. As a consequence, it seems reasonable to postpone screening of asymptomatic family members until puberty, unless requested by families. Furthermore, it should only be done if the results are likely to change medical management.

Disadvantages of testing for thrombophilia in children with venous thromboembolic disease include the costs of testing, the psychological impact of knowing that one is a carrier of a congenital prothrombotic disorder and potential problems with health insurance (81,82). In adults, some studies have been performed to investigate the cost-effectiveness of testing for thrombophilia. One study showed that testing for double heterozygosity of factor V and factor II mutation in patients with thrombosis followed by prolongation of therapy in those tested positive for both mutations appeared cost-effective (83). Conversely, screening for thrombophilia in certain populations (for example, all women at the onset of pregnancy) is unlikely to be cost-effective. Selective screening based on the presence of personal or family history of venous thrombosis may improve the potential cost-effectiveness (84).

DIAGNOSIS

Clinical diagnosis

The clinical presentation of venous thromboembolism depends on the location of the thrombi. The majority of paediatric venous thrombi are catheter related and therefore situated in the upper venous system (Figure 17.2). Many of these thrombi are asymptomatic. When symptomatic, symptoms include swelling, pain and discoloration of the upper extremity, superior vena cava syndrome (swelling of the face and neck, distended veins in the skin over the chest), chylothorax and chylopericardium (85,86). In general, sepsis and repeated loss of patency of the catheter raise the suspicion of catheter-related thrombosis. Chronic catheter-related thrombosis often presents with collateral circulation in the skin (26). Venous thrombosis in the lower extremity usually causes abdominal, inguinal or leg pain, swelling of the abdomen or leg and reddish or blue–purple

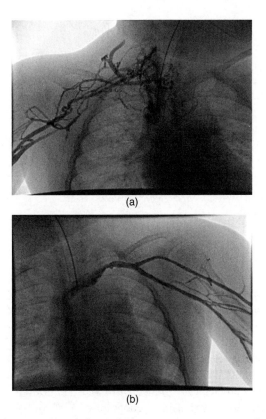

(a)

(b)

Figure 17.2 (a) Abnormal venogram of the right upper venous system after catheter-related venous thrombosis in a 1-year-old girl with intestinal failure and long-term total parenteral nutrition since the age of 3 months. (b) Normal venogram of the left upper venous system of the same patient.

discoloration of the lower extremity. In some neonates, sudden thrombocytopenia appears to be the only sign of thrombosis due to consumption of platelets.

The clinical diagnosis of PE is confounded by a clinical presentation that may be very subtle, mimics many other diseases or is obscured by an underlying clinical condition. Increased clinical suspicion is needed to prevent delay in diagnosis. In teenagers, pleuritic chest pain appeared to be the most common presenting complaint, mentioned in 84% of the patients (87). Other complaints included dyspnea (58%), cough (47%) and haemoptysis (32%). Presenting signs in teenagers were arterial hypoxaemia, physical signs of a DVT of the lower extremity, abnormal chest radiograph, tachypnea and fever. Unexplained persistent tachypnea can be an important indication of PE in paediatric patients of all age categories (88,89). In children receiving artificial ventilation, an increase in oxygen requirement may be a sign of PE. Other signs and symptoms that have been reported to occur in children with acute PE include acute right heart failure, cyanosis, hypotension, arrhythmia, pallor, syncope or sudden death.

In adults, the combination of clinical signs and symptoms and the presence of risk factors are used to assess the pre-test probability of VTE. During the last decade, several sets of prediction rules have been published, which varied in complexity (see Chapter 5) (90–93). These prediction rules classify patients in two or three clinical probability categories. The combined use of the clinical probability and the results of one or more laboratory or radiographic tests improve the precision of diagnosis for venous thromboembolism compared with assessment alone. In children, clinical prediction rules have yet to be validated.

D-dimer test

D-dimer is a marker of endogenous fibrinolysis and should therefore be detectable in patients with VTE (see Chapter 6). Venous thromboembolism can be ruled out in adult patients who are considered low risk clinically and who have a negative D-dimer test. Ultrasound testing can be safely omitted in such patients (92,94). The usefulness of the D-dimer test as a screening test in children with suspected VTE has not been studied. Due to a lack of available data, one cannot exclude VTE even if the level of D-dimer is very low. Furthermore, the majority of children with VTE have serious systemic illnesses such as cancer or cardiac disease, which are usually associated with elevated D-dimer levels. Radiographic tests remain required in case of clinical suspicion of VTE in children.

Radiographic diagnosis

Individual radiographic tests that are used to diagnose venous thromboembolic disease are the same as those used in adults (for a more detailed description, see the relevant chapters elsewhere in this book). All tests have advantages and disadvantages in paediatric patients, as shown in Table 17.2.

For evaluation of the upper venous system, both ultrasonography and venography are required. This has become apparent in the PARKAA study, a prospective diagnostic study in 66 children with ALL and a central venous catheter (95). Nineteen of the 66 children developed catheter-related thrombosis. Thrombi were diagnosed using venography in 15 of 19 patients (sensitivity 79%) and ultrasonography in seven of 19 patients (sensitivity 37%). Three of four thrombi detected by ultrasonography but not by venography were located in the jugular veins. Venography is not effective in the jugular veins as the dye cannot flow in a retrograde way. Therefore, venography is

Table 17.2 Advantages and Disadvantages of Diagnostic Tests for Venous Thromboembolic Disease in Childhood

Diagnostic test	Disadvantages	Advantages
Venography	Invasive	Reference standard for diagnosis in upper and lower venous system, except in jugular vein
	Unavailable in some centres	
	Requires expertise in performance and interpretation	
	Expensive	
	Use of iodinated contrast media	
	Radiation exposure	
Ultrasonography	Low sensitivity in upper venous system (except in jugular vein)	Non-invasive
	Difficulty in obese patients	In adults excellent sensitivity and specificity compared with venography for diagnosis of thrombosis in lower venous system (in children not studied)
		Inexpensive
		Easy to perform and interpret (in pre-term neonates also)
		Universally available
Ventilation–perfusion lung scanning	High percentage of non-diagnostic (i.e., low or intermediate probability) scans	Relatively easy to perform, even in small children
	Underlying diseases may hamper the interpretation of scans	Low radiation exposure

(continued overleaf)

Table 17.2 Continued

Diagnostic test	Disadvantages	Advantages
Multi-detector computed tomography	Significant radiation exposure Use of iodinated contrast media	Identification of other chest/pulmonary disorders Relatively easy to perform in critically ill patients
Pulmonary angiography	Invasive Unavailable in some centres Requires expertise in performance and interpretation Expensive Use of iodinated contrast media Radiation exposure	Reference standard for diagnosis of PE
Magnetic resonance venography and pulmonary angiography	Requirement for anaesthesia in small children Expensive Unavailable in some centres Sensitivity and specificity unknown	Absence of radiation exposure Minimal invasiveness Contrast media well tolerated

recommended for the detection of thrombosis in the central veins and ultrasonography for the jugular veins. Echocardiography can be a useful diagnostic method to detect thrombi in the right atrium.

To detect lower extremity thrombosis, ultrasonography is usually an adequate method. The sensitivity of this diagnostic method has not been investigated in paediatric patients and therefore adult guidelines are followed. If clinical suspicion is high, but the ultrasonography result is negative, it is advised to repeat ultrasonography after 5–7 days or to perform venography (96).

Pulmonary embolism can be diagnosed by multidetector computed tomography (CT) or ventilation–perfusion lung scintigraphy (97,98). CT is becoming the first-choice diagnostic test in many centres. In addition to visualization of the emboli, it can also identify other chest and pulmonary disorders, which should be differentiated from PE. Important disadvantages are the use of iodinated contrast media and, especially in children, the significant radiation exposure. Ventilation–perfusion lung scintigraphy is a valuable test when the results are definitive. A normal perfusion scan rules out the diagnosis of a clinically relevant recent PE, and if a patient has a high-probability lung scan (mismatched perfusion defects that are segmental or larger), there is a more than 85% chance that the patient has PE. However, the majority of patients have low- or intermediate-probability scans which are non-diagnostic. An increase in definitive diagnosis can be achieved in the presence of a normal chest radiograph when deciding to proceed with ventilation–perfusion lung scanning instead of CT (99).

PROPHYLAXIS

In children, the risk of VTE is much lower than in adults and, consequently, indications for primary prophylaxis in the paediatric population are fewer. To prevent thrombosis in children, it seems to be logical to focus on patients with central venous catheters as they are the most frequent risk factors in children with venous thrombosis. Several measures are available to prevent catheter-related thrombosis, including prophylactic doses of anticoagulation and heparin-bonded catheters. A few studies evaluated these measures in children.

Recently, a randomized, placebo-controlled study showed that very low doses of unfractionated heparin (UFH) (0.5 U/kg/h) prolonged the duration of stay of peripherally inserted central venous catheters and decreased the incidence of catheter occlusion in neonates. Unfortunately, heparin did not influence the incidence of venous thrombosis and catheter-related infection (100). In children more than 3 months old, one study has been performed to assess the efficacy and safety of low molecular weight heparin (LMWH) (reviparin) compared with standard care to prevent clinically and venography-proven catheter-related thrombosis in the first 30 days after insertion (25). Eleven of 78 patients (14.1%) with reviparin and 10 of 80 patients (12.5%) with standard care developed thrombosis. One patient in the standard care group had a major bleed. However, due to slow accrual, the PROTEKT study was closed prematurely and the efficacy of LMWH remained unclear. Hence available studies do not allow definitive recommendations for catheter-related thromboprophylaxis in children.

Nevertheless, despite the lack of randomized controlled trials, in some patient groups with central venous catheters antithrombotic prophylaxis should be considered. For example, children using the catheter for long-term parenteral nutrition are at increased risk of venous thrombosis. The incidence of thrombosis in this patient group ranges from 4 to 75% with a median of 11.4%, depending on the different types of studies and diagnostic methods (101). Prospective and cross-sectional studies that routinely screened for venous thrombosis reported increased incidence rates (median 35.3%). For these children, the venous catheter is a 'life line' and preventing thrombosis is extremely important. A study by Newall *et al.* demonstrated that in eight children with short-gut syndrome or small intestine anomalies, warfarin therapy increased the mean catheter duration from 160.9 to 351.7 days. There were no major bleedings and no clinical extension of thrombosis was observed (102).

Many short-term venous catheters in critically ill paediatric patients are situated in the femoral vein. The incidence of catheter-related thrombosis in these patients varies between 0 and 50%. Most thrombi are asymptomatic and remain unobserved. Two prospective randomized studies showed that heparin-bonded catheters may reduce the incidence of catheter-related thrombosis and catheter-related infection (23,103). In these studies, patients were examined with routine ultrasonography. In the largest study, by Pierce *et al.*, catheter-related thrombosis developed in 0 of 97 (0%) patients with heparin-bonded catheters and eight of 103 (8%) patients with non-heparin-bonded catheters. Catheter-related infection was observed in 4 and 33%, respectively (23). On the other hand, one randomized controlled trial in infants (<1 year old) who were post-surgery for congenital heart disease, revealed no benefit of using heparin-bonded catheters for the prevention of thrombosis (104). A Cochrane review included both studies in its analysis and concluded that heparin-bonded catheters do not prevent catheter-related thrombosis [relative risk (RR) 0.71; 95% CI: 0.44 to 1.15], but might play a role in reducing catheter-related infections (RR 0.06; 95% CI: 0.01 to 0.41) and colonization of the catheter (RR 0.21; 95% CI: 0.06 to 0.71) (105).

In children with ALL, central venous catheters are used for the administration of cytostatic drugs, blood products and sometimes parenteral nutrition. Asparaginase is an important component of ALL treatment. As a side effect, asparaginase can reduce the synthesis of several coagulation factors and inhibitors, including antithrombin. In the PARKAA study, the efficacy and safety of antithrombin supplementation were investigated in reducing thrombosis incidence in children with ALL and a central venous catheter (106). It showed a trend that antithrombin supplementation may decrease the incidence of thrombi in children with ALL treated with asparaginase. Another randomized study of low-dose oral anticoagulation for the prevention of catheter-related thrombosis in children with cancer did not show any benefit of warfarin adjusted to maintain an international normalized ratio (INR) between 1.3 and 1.9 (107). One prospective cohort study reported the use of prophylactic therapy with LMWH (enoxaparin) in 41 children with ALL during asparaginase treatment. None of the children developed symptomatic thrombosis during 76 courses of asparaginase (108). In addition to prophylactic doses of anticoagulant drugs, the choice of location of a catheter may also be important to prevent catheter-related thrombosis. Male *et al.* showed that the risk of thrombosis was significantly higher when the catheter was placed on the left side of the body (OR 2.5; 95% CI: 1.0 to 6.4) and in the subclavian vein (OR 3.1; 95% CI: 1.2 to 8.5) than on the right side and in the jugular vein (21).

TREATMENT

Initial treatment

Treatment regimens for DVT and PE are similar because the two conditions are manifestations of the same disease process. Anticoagulation, including LMWH subcutaneously or UFH intravenously, is the main therapy for acute VTE in paediatric patients. The aims of anticoagulant therapy are to prevent thrombus extension, embolization and early and late recurrent thrombosis. In selected patients, thrombolytic therapy can be administered.

Low molecular weight heparin

As venous thrombosis occurs infrequently in children, treatment has always been extrapolated from treatment of adults with thrombotic events. When LMWHs were introduced in the mid-1990s and appeared to be as effective and safe as UFH in adults for the initial therapy of thrombosis (109), it did not take long before paediatric patients with venous thrombosis were also treated with

LMWHs. Whereas in 1994 none of the 137 patients in the Canadian paediatric venous thrombosis registry received LMWH, 10 years later more than 60% of the 200 paediatric patients in the British registry were treated with LMWHs (1,110). Especially in children, LMWHs have many advantages over UFH. LMWHs have a greater bioavailability, a more predictable anticoagulant response and longer half-life. Hence LMWHs can be given subcutaneously, once or twice daily, with limited laboratory monitoring. This is an important advantage in neonates and infants in whom intravenous access can be very difficult. Furthermore, as a result of reduced binding to platelet factor 4 or osteoblasts, the risk of heparin-induced thrombocytopenia (HIT) and osteopenia is decreased.

In children, only one randomized controlled trial (REVIVE) has been performed to assess the efficacy and safety of LMWH (reviparin) compared with UFH and vitamin K antagonists for the treatment of VTE (111). At 6 months, the risk of recurrent thrombosis was 12.5%, identical with the risk of major bleeding for UFH/vitamin K antagonists, compared with 5.6% for recurrent thrombosis and 5.6% for major bleeding for LMWH. This study, however, was underpowered as the result of premature closure. Small case series, evaluating the efficacy and safety of enoxaparin, reviparin, nadroparin, tinzaparin and dalteparin, showed that LMWH appeared to be an efficient and safe anticoagulant for treatment and prophylaxis of VTE in children, including prematurely born neonates (112–117). In these cohort studies, recurrent thrombosis and major bleedings occurred in 0–5 and 0–8% of patients, respectively (118).

Monitoring of LMWH should be done by using the anti-Xa assay. The paediatric therapeutic range is extrapolated from the adult therapeutic range and is 0.5–1.0 U/mL 4 h post-LMWH dose (Table 17.3). In contrast to adults, it is advised to measure anti-Xa levels in children until these levels have reached therapeutic ranges, especially in young children. Young children need a higher dose to reach therapeutic range than older children (118). A similar age-dependent response has been found for unfractionated heparin and vitamin K antagonists (119,120). The mechanisms responsible for this observation are not entirely clear. An important causative factor in the need for higher doses of LMWH in younger patients is the increased clearance. For a 10 kg child, Laporte et al. estimated the nadroparin clearance at 37 mL/h/kg (121). In adults, the clearance is estimated at about 12.5 mL/h/kg in healthy volunteers and 11.6 mL/h/kg in patients with VTE (122). Pre-term neonates seem to require the highest doses. Whereas in infants weighing <5 kg and younger than 2 months the recommended starting dose of enoxaparin is 1.5 mg/kg per 12 h, in the study by Michaels et al. pre-term neonates needed 2.27 mg/kg per 12 h to reach the therapeutic target range (115). Another reason to check anti-Xa levels in paediatric patients is the presence of severe underlying diseases, which may cause an increased risk of bleeding (malignancy) or accumulation (renal insufficiency). One pharmacokinetic study showed that in children younger than 5 years of age, peak anti-Xa levels of tinzaparin were reached after 2–3 h. This indicates that in this age category anti-Xa levels need to be taken after 2 h instead of 4 h. More studies are needed to confirm this finding (112).

Unfractionated heparin

UFH is a reasonable alternative for LMWH as the initial therapy for venous thrombosis, especially in critically ill patients. It has a fast onset of action and a short half-life and consequently its action can be reversed relatively rapidly. Furthermore, an effective antidote is available. So far, only one prospective study has been performed in which the effect of UFH in children has been evaluated (120). A loading dose of 75–100 U/kg is necessary to reach therapeutic levels of activated partial thromboplastin time (aPTT) in 90% of patients. The maintenance dose is age dependent: 28 U/kg for infants younger than 1 year and 20 U/kg for infants older than 1 year. The recommended therapeutic aPTT range is extrapolated from the adult therapeutic range and is an aPTT that corresponds to an anti-Xa level of 0.3–0.7 U/mL (Table 17.3). Recently, the in vivo response to

Table 17.3 Heparin Therapy in Children with Venous Thromboembolic Disease
(112–114,116,117,120)[a]

Drug	Dosage	Monitoring
Low molecular weight heparin		
	120 U/kg/dose every 12 h sc	Anti-Xa level, platelets
Nadroparin		Target anti-Xa level: 0.5–1.0 U/mL
0–2 m	85.5 U/kg/dose every 12 h sc	
>2 m		
Enoxaparin	1.5 mg/kg/dose every 12 h sc	
0–2 m		
>2 m	1.0 mg/kg/dose every 12 h sc	
Dalteparin		
0–16 y	129 ± 43 U/kg/dose every 24 h sc	
Tinzaparin		
0–2 m	275 U/kg/dose every 24 h sc	
2–12 m		
1–5 y	250 U/kg/dose every 24 h sc	
5–10 y		
10–16 y	240 U/kg/dose every 24 h sc	
Reviparin		
<5 kg	200 U/kg/dose every 24 h sc	
>5 kg		
	175 U/kg/dose every 24 h sc	
	150 U/kg/dose every 12 h sc	
	100 U/kg/dose every 12 h sc	
Unfractionated heparin		
Loading dose	75 U/kg in 10 min iv	aPTT and platelets
Maintenance dose	28 U/kg/h iv	Therapeutic aPTT level: aPTT prolongation corresponding to plasma heparin levels from 0.3 to 0.7 U/mL anti-Xa activity by the amidolytic assay
<1 y	20 U/kg/h iv	
>1 y		

[a]Abbreviations: m, month; y, year; sc, subcutaneously; iv, intravenously; aPTT, activated partial thromboplastin time.

UFH was examined in children who received UFH for various reasons in a paediatric intensive care unit. This study showed that there was little agreement between UFH dose, aPTT and anti-Xa activity. Most clinicians who routinely use the aPTT to monitor UFH in children will frequently adjust UFH doses down, based on the aPTT results, causing subtherapeutic heparinization as defined by an appropriate anti-Xa range (123).

The most common complication of UFH is bleeding. Andrew *et al*. reported bleeding complications in about 2% of the paediatric patients in a prospective cohort study (120). However, many children were treated suboptimally. In critically ill patients, the incidence of bleeding seems to be higher. Recently, Kuhle *et al*. showed that major bleeding events occurred in nine of the 38 children (24%; 95% CI: 11 to 40%) in the critical care unit. In this study, 28 patients were missed for enrolment. Even after inclusion of the 28 missed patients with the assumption of no bleedings, the bleeding rate would still be as high as 14% (124). Another complication is heparin-induced thrombocytopenia (HIT), a potentially severe complication which occurs in 1–2% of children receiving UFH (125).

Thrombolytic therapy

The decision to use thrombolytic agents in paediatric patients with VTE should be very much individualized. In general, these agents should be considered in children with large, new PE, particularly if the embolism is haemodynamically compromising or in children with extensive venous thrombosis in a threatened organ or extremity and a low bleeding risk. Recently, Goldenberg *et al*. showed that there may be a new indication for thrombolysis in children (126). In a small retrospective analysis of 22 children with acute occlusive DVT, they showed that the post-thrombotic syndrome (PTS) occurred in two of nine (23%) patients with a thrombolytic regime and in 10 of 13 (77%) patients with standard anticoagulation (UFH or LMWH followed by vitamin K antagonists). Disadvantages of this study are the retrospective design, the small number of patients, which makes the assessment of efficacy and safety impossible, and the heterogeneity of the thrombolytic regime. Furthermore, PTS in four of the 10 patients in the standard group consisted of increased circumference of the leg without pain or activity limitations. The question is whether thrombolysis with increased risk of bleeding complications is warranted to prevent an increased circumference of the leg. To answer this question, a prospective multicentre study is in development.

Thrombolytic agents are plasminogen activators and include urokinase, streptokinase and tissue plasminogen activator (tPA) (Table 17.4). In most centres, tPA is favoured over the other thrombolytic agents as a result of fibrin specificity and affinity and low immunogenicity (127,128). Although several case reports and small case series have reported successful thrombolysis in children, large clinical trials assessing the efficacy and safety of thrombolytic agents compared with other antithrombotic agents are lacking. The major drawback of thrombolytic therapy is the increased number of major bleeding complications. Retrospective case series revealed these complications to occur in up to 40% of the children treated with tPA (129–132). The optimal dose and duration of thrombolytic therapy in children are unknown. The recommended dose of tPA is 0.1–0.6 mg/kg/h for 6 h (127). However, lower doses of tPA also appear to be effective. In a recent study, complete clot resolution was achieved in 17 children with acute thrombosis treated with low-dose infusions of tPA (0.01–0.06 mg/kg/h) for total infusion durations of up to 96 h. Major bleeding occurred in one patient (133).

Table 17.4 Thrombolytic Therapy in Children with Venous Thromboembolic Disease (127)[a]

Drug	Loading dose	Maintenance dose	Monitoring
tPA	–	0.1 – 0.6 mg/kg/h iv for 6 h	Fibrinogen, aPTT, PT, TCT, D-dimer
Urokinase	4.400 U/kg	4.400 U/kg/h iv for 6–12 h	
Streptokinase	2.000 U/kg	2.000 U/kg/h iv for 6–12 h	

[a]Abbreviations: aPTT, activated partial thromboplastin time; PT, prothrombin time; TCT, thrombin clotting time; iv, intravenously.

Long-term treatment

Paediatric patients with acute VTE require long-term anticoagulant treatment to prevent symptomatic extension of thrombosis and/or recurrent thrombosis. Both vitamin K antagonists and LMWH can be used for long-term anticoagulant treatment in paediatric patients.

Treatment with *vitamin K antagonists* can be initiated together with UFH or LMWH (Table1 17.5). The duration of the initial therapy with heparin should be a minimum of 5 days. Heparin can be discontinued when the INR is stable and >2.0. In general, three vitamin K antagonists are available: warfarin ($t_{1/2} = 36-42$ h), acenocoumarol ($t_{1/2} = 8$ h) and phenprocoumon ($t_{1/2} = 157$ h). The vitamin K antagonist of choice is usually influenced by availability and previous experience within a region or country. Warfarin is the most commonly used vitamin K antagonist worldwide. In children, only a few studies have established the doses of warfarin and acenocoumarol required for long-term treatment in children (119,134). No studies about phenprocoumon in paediatric patients have been published. The initial dose of warfarin is 0.2 mg/kg, with subsequent dose adjustments according to a nomogram (119). One large cohort study of 319 patients showed that in order to maintain a target INR of 2–3, infants and adolescents needed 0.33 and 0.09 mg/kg/day of warfarin, respectively (135). The same age dependency was found for acenocoumarol by Bonduel *et al*. (134). Therefore, they proposed an age-adjusted loading dose regimen for acenocoumarol. This regimen allowed most children to achieve a target range within 1 week of commencing acenocoumarol. None of the children achieved an INR >4. The incidences of bleeding or recurrence were the same as those seen in children taking warfarin therapy: major bleeding in 0–0.5% and recurrent thrombosis in 1.3% of patients (134,135).

Frequent monitoring of the INRs via venepuncture can be technically difficult and traumatic for the child. This can be resolved by using whole-blood prothrombin time/INR monitors, applying capillary blood (136,137). These monitors appeared to be acceptable and reliable for children in the outpatient laboratory and home settings.

Maintenance of stable therapeutic INR levels is difficult in children, because of differences in diet, medication and primary underlying clinical conditions. Breast-fed babies are very sensitive to vitamin K antagonists, as they ingest low concentrations of vitamin K in breast milk. In contrast, other children are relatively resistant to vitamin K antagonists as a result of impaired absorption, total parenteral nutrition or formula containing high concentrations of vitamin K. Especially patients younger than 1 year have fewer INR values in the target range and require more frequent INR testing and dose adjustments. In young infants and in children with malignancies, who require frequent lumbar punctures and develop thrombocytopenia due to cytostatic therapy, *LMWH* is a good alternative to vitamin K antagonists for long-term treatment of venous thrombosis. It is

Table 17.5   Vitamin K Antagonists in Children with Venous Thromboembolic Disease(119;134;135)

Vitamin K antagonist	Age (years)	Loading dose (mg/kg)	Monitoring[a]
Warfarin	All ages	0.2 orally	INR Dose adjustments according to nomogram
Acenocoumarol	<1 1–5 >5	0.15 orally 0.1 orally 0.05 orally	INR Dose adjustments according to nomogram

[a]Abbreviation: INR, international normalized ratio.

advised to measure anti-Xa levels monthly in neonates and children with kidney disease, as a result of increasing body weight and accumulation of the drug, respectively.

Little is known about the optimal duration of antithrombotic therapy in children with venous thrombosis. Guidelines for paediatric patients are extrapolated from guidelines for adult patients with VTE (138). In the individual patient, the risk of bleeding should be balanced against the risk of recurrence. Paediatric patients with a first episode of venous thrombosis secondary to a transient risk factor are usually treated for 3 months. In the presence of an ongoing risk factor, such as nephrotic syndrome or central venous catheter, antithrombotic prophylaxis until the risk factor has resolved is suggested in order to prevent recurrent thrombosis. Patients with a first episode of idiopathic VTE with or without thrombophilia are treated for at least 6 months. A longer duration is suggested if the risk of recurrence is felt to be high, such as in patients with persistent antiphospholipid antibodies and in patients with recurrent thrombosis. In these patients, the need for secondary prophylaxis should be continually evaluated, as the risk of recurrent thrombosis decreases and the risk of anticoagulant-related bleeding may vary over time.

New anticoagulant therapy

UFH and vitamin K antagonists have been used as the anticoagulants of choice for over five decades. Subsequently, LMWHs became widely available and have provided several advantages, especially in paediatric patients. However, LMWHs still possess some of the shortcomings of UFH, such as the inability to bind to and to inactivate cell membrane- and clot-bound thrombin and platelet-bound factor Xa, lack of oral bioavailability and the lack of general availability of assays to monitor their effects. Furthermore, the costs of LMWHs are higher than those of UFH. On the other hand, costs of hospital admissions have decreased. Disadvantages of vitamin K antagonists include a narrow therapeutic window leading to potentially fatal bleeding, large inter-individual dosing differences, interactions with diet and medication and the need for close monitoring. During the last decade, new anticoagulant drugs have been developed with better efficacy and fewer side-effects (139,140). A large number of these drugs have been tested in phase II and III clinical trials and some of them have already been approved as alternatives to current therapies in adults with VTE. Regrettably, no large clinical trials have been performed in paediatric patients. As a result of advances in paediatric tertiary care, more and more children will need anticoagulant therapy and as a consequence clinical trials with the new anticoagulant drugs are needed. It is hoped that new legislation and multinational collaborations will encourage the performance of randomized controlled trials assessing specific paediatric aspects of anticoagulant therapy in order to develop validated guidelines for antithrombotic therapy in children.

Thrombin inhibitors

Direct thrombin inhibitors inhibit thrombin without binding to antithrombin and are therefore unaffected by low or fluctuating concentrations of antithrombin and thus of important advantage in neonates and infants. Furthermore, thrombin inhibitors do not bind to platelet factor 4 and as a consequence do not cause HIT. Finally, in contrast to heparin, they inactivate fibrin-bound thrombin, and also fluid-phase thrombin, which may lead to improved efficacy. A disadvantage of direct thrombin inhibitors is lack of antidote.

Lepirudin is the most potent direct thrombin inhibitor, is approved for the treatment of thrombosis in the presence of HIT in adults and has been reported to be used in about 15 paediatric patients with HIT. No formal dose-finding studies have been performed in children. In a review of paediatric patients with HIT, it has been suggested to start lepirudin as a continuous infusion of 0.03–0.05 mg/kg/h for neonates and 0.1 mg/kg/h for older children without a preceding bolus. It can be monitored by aPTT, with a target range of 1.5–2.5 times the patient's baseline value (141). Disadvantages of lepirudin are increased bleeding due to lack of antidote, formation of antihirudin antibodies and anaphylaxis after re-exposure.

Argatroban is a rapidly active, parenteral direct thrombin inhibitor. It is predominantly metabolized by the liver and dose reductions should be considered in patients with impaired liver function and also in critically ill patients. In North America, argatroban is indicated in adults for prophylaxis or treatment of thrombosis in HIT. In children, a systematic review of the literature described 34 paediatric patients treated with argatroban for indications such as prophylaxis or treatment of HIT or cardiac catheterization (142). These patients received a wide range of doses from 0.1 to 12μg/kg/min without an obvious relationship between patient age and dosage requirement. In general, most of these patients achieved therapeutic levels of anticoagulation despite the various dosages used. A study to establish the pharmacokinetics of argatroban in children is under way.

Bivalirudin, another direct inhibitor of thrombin, has been studied in children <6 months of age as a primary treatment for venous or arterial thrombosis. Based on this study, the suggested bolus dose and initial infusion rates for these patients are 0.125 mg/kg and 0.125 mg/kg/h, respectively (143). These were the lowest doses required to achieve therapeutic aPTT levels. Six of 16 patients (37%) had either complete or partial resolution of their thrombi by 48–72 h. Two patients had major bleedings, i.e., gross haematuria, which resolved with a reduction in the bivalirudin infusion rate. It can be used in patients with renal insufficiency.

Finally, *dabigatran* is an oral thrombin inhibitor. It has been evaluated in phase III adult trials for the prevention of VTE after orthopaedic surgery (144). Reports on the use of dabigatran in children are not available.

Factor Xa inhibitors

Fondaparinux is an indirect factor Xa inhibitor, a synthetic pentasaccharide, an analogue of the unique pentasaccharide sequence of heparin (145). Its advantages over other anticoagulants are its predictable linear pharmacokinetics requiring no therapeutic monitoring, a half-life of 12–17 h requiring once-daily dosing subcutaneously and the lack of cross-reactivity with heparin-induced antibodies. Renal excretion accounts for 55–85% of its clearance. It has been approved by the FDA for the initial treatment and prevention of VTE in adults. A few paediatric case reports about the use of fondaparinux in children with HIT have been published (146).

Idraparinux is a long-acting synthetic pentasaccharide with an expected half-life of approximately 4 days, which allows stable anticoagulation with once-weekly subcutaneous injections. The Van Gogh study showed that in adult patients with DVT, once-weekly subcutaneous idraparinux for 3 or 6 months had an efficacy similar to that of LMWH or UFH plus a vitamin K antagonist. However, in patients with PE, idraparinux was less efficacious than standard therapy (147). During a 6 month extension of prophylaxis, idraparinux was effective in preventing recurrent VTE but was associated with an increased risk of a major haemorrhage (148). To date, no studies in children have been performed.

Rivaroxaban and *apixaban* are both oral direct factor Xa inhibitors. Rivaroxaban has already been studied in adult phase III trials as antithrombotic prophylaxis in orthopaedic surgery (149). Adult phase III trials with apixaban have just started (150).

OUTCOME

Mortality

The all-cause mortality rate in paediatric patients with VTE is high and ranges from 7 to 23% (Table 17.6). In contrast, mortality directly as a result of VTE is lower at 0–4.2%. PE is the most common cause of direct mortality. The difference between all-cause and direct mortality reflects the severe underlying diseases of the children with venous thrombosis.

Recurrent thrombosis

In general, the risk of recurrent thrombosis in children is lower than reported in adult studies. In both children and adults, the recurrence rate seems to increase with increasing duration of follow-up. In adults, the risk of recurrent thrombosis is about 6–10% during the first year, but increases to about 30% at 8–10 years after the initial event (151). In children, a single-centre outcome study reported the cumulative recurrence-free survival to be 92% after 1 year and 82% after 7 years of follow-up (Figure 17.3) (15). The lower recurrence risk in children is probably caused by the high incidence of transient acquired risk factors, such as central venous catheters.

It is important to identify paediatric patients with increased risk of recurrent thrombosis, as these patients could be candidates for prolonged anticoagulant treatment or intermittent antithrombotic prophylaxis in high-risk situations. However, limited data are available on the risk factors of recurrent thrombosis, especially due to the low numbers of patients and inadequate duration of follow-up in most studies. One German study reported that in paediatric patients with a spontaneous first thrombotic event, the risk of recurrent thrombosis was significantly lower in patients carrying a single (OR 4.6; 95% CI: 2.3 to 9.0) compared with a combined (OR 24.0; 95% CI: 5.3 to 108.7) congenital prothrombotic risk factor (66). Age at the first thrombotic event may also be an important risk factor. In both the Canadian and Dutch outcome studies, children with recurrent thrombosis were older at the time of their first event than children who did not develop recurrent thrombosis (15,152).

Catheter-related complications

In some paediatric patients, treatment depends on the insertion of a central venous catheter such as for chemotherapy for children with malignancy and total parenteral nutrition for children with intestinal failure. Loss of catheter patency is an important complication in these patients. In most patients, patency can be restored with unfractionated heparin or low-dose thrombolytic therapy (153). In approximately 10% of the patients with loss of patency, clinically important catheter-related thrombosis can be detected (154).

There seems to be a close association of catheter-related thrombosis and infection, especially in patients with malignancies, who suffer long periods of neutropenia. The formation of a thin biofilm, which is commonly observed after catheterization, may play an important role in the development of certain catheter-related infections. This biofilm consists of several proteins such as fibrin, fibronectin, collagen, laminin and several types of immunoglobulins. Microorganisms, especially *Staphylococcus aureus* and certain types of coagulase-negative *Staphylococcus*, easily adhere to these thrombin sheets. This association was first suggested by Press *et al.* in 1984, based on observations from a review of the literature (155). Recently, van Rooden *et al.* showed that the risk of clinically manifest thrombosis is increased after an episode of catheter-related infection (RR

Table 17.6 Outcome of Venous Thromboembolic Disease in Childhood[a]

Study	Study design	No. of patients	Age at time of VTE	Follow-up period	Type of VTE	All-cause mortality	Direct mortality	Recurrent VTE
Andrew (1994) (1)	Registry	137	1 m–18 y	6 m–3 y (median 18 m)	DVT and PE	$n=13$ (9.5%)	$n=3$ (2.2%)	$n=23$ (17%)
Massicotti (1998)(163)	Prospective cohort	244	1 m–18 y	3 m–7 y (median 2 y)	Catheter-related VTE	$n=57$ (23%)	$n=9$ (3.7%)	$n=16$ (6.5%)
Monagle (2000)(152)	Prospective cohort	405	1 m–18 y	2 w–6 y (median 2.9 y)	DVT and PE	$n=65$ (16%)	$n=9$ (2.2%)	$n=33$ (8%)
Gurgey (2001)(164)	Retrospective	95	1 m–17 y	12 m–41 m (mean 3 y)	Non-catheter-related VTE	$n=19$ (20%)	$n=4$ (4.2%)	$n=3$ (3.1%)
Hausler (2001)(165)	Retrospective	21	0 m–13 y	3 m–18 y (median 10.2 y)	Inferior caval vein thrombosis	$n=3$ (14%)	$n=0$ (0%)	–
Nowak-Göttl (2001) (66)	Prospective cohort	301	0 m–18 y	6 m–15 y (median 7 y)	Spontaneous VTE	–	–	$n=64$ (21.3%)
van Ommen (2001) (4)	Registry	99	0 m–18 y	1 m–1 y (median 6 m)	All VTE	$n=16$ (16%)	$n=2$ (2%)	$n=7$ (7%)
Massicotti (2003) (111)	RCT	76	2 m–18 y	6 m	DVT and PE	$n=5$ (7%)	$n=0$ (0%)	$n=7$ (9.2%)
van Ommen (2003) (15)	Prospective cohort	100	0 m–18 y	1 m–12 y (median 4 y)	All VTE	$n=20$ (20%)	$n=1$ (1%)	$n=11$ (11%)

[a]Abbreviations: VTE, venous thromboembolic disease; m, month; y, year; w, week; DVT, deep vein thrombosis; PE, pulmonary embolism; CNS, central nervous system; RCT, randomized controlled trial.

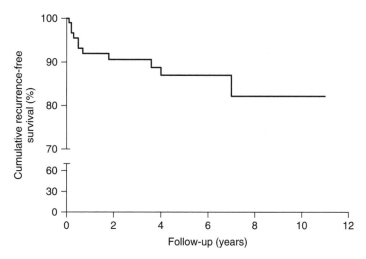

Figure 17.3 The cumulative recurrence-free survival of 100 paediatric patients with venous thromboembolism in one tertiary centre in The Netherlands. Reprinted from van Ommen CH, Heijboer H, van den Dool EJ, Hutten BA, Peters M. Paediatric venous thromboembolic disease in one single centre: congenital prothrombotic disorders and the clinical outcome. J Thromb Haemost 2003; 1:2516–22, with permission of Blackwell Publishing.

17.6; 95% CI: 4.1 to 74.1) in adult patients undergoing intensive chemotherapy (156). In children, two studies performed in the intensive care unit demonstrated that heparin-bonded catheters not only decreased the presence of clinical and subclinical thrombosis detected by routine Doppler ultrasound, but also reduced the incidence of catheter-related infection (23,103). In children with cancer, a retrospective cohort study revealed that children with catheter-related thrombosis had a higher rate of infection (2.7 vs 1.2 episodes per 1000 catheter days) and catheter occlusion (6.2 vs 1.6 episodes per 1000 catheter days) than those without thrombosis (19). These data suggest that (sub)clinical thrombosis might contribute to catheter infection, an important cause of morbidity and mortality in sick patients with central venous catheters.

Post-thrombotic syndrome (PTS)

PTS is a potentially disabling complication. Its symptoms and signs may vary from mild leg heaviness or aching, dilated veins and/or oedema to severe lipodermatosclerosis and ulceration (Figure 17.4). Typically, the symptoms worsen on standing and walking and improve with rest and leg elevation. PTS is most likely caused by venous hypertension, which is the result of persistent outflow obstruction and/or valvular insufficiency. Venous hypertension causes capillary leakage of water, large proteins, including fibrinogen, erythrocytes and leukocytes, and it hampers lymphatic flow, producing oedema, tissue hypoxia, inflammation and sometimes ulceration.

There is no gold standard test for the diagnosis of PTS. In patients with objectively confirmed venous thrombosis, diagnosis of PTS is usually based on the presence of typical symptoms and signs. Diagnosis of PTS can be made from 3 to 6 months after the acute thrombotic event as it takes that period for the initial pain and swelling to disappear. In children, various definitions of PTS have been reported. In some paediatric outcome studies, children were systematically screened for PTS using standardized criteria, which are shown in Table 17.7 (15,126,157). One paediatric PTS scale has been validated in children. This scoring system encompassed the assessment of both physical examination findings and functional limitations and was adapted from the validated

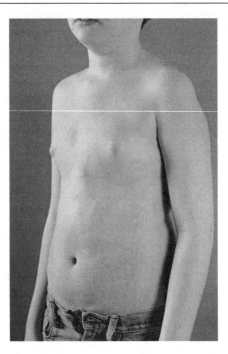

Figure 17.4 Extended collateral circulation in the skin after venous thromboembolic disease of both legs. A full colour version of this image appears in the plate section of this book. Reprinted from van Ommen CH, Peters M. A new diagnosis in children: the post-thrombotic syndrome. Progr Pediatr Cardiol 2005; 21:23–9, with permission of Elsevier.

international adult PTS scale, the Clinical–Aetiology–Anatomic–Pathophysiologic (CEAP) classification. In this paediatric PTS scale, the validated Wong–Baker Faces Pain Scale was used for pain assessment (126).

It is possible to confirm the clinical diagnosis of PTS objectively by diagnostic methods such as plethysmography or duplex ultrasonography, showing the presence and extent of obstructed and/or valvular reflux flow and collateral circulation (158). In paediatric studies, these methods have not been used frequently. Because of the poor specificity of these methods, the diagnosis of PTS should be based on the typical clinical signs and symptoms. Patients who have been objectively diagnosed with venous reflux but who are asymptomatic do not have PTS.

Relatively few studies have evaluated children after venous thrombosis for the presence of PTS. The prevalence ranged from 3.1 to 70%, as a result of a difference in patient population, study design, number of patients investigated, length of follow-up period and definition of PTS (Table 17.8). In the Canadian and Dutch paediatric cohort studies evaluating PTS with standardized scorings systems, PTS occurred in 63–70% of children after symptomatic venous thrombosis (15,157). This is the same incidence as in adult patients without PTS prophylaxis (compression stockings). As opposed to adults, the syndrome in paediatric patients is usually mild. In both the Canadian and Dutch studies, the most frequent objective signs were increased limb circumference and presence of collateral veins. Moderate post-thrombotic signs and symptoms were present in about 10% of the paediatric patients. These included increased limb circumference, collateral veins, telangiectases, malleolar flaring, pigmentation of the skin and complaint of heaviness or pain in the affected leg while standing or walking. None of the paediatric patients had venous ulceration, but longer follow-up is needed to investigate whether these patients with mild and moderate PTS will eventually develop ulcerations.

Table 17.7 Clinical Scales used for the Diagnosis of Post-thrombotic Syndrome (PTS) in Childhood

PTS scale	Criteria used to diagnose PTS
Paediatric PTS score based on Villalta score (157)	2 Subjective symptoms: Pain or abnormal use, swelling 9 Objective symptoms: Change in skin colour, increase in limb circumference, pitting oedema, collateral vessels, pigmentation, tenderness on palpation, oedema of the head, varicosities and ulceration Each rated as 0=absent, 1=present, except oedema of the head and varicosities, which are rated as 0=absent, 1=moderate, 2=severe and ulceration, which is rated as 0=absent and>8=present *Total score:* 0=no PTS, 1–3=mild PTS, 4–8=moderate PTS,>8=severe PTS
CEAP-classification (15)	Class 0. No clinical signs of venous disease Class 1. Telangiectasias, reticular veins, malleolar flaring Class 2. Varicose veins Class 3. Oedema, no skin changes Class 4. Skin changes, such as pigmentation, eczema, lipodermatosclerosis Class 5. Skin changes with healed ulcer Class 6. Skin changes with active ulcer

Paediatric PTS score based on CEAP classification and Wong–Baker Faces pain score (126)	1. Physical findings
	  (a) No visible or palpable signs of venous disease
	  (b) Swelling, with or without pitting oedema
	  (c) Dilated collateral circulation of extremity only
	  (d) Skin changes such as pigmentation, eczema, lipodermatosclerosis
	  (e) Skin changes as in 4 with healed or active ulcer
	  Individual findings were each rated with 1 point, for a maximum score of 4
	2. Functional limitation due to pain was assessed for the affected and contralateral limb for each level of activity (at rest, activities of daily living, aerobic exercise only) Each pain limitation was rated with 1 point PTS was defined as a composite score of 1 or more

Table 17.8 Prevalence of Post-thrombotic Syndrome (PTS) in Children after an Episode of Venous Thrombosis[a]

Study	No. (n)	Age at time of onset of thrombosis	Follow-up period	Type of thrombosis	Definition of PTS	PTS (%)
Massicotti (1998) (26)	244	1 m–18 y	3 m–7 y (mean 2 y)	Catheter-related VTE	Swelling, discoloration, obvious collateral circulation or pain 3 months after VTE	n = 23 (9.4%)
Monagle (2000) (152)	356	1 m–18 y	2 w–6 y (mean 3.1 y)	Extremity VTE	Pain, swelling, browny discoloration of limb	n = 50 (14%)
Manco-Johnson (2000) (166)	27	1 m–18 y	1–10 y (median 4.5 y)	Extremity VTE	Discoloration, swelling, pain with activities	n = 5 (19%)
Gurgey (2001) (164)	95	1 m–17 y	12–41 m (mean 36 m)	All VTE	Pain, discoloration, induration of skin, swelling	n = 3 (3.1%)
Häusler (2001) (165)	21	0 m–13 y	3 m–18 y (median 10.2 y)	Extensive inferior caval vein thrombosis	Exanthema, ulcers, oedema, phlebothrombosis	n = 7 (33%)
van Ommen (2002)(167)	28	0 m–16 y	7–10 y (mean 8.9 y)	Asymptomatic catheter-related VTE in lower extremity	CEAP classification	n = 14 (50%)
van Ommen (2003) (15)	33	0 m–17 y	1 m–12 y (median 4.0 y)	Lower extremity VTE	CEAP classification	n = 23 (70%)
Kuhle (2003) (157)	153	0 m–193 m	1–159 m (median 16 m)	Extremity VTE	Paediatric PTS score based on Villalta score	n = 96 (63%)
Goldenberg (2007) (126)	22	0.7 y–19 y	18–24 m	Lower extremity VTE treated with thrombolysis (n = 9) or standard anticoagulation (n = 13)	CEAP classification and Wong–Baker Faces pain rating scale	n = 2 (22.2%) thrombolysis n = 10 (76.9%) standard anticoagulation

[a] Abbreviations: w, week; m, month; y, year; VTE, venous thromboembolic disease; CEAP, Clinical–Aetiology–Anatomic–Pathophysiologic.

Little information is available on the risk factors for the development of PTS both in adults and in children. In adults, the only clearly identified risk factor is recurrent, ipsilateral DVT (151,159). Recurrence has not been investigated in children as a potential predictor of PTS due to the small number of children with recurrent thrombosis in paediatric studies. In children, a potential risk factor is the size of the initial thrombus. A Canadian paediatric cohort study showed that the chance of having a higher PTS score increased by a factor of 2.1 for every additional vessel involved (157). Furthermore, children with no resolution or extension of thrombi as assessed by radiographic tests were four times more likely to develop PTS than children with resolution of their trombi. In the study by Goldenberg *et al*., elevated levels of factor VIII and/or D-dimers at the time of presentation and at 3–6 months of follow-up also appeared to be predictors of an adverse thrombotic outcome, including PTS (160).

In adults, prevention of PTS after developing a thrombotic event can be achieved by below-knee elastic compression stockings, worn for at least 2 years. Two randomized controlled trials, evaluating the efficacy of these stockings showed that PTS developed in about half of the controls without stockings and in about one-quarter of the patients wearing elastic stockings (159,161). The efficacy of elastic stockings in children after DVT has not been investigated. As mentioned above, a thrombolysis regimen may reduce the risk of PTS in children with occlusive lower-extremity high-risk acute venous thrombosis. A prospective multicentre clinical trial is in development.

REFERENCES

1. Andrew M, David M, Adams M, Ali K, Anderson R, Barnard D, *et al*. Venous thromboembolic complications (VTE) in children: first analyses of the Canadian Registry of VTE. *Blood* 1994; **83**: 1251–7.
2. Nordström M, Lindblad B, Bergqvist D, Kjellström T. A prospective study of the incidence of deep-vein thrombosis within a defined urban population. *J Intern Med* 1992; **232**:155–60.
3. Schmidt B, Andrew M. Neonatal thrombosis: report of a prospective Canadian and international registry. *Paediatrics* 1995; **96**:939–43.
4. van Ommen CH, Heijboer H, Büller HR, Hirasing RA, Heijmans HS, Peters M. Venous thromboembolism in childhood: a prospective two-year registry in The Netherlands. *J Pediatr* 2001; **139**:676–81.
5. Heit JA. Venous thromboembolism: disease burden, outcomes and risk factors. *J Thromb Haemost* 2005; **3**: 1611–7.
6. Buck JR, Connors RH, Coon WW, Weintraub WH, Wesley JR, Coran AG. Pulmonary embolism in children. *J Pediatr Surg* 1981; **16**:385–91.
7. Andrew M, Vegh P, Johnston M, Bowker J, Ofosu F, Mitchell L. Maturation of the hemostatic system during childhood. *Blood* 1992; **80**:1998–2005.
8. White RH. The epidemiology of venous thromboembolism. *Circulation* 2003; **107** (Suppl 1):I4–I8.
9. Chalmers EA. Epidemiology of venous thromboembolism in neonates and children. *Thromb Res* 2006; **118**:3–12.
10. Virchow R. Phlogose and Thrombose im Gefässsystem. In Virchow R (ed), *Gesammelte Abhandlungen zur Wissenschaftlichen Medizin*. Von Meidinger Sohn, Frankfurt, 1856, pp. 458–636.
11. Silverstein MD, Heit JA, Mohr DN, Petterson TM, O'Fallon WM, Melton LJ III. Trends in the incidence of deep vein thrombosis and pulmonary embolism: a 25-year population-based study. *Arch Intern Med* 1998; **158**:585–93.
12. White RH, Zhou H, Romano PS. Incidence of idiopathic deep venous thrombosis and secondary thromboembolism among ethnic groups in California. *Ann Intern Med* 1998; **128**:737–40.
13. Manco-Johnson MJ. Etiopathogenesis of paediatric thrombosis. *Hematology* 2005; **10**(Suppl 1):167–70.
14. Nowak-Göttl U, von Kries R, Göbel U. Neonatal symptomatic thromboembolism in Germany: two year survey. *Arch Dis Child Fetal Neonatal Ed* 1997; **76**:F163–F167.
15. van Ommen CH, Heijboer H, van den Dool EJ, Hutten BA, Peters M. Paediatric venous thromboembolic disease in one single centre: congenital prothrombotic disorders and the clinical outcome. *J Thromb Haemost* 2003; **1**:2516–22.

16. Journeycake JM, Buchanan GR. Thrombotic complications of central venous catheters in children. *Curr Opin Hematol* 2003; **10**:369–74.

17. Andrew M, Marzinotto V, Pencharz P, Zlotkin S, Burrows P, Ingram J, *et al*. A cross-sectional study of catheter-related thrombosis in children receiving total parenteral nutrition at home. *J Pediatr* 1995; **126**:358–63.

18. Miga DE, McKellar LF, Denslow S, Wiles HB, Case CL, Gillette PC. Incidence of femoral vein occlusion after catheter ablation in children: evaluation with magnetic resonance angiography. *Pediatr Cardiol* 1997; **18**:204–7.

19. Journeycake JM, Buchanan GR. Catheter-related deep venous thrombosis and other catheter complications in children with cancer. *J Clin Oncol* 2006; **24**:4575–80.

20. Ingram J, Weitzman S, Greenberg ML, Parkin P, Filler R. Complications of indwelling venous access lines in the paediatric hematology patient: a prospective comparison of external venous catheters and subcutaneous ports. *Am J Pediatr Hematol Oncol* 1991; **13**:130–6.

21. Male C, Chait P, Andrew M, Hanna K, Julian J, Mitchell L. Central venous line-related thrombosis in children: association with central venous line location and insertion technique. *Blood* 2003; **101**:4273–8.

22. Mitchell LG, Andrew M, Hanna K, Abshire T, Halton J, Anderson R, *et al* A prospective cohort study determining the prevalence of thrombotic events in children with acute lymphoblastic leukemia and a central venous line who are treated with L-asparaginase – Results of the Prophylactic Antithrombin Replacement in Kids with Acute Lymphoblastic Leukemia Treated with Asparaginase (PARKAA) study. *Cancer* 2003; **97**:508–16.

23. Pierce CM, Wade A, Mok Q. Heparin-bonded central venous lines reduce thrombotic and infective complications in critically ill children. *Intensive Care Med* 2000; **26**:967–72.

24. Ruud E, Natvig S, Holmstrom H, Wesenberg F. Low prevalence of femoral venous thrombosis after cardiac catheterizations in children: a prospective study. *Cardiol Young* 2002; **12**:513–8.

25. Massicotte P, Julian JA, Gent M, Shields K, Marzinotto V, Szechtman B, *et al*. An open-label randomized controlled trial of low molecular weight heparin for the prevention of central venous line-related thrombotic complications in children: the PROTEKT trial. *Thromb Res* 2003; **109**:101–8.

26. Massicotte MP, Dix D, Monagle P, Adams M, Andrew M. Central venous catheter related thrombosis in children: analysis of the Canadian Registry of Venous Thromboembolic Complications. *J Pediatr* 1998; **133**:770–6.

27. Perloff JK. Longevity in congenital heart disease: a tribute to paediatric cardiology. *J Pediatr* 1993; **122**:S49–S58.

28. Petaja J, Lundstrom U, Sairanen H, Marttinen E, Griffin JH. Central venous thrombosis after cardiac operations in children. *J Thorac Cardiovasc Surg* 1996; **112**:883–9.

29. Monagle P, Karl TR. Thromboembolic problems after the Fontan operation. *Semin Thorac Cardiovasc Surg Pediatr Card Surg Annu* 2002; **5**:36–47.

30. Berman W Jr, Fripp RR, Yabek SM, Wernly J, Corlew S. Great vein and right atrial thrombosis in critically ill infants and children with central venous lines. *Chest* 1991; **99**:963–7.

31. Monagle P, Cochrane A, McCrindle B, Benson L, Williams W, Andrew M. Thromboembolic complications after fontan procedures – the role of prophylactic anticoagulation. *J Thorac Cardiovasc Surg* 1998; **115**:493–8.

32. Cromme-Dijkhuis AH, Henkens CM, Bijleveld CM, Hillege HL, Bom VJ, van der Meer J. Coagulation factor abnormalities as possible thrombotic risk factors after Fontan operations. *Lancet* 1990; **336**:1087–90.

33. Jahangiri M, Shore D, Kakkar V, Lincoln C, Shinebourne E. Coagulation factor abnormalities after the Fontan procedure and its modifications. *J Thorac Cardiovasc Surg* 1997; **113**:989–92.

34. Odegard KC, McGowan FX Jr, DiNardo JA, Castro RA, Zurakowski D, Connor CM, *et al*. Coagulation abnormalities in patients with single-ventricle physiology precede the Fontan procedure. *J Thorac Cardiovasc Surg* 2002; **123**:459–65.

35. Odegard KC, McGowan FX Jr, Zurakowski D, DiNardo JA, Castro RA, del Nido PJ, *et al*. Procoagulant and anticoagulant factor abnormalities following the Fontan procedure: increased factor VIII may predispose to thrombosis. *J Thorac Cardiovasc Surg* 2003; **125**:1260–7.

36. Giannakopoulos B, Passam F, Rahgozar S, Krilis SA. Current concepts on the pathogenesis of the antiphospholipid syndrome. *Blood* 2007; **109**:422–30.

37. Male C, Foulon D, Hoogendoorn H, Vegh P, Silverman E, David M, *et al*. Predictive value of persistent versus transient antiphospholipid antibody subtypes for the risk of thrombotic events in paediatric patients with systemic lupus erythematosus. *Blood* 2005; **106**:4152–8.

38. Levy DM, Massicotte MP, Harvey E, Hebert D, Silverman ED. Thromboembolism in paediatric lupus patients. *Lupus* 2003; **12**:741–6.
39. Berkun Y, Padeh S, Barash J, Uziel Y, Harel L, Mukamel M, *et al*. Antiphospholipid syndrome and recurrent thrombosis in children. *Arthritis Rheum* 2006; **55**:850–5.
40. Campos LM, Kiss MH, D'Amico EA, Silva CA. Antiphospholipid antibodies in 57 children and adolescents with systemic lupus erythematosus. *Rev Hosp Clin Fac Med Sao Paulo* 2003; **58**:157–62.
41. Knöfler R, Siegert E, Lauterbach I, Taut-Sack H, Siegert G, Gehrisch S, *et al*. Clinical importance of prothrombotic risk factors in paediatric patients with malignancy – impact of central venous lines. *Eur J Pediatr* 1999; **158**:S147–S150.
42. Wermes C, von Depka P, Lichtinghagen R, Barthels M, Welte K, Sykora KW. Clinical relevance of genetic risk factors for thrombosis in paediatric oncology patients with central venous catheters. *Eur J Pediatr* 1999; **158**:S143–S146.
43. Glaser DW, Medeiros D, Rollins N, Buchanan GR. Catheter-related thrombosis in children with cancer. *J Pediatr* 2001; **138**:255–9.
44. Ruud E, Holmstrom H, Natvig S, Wesenberg F. Prevalence of thrombophilia and central venous catheter-associated neck vein thrombosis in 41 children with cancer–a prospective study. *Med Pediatr Oncol* 2002; **38**:405–10.
45. Santoro N, Giordano P, Del Vecchio GC, Guido G, Rizzari C, Varotto S, *et al*. Ischemic stroke in children treated for acute lymphoblastic leukemia: a retrospective study. *J Pediatr Hematol Oncol* 2005; **27**:153–7.
46. Caruso V, Iacoviello L, Di Castelnuovo A, Storti S, Mariani G, de Gaetano G, *et al*. Thrombotic complications in childhood acute lymphoblastic leukemia: a meta-analysis of 17 prospective studies comprising 1752 paediatric patients. *Blood* 2006; **108**:2216–22.
47. Athale UH, Chan AK. Thrombosis in children with acute lymphoblastic leukemia. Part II. Pathogenesis of thrombosis in children with acute lymphoblastic leukemia: effects of the disease and therapy. *Thromb Res* 2003; **111**:199–212.
48. Weimann E, Brack C. Severe thrombosis during treatment with ethinylestradiol for tall stature. *Horm Res* 1996; **45**:261–3.
49. Werder EA, Waibel P, Sege D, Flury R. Severe thrombosis during oestrogen treatment for tall stature. *Eur J Pediatr* 1990; **149**:389–90.
50. van Ommen CH, Fijnvandraat K, Vulsma T, Delemarre-Van De Waal HA, Peters M. Acquired protein S deficiency caused by estrogen treatment of tall stature. *J Pediatr* 1999; **135**:477–81.
51. D'Angelo A, Mazzola G, Vigano D'Angelo S. High prevalence of severe, transient autoimmune protein s deficiency in young patients with purpura fulminans or extensive venous thromboembolism associated with varicella infection. *Thromb Haemost* 1999; **80**(Suppl):427.
52. Levin M, Eley BS, Louis J, Cohen H, Young L, Heyderman RS. Postinfectious purpura fulminans caused by an autoantibody directed against protein S. *J Pediatr* 1995; **127**:355–63.
53. van Ommen CH, van Wijnen M, de Groot FG, van der Horst CM, Peters M. Postvaricella purpura fulminans caused by acquired protein s deficiency resulting from antiprotein s antibodies: search for the epitopes. *J Pediatr Hematol Oncol* 2002; **24**:413–6.
54. Arnoux JB, Boddaert N, Valayannopoulos V, Romano S, Bahi-Buisson N, Desguerre I, *et al*. Risk assessment of acute vascular events in congenital disorder of glycosylation type Ia. *Mol Genet Metab* 2008; **93**:444–9.
55. Fiumara A, Barone R, Buttitta P, Musso R, Pavone L, Nigro F, *et al*. Haemostatic studies in carbohydrate-deficient glycoprotein syndrome type I. *Thromb Haemost* 1996; **76**:502–4.
56. Young G, Driscoll MC. Coagulation abnormalities in the carbohydrate-deficient glycoprotein syndrome: case report and review of the literature. *Am J Hematol* 1999; **60**:66–9.
57. van Ommen CH, Peters M, Barth PG, Vreken P, Wanders RJ, Jaeken J. Carbohydrate-deficient glycoprotein syndrome type 1a: a variant phenotype with borderline cognitive dysfunction, cerebellar hypoplasia and coagulation disturbances. *J Pediatr* 2000; **136**:400–3.
58. Egeberg O. Inherited antithrombin deficiency causing thrombophilia. *Thromb Diath Haemorrh* 1965; **13**:516–30.
59. Heit JA. Thrombophilia: common questions on laboratory assessment and management. *Hematology Am Soc Hematol Educ Program* 2007; **2007**:127–35.
60. Bonduel M, Hepner M, Sciuccati G, Torres AF, Pieroni G, Frontroth JP. Prothrombotic abnormalities in children with venous thromboembolism. *J Pediatr Hematol Oncol* 2000; **22**:66–72.
61. Bonduel M, Hepner M, Sciuccati G, Pieroni G, Feliu-Torres A, Mardaraz C, *et al*. Factor V Leiden and prothrombin gene G20210A mutation in children with venous thromboembolism. *Thromb Haemost* 2002; **87**:972–7.

62. Ehrenforth S, Junker R, Koch HG, Kreuz W, Münchow N, Scharrer I,*et al*. Multicentre evaluation of combined prothrombotic defects associated with thrombophilia in childhood. Childhood Thrombophilia Study Group. *Eur J Pediatr* 1999; **158**:S97–S104.

63. Junker R, Koch HG, Auberger K, Münchow N, Ehrenforth S, Nowak-Göttl U. Prothrombin G20210A gene mutation and further prothrombotic risk factors in childhood thrombophilia. *Arterioscler Thromb Vasc Biol* 1999; **19**:2568–72.

64. Kosch A, Junker R, Kurnik K, Schobess R, Günther G, Koch H,*et al*. Prothrombotic risk factors in children with spontaneous venous thrombosis and their asymptomatic parents: a family study. *Thromb Res* 2000; **99**:531–7.

65. Lawson SE, Butler D, Enayat MS, Williams MD. Congenital thrombophilia and thrombosis: a study in a single centre. *Arch Dis Child* 1999; **81**:176–8.

66. Nowak-Göttl U, Junker R, Kreuz W, von Eckardstein A, Kosch A, Nohe N,*et al*. Risk of recurrent venous thrombosis in children with combined prothrombotic risk factors. *Blood* 2001; **97**:858–62.

67. Salonvaara M, Riikonen P, Kekomäki R, Heinonen K. Clinically symptomatic central venous catheter-related deep venous thrombosis in newborns. *Acta Paediatr* 1999; **88**:642–6.

68. Schobess R, Junker R, Auberger K, Münchow N, Burdach S, Nowak-Göttl U. Factor V G1691A and prothrombin G20210A in childhood spontaneous venous thrombosis – evidence of an age-dependent thrombotic onset in carriers of factor V G1691A and prothrombin G20210A mutation. *Eur J Pediatr* 1999; **158**:S105–S108.

69. Koster T, Rosendaal FR, Reitsma PH, van der Velden, Briët E, Vandenbroucke JP. Factor VII and fibrinogen levels as risk factors for venous thrombosis. A case–control study of plasma levels and DNA polymorphisms – the Leiden Thrombophilia Study (LETS). *Thromb Haemost* 1994; **71**:719–22.

70. Koster T, Blann AD, Briët E, Vandenbroucke JP, Rosendaal FR. Role of clotting factor VIII in effect of von Willebrand factor on occurrence of deep-vein thrombosis. *Lancet* 1995; **345**:152–5.

71. Meijers JCM, Tekelenburg WLH, Bouma BN, Bertina RM, Rosendaal FR. High levels of coagulation factor XI as a risk factor for venous thrombosis. *N Engl J Med* 2000; **342**:696–701.

72. van Hylckama Vlieg A, van der Linden IK, Bertina RM, Rosendaal FR. High levels of factor IX increase the risk of venous thrombosis. *Blood* 2000; **95**:3678–82.

73. van Tilburg NH, Rosendaal FR, Bertina RM. Thrombin activatable fibrinolysis inhibitor and the risk for deep vein thrombosis. *Blood* 2000; **95**:2855–9.

74. den Heyer M, Lewington S, Clarke R. Homocysteine, MTHFR and risk of venous thrombosis: a meta-analysis of published epidemiological studies. *J Thromb Haemost* 2005; **3**:292–9.

75. Bezemer ID, Bare LA, Doggen CJ, Arellano AR, Tong C, Rowland CM,*et al*. Gene variants associated with deep vein thrombosis. *JAMA* 2008; **299**:1306–14.

76. Revel-Vilk S, Chan A, Bauman M, Massicotte P. Prothrombotic conditions in an unselected cohort of children with venous thromboembolic disease. *J Thromb Haemost* 2003; **1**:915–21.

77. Middeldorp S, Henkens CM, Koopman MM, van Pampus EC, Hamulyak K, van der Meer J, *et al*. The incidence of venous thromboembolism in family members of patients with factor V Leiden mutation and venous thrombosis. *Ann Intern Med* 1998; **128**:15–20.

78. Middeldorp S, Meinardi JR, Koopman MM, van Pampus EC, Hamulyak K, van der Meer J,*et al*. A prospective study of asymptomatic carriers of the factor V Leiden mutation to determine the incidence of venous thromboembolism. *Ann Intern Med* 2001; **135**:322–7.

79. Simioni P, Sanson BJ, Prandoni P, Tormene D, Friederich PW, Girolami B, *et al*. Incidence of venous thromboembolism in families with inherited thrombophilia. *Thromb Haemost* 1999; **81**:198–202.

80. Tormene D, Simioni P, Prandoni P, Franz F, Zerbinati P, Tognin G, *et al*. The incidence of venous thromboembolism in thrombophilic children: a prospective cohort study. *Blood* 2002; **100**:2403–5.

81. Bank I, Scavenius MP, Büller HR, Middeldorp S. Social aspects of genetic testing for factor V Leiden mutation in healthy individuals and their importance for daily practice. *Thromb Res* 2004; **113**:7–12.

82. Legnani C, Razzaboni E, Gremigni P, Ricci Bitti PE, Favaretto E, Palareti G. Psychological impact of testing for thrombophilic alterations. *Thromb Haemost* 2006; **96**:348–55.

83. Marchetti M, Quaglini S, Barosi G. Cost-effectiveness of screening and extended anticoagulation for carriers of both factor V Leiden and prothrombin G20210A. *QJM* 2001; **94**:365–72.

84. Wu O, Robertson L, Twaddle S, Lowe GD, Clark P, Greaves M, *et al*. Screening for thrombophilia in high-risk situations: systematic review and cost-effectiveness analysis. The Thrombosis: Risk and Economic Assessment of Thrombophilia Screening (TREATS) study. *Health Technol Assess* 2006; **10**:1–110.

85. Kurekci E, Kaye R, Koehler M. Chylothorax and chylopericardium: a complication of a central venous catheter. *J Pediatr* 1998; **132**:1064–6.

86. Mulvihill SJ, Fonkalsrud EW. Complications of superior versus inferior vena cava occlusion in infants receiving central total parenteral nutrition. *J Pediatr Surg* 1984; **19**:752–7.

87. Bernstein D, Coupey S, Schonberg SK. Pulmonary embolism in adolescents. *Am J Dis Child* 1986; **140**:667–71.

88. van Ommen CH, Heyboer H, Groothoff JW, Teeuw R, Aronson DC, Peters M. Persistent tachypnea in children: keep pulmonary embolism in mind. *J Pediatr Hematol Oncol* 1998; **20**:570–3.

89. Derish MT, Smith DW, Frankel LR. Venous catheter thrombus formation and pulmonary embolism in children. *Pediatr Pulmonol* 1995; **20**:349–54.

90. Miniati M, Prediletto R, Formichi B, Marini C, Di Ricco G, Tonelli L, *et al*. Accuracy of clinical assessment in the diagnosis of pulmonary embolism. *Am J Respir Crit Care Med* 1999; **159**:864–71.

91. Wells PS, Anderson DR, Rodger M, Ginsberg JS, Kearon C, Gent M, *et al*. Derivation of a simple clinical model to categorize patients probability of pulmonary embolism: increasing the models utility with the SimpliRED D-dimer. *Thromb Haemost* 2000; **83**:416–20.

92. Wells PS, Anderson DR, Rodger M, Stiell I, Dreyer JF, Barnes D, *et al*. Excluding pulmonary embolism at the bedside without diagnostic imaging: management of patients with suspected pulmonary embolism presenting to the emergency department by using a simple clinical model and D-dimer. *Ann Intern Med* 2001; **135**:98–107.

93. Wicki J, Perneger TV, Junod AF, Bounameaux H, Perrier A. Assessing clinical probability of pulmonary embolism in the emergency ward: a simple score. *Arch Intern Med* 2001; **161**:92–7.

94. de Groot MR, van Marwijk Kooy M, Pouwels JG, Engelage AH, Kuipers BF, Büller HR. The use of a rapid D-dimer blood test in the diagnostic work-up for pulmonary embolism: a management study. *Thromb Haemost* 1999; **82**:1588–92.

95. Male C, Chait P, Ginsberg JS, Hanna K, Andrew M, Halton J, *et al*. Comparison of venography and ultrasound for the diagnosis of asymptomatic deep vein thrombosis in the upper body in children: results of the PARKAA study. Prophylactic Antithrombin Replacement in Kids with ALL treated with Asparaginase. *Thromb Haemost* 2002; **87**:593–8.

96. Goodacre S, Sampson F, Thomas S, van Beek E, Sutton A. Systematic review and meta-analysis of the diagnostic accuracy of ultrasonography for deep vein thrombosis. *BMC Med Imaging* 2005; **5**:6.

97. Miniati M, Pistolesi M, Marini C, Di RG, Formichi B, Prediletto R, *et al*. Value of perfusion lung scan in the diagnosis of pulmonary embolism: results of the Prospective Investigative Study of Acute Pulmonary Embolism Diagnosis (PISA-PED). *Am J Respir Crit Care Med* 1996; **154**:1387–93.

98. Moores LK, Jackson WL Jr, Shorr AF, Jackson JL. Meta-analysis: outcomes in patients with suspected pulmonary embolism managed with computed tomographic pulmonary angiography. *Ann Intern Med* 2004; **141**:866–74.

99. Daftary A, Gregory M, Daftary A, Seibyl JP, Saluja S. Chest radiograph as a triage tool in the imaging-based diagnosis of pulmonary embolism. *AJR Am J Roentgenol* 2005; **185**:132–4.

100. Shah PS, Kalyn A, Satodia P, Dunn MS, Parvez B, Daneman A, *et al*. A randomized, controlled trial of heparin versus placebo infusion to prolong the usability of peripherally placed percutaneous central venous catheters (PCVCs) in neonates: the HIP (Heparin Infusion for PCVC) study. *Paediatrics* 2007; **119**:e284–e291.

101. Kakzanov V, Monagle P, Chan AK. Thromboembolism in infants and children with gastrointestinal failure receiving long-term parenteral nutrition. *JPEN J Parenter Enteral Nutr* 2008; **32**:88–93.

102. Newall F, Barnes C, Savoia H, Campbell J, Monagle P. Warfarin therapy in children who require long-term total parenteral nutrition. *Paediatrics* 2003; **112**:e386–e388.

103. Krafte-Jacobs B, Sivit CJ, Mejia R, Pollack MM. Catheter-related thrombosis in critically ill children: comparison of catheters with and without heparin bonding. *J Pediatr* 1995; **126**:50–4.

104. Anton N, Cox P, Massicotte P, Dinyari M, Vegh P, Mitchell LG. No difference in incidences of thrombosis between heparin bonded catheters and non heparin bonded catheters in infants in the critical care unit following surgery for congenital heart disease: a randomised controlled triple blind study (abstract). *J Thromb Haemost* 2005; **3** (Suppl 1):P1726.

105. Shah PS, Shah N. Heparin-bonded catheters for prolonging the patency of central venous catheters in children. *Cochrane Database Syst Rev* 2007; (4):CD005983.

106. Mitchell L, Andrew M, Hanna K, Abshire T, Halton J, Wu J, *et al*. Trend to efficacy and safety using antithrombin concentrate in prevention of thrombosis in children receiving l-asparaginase for acute lymphoblastic leukemia – Results of the PARKAA study. *Thromb Haemost* 2003; **90**:235–44.

107. Ruud E, Holmstrom H, de Lange C, Hogstad EM, Wesenberg F. Low-dose warfarin for the prevention of central line-associated thromboses in children with malignancies – a randomized, controlled study. *Acta Paediatr* 2006; **95**:1053–9.

108. Elhasid R, Lanir N, Sharon R, Weyl Ben AM, Levin C, Postovsky S, *et al*. Prophylactic therapy with enoxaparin during L-asparaginase treatment in children with acute lymphoblastic leukemia. *Blood Coagul Fibrinol* 2001; **12**:367–70.

109. Hettiarachchi RJ, Prins MH, Lensing AW, Büller HR. Low molecular weight heparin versus unfractionated heparin in the initial treatment of venous thromboembolism. *Curr Opin Pulm Med* 1998; **4**:220–5.

110. Gibson BE, Chalmers E, Bolton-Maggs P, Henderson DJ, Lynn R. Thromboembolism in childhood: a prospective two year BPSU study in the United Kingdom. February 2001–February 2003. *J Thromb Haemost* 2003 **1** (Suppl.1):OC422.

111. Massicotte P, Julian JA, Gent M, Shields K, Marzinotto V, Szechtman B, *et al*. An open-label randomized controlled trial of low molecular weight heparin compared to heparin and coumadin for the treatment of venous thromboembolic events in children: the REVIVE trial. *Thromb Res* 2003; **109**:85–92.

112. Kuhle S, Massicotte P, Dinyari M, Vegh P, Mitchell D, Marzinotto V, *et al*. Dose-finding and pharmacokinetics of therapeutic doses of tinzaparin in paediatric patients with thromboembolic events. *Thromb Haemost* 2005; **94**:1164–71.

113. Massicotte P, Adams M, Marzinotto V, Brooker LA, Andrew M. Low-molecular-weight heparin in paediatric patients with thrombotic disease: a dose finding study. *J Pediatr* 1996; **128**:313–8.

114. Massicotte P, Julian JA, Marzinotto V, Gent M, Shields K, Chan AK, *et al*. Dose-finding and pharmacokinetic profiles of prophylactic doses of a low molecular weight heparin (reviparin-sodium) in paediatric patients. *Thromb Res* 2003; **109**:93–9.

115. Michaels LA, Gurian M, Hegyi T, Drachtman RA. Low molecular weight heparin in the treatment of venous and arterial thromboses in the premature infant. *Paediatrics* 2004; **114**:703–7.

116. Nohe N, Flemmer A, Rumler R, Praun M, Auberger K. The low molecular weight heparin dalteparin for prophylaxis and therapy of thrombosis in childhood: a report on 48 cases. *Eur J Paediatr* 1999; **158**:S134–S139.

117. van Ommen CH, van den Dool EJ, Peters M. Nadroparin therapy in paediatric patients with venous thromboembolic disease. *J Pediatr Hematol Oncol* 2008; **30**:230–4.

118. Sutor AH, Chan AKC, Massicotte P. Low-molecular-weight heparin in paediatric patients. *Semin Thromb Hemost* 2004; **30**:31–9.

119. Andrew M, Marzinotto V, Brooker LA, Adams M, Ginsberg J, Freedom R, *et al*. Oral anticoagulation therapy in paediatric patients: a prospective study. *Thromb Haemost* 1994; **71**:265–9.

120. Andrew M, Marzinotto V, Massicotte P, Blanchette V, Ginsberg J, Brill-Edwards P, *et al*. Heparin therapy in paediatric patients: a prospective cohort study. *Pediatr Res* 1994; **35**:78–83.

121. Laporte S, Mismetti P, Piquet P, Doubine S, Touchot A, Decousus H. Population pharmacokinetic of nadroparin calcium (Fraxiparine) in children hospitalised for open heart surgery. *Eur J Pharm Sci* 1999; **8**:119–25.

122. Mismetti P, Laporte-Simitsidis S, Navarro C, Sie P, d'Azemar P, Necciari J, *et al*. Aging and venous thromboembolism influence the pharmacodynamics of the anti-factor Xa and anti-thrombin activities of a low molecular weight heparin (nadroparin). *Thromb Haemost* 1998; **79**:1162–5.

123. Ignjatovic V, Summerhayes R, Than J, Gan A, Monagle P. Therapeutic range for unfractionated heparin therapy: age-related differences in response in children. *J Thromb Haemost* 2006; **4**:2280–2.

124. Kuhle S, Eulmesekian P, Kavanagh B, Massicotte P, Vegh P, Mitchell LG. A clinically significant incidence of bleeding in critically ill children receiving therapeutic doses of unfractionated heparin: a prospective cohort study. *Haematologica* 2007; **92**:244–7.

125. Risch L, Huber AR, Schmugge M. Diagnosis and treatment of heparin-induced thrombocytopenia in neonates and children. *Thromb Res* 2006; **118**:123–35.

126. Goldenberg NA, Durham JD, Knapp-Clevenger R, Manco-Johnson MJ. A thrombolytic regimen for high-risk deep venous thrombosis may substantially reduce the risk of postthrombotic syndrome in children. *Blood* 2007; **110**:45–53.

127. Monagle P, Chan A, Massicotte P, Chalmers E, Michelson AD. Antithrombotic therapy in children: the Seventh ACCP Conference on Antithrombotic and Thrombolytic Therapy. *Chest* 2004; **126** (3 Suppl):645S–687S.

128. Ouriel K. Comparison of safety and efficacy of the various thrombolytic agents. *Rev Cardiovasc Med* 2002; **3** (Suppl 2):S17–S24.

129. Chalmers EA, Gibson BE. Thrombolytic therapy in the management of paediatric thromboembolic disease. *Br J Haematol* 1999; **104**:14–21.

130. Gupta AA, Leaker M, Andrew M, Massicotte P, Liu L, Benson LN, *et al*. Safety and outcomes of thrombolysis with tissue plasminogen activator for treatment of intravascular thrombosis in children. *J Pediatr* 2001; **139**:682–8.

131. Knöfler R, Dinger J, Kabus M, Müller D, Lauterbach I, Rupprecht E, *et al*. Thrombolytic therapy in children – clinical experiences with recombinant tissue-plasminogen activator. *Semin Thromb Hemost* 2001; **27**:169–74.

132. Nowak-Gottl U, Auberger K, Halimeh S, Junker R, Klinge J, Kreuz WD, *et al*. Thrombolysis in newborns and infants. *Thromb Haemost* 1999; **82**(Suppl 1):112–6.

133. Wang M, Hays T, Balasa V, Bagatell R, Gruppo R, Grabowski EF, *et al*. Low-dose tissue plasminogen activator thrombolysis in children. *J Pediatr Hematol Oncol* 2003; **25**:379–86.

134. Bonduel M, Sciuccati G, Hepner M, Torres AF, Pieroni G, Frontroth JP, *et al*. Acenocoumarol therapy in paediatric patients. *J Thromb Haemost* 2003; **1**:1740–3.

135. Streif W, Andrew M, Marzinotto V, Massicotte P, Chan AKC, Julian JA, *et al*. Analysis of warfarin therapy in paediatric patients: a prospective cohort study of 319 patients. *Blood* 1999; **94**:3007–14.

136. Marzinotto V, Monagle P, Chan A, Adams M, Massicotte P, Leaker M, *et al*. Capillary whole blood monitoring of oral anticoagulants in children in outpatient clinics and the home setting. *Pediatr Cardiol* 2000; **21**:347–52.

137. Massicotte P, Marzinotto V, Vegh P, Adams M, Andrew M. Home monitoring of warfarin therapy in children with a whole blood prothrombin time monitor. *J Pediatr* 1995; **127**:389–94.

138. Büller HR, Agnelli G, Hull RD, Hyers TM, Prins MH, Raskob GE. Antithrombotic therapy for venous thromboembolic disease: the Seventh ACCP Conference on Antithrombotic and Thrombolytic Therapy. *Chest* 2004; **126** (3 Suppl):401S–428S.

139. Weitz JI, Linkins LA. Beyond heparin and warfarin: the new generation of anticoagulants. *Expert Opin Invest Drugs* 2007; **16**:271–82.

140. Gross PL, Weitz JI. New anticoagulants for treatment of venous thromboembolism. *Arterioscler Thromb Vasc Biol* 2008; **28**:380–6.

141. Risch L, Fischer JE, Herklotz R, Huber AR. Heparin-induced thrombocytopenia in paediatrics: clinical characteristics, therapy and outcomes. *Intensive Care Med* 2004; **30**:1615–24.

142. Hursting MJ, Dubb J, Verme-Gibboney CN. Argatroban anticoagulation in paediatric patients: a literature analysis. *J Pediatr Hematol Oncol* 2006; **28**:4–10.

143. Young G, Tarantino MD, Wohrley J, Weber LC, Belvedere M, Nugent DJ. Pilot dose-finding and safety study of bivalirudin in infants<6 months of age with thrombosis. *J Thromb Haemost* 2007; **5**:1654–9.

144. Martins HS, Scalabrini-Neto A, Velasco IT. Dabigatran versus enoxaparin after total hip replacement. *Lancet* 2007; **370**:2002–3.

145. Linkins LA, Weitz JI. New anticoagulants. *Semin Thromb Hemost* 2003; **29**:619–31.

146. Mason AR, McBurney PG, Fuller MP, Barredo JC, Lazarchick J. Successful use of fondaparinux as an alternative anticoagulant in a 2-month-old infant. *Pediatr Blood Cancer* 2008; **50**:1084–5.

147. Büller HR, Cohen AT, Davidson B, Decousus H, Gallus AS, Gent M, *et al*. Idraparinux versus standard therapy for venous thromboembolic disease. *N Engl J Med* 2007; **357**:1094–104.

148. Büller HR, Cohen AT, Davidson B, Decousus H, Gallus AS, Gent M, *et al*. Extended prophylaxis of venous thromboembolism with idraparinux. *N Engl J Med* 2007; **357**:1105–12.

149. Agnelli G, Gallus A, Goldhaber SZ, Haas S, Huisman MV, Hull RD, *et al*. Treatment of proximal deep-vein thrombosis with the oral direct factor Xa inhibitor rivaroxaban (BAY 59-7939): the ODIXa-DVT (Oral Direct Factor Xa Inhibitor BAY 59-7939 in Patients With Acute Symptomatic Deep-Vein Thrombosis) study. *Circulation* 2007; **116**:180–7.

150. Lassen MR, Davidson BL, Gallus A, Pineo G, Ansell J, Deitchman D. The efficacy and safety of apixaban, an oral, direct factor Xa inhibitor, as thromboprophylaxis in patients following total knee replacement. *J Thromb Haemost* 2007; **5**:2368–75.

151. Prandoni P, Lensing AWA, Cogo A, Cuppini S, Villalta S, Carta M, *et al*. The long-term clinical course of acute deep venous thrombosis. *Ann Intern Med* 1996; **125**:1–7.

152. Monagle P, Adams M, Mahoney M, Ali K, Barnard D, Bernstein M, *et al*. Outcome of paediatric thromboembolic disease: a report from the Canadian Childhood Thrombophilia Registry. *Pediatr Res* 2000; **47**:763–6.

153. Choi M, Massicotte MP, Marzinotto V, Chan AK, Holmes JL, Andrew M. The use of alteplase to restore patency of central venous lines in paediatric patients: a cohort study. *J Pediatr* 2001; **139**:152–6.

154. Andrew M. Epidemiology of venous thromboembolic events. In Andrew M, Monagle P, Brooker L (eds), *Thromboembolic Complications During Infancy and Childhood*, 1st edn. BC Decker, Hamilton, ON, 2000, pp. 111–46.

155. Press OW, Ramsey PG, Larson EB, Fefer A, Hickman RO. Hickman catheter infections in patients with malignancies. *Medicine* 1984; **63**:189–200.
156. van Rooden CJ, Schippers EF, Barge RMY, Rosendaal FR, Guiot HFL, van der Meer FJM, *et al*. Infectious Complications of central venous catheters increase the risk of catheter-related thrombosis in hematology patients: a prospective study. *J Clin Oncol* 2005; **23**:2655–60.
157. Kuhle S, Koloshuk B, Marzinotto V, Bauman M, Massicotte P, Andrew M, *et al*. A cross-sectional study evaluating post-thrombotic syndrome in children. *Thromb Res* 2003; **111**:227–33.
158. Janssen MCH, Wollersheim H, van Asten WN, de Rooij MJ, Nováková IR, Thien Th. The post-thrombotic syndrome: a review. *Phlebology* 1996; **11**:86–94.
159. Prandoni P, Lensing AW, Prins MH, Frulla M, Marchiori A, Bernardi E, *et al*. Below-knee elastic compression stockings to prevent the post-thrombotic syndrome: a randomized, controlled trial. *Ann Intern Med* 2004; **141**:249–56.
160. Goldenberg NA, Knapp-Clevenger R, Manco-Johnson MJ. Elevated plasma factor VIII and D-dimer levels as predictors of poor outcomes of thrombosis in children. *N Engl J Med* 2004; **351**:1081–8.
161. Brandjes DPM, Büller HR, Heijboer H, Huisman MV, de Rijk M, Jagt H, *et al*. Randomised trial of effect of compression stockings in patients with symptomatic proximal-vein thrombosis. *Lancet* 1997; **349**:759–62.
162. van Ommen CH, Peters M. A new diagnosis in children: the post-thrombotic syndrome. *Progr Pediatr Cardiol* 2005; **21**:23–9.
163. Massicotte MP, Dix D, Monagle P, Adams M, Andrew M. Central venous catheter related thrombosis in children: analysis of the Canadian Registry of Venous Thromboembolic Complications. *J Pediatr* 1998; **133**:770–6.
164. Gurgey A, Aslan D. Outcome of noncatheter-related thrombosis in children: influence of underlying or coexisting factors. *J Pediatr Hematol Oncol* 2001; **23**: 159–64.
165. Häusler M, Hübner D, Delhaas T, Mühler EG. Long term complications of inferior vena cava thrombosis. *Arch Dis Child* 2001; **85**:228–33.
166. Manco-Johnson MJ, Nuss R, Hays T, Krupski W, Drose J, Manco-Johnson ML. Combined thrombolytic and anticoagulant therapy for venous thrombosis in children. *J Pediatr* 2000; **136**:446–53.
167. van Ommen CH, Ottenkamp J, Lam J, Brennickmeier M, Heijmans HS, Büller HR, *et al*. The risk of postthrombotic syndrome in children with congenital heart disease. *J Pediatr* 2002; **141**:582–6.

CHAPTER 18

Management of Suspected Chronic Thromboembolic Pulmonary Hypertension

Robin Condliffe, Charlie A. Elliot and David G. Kiely

Pulmonary Vascular Disease Unit, Royal Hallamshire Hospital, Sheffield, UK

INTRODUCTION

Chronic thromboembolic pulmonary hypertension (CTEPH) is thought to occur in up to 3.8% of patients who survive an acute pulmonary embolism (PE), although in a significant minority of cases there is no history of a previous PE or deep vein thrombosis (DVT) (1). Figure 18.1 gives an overview of the main topics that are involved in dealing with this disease process. It is hypothesized that incomplete thrombus lysis occurs with subsequent organization of the thrombus into the vessel wall. Pathological changes identical with those seen in other forms of pulmonary arterial hypertension (PAH) can then occur in areas distal to both affected and non-affected portions of the proximal pulmonary arterial tree (2). As a consequence of pulmonary arterial obstruction, pulmonary vascular resistance increases with a resultant increase in pulmonary artery pressure. If this process proceeds unchecked it results in right heart failure which can lead to death.

Studies of patients diagnosed with CTEPH prior to the availability of specific pulmonary vascular treatments suggested a poor outcome. Riedel *et al.*, in a study involving 26 patients with CTEPH, found that 2 year survival was <20% in patients with a mean pulmonary artery pressure (mPAP) >50 mmHg (3). A second study involving 49 patients demonstrated a 3 year survival of 10% in patients with a mPAP >30 mmHg (4). Over recent years, in association with the availability of new treatment options, this outlook appears to have improved.

Pulmonary endarterectomy (PEA) is now recognized as the gold-standard treatment in patients with surgically accessible disease (see Chapter 25). When surgery is successful, patients have excellent symptomatic and haemodynamic response while overall the 6 year survival of patients undergoing PEA is 75% (5). In a proportion of CTEPH patients, however, the severity of pulmonary hypertension is out of keeping with the degree of radiologically demonstrable thromboembolic load. In these patients, less satisfactory results from surgery are obtained and the risk of peri-operative mortality is considerable. Dartevelle *et al.* found that in patients with a pulmonary

Deep Vein Thrombosis and Pulmonary Embolism Edited by Edwin J.R. van Beek, Harry R. Büller and Matthijs Oudkerk
© 2009 John Wiley & Sons, Ltd

- Chronic thromboembolic pulmonary hypertension (CTEPH) is an underdiagnosed condition which historically had a poor outcome.
- Pulmonary endarterectomy leads to improved survival and functional status in those with suitable disease.
- There is increasing evidence that medical therapies may improve the outcome in those with distal, non-surgical disease.
- In the light of these therapeutic advances effective and timely diagnosis is therefore essential.
- Clinical history, ECG and CXR may suggest the diagnosis but are not sensitive enough to exclude CTEPH.
- A systematic diagnostic evaluation of all patients with risk factors, unexplained symptoms or pulmonary hypertension of unknown aetiology is therefore crucial.
- Echocardiography is the initial investigation of choice in those with suspected pulmonary hypertension.
- In previously healthy individuals the right ventricle is only capable of generating a right ventricular systolic pressure of 50 mmHg. In patients presenting acutely with pressures in excess of this CTEPH should be suspected.
- A combination of CT, MR and isotope perfusion scanning together with right heart catheterisation will confidently diagnose or exclude CTEPH in the vast majority of cases. Where CTEPH is excluded this combination of investigations will usually suggest an alternative diagnosis.
- Screening of patients following an acute pulmonary embolism for evidence of CTEPH may be feasible and effective but this strategy requires further evaluation.

Figure 18.1 Overview of the main topics related to chronic thromboembolic pulmonary hypertension.

vascular resistance (PVR) $<900 \, \text{dyn s cm}^{-5}$ perioperative mortality was 4% but that this rose to 20% in patients with a PVR$>1200 \, \text{dyn s cm}^{-5}$(6).

In those patients with a non-surgical distribution of thromboembolic disease, the disease-modifying therapies used in other forms of pulmonary arterial hypertension have been used. A retrospective study of 27 patients with inoperable CTEPH treated with prostacyclin (epoprostenol) observed that after 3 months of treatment the mean pulmonary artery pressure decreased by 5 mmHg, cardiac index increased by 0.4 L min m^{-2} and 6 minute walk distance increased by 66 m (all $p < 0.001$) (7). In an uncontrolled study of 25 patients treated with the prostacyclin analogue treprostinil, significant improvements in pulmonary haemodynamics, exercise tolerance and functional class were also noted (8). An open-label study involving 104 patients treated with the phosphodiesterase-5 inhibitor sildenafil demonstrated that both pulmonary vascular resistance and exercise tolerance improved after 3 months of treatment (9). A recent small randomized controlled trial of sildenafil has subsequently been published (10). In this study, involving 19 patients with non-surgical disease, significant improvements in pulmonary vascular resistance and functional class were noted at 3 months in those patients receiving sildenafil. No treatment effect on the 6 minute walk distance was noted at that stage. After 12 months of open-label treatment, however, significant improvements in exercise tolerance were observed.

Finally, three observational papers noted that the endothelin-1 receptor antagonist bosentan improved pulmonary haemodynamics, exercise tolerance and B-type brain natriuretic peptide levels after between 3 and 12 months of treatment (11–13). The results of a randomized controlled trial of bosentan have recently been reported (14). A study evaluated 157 patients with inoperable CTEPH or persistent pulmonary hypertension following PEA who were randomized to receive bosentan or placebo for 16 weeks. Although a significant improvement in pulmonary vascular resistance

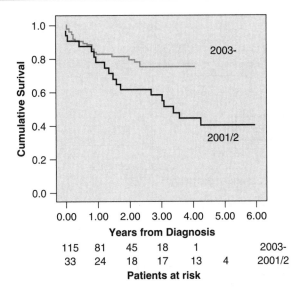

Figure 18.2 Survival of patients with non-surgical CTEPH in the UK ($p = 0.023$). Survival improved in those diagnosed from 2003 onwards (16). Reproduced from Condliffe R, Kiely DG, Gibbs JSR, *et al*. Improved outcomes in medically and surgically treated chronic thromboembolic pulmonary hypertension. Am J Respir Crit Care Med 2008; 177:1122–1127, by permission of the American Journal of Respiratory and Critical Care Medicine, official publication of the American Thoracic Society.

was noted, no such improvement was observed in the other co-primary endpoint, 6 minute walk distance. All patients diagnosed with CTEPH receive life-long anticoagulation to prevent recurrent thromboembolic events, although improvements in established CTEPH are not usually seen with this treatment alone (15).

Data reflecting the management and outcome of patients with non-surgical disease in a nation-wide setting has recently been published (16). In 148 such patients consecutively diagnosed in the UK, 1 and 3 year survival was 82 and 70%, respectively, better than that seen in historical series. A higher proportion of those patients diagnosed later in the study period received disease-modifying therapies (70 vs 90%, $p = 0.005$). Furthermore, of those receiving monotherapy, 83% of the earlier group received prostanoids whereas 89% in the later group received oral therapies ($p < 0.05$). As shown in Figure 18.2, the survival in this later group was significantly improved, suggesting that oral therapies (bosentan and sildenafil) are at least as efficacious as parenteral prostanoid therapy. Given their easier administration, they may also be introduced earlier, which may in part explain the improved survival observed in the later patients in this study.

In the light of the treatments which are now available, it is therefore important to identify and investigate properly patients who may have CTEPH. The various clinical features and investigations which are important in this process will be described below.

CLINICAL ASSESSMENT

Clinical history

Patients who receive a diagnosis of CTEPH may present in a variety of ways (Figure 18.3). Patients may presents with symptoms of breathlessness, right heart failure and collapse months to years following an acute PE (pathway A). Alternatively, patients with CTEPH may present with

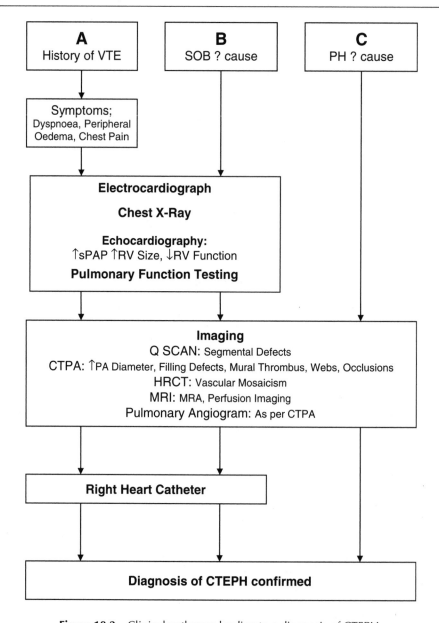

Figure 18.3 Clinical pathways leading to a diagnosis of CTEPH.

either dyspnoea of unknown cause (pathway B) or with pulmonary hypertension of unknown origin (pathway C). It is important to realize that a significant proportion of patients eventually diagnosed with CTEPH do not have a previously diagnosed PE. Between 40 and 50% of patients with an acute DVT have evidence of a silent PE on perfusion lung scan (17). Therefore, patients with a history of previous DVT, but no PE, may still be at increased of developing CTEPH. Furthermore, a previous history of a VTE was absent in almost half of all CTEPH patients presenting to a single centre (18). It is therefore important to consider CTEPH as a potential cause in all breathless patients whose investigations and history do not fit with a more common cause of dyspnoea and also in all patients found to have pulmonary hypertension.

Certain groups of patients have been identified as being at higher risk of developing CTEPH. Previous splenectomy, ventriculo-atrial shunts and the chronic inflammatory states of osteomyelitis and inflammatory bowel disease have been shown to be independent risk factors for developing CTEPH (18). The inherited thrombophilias which are associated with an increased risk of acute VTE do not appear to increase the risk of developing CTEPH. Interestingly, however, antiphospholipid antibody levels are higher in CTEPH patients than in idiopathic PAH patients or healthy controls (19).

Examination

Clinical signs consistent with pulmonary hypertension, such as a loud second heart sound, a right ventricular heave or systolic murmur of tricuspid regurgitation, may be present. Evidence of right heart failure with an elevated jugular venous pressure, peripheral oedema and engorged liver may also be seen. The presence of these signs suggests more advanced pulmonary hypertension and so their absence does not exclude CTEPH. It should be emphasized that the clinical signs of pulmonary hypertension can be subtle even in the presence of significantly elevated pulmonary pressures. In a minority of patients bruits can be heard peripherally in the lung fields due to turbulent blood flow through partially occluded pulmonary vessels. This is a relatively specific but insensitive sign of CTEPH (20).

Investigations

Lung function

Although CTEPH patients will often have a reduction in gas transfer, this is typically mild. In patients with surgically accessible disease from the UK national CTEPH registry, mean gas transfer was 69% ($\pm$17%) of predicted and 73% of patients had a gas transfer <80% predicted (16). A gas transfer within normal limits therefore does not exclude CTEPH. Spirometry is usually unremarkable, although a minority of patients have a mild restrictive pattern thought to be related to scarring secondary to pulmonary infarcts (21).

Electrocardiography

Signs of right heart strain such as right axis deviation, right bundle-branch block, p-pulmonale and T-wave inversion in the anterior and inferior leads may be present. Although highly specific for pulmonary hypertension in patients without concomitant cardio-respiratory disease, these electrocardiographic signs were found to be only 40–50% sensitive for the diagnosis of pulmonary hypertension in a study of 44 patients with chronic thromboembolic disease (22).

Chest X-ray

Especially in milder disease, the chest X-ray may be unremarkable. Cardiomegaly is the commonest abnormality seen but other, more subtle changes may be present (23). These include pulmonary artery enlargement and asymmetry, abrupt truncation of vessels, oligaemia and peripheral atelactasis.

Echocardiography

Transthoracic echocardiography provides a means of non-invasive assessment of cardiac chamber size and function. It can also provide an estimation of systolic pulmonary artery pressure in the majority of patients. Using the peak tricuspid regurgitant jet velocity (V) as assessed by continuous-wave Doppler echocardiography, the modified Bernoulli equation can be used to estimate systolic pulmonary artery pressure:

$$(sPAP = 4V^2) + \text{ right atrial pressure}$$

In some subjects, the diastolic pulmonary artery pressure can also be estimated from the pulmonary valve regurgitant jet (24). The right atrial pressure can be assigned an assumed value or can be estimated by visualizing the inferior vena cava. In normality the diameter of the inferior cava should reduce by >50% during inspiration as the venous return increases. Higher right atrial pressures are suggested in patients where this does not occur (25). It has been shown that the majority of patients with severe baseline tricuspid regurgitation who undergo PEA demonstrate a marked improvement on postoperative echocardiography (26).

In addition to estimating pressures, echocardiography also allows the assessment of the cardiac chambers, valves and interventricular and interatrial septa. Due its complex geometry, size and function of the right ventricle are normally assessed qualitatively. Right ventricular ejection fractions can, however, be estimated using planimetry of the four-chamber view (27):

$$\text{right ventricular ejection fraction} = \frac{100 \times (\text{end diastolic area} - \text{end systolic area})}{\text{end diastolic area}}$$

Over recent years, the development of three-dimensional echocardiography has provided the ability to measure actual end-diastolic and end-systolic volumes of the right ventricle. The ejection fractions calculated using this method were noted to improve significantly in nine patients following PEA (28). Left ventricular diastolic filling may also be affected in patients with CTEPH. Initially this was thought to be a result of direct compressive effects of the right ventricle and interventricular septum on the left ventricle (29,30). Subsequent studies have suggested that the abnormal left ventricular filling seen in CTEPH patients is actually due to a low left ventricular preload (31,32).

Although a very useful tool in the assessment of patients with suspected CTEPH, echocardiography does have several limitations. A proportion of patients, for example those with a large body habitus, provide poor echo windows. The technique probably has more inter-observer variability than other imaging modalities, such as computed tomography (CT).

Right Heart Catheterization

Pulmonary haemodynamics obtained during right heart catheterization are not only essential in confirming the diagnosis of pulmonary hypertension but also provide useful prognostic information. As has already been discussed, Dartevelle *et al.* found that perioperative mortality in patients undergoing PEA rose dramatically in patients with a PVR >1200 dyn s cm^{-5} (6). It is hypothesized that these patients with a PVR out of keeping with the degree of radiologically demonstrable thromboembolic load have a significant distal vasculopathy and so are at greater risk of reperfusion oedema and persistent pulmonary hypertension. A more complex model has therefore been developed to attempt to partition the contribution to the total PVR into proximal 'upstream' or distal 'downstream' locations (33). In this technique, the rate of decay of pressure from the point of occluding the pulmonary artery (P_{occl}, occlusion pressure) to the steady-state pulmonary artery occluded pressure (P_{PAO}) is measured. When this decay is rapid, it is postulated that there is relatively little contribution to the total PVR from distal vessels, i.e., high upstream resistance (R_{up}). Conversely when R_{up} is low, it is hypothesized that a significant proportion of the total PVR is caused by distal disease. In a study of 26 patients undergoing PEA, Kim *et al.* found that lower R_{up} correlated with worse postoperative pulmonary haemodynamics (34). Furthermore, patients with a R_{up} <60% appeared to be at the highest risk of death. An alternative derived parameter which has been studied in CTEPH patients is the ratio of pulmonary artery pulse pressure and mean pulmonary artery pressure – the fractional pulse pressure (P_{Pf}). It has been hypothesized that stiffness of the proximal vessel wall due to thrombus would lead to an increased pulse pressure whereas stiffness of the distal vessel wall due to either distal thrombus or distal vasculopathy would lead to increased mean arterial pressure. To investigate this, 32 patients with CTEPH were compared with 18 patients with idiopathic PAH (35). P_{Pf} was significantly higher in CTEPH than in idiopathic PAH. Furthermore, P_{Pf} was significantly higher in survivors than in non-survivors of PEA. A possible problem with using this technique in patients with severely reduced cardiac index is that the pulse pressure can be influenced by right ventricular function.

Isotope ventilation–perfusion Scan

An entirely normal isotope ventilation–perfusion (V/Q) scan effectively excludes the diagnosis of CTEPH. In a study of 75 patients with pulmonary hypertension, which included 25 patients with angiographically confirmed CTEPH, no CTEPH patients had a normal or low-probability V/Q scan (36). In patients with proven PH, at least one segmental or lobar mismatched defect indicates CTEPH whereas multiple subsegmental defects suggest another cause, including idiopathic PAH (37,38). Although V/Q scans have been shown to be highly sensitive for CTEPH, in a study of 25 CTEPH patients the extent of perfusion defects consistently underestimated both the degree of obstruction demonstrated angiographically and the severity of pulmonary haemodynamics (39).

Computed tomography

Multidetector row computed tomography pulmonary angiography (CTPA) has become integral to the assessment of patients with suspected CTEPH (see Chapter 7). Not only does it provide excellent imaging of the pulmonary arterial tree but it also provides substantial information regarding cardiac and pulmonary structure and function (Figure 18.4). Diagnostic findings in patients with chronic pulmonary emboli include peripheral intraluminal filling defects which form obtuse angles with vessel walls, webs within contrast-filled arteries, contrast flowing through thickened and recanalized vessels and complete occlusions (40). A large amount of other supportive information can be gained from both CTPA and high-resolution computed tomography (HRCT). Cardiac chamber size and the position of the interventricular septum can be assessed. Enlargement of the main pulmonary artery to greater than the accompanying aorta or 33 mm suggests pulmonary hypertension (41). The presence or absence of right ventricular or outflow tract hypertrophy can also be noted. Pericardial or pleural effusions are well visualized and the presence of significant tricuspid regurgitation is demonstrated by contrast refluxing into the inferior vena cava. Enlarged bronchial arteries strongly suggest CTEPH as opposed to other causes of pulmonary hypertension (42). A mosaic perfusion pattern with smaller pulmonary vessels in the darker, hypoperfused areas than in the normal areas of the lung is frequently seen on HRCT slices (43). Finally, evidence of previous infarcts in the form of peripheral atelectasis, scarring or cavitation can also be present (Figure 18.5). CT may be especially helpful in patients presenting with persistent symptoms following a PE where echocardiography is non-diagnostic.

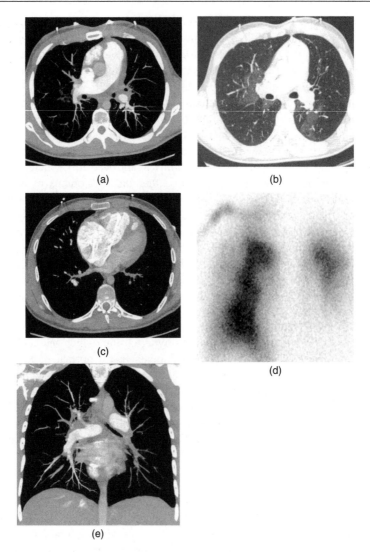

Figure 18.4 Images from a 20-year-old man with breathlessness and a previous DVT: (a) CTPA showed lobar and segmental disease; (b) HRCT shows mosaicism with dark hypoperfused areas; (c) CTPA through cardiac chambers shows dilated right-sided chambers and underfilled left-sided chambers; (d) AP perfusion scan shows segmental defects in the right lung and lack of perfusion to the left lower lobe; (e) maximum intensity projection CT image shows webs and occlusions on the right and complete occlusion to the left lower lobe pulmonary artery.

The sensitivity of CTPA in diagnosing CTEPH has recently been compared with that of V/Q scanning (44). In a study involving 227 patients with suspected VTE, non-selective pulmonary angiography was performed if abnormalities had been seen on V/Q or CTPA. Seventy-eight individuals were given a final diagnosis of CTEPH based on the appearances of angiography. When compared with the angiographic findings, V/Q scanning was found to have a sensitivity of >95% whereas CTPA had a sensitivity of only 51%. However, the multislice CT scanners used in that study were relatively early models with either 4 × 3 mm collimation and 2.5 mm reconstruction or 8 × 1.25 mm collimation and 1.25 mm reconstruction. It is possible that a much greater

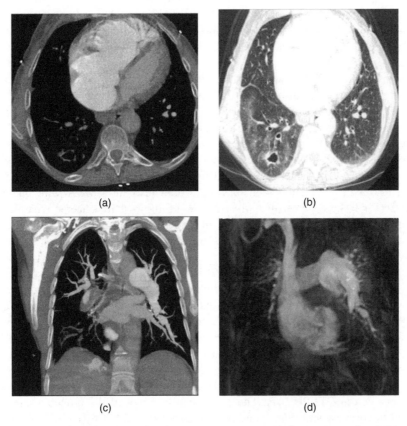

(a) (b)

(c) (d)

Figure 18.5 Patient with cavitation of unknown cause: (a) and (b) CTPA and HRCT show dilated right-sided chambers and cavitation in right lower lobe; (c) maximum intensity projection CT shows significant thromboembolic material in the right lower lobe artery together with webs in both upper lobe and left lower lobe arteries; (d) MRA in the same patient shows a similar pattern but also can demonstrate dynamic perfusion.

sensitivity of CTPA may have been observed if the latest multislice scanners had been used where the resolution now matches that obtained with conventional pulmonary angiography (45).

Magnetic resonance imaging

Magnetic resonance imaging (MRI) is an increasingly used modality for the assessment of patients with potential CTEPH (see Chapter 9). Gadolinium-enhanced magnetic resonance angiography (MRA) has enabled the pulmonary macrocirculation to be visualized. The largest study to date involving patients with suspected acute PE demonstrated that, compared with conventional pulmonary angiography, MRA detected PE with a sensitivity of 77% and a specificity of 98% (46). The sensitivity was excellent in lobar PE (100%) but poor in subsegmental PE (40%). A similar finding was observed in a study of 34 patients who subsequently underwent PEA. Kreitner *et al*. found that typical findings of CTEPH, such as intraluminal webs and vessel cut-offs, were observed in all patients (47). However, although MRA demonstrated all vessels up to the segmental level, only 681 subsegmental arteries were seen compared with 733 with digital subtraction angiography (DSA). It was noted that MRA was superior to DSA at assessing the proximal starting point of thromboembolic disease. This is seen in clinical practice, where DSA can underestimate the degree of laminated thrombus seen at surgery in the main and lobar pulmonary arteries. Finally, when compared with CTPA, in a study involving 32 patients MRA once again performed well at visualizing lobar and segmental arteries (366 vs 357) but less well in subsegmental arteries (627 vs 834) (48).

The development of parallel imaging has permitted the clinical utilization of both time-resolved magnetic resonance (MR) perfusion-weighted images of the lung parenchyma and high spatial resolution MRA. In a group of iPAH and CTEPH patients, MR perfusion imaging showed a 79% agreement with V/Q scanning whereas high spatial resolution MRA demonstrated 86% agreement with the results of CTPA and/or DSA (49). The combination of both modalities allowed the correct diagnosis to be assigned in 90% of patients. Work is ongoing on the development of time-resolved MR perfusion imaging to produce regional quantitative perfusion images. It is conceivable that the matching of vessel obstruction seen on high spatial resolution MRA with quantitative MR perfusion defects may be a powerful tool in predicting the potential haemodynamic benefit and also perioperative risk from PEA. A large quantitative perfusion defect present in an area with minimal vascular obstruction would suggest a significant degree of distal thromboembolic load or vasculopathy.

A further use of MRI in patients with CTEPH is the assessment of cardiac function. Cine-MRI provides an excellent way of assessing both right and left cardiac size and function. Ventricular or outflow tract hypertrophy can be measured while ventricular function can be qualitatively assessed. Alternatively, ventricular end-diastolic and end-systolic volumes can be measured from which cardiac output, ejection fraction and ventricular mass can be then calculated (50). An alternative method of calculating cardiac output is to use velocity-encoded phase contrast flow images of the pulmonary artery and aorta. Any difference between pulmonary and systemic blood flow may be related to the increased broncho-systemic shunting that occurs through the enlarged bronchial arteries that are seen in CTEPH (47). The cross-sectional area of the bronchial arteries seen on CT was found to correlate with this shunt volume as calculated by MRI flow volumes (51). Following PEA, this broncho-systemic shunt volume disappeared. The relationship between several parameters obtained via phase contrast MRI, including pulmonary acceleration and ejection times and pulse wave velocity and pulmonary haemodynamics measured at right heart catheter, have been assessed (47,52). Only weak correlations were found, suggesting that at present haemodynamic measurements made with MRI cannot replace those obtained at right heart catheter. It is possible that these weak correlations were due to limited temporal resolutions and with technical improvements more accurate measures of pulmonary haemodynamics may be possible (53).

Hyperpolarized noble gas MRI

This imaging modality has an exciting potential in the further assessment of patients with CTEPH. Regional ventilation can be quantified using inhaled hyperpolarized ^{3}He or ^{129}Xe. These images can then be compared with MRA perfusion images to assess V/Q mismatching. Furthermore, the rate of decay of the hyperpolarized state of the inhaled gas is inversely proportional to the intra-alveolar PO_2 (54). This raises the possibility of developing a clinical technique whereby localised ventilation and perfusion can be accurately matched. This could be an extremely useful tool in predicting potential benefit from disobliteration of the pulmonary vascular tree by PEA (53).

Pulmonary angiography

Before the advent of cross-sectional imaging, pulmonary angiography was the technique of choice to demonstrate the morphology of pulmonary vascular obstruction (see Chapter 10). The risks associated with pulmonary angiography may have been overstated; in a review of 67 consecutive selective left and right pulmonary angiograms performed in patients with severe pulmonary hypertension, there were no cases of death or significant cardiovascular compromise (55). Although a later study involving 200 patients with pulmonary hypertension did report a mortality rate of 1.5%, of the three patients who died one had a massive acute PE, one had massive intravascular metastases and one had severe pulmonary hypertension associated with pregnancy (56). Furthermore, no significant pulmonary haemodynamic effects from non-ionic contrast were seen during pulmonary angiograms performed on 33 CTEPH patients (57). Nonetheless, due to the improved availability and accuracy of the non-invasive modalities, pulmonary angiography in our institution is now usually performed only when other forms of imaging have either not adequately demonstrated the extent of any thromboembolic material present or where their findings do not agree. In other centres with poorer access to the most up-to-date CT or MRI techniques, however, pulmonary angiography still retains a central role in radiological evaluation.

Pulmonary angioscopy

Prior to the development of other imaging techniques, angioscopy was used in some centres to visualize endovascular abnormalities such as intimal thickening and webs (58). The technique is both invasive and highly specialized and with the advent of improved cross-sectional imaging techniques the role of pulmonary angioscopy in the diagnosis and surgical assessment of CTEPH patients is likely to be limited to a highly selected group of patients.

CLINICAL APPROACH

So far we have reviewed the various clinical features and investigations which can be utilized to arrive at a diagnosis of CTEPH and to assess for surgical operability. The possible clinical pathways leading to an eventual diagnosis of CTEPH, together with appropriate investigations, have already been highlighted in Figure 18.3.

The majority of patients referred to our unit are suspected of having pulmonary hypertension but in many cases the underlying cause is unknown. Although it is not common, we do occasionally find evidence of chronic thromboembolic disease in patients with other possible causes for pulmonary hypertension, such as hypoxic lung disease. As part of our systematic diagnostic evaluation, we therefore perform investigations to exclude CTEPH in all patients suspected of having pulmonary hypertension. A suggested diagnostic protocol is shown in Figure 18.6. In patients in whom pulmonary hypertension is suspected, we perform perfusion scans, CT and MRI as additional and complementary information can be gained from all three techniques. An isotope perfusion scan, in addition to demonstrating perfusion defects consistent with CTEPH, can also quantify renal isotope uptake due to a right–left shunt. This information can be useful in explaining unexpected hypoxia in pulmonary hypertension of all causes. On the other hand, CT scanning can demonstrate not only abnormalities within the pulmonary vascular tree suggestive of CTEPH but also associated features supportive of this diagnosis such as bronchial artery dilatation, vascular pattern mosaicism and peripheral infarcts. In cases of pulmonary hypertension due to causes other than CTEPH, CT can provide other diagnostic clues such as significant emphysema or fibrosis in respiratory disease-associated pulmonary hypertension or interlobular septal thickening, pleural effusions and ground glass opacities in the rare conditions of veno-occlusive disease or pulmonary capillary haemangiomatosis. As already discussed, MRI is proving increasingly useful in demonstrating not only the pulmonary vasculature and perfusion but also cardiac structure and function.

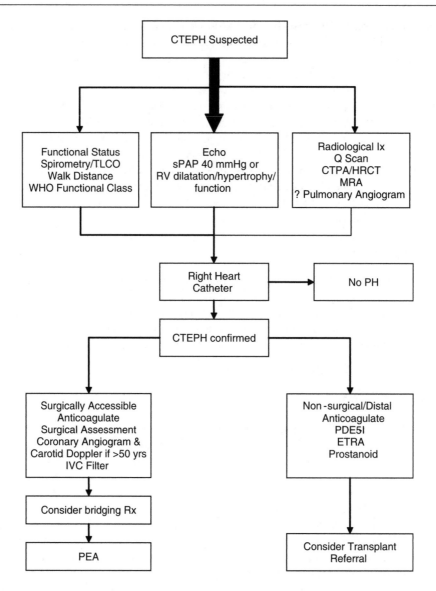

Figure 18.6 Diagnostic approach to CTEPH.

In all cases where CTEPH is diagnosed, imaging and clinical parameters should be reviewed in a multidisciplinary fashion to assess potential operability. Two imaging modalities are normally required to provide a 'road map' for surgery. Normally CTPA and MRA are sufficient but in some circumstances, for example poor breath holding during MRA, a selective pulmonary angiogram may still be needed. In patients >50 years old, both carotid Doppler and coronary angiogram are also performed prior to surgery to assess for the presence of vascular disease. If significant coronary artery disease is present then coronary artery bypass grafting is performed at the time of PEA; this procedure is not felt to increase the surgical risk. For a detailed discussion on surgical and perioperative management of these patients, see Chapter 25.

In patients with either surgically inaccessible disease or who have pulmonary haemodynamics that outweigh the degree of thromboembolic load, the potential benefits from PEA are far outweighed by the increased risk of perioperative complications and persistent postoperative pulmonary hypertension. As discussed, these patients are increasingly treated with the disease-modifying therapies originally used in other forms of pulmonary hypertension. In highly selected cases, referral for lung transplant assessment is indicated.

SCREENING

An important and as yet unanswered question is whether the most obvious group of patients at risk of developing CTEPH, i.e., those with an acute PE, should be routinely screened. The incidence of CTEPH in patients following an acute PE has been estimated in recent studies to be between 1 and 5% (1,59–61). It is therefore likely that a significant number of cases of CTEPH are undiagnosed. In our institution, a quaternary referral centre for pulmonary hypertension covering a population of 15 million and which also serves a local population of approximately 600 000, 200–250 patients present annually with an acute PE. Given a 30 day mortality of 10–15%, approximately 200 patients per year therefore survive an acute PE and may be at risk of developing CTEPH (62,63). Using the incidence of CTEPH of 3.8% as calculated by Pengo *et al.*, one would therefore expect around eight patients per year to develop CTEPH in our population (1).

In a follow-up study of 78 selected patients, many with large PE, 90% of patients had normalization of their systolic pulmonary artery pressure and right ventricular function within 30 days (61), with pressure falling exponentially in the first week. Patients identified as having persistent elevation of pulmonary artery pressure at 4–6 weeks were at higher risk of developing CTEPH. Furthermore, the presence of a systolic pulmonary artery pressure >50 mmHg at the time of acute presentation strongly predicted persistence of elevated pressures at 1 year. This is consistent with the observation that the right ventricle is only able to generate acutely a right ventricular systolic pressure of 50 mmHg.

These data suggest that routine screening with echocardiography of patients at around 12 weeks after a diagnosis of acute PE would be capable of identifying patients with an increased risk of CTEPH. Patients with elevated systolic artery pressures at that time could then either be followed closely to assess for evidence of subsequent improvement or be investigated as suggested in Figure 18.6. Also, in patients who remain symptomatic at follow-up in the absence of elevated pulmonary artery pressures on echocardiography, CT may provide important information as to the cause of their symptomatic limitations. The direct evidence for the clinical and financial effectiveness of this approach is, however, lacking.

CONCLUSION

CTEPH can present as persistent breathlessness in patients following an acute PE; however, it can also develop in patients with no previous history of VTE. A high index of suspicion should be maintained in patients with persistent breathlessness in addition to those being investigated for suspected pulmonary hypertension. To ensure that the diagnosis is not missed, a systematic diagnostic evaluation is essential in all these groups. CT scanning is central to this process; although an entirely normal V/Q scan excludes the diagnosis, CT imaging provides significant additional information regarding other potential diagnoses and also is vital in planning surgery should CTEPH be demonstrated. MRI is increasingly being used to image the pulmonary vascular tree and also to assess cardiac function. Future developments in imaging include the potential of hyperpolarized noble gas MRI in conjunction with MRA perfusion providing an accurate assessment of regional perfusion and ventilation which could be used to assess more effectively the likely benefit of PEA. A strong argument for the routine screening of patients following an acute PE exists, although the cost-effectiveness of this approach is yet to be assessed.

ACKNOWLEDGEMENTS

The authors would like to thank Christine Davies, Rhona Maclean and Neil Woodhouse for their help in preparing this chapter.

REFERENCES

1. Pengo V, Lensing AW, Prins MH,. et al Incidence of chronic thromboembolic pulmonary hypertension after pulmonary embolism. N Engl J Med 2004; 350:2257–2264.
2. Auger WR, Kim NH, Kerr KM,. et al Chronic thromboembolic pulmonary hypertension. Clin Chest Med 2007; 28:255–269.
3. Riedel M, Stanek V, Widimisky J,. et al Longterm follow-up of patients with pulmonary thromboembolism: late prognosis and evolution of hemodynamic and respiratory data. Chest 1982; 81:151–158.
4. Lewczuk J, Piszko P, Jagas J,. et al Prognostic factors in medically treated patients with chronic pulmonary embolism. Chest 2001; 119:818–823.
5. Thistlethwaite PA, Madani M, Jamieson SW. Outcomes of pulmonary endarterectomy surgery. Semin Thorac Cardiovasc Surg 2006; 18:257–264.
6. Dartevelle P, Fadel E, Mussot S,. et al Chronic thromboembolic pulmonary hypertension. Eur Respir J 2004; 23:637–648.
7. Cabrol S, Souza R, Jais X,. et al Intravenous epoprostenol in inoperable chronic thromboembolic pulmonary hypertension. J Heart Lung Transplant 2007; 26:357–362.
8. Skoro-Sajer N, Bonderman D, Wiesbauer F,. et al Treprostinil for severe inoperable chronic thromboembolic pulmonary hypertension. J Thromb Haemost 2007; 5:483–489.
9. Reichenberger F, Voswinckel R, Enke B,. et al Long-term treatment with sildenafil in chronic thromboembolic pulmonary hypertension. Eur Respir J 2007; 30:922–927.
10. Suntharalingam J, Treacy CM, Doughty N,. et al Long term use of sildenafil in inoperable chronic thromboembolic pulmonary hypertension. Chest. 2008; In Press.
11. Bonderman D, Nowotny R, Skoro-Sajer N,. et al Bosentan therapy for inoperable chronic thromboembolic pulmonary hypertension. Chest 2005; 128:2599–2603.
12. Hoeper MM, Kramm T, Wilkens H,. et al Bosentan therapy for inoperable chronic thromboembolic pulmonary hypertension. Chest 2005; 128:2363–2367.
13. Hughes RJ, Jais X, Bonderman D,. et al The efficacy of bosentan in inoperable chronic thromboembolic pulmonary hypertension: a 1-year follow-up study. Eur Respir J 2006; 28:138–143.
14. Jais X, Ghofrani A, Hoeper MM,. et al Bosentan for inoperable chronic thromboembolic pulmonary hypertension (CTEPH): a randomized, placebo-controlled trial – BENEFIT. Am J Respir Crit Care Med 2007; 175:A896.
15. Hoeper MM, Mayer E, Simonneau G,. et al Chronic thromboembolic pulmonary hypertension. Circulation 2006; 113:2011–2020.
16. Condliffe R, Kiely DG, Gibbs JSR,. et al Improved outcomes in medically and surgically treated chronic thromboembolic pulmonary hypertension. Am J Respir Crit Care Med 2008; 177:1122–1127.
17. Meignan M, Rosso J, Gauthier H,. et al Systematic Lung scans reveal a high frequency of silent pulmonary embolism in patients with procximal deep venous thrombosis. Arch Intern Med 2000; 160:159–164.
18. Bonderman D, Jakowitsch J, Adlbrecht C,. et al Medical conditions increasing the risk of chronic thromboembolic pulmonary hypertension. Thromb Haemost 2005; 93:512–516.
19. Wolf M, Boyer-Neumann C, Parent F,. et al Thrombotic risk factors in pulmonary hypertension. Eur Respir J 2000; 15:395–399.
20. ZuWallack R, Liss J, Lahiri B. Acquired continuous murmur associated with acute pulmonary thromboembolism. Chest 1976; 70:557–559.

21. Morris TA, Auger WR, Ysrael MZ,. *et al* Parenchymal scarring is associated with restrictive spirometric defects in patients with chronic thromboembolic pulmonary hypertension. *Chest* 1996; **110**:399–403.

22. Lewczuk J, Ajlan AW, Piszko P,. *et al* Electrocardiographic signs of right ventricular overload in patients who underwent pulmonary embolism event (s). Are they useful in diagnosis of chronic thromboembolic pulmonary hypertension? *J Electrocardiol* 2004; **37**:219–225.

23. Woodruff W III, Hoeck B, Chitwood W Jr, *et al*. Radiographic findings in pulmonary hypertension from unresolved embolism. *Am J Roentgenol* 1984; **144**:681–686.

24. Masuyama T, Kodama K, Kitabatake A. Continuous-wave Doppler echocardiographic detection of pulmonary regurgitation and its application to noninvasive estimation of pulmonary artery pressure. *Circulation* 1986; **74**:484–492.

25. Pepi M, Tamborini G, Galli C,. *et al* A new formula for echo-Doppler estimation of right ventricular systolic pressure. *J Am Soc Echocardiogr* 1994; **7**:20–26.

26. Thistlethwaite PA, Jamieson SW. Tricuspid valvular disease in the patient with chronic pulmonary thromboembolic disease. *Curr Opin Cardiol* 2003; **18**:111–116.

27. Lang R, Biering M, Devereux R. Recommendations for chamber quantification. *Eur J Echocardiogr* 2006; **7**:79–108.

28. Menzel T, Kramm T, Bruckner A,. *et al* Quantitative assessment of right ventricular volumes in severe chronic thromboembolic pulmonary hypertension using transthoracic three-dimensional echocardiography: changes due to pulmonary thromboendarterectomy. *Eur J Echocardiogr* 2002; **3**:67–72.

29. Louie EK, Rich S, Brundage BH. Doppler echocardiographic assessment of impaired left ventricular filling in patients with right ventricular pressure overload due to primary pulmonary hypertension. *J Am Coll Cardiol* 1986; **8**:1298–1306.

30. Alpert J. Effect of right ventricular dysfunction on left ventricular function. *Adv Cardiol* 1986; **34**:25–34.

31. Mahmud E, Raisinghani A, Hassankhani A,. *et al* Correlation of left ventricular diastolic filling characteristics with right ventricular overload and pulmonary artery pressure in chronic thromboembolic pulmonary hypertension. *J Am Coll Cardiol* 2002; **40**:318–324.

32. Gurudevan SV, Malouf PJ, Auger WR,. *et al* Abnormal left ventricular diastolic filling in chronic thromboembolic pulmonary hypertension: true diastolic dysfunction or left ventricular underfilling? *J Am Coll Cardiol* 2007; **49**:1334–1339.

33. Fesler P, Pagnamenta A, Vachiery JL,. *et al* Single arterial occlusion to locate resistance in patients with pulmonary hypertension. *Eur Respir J* 2003; **21**:31–36.

34. Kim NH, Fesler P, Channick RN,. *et al* Preoperative partitioning of pulmonary vascular resistance correlates with early outcome after thromboendarterectomy for chronic thromboembolic pulmonary hypertension. *Circulation* 2004; **109**:18–22.

35. Tanabe N, Okada O, Abe Y,. *et al* The influence of fractional pulse pressure on the outcome of pulmonary thromboendarterectomy. *Eur Respir J* 2001; **17**:653–659.

36. Worsley D, Palevsky H, Alavi A. Ventilation–perfusion lung scanning in the evaluation of pulmonary hypertension. *J Nucl Med* 1994; **35**:793–796.

37. Fishman A, Moser K, Fedullo PF. Perfusion lung scans vs pulmonary angiography in evaluation of suspected pulmonary hypertension. *Chest* 1983; **84**:679–683.

38. Lisbona R, Kreisman H, Novales-Diaz J,. *et al* Perfusion lung scanning: differentiation of primary from thromboembolic pulmonary hypertension. *AJR Am J Roentgenol* 1985; **144**:27–30.

39. Ryan KL, Fedullo PF, Davis GB,. *et al* Perfusion scan findings understate the severity of angiographic and hemodynamic compromise in chronic thromboembolic pulmonary hypertension. *Chest* 1988; **93**:1180–1185.

40. Washington L, Goodman L, Sostman H. CT for thromboembolic disease. *Radiol Clin North Am* 2002; **2002**:1886–1905.

41. Edwards P, Bull R, Coulden R. CT measurement of main pulmonary artery diameter. *Br J Radiol* 1998; **1998**:10810–11020.

42. Remy-Jardin M, Duhamel A, Deken V,. *et al* Systemic collateral supply in patients with chronic thromboembolic and primary pulmonary hypertension: assessment with multi-detector row helical CT angiography. *Radiology* 2005; **235**:274–281.

43. Sherrick A, Swensen S, Hartman T. Mosaic pattern of lung attenuation on CT scans: frequency among patients with pulmonary artery hypertension of different causes. *Am J Roentgenol* 1997; **169**:79–82.

44. Tunariu N, Gibbs SJR, Win Z,. *et al* Ventilation–perfusion scintigraphy is more sensitive than multidetector CTPA in detecting chronic thromboembolic pulmonary disease as a treatable cause of pulmonary hypertension. *J Nucl Med* 2007; **48**:680–684.

45. Coulden R. State-of-the-art imaging techniques in chronic thromboembolic pulmonary hypertension. *Proc Am Thorac Soc* 2006; **3**:577–583.

46. Ouderk M, Van Beek EJ, Wielopoloski P. Comparison of contrast-enhanced magnetic resonance angiography and conventional pulmonary angiography for the diagnosis of pulmonary embolism: a prospective study. *Lancet* 2002; **359**:1643–1647.
47. Kreitner KF, Ley S, Kauczor HU,. *et al* Chronic thromboembolic pulmonary hypertension: pre- and postoperative assessment with breath-hold MR imaging techniques. *Radiology* 2004; **232**:535–543.
48. Ley S, Kauczor HU, Heussel CP,. *et al* Value of contrast-enhanced MR angiography and helical CT angiography in chronic thromboembolic pulmonary hypertension. *Eur Radiol* 2003; **13**:2365–2371.
49. Nikolaou K, Schoenberg S, Attenberger U,. *et al* Pulmonary arterial hypertension: diagnosis with fast perfusion MR imaging and high-spatial-resolution MR angiography-preliminary experience. *Radiology* 2005; **236**:694–703.
50. Wolferen S, Marcus J, Boonstra A,. *et al* Prognostic value of right ventricular mass, volume and function in idiopathic pulmonary arterial hypertension. *Eur Heart J* 2007; **28**:1250–1257.
51. Ley S, Kreitner KF, Morgenstern I,. *et al* Bronchopulmonary shunts in patients with chronic thromboembolic pulmonary hypertension: evaluation with helical CT and MR imaging. *Am J Roentgenol* 2002; **179**:1209–1215.
52. Roeleveld RJ, Marcus JT, Boonstra A,. *et al* A comparison of noninvasive MRI-based methods of estimating pulmonary artery pressure in pulmonary hypertension. *J Magn Reson Imaging* 2005; **22**:67–72.
53. Kreitner KF, Kunz RP, Ley S,. *et al* Chronic thromboembolic pulmonary hypertension – assessment by magnetic resonance imaging. *Eur Radiol* 2007; **17**:11–21.
54. Wild JM, Fichele S, Woodhouse N,. *et al* 3D volume-localised pO_2 measured in the human lung with ^{3}He MRI. *Magn Reson Med* 2005; **53**:1055–1064.
55. Nicod P, Peterson K, Levine M,. *et al* Pulmonary angiography in severe chronic pulmonary hypertension. *Ann Intern Med* 1987; **107**:565–568.
56. Hofmann LV, Lee DS, Gupta A,. *et al* Safety and hemodynamic effects of pulmonary angiography in patients with pulmonary hypertension: 10-year single-center experience. *Am J Roentgenol* 2004; **183**:779–786.
57. Pitton MB, Duber C, Mayer E,. *et al* Hemodynamic effects of nonionic contrast bolus injection and oxygen inhalation during pulmonary angiography in patients with chronic major-vessel thromboembolic pulmonary hypertension. *Circulation* 1996; **94**:2485–2491.
58. Shure D, Gregoratos G, Moser KM. Fiberoptic angioscopy: role in the diagnosis of chronic thromboembolic pulmpnary arterial obstruction. *Ann Intern Med* 1985; **103**:844–850.
59. Becattini C, Agnelli G, Pesavento R,. *et al* Incidence of chronic thromboembolic pulmonary hypertension after a first episode of pulmonary embolism. *Chest* 2006; **130**:172–175.
60. Miniati M, Monti S, Bottai M,. *et al* Survival and restoration of pulmonary perfusion in a long-term follow-up of patients after acute pulmonary embolism. *Medicine* 2006; **85**:253–262.
61. Ribiero A, Lindmaker P, Johnsson H,. *et al* Pulmonary embolism: one-year follow-up with echocardiography doppler and five-year survival analysis. *Circulation* 1999; **99**:1325–1330.
62. Naess I, Christiansen S, Romundstad P,. *et al* Incidence and mortality of venous thrombosis: a population-based study. *J Thromb Haemost* 2007; **5**:692–699.
63. Goldhaber S, Visani L, De Rosa M. Acute pulmonary embolism: clinical outcomes in the International Cooperative Pulmonary Embolism Register (ICOPER). *Lancet* 1999; **353**:1386–1389.

PART V

Prevention of VTE

CHAPTER 19

Mechanical Prevention of Venous Thromboembolism

Juan I. Arcelus[1] and Joseph A. Caprini[2]

[1]Department of Surgery, University of Granada Medical School, Granada, Spain

[2]Louis W. Biegler Professor of Surgery and Bioengineering Robert R. McCormick School of Engineering and Applied Sciences, Department of Surgery, NorthShore University HealthSystem, Evanston and Northwestern University Feinberg School of Medicine, Glenbrook Hospital, Illinois, USA

INTRODUCTION

Venous thromboembolism (VTE) represents a major health problem, with hundreds of thousands of new cases occurring every year in Europe and the USA (1,2). The high prevalence and frequently silent onset of VTE, with serious short- and long-term consequences, underscores the need for appropriate prophylaxis for this condition. Hypercoagulability, venous stasis and vein wall injury are the main risk factors to develop VTE, which includes both deep vein thrombosis (DVT) and pulmonary embolism (PE). For this reason, methods used to prevent VTE are either mechanical, aiming to reduce vein dilatation and improve venous flow, or pharmacological, based on anticoagulants to neutralize hypercoagulability. This chapter focuses on the rationale and clinical results of mechanical methods in the prevention of VTE, used alone or in combination with anticoagulants.

PATHOGENESIS OF VTE

The pathogenesis of VTE is multifactorial, as proposed by Rudolph Virchow more than 150 years ago in his classical triad–namely, blood hypercoagulability, endothelial damage and venous stasis. Venous stasis is very important in the development of venous thrombosis for several reasons. First, stasis prevents the local clearance of activated coagulation factors and their mixing with their physiological inhibitors. Also, in situations of venous stasis there is local accumulation of ADP derived from red blood cells and leukocytes that stimulates platelet adhesion and aggregation. In addition, venous stasis might reduce the release of fibrinolytic activators from the endothelium, such as tissue-type plasminogen activator (t-PA) and urokinase-type plasminogen activator (u-PA). Likewise, venous dilatation may disturb the normal linear blood flow and cause endothelial tears

Deep Vein Thrombosis and Pulmonary Embolism   Edited by Edwin J.R. van Beek, Harry R. Büller and Matthijs Oudkerk
© 2009 John Wiley & Sons, Ltd

and intimal damage, allowing platelets, red blood cells and leukocytes to contact the damaged endothelium and the exposed basement membrane and sub-endothelial collagen. In several elegant pioneering studies, Stewart established the relationship between operative vein dilatation, inflammation and thrombosis (3). More recent studies have investigated the role of inflammation in the pathogenesis and outcome of venous thrombosis (4). Under physiological conditions, endothelial cells prevent thrombosis by several mechanisms, including production of thrombomodulin which activates protein C, the expression of heparan and dermatan sulfate, which accelerate antithrombin activity, release of tissue factor pathway inhibitor (TFPI) which will inhibit factor VII, local expression of t-PA and u-PA and production of platelet inhibitors nitric oxide (NO), prostacyclin and Il-10. In contrast, situations of endothelial dysfunction, such as the above-mentioned venous dilatation and stasis associated with the perioperative period, result in the release of prothrombotic and proinflammatory molecules, such as platelet activating factor, von Willebrand's factor, tissue factor, plasminogen activator inhibitor (PAI-1) and factor V. Moreover, in response to injury, endothelial cells express surface adhesion molecules (P-selectin and E-selectin), which promote adhesion to leukocytes and platelets and their activation (5).

A correlation between venous dilatation and thrombosis was first documented in experimental animal models by Schaub *et al*. (6). These investigators also showed that intraoperative distension of the arm veins correlated with DVT in the lower extremities in patients undergoing total hip replacement (7). Subsequently, Coleridge-Smith *et al*. reported a significant dilatation of the deep calf veins documented by duplex imaging in patients undergoing abdominal surgery (8).

These findings provide a better understanding of the consequences of venous stasis and dilatation as a key factor leading to an increased risk to develop DVT in immobilized patients. Therefore, several physical and mechanical methods have been proposed to overcome venous stasis and prevent VTE.

MECHANICAL METHODS FOR VTE PREVENTION

Physical and mechanical methods may be divided into two main categories: passive and active, based on their mechanism of action (Table 19.1). Among the passive methods, elastic stockings have been extensively investigated for VTE prophylaxis, especially in surgical patients. Regarding active methods, most studies have been done with intermittent pneumatic compression (IPC) and, in recent years, impulse foot compression has been investigated, mainly in patients undergoing orthopaedic surgery.

Table 19.1   Mechanical and physical methods for VTE prevention

Passive
Leg elevation
Bandages
Elastic stockings:
Uniform compression
Graduated compression
Active
Intermittent pneumatic compression of the legs:
Uniform compression
Sequential compression
Impulse foot compression

Compression stockings

Description

Elastic compression stockings of the legs reduce the cross-sectional area of the veins and, as a result, increase the velocity of blood flow, depending on the pressure gradient applied to the limb. Sigel *et al*. demonstrated that graduated compression stockings (GCS) significantly increased the blood velocity around 30% at the femoral vein during recumbence as detected by Doppler ultrasound (9). They also found that the optimal pressure profile consisted of 18 mmHg at the ankle, decreasing to 8 mmHg in the upper thigh.

The acceleration of blood flow in the deep veins of the leg reduces venous stasis and decreases the risk of thrombus formation by decreasing vein wall distension, which results in less endothelial cracking (7). In addition, compression reduces the contact time between blood and endothelium and improves the emptying of valvular cusps, where many thrombi start in immobilized patients.

In patients undergoing surgery with general anaesthesia, Coleridge-Smith *et al*. measured by duplex ultrasonography the diameter of gastrocnemius veins before and after the operation in a control group and in patients with GCS (10). Application of the stockings reduced the average vein diameter by 32% before induction of anaesthesia. At the end of surgery, the vein diameter in the GCS group experienced an additional 5.5% reduction, while the diameter increased by 19% in the control group. These results indicate that GCS can prevent venous distension that occurs in deep veins of the leg over the course of surgery. We found similar results in healthy volunteers placed in a reverse Trendelenburg position, as GCS were able to reduce calf vein distension compared with controls (11). In the same study, we also showed that tissue factor pathway inhibitor (TFPI) levels were significantly increased after tilting when GCS were used compared with controls in the same tilting position.

Efficacy for VTE prevention

Several trials have investigated the efficacy of GCS for VTE prevention in different surgical populations, with most studies focusing on general surgical patients. A meta-analysis of the literature reviewed 11 studies investigating the efficacy of GCS in 1800 moderate-risk patients undergoing mostly general surgery. The results showed a significant 68% reduction in the incidence of postoperative DVT in patients with stockings [odds ratio (OR) 0.28; 95% confidence interval (CI) 0.23 to 0.48; $p < 0.0001$] (12).

A review from the Cochrane Collaboration analysed seven randomized controlled trials in general, gynaecological, orthopaedic and neurosurgical patients (13). The incidence of postoperative DVT detected by objective diagnostic methods was significantly reduced, from 29% in the control group to 15% in the GCS group (OR 0.33; 95% CI 0.26 to 0.49; $p < 0.0001$). Another more recent systematic review of the literature evaluated the results of 17 trials assessing GCS in more than 2400 patients. In nine trials in which GCS were used as monotherapy, there was a 66% reduction in the incidence of DVT, from 21% (133/627) in the controls to 8.6% (57/665) in the GCS group ($p < 0.001$) (Table 19.2) (14).

Current evidence suggests that GCS, used as monotherapy, are effective for DVT prevention in moderate-risk surgical patients, but there is a lack of data in high-risk patients, such as those undergoing cancer or orthopaedic surgery. Likewise, there is no evidence that GCS used alone reduce the incidence of PE in medical or surgical patients.

Table 19.2 Efficacy of GCS used as monotherapy for the prevention of DVT in different patient populations[a]

Study	DVT			OR (%)
	Patients	**GCS**	**Control**	
Allan, 1983 (49)	GS	15/97	37/103	65
Barnes, 1978 (50)	THR	0/8	5/10	100
Holford, 1976(51)	GS	11/50	23/48	68
Inada, 1983 (52)	GS	4/110	16/110	73
Rosengarten, 1970 (53)	GS	8/25	8/25	–
Muir, 2000 (54)	Stroke	7/65	7/32	–
Shirai, 1985(55)	GS	5/126	17/126	70
Turner, 1984 (56)	GYN	0/104	4/92	–
Turpie, 1989 (57)	NEU	7/80	16/81	59
Total		57/665	133/627	66
		(8.6%)	(21.2%)	$p < 0.0001$

[a]Abbreviations: GS, general surgery; THR, total hip replacement; GYN, gynaecology; NEU, neurosurgery; OR, odds reduction.

Thigh-length versus knee-length stockings

Regarding their length, GCS used for VTE prevention may be classified into thigh-length and knee-length stockings. A few studies have compared the haemodynamic effects and patient compliance for both types. In a group of orthopaedic surgical patients, knee-length and thigh-length stockings were similarly effective in decreasing venous stasis (15). Although thigh-length stockings are widely perceived to be more effective for VTE prophylaxis, data to support that conclusion are not available. A systematic review of the literature has identified two trials comparing thigh-length and knee-length stockings and the incidence of DVT was 8.7% (9/104) and 8.3% (9/108). These results are considered inconclusive due to the small number of patients and the low DVT rate (15,16).

On the other hand, knee-length stockings are easier to apply and maintain, wrinkle less often and are better tolerated by patients, whereas thigh-length stockings often roll down at the thigh, either hanging loosely around the knee or causing a tourniquet effect (17). Other studies suggest that knee-length stockings are more likely to be correctly applied than thigh-length and are less expensive, therefore increasing the level of compliance by patients and nurses (18–20).

Limitations and advantages of compression stockings

The main limitations of GCS include the lack of international standardization of their pressure profiles and the difficulty in fitting patients with unusual leg sizes or shapes. Patient compliance may be another limiting issue, especially with thigh-length stockings, as discussed above. According to one study, the most common reasons for non-compliance by patients and nurses were that stockings were not reapplied after cleaning or bathing or were removed because patients complained from itching or heat (19). Compression stockings should not be used in patients with peripheral arterial disease. Therefore, lack of foot pulses or an ankle–brachial index lower than 0.8 should be considered contraindications for their use, and also in patients with massive leg oedema associated with cardiac failure. Infectious dermatitis and fragile skin secondary to diabetes are other contraindications to the use of GCS.

Apart from their proven efficacy in preventing VTE, stockings are safe, relatively easy to apply and inexpensive. Another important benefit of GCS that will be discussed in another section is the possibility of combining them with pharmacological prophylaxis in patients at very high risk of developing VTE.

Intermittent pneumatic compression

Description

IPC is the most extensively studied of the mechanical methods of thromboprophylaxis and is considered the most effective of these methods. Basically, this method avoids venous stasis by intermittent pumping of the leg veins. Most IPC models consist of a pneumatic boot or sleeve that is fitted on the leg. The boot is connected to an electrical compressor that insufflates air to a preselected pressure. The sleeves are intermittently inflated and emptied to allow the veins to refill with blood between compression cycles. These devices may compress the pneumatic chambers sequentially from the foot or ankle proximally to the knee or thigh or they may have a single chamber, providing uniform compression. As for stockings, IPC sleeves may extend up to the knee or to the upper thigh.

Different pressure profiles and compression can be used, depending on the IPC model. The maximum pressures investigated for VTE prevention range from 35 to 55 mmHg at the ankle. Insufflation times vary from 10 to 35 s with a deflation period of approximately 1 min to allow blood to refill the veins of the legs. In recent years, an IPC device has been designed which detects the post-compression refill of the leg veins, thereby increasing by 75% the total volume of blood expelled per hour (21). Apart from preserving venous capacitance and outflow, IPC improves flow velocity and clearance of the venous system of the legs, resulting in a reversible increase of preload (22). Another important effect of IPC for VTE prevention is the stimulation of fibrinolysis and coagulation physiological inhibitors by different mechanisms, including the increase in plasma levels of prostacyclin (23), t-PA (24) and tissue factor pathway inhibitor (TFPI). In addition, IPC has been shown to reduce the plasma levels of a plasminogen activator inhibitor (PAI-1) (25) and to reduce platelet activation (26).

Efficacy for VTE prevention

The results of IPC have been variable, depending on the type of surgery, patients' risk factors and endpoints used to detect DVT. Overall, most studies show that IPC reduces the incidence of DVT in general surgery, urology, neurosurgery and orthopaedic surgery. A systematic review by Roderick *et al.* (14) identified 19 trials assessing IPC as monotherapy in 2255 patients undergoing different types of surgery. The results show that IPC significantly reduced the incidence of DVT from 23.4% (268/1147) in the control group to 10.1% (112/1108) in the IPC group, a 66% odds reduction ($p < 0.0001$) (Table 19.3). There was no evidence that sequential compression devices were more protective than uniform compression machines, as their odds reductions were 65% (six trials) and 66% (12 trials), respectively.

A meta-analysis of the literature reviewed 15 randomized controlled trials with a total of 16 treatment groups comparing IPC with controls in 2270 surgical patients with objective diagnosis of DVT by imaging techniques (27). In comparison with no prophylaxis, IPC reduced the risk of DVT by 60% [relative risk (RR) 0.40; 95% CI 0.29 to 0.56; $p < 0.001$).

Limitations and advantages

A limitation of these studies is related to possible diagnostic bias, since most trials used the fibrinogen uptake test and impedance plethysmography to detect DVT; these have been replaced

Table 19.3   Efficacy of IPC used as monotherapy for the prevention of postoperative DVT[a]

Study	DVT			OR (%)
	Patients	GCS	Control	
Bachman, 1976 (58)	THR/TKR	4/26	13728	76
Blackshear, 1987 (59)	GS	0/20	0/20	–
Butson, 1981(60)	GS	4/62	4/57	–
Bynke, 1987 (61)	NEU	0/31	6/31	100
Clark, 1974 (62)	GS	0/36	7/36	100
Clarke-Pearson,1984 (63)	GYN	5/59	17/57	75
Clarke-Pearson,1984 (64)	GYN	14/104	11/105	–
Coe, 1978 (65)	URO	1/35	5/24	–
Fisher, 1995 (66)	HF	4/145	9/159	–
Gallus, 1983 (67)	THR	15/43	25/47	52
Hills, 1972 (68)	GS	7/70	23/70	74
Hull, 1979 (69)	TKR	2/32	19/29	92
Hull, 1990 (70)	THR	36/152	77/158	66
Knudson, 1994 (71)	TRA	0/26	5/39	–
Kosir, 1986 (72)	GS	0/25	0/45	–
Skillman, 1978 (73)	NEU	4/47	12/48	69
Turpie, 1977 (74)	NEU	8/82	13/79	–
Turpie, 1979 (75)	NEU	8/112	20/106	65
Weitz, 1986 (76)	NEU	0/5	2/9	–
Total		112/1108	268/1147	66
		(10.1%)	(23.3%)	$p < 0.0001$

[a]Abbreviations: GS, general surgery; THR, total hip replacement; TKR, total knee replacement; GYN, gynaecology; URO, urology; NEU, neurosurgery; TRA, trauma; OR, odds reduction.

by other tests such as ultrasonography, because of their low sensitivity. Besides, most studies had a very short follow-up period, between 3 and 14 days, and very probably some DVTs developed after hospital discharge and, therefore, were missed for the analysis.

The issue of whether above-knee IPC devices are more effective than calf-length devices remains unclear in the absence of large-scale trials. The choice between the two alternatives should be made on practical grounds, depending on their availability and cost.

As with GCS, another important issue regarding IPC is compliance and adequate implementation. Studies have documented effective implementation of IPC between 50% (19) and 78% (28). Although compliance seems to be better in the ICU setting than in the general wards, as shown by Comerota *et al.* (29), there is an urgent need to improve patient and nursing staff education on the appropriate use of IPC for VTE prophylaxis in order to optimize implementation (30).

COMBINATION OF PHYSICAL AND PHARMACOLOGICAL METHODS

Rationale

The combination of an anticoagulant and passive or active compression of the legs is an attractive approach since venous stasis, venous dilatation with endothelial cracking and hypercoagulability are all addressed.

Combination of mechanical methods and anticoagulants

Amaragiri, in a Cochrane analysis, identified in seven randomized controlled trials (RCTs) that the combination of GCS in addition to another prophylactic method was significantly more effective than GCS alone (31). DVT was seen in only 2% of the patients in the combined group compared with 15% in the control group. A large multicentre trial comparing aspirin with placebo for orthopaedic patients contained a group receiving aspirin plus GCS which showed a statistically significant reduction in pulmonary emboli compared with the control group (32). Another Cochrane analysis documented that the combination of heparin and GCS was better than heparin alone following colorectal surgery (33).

Most studies using combined modalities involve the use of intermittent IPC in conjunction with various anticoagulants. One of the earliest investigations showed that, using the combination of aspirin, heparin or coumadin in conjunction with IPC, DVT was virtually eliminated in a group of 328 patients. There was only a 1.5% incidence of DVT in the treated population compared with 26.8% in the control group (34).

Woolson and Watt randomized patients undergoing total hip replacement (THR) to intermittent pneumatic compression alone, intermittent pneumatic compression and aspirin or intermittent pneumatic compression and low-dose warfarin (35). The incidence of ultrasound-detected VTE was 10% in each of the groups. In this study, the combination prophylaxis was not better than IPC although the ultrasonic endpoint and small size of the study (196 patients) make it difficult to conclude that combination prophylaxis is not valuable. In another small study, the effectiveness of the plantar venous plexus foot pump combined with unfractionated heparin in patients having THR showed a 6.6% venographic DVT rate compared with 27.% in the non-pumped group ($p < 0.025$). The authors concluded that chemical prophylaxis plus the use of GCS stockings, pneumatic compression and the arteriovenous impulse system reduces the incidence of thromboembolic complications further than chemical prophylaxis alone (36). The incidence of pulmonary emboli was investigated in 2551 patients having coronary artery bypass surgery (CABG) over a 10 year period. Patients received either 5000 units of UFH daily alone or in combination with long-leg sequential IPC. The incidence of imaging-proven PE was 4.0% in the heparin group and 1.5% in the combination prophylaxis group ($p < 0.001$) (37). A prospective randomized study in 139 patients following THR or total knee replacement (TKR), LMWH in combination with IPC compression and monitored by ultrasonography showed no evidence of thrombosis, whereas the group receiving LMWH and compression stockings revealed a DVT incidence of 28.6% (40% after TKR, 14% after THR) ($p < 0.0001$) (38). The combination of a foot pump and either LMWH or aspirin was studied in 275 TKR patients and the incidence of ultrasound DVT was 14.1% using LMWH and the foot pump and 17.8% with aspirin and the foot pump (39). Similarly, 1803 orthopaedic patients were prospectively randomized to receive either LMWH alone or in combination with IPC. In the LMWH group, 15 patients (1.7%) had a DVT and in the combined group four patients (0.4%) had a DVT ($p = 0.007$). In the combined prophylaxis group no DVTs were found in patients who received more than 6 h of intermittent pneumatic compression daily (40). The most recent study was conducted in 1309 patients having abdominal surgery, all of whom received IPC according to hospital protocols. These patients were randomized to receive either a placebo saline injection daily or 2.5 mg of fondaparinux, a selective inhibitor of factor Xa, daily for 7 days. The venographic incidence of DVT in the placebo group was 5.3% and in the fondaparinux group 1.7% (41). It is interesting that this large series in general surgery shows a similar VTE rate to the Borow studies 25 years ago, in a similar group of patients in 1983 using a variety of anticoagulants. Overall, it appears that the combination of anticoagulants and IPC statistically improves VTE prevention rates compared with single-modality prophylaxis.

Current recommendations for combined prophylaxis

The latest guidelines (8th edition) from the American College of Chest Physicians (ACCP) recommend mechanical methods of prophylaxis primarily in patients at high risk for bleeding (grade 1A) or as an option in conjunction with heparin or LMWH, in patients in the highest risk category for VTE (42). The combination of mechanical methods and these anticoagulants is listed as a grade 2A suggestion. These guidelines also recommend careful attention to ensure proper use of and optimal adherence to these methods (grade 1A).

The large general surgery trial which was randomized, double blinded and used a venographic endpoint combining IPC with either saline placebo or fondaparinux had not been published until 2007 (41). It remains to be seen if the new guidelines are modified as a result of these new data. Previously, the ACCP authors were concerned that many of the trials involving mechanical methods were unblinded and lacked a venographic endpoint. These objections were overcome in the latest trial involving combined prophylaxis. The International Consensus guidelines also recommend UFH, LMWH or fondaparinux in conjunction with mechanical methods in the high-risk patient group (grade B) (43).

CURRENT USE OF MECHANICAL PROPHYLAXIS IN THE REAL WORLD

We surveyed 3500 North American general surgeons in 1992 and found that 86% used some form of specific thrombosis prophylaxis other than early ambulation in their patients. IPC was the preferred modality followed by UFH and elastic stockings. Combined mechanical and pharmacological modalities were used by 26% of the respondents (44).

A follow-up survey after the introduction of LMWH for prophylaxis in the USA found that most (96%) of the respondents used prophylaxis against VTE (45). Although LMWHs were rated first regarding efficacy and second regarding simplicity of use, conventional unfractionated heparin at fixed doses remained the preferred pharmacological agent for VTE prevention (74%), followed by two LMWHs, enoxaparin (34%) and dalteparin (16%). Overall, 52% of surgeons preferred physical methods over pharmacological methods when used separately and 26% of surgeons utilized combined physical–pharmacological modalities. This percentage had not changed since the previous survey in 1992. The survey concluded that although physical methods and unfractionated heparin remained the preferred prophylactic modalities, LMWHs have gained in popularity only over the last 4 years in the USA.

A multinational cross-sectional study recently completed, involving 68 183 patients representing 352 hospitals from 32 countries, revealed that the use of IPC was 10% in surgical patients and 4% in medical patients, with GCS use in 19% of surgical and 5% of medical patients. The use of combined modalities is not apparent from the reported data, but that might relate to the lack of widespread availability of IPC worldwide. It is interesting that 10% of patients at high risk of VTE had some contraindication to the use of pharmacological prophylaxis (46).

Recently, Warwick et al. reported findings from the Global Orthopedic Registry (GLORY) regarding the time courses of both the incidence of VTE and effective prophylaxis (47). Overall, 95% of the 15 000 patients received anticoagulant or mechanical prophylaxis following THR or TKR. IPC was used in combination with either warfarin or LMWH depending on the country involved. LMWH combined with IPC was used in 17.4% of TKR patients outside the USA and in 25% of TKR patients in the USA. That same combination was used in 11.4% THR patients outside the USA and 24.6% of patients in the USA. Warfarin plus IPC was rare outside the USA (0.2%) following either THR or TKR, but in the USA IPC plus warfarin was used in 33.5% of

THR patients and 18.0% of TKR patients. These data support the concept that many surgeons use combined modalities in the highest risk patients rather than relying on anticoagulants alone (47).

Amin *et al*. performed a database review of data from 227 hospitals over a 3.5 year period involving nearly 200 000 patients looking at thrombosis prophylaxis rates in US hospitals (48). Overall, they found that although the thrombosis prophylaxis rate was 66.8%, only 33.9% received appropriate prophylaxis according to the ACCP guidelines. They noted that 26.8% of the patients received mechanical prophylaxis alone in cases where there was no contraindication because of bleeding. Inappropriate prophylaxis post-discharge was seen in two-thirds of the patients, including 4.7% who received mechanical prophylaxis alone.

CONCLUSIONS

Compression stockings and IPC devices are important modalities in the prevention of VTE. The mechanism of action of these modalities helps neutralize all of the elements of Virchow's triad. Venous stasis is minimized, thus inhibiting over-distension of the leg veins and preventing endothelial cracks that frequently accompany venous dilatation. Specific fibrinolytic blood elements are activated, which helps limit hypercoagulability that accompanies surgery, infection, cancer, trauma and other conditions.

The use of IPC during operating procedures can limit the formation of intraoperative thrombi that occur, especially during long operating procedures for cancer or when the legs are in stirrups or a dependent position that fosters over-distension of the leg veins. Postoperatively these devices provide a certain degree of thrombosis prophylaxis until anticoagulants are started in patients where there is a concern about using the drugs soon after the operation because of increased bleeding risk. Mechanical devices are most valuable in situations where anticoagulants are contraindicated due to active bleeding or very high bleeding risk.

The combination of physical and pharmacological prophylaxis has been shown to provide the greatest level of protection against thrombosis in both medical and surgical patients, which makes this approach ideal in those with the greatest risk of VTE.

Finally, it should be noted that in order to be effective, these mechanical devices must be functioning properly and connected correctly to the patient. They must be in place at all times when the patient is in bed or a chair. Lack of compliance has been a major problem in the past but with the newer devices that sense leg pressure, electronic alerts and timers can document and foster appropriate compliance. If this goal is accomplished, the value of IPC devices will be greatly enhanced.

REFERENCES

1. Cohen AT, Agnelli G, Anderson FA,. *et al*. Venous thromboembolism (VTE) in Europe. The number of VTE events and associated morbidity and mortality. *Thromb Haemost* 2007; **98**:756–64.
2. Heit JA. The epidemiology of venous thromboembolism in the community. *Arteriosclerosis, Thromb Vasc Biol* 2008; **28**:370–2.
3. Stewart GJ. Neutrophils and deep venous thrombosis. *Haemostasis* 1993; **23** (Suppl 1):127–40.
4. Wakefield TW, Myers DD, Henke PK. Mechanisms of venous thrombosis and resolution. *Arteriosclerosis, Thromb Vasc Biol* 2008; **28**:387–91.
5. Myers DD, Wakefield TW. Inflammation-dependent thrombosis. *Frontiers Biosci* 2005; **10**:2750–7.
6. Schaub RG, Lynch PR, Stewart GJ. The response of canine veins to three types of abdominal surgery: a scanning and transmission electron microscopic study. *Surgery* 1978; **83**:411–24.
7. Comerota AJ, Stewart GJ, Alburger PD,. *et al*. Operative venodilation: a previously unsuspected factor in the cause of postoperative deep vein thrombosis. *Surgery* 1989; **106**:301–8.

8. Coleridge-Smith PD, Hasty JH, Scurr JH. Venous stasis and vein lumen changes during surgery. *Br J Surg* 1990; **77**:1055–9.
9. Sigel B, Edelstein AL, Felix WR Jr, *et al.*. Compression of the deep venous system of the lower leg during inactive recumbency. *Arch Surg* 1973; **106**:38–43.
10. Coleridge-Smith PD, Hasty JH, Scurr JH. Deep vein thrombosis: effect of graduated compression stockings on distension of the deep veins of the calf. *Br J Surg* 1991; **78**:724–6.
11. Arcelus JI, Caprini JA, Hoffman KN,. *et al.* Modifications of plasma levels of tissue factor pathway inhibitor and endothelin-1 induced by a reverse Trendelenburg position: influence of elastic compression – preliminary results. *J Vasc Surg* 1995; **22**:568–72.
12. Wells PS, Lensing AW, Hirsh J. Graduated compression stockings in the prevention of postoperative venous thromboembolism. A meta-analysis. *Arch Intern Med* 1994; **154**:67–72.
13. Amaragiri SV, Lees TA. Elastic compression stockings for prevention of deep vein thrombosis. *Cochrane Database Syst Rev* 2000; (1):CD001484.
14. Roderick P, Ferris G, Wilson K,. *et al.* Towards evidence-based guidelines for the prevention of venous thromboembolism: systematic reviews of mechanical methods, oral anticoagulation, dextran and regional anaesthesia as thromboprophylaxis. *Health Technol Assess* 2005; **9**:iii–iv.
15. Benko T, Cooke EA, McNally MA,. *et al.* Graduated compression stockings: knee length or thigh length. *Clin Orthop* 2001; **383**:197–203.
16. Roderick P, Ferris G, Wilson K,. *et al.* Towards evidence-based guidelines for the prevention of venous thromboembolism: systematic reviews of mechanical methods, oral anticoagulation, dextran and regional anaesthesia as thromboprophylaxis. *Health Technology Assess* 2005; **9**:iii–iv.
17. Byrne B. Deep vein thrombosis prophylaxis: the effectiveness and implications of using below-knee or thigh-length graduated compression stockings. *Heart Lung* 2001; **30**:277–84.
18. Hameed MF, Browse DJ, Immelman EJ,. *et al.* Should knee-length replace thigh-length graduated compression stockings in the prevention of deep-vein thrombosis? *S Afr J Surg* 2002; **40**:15–6.
19. Brady D, Raingruber B, Peterson J,. *et al.* The use of knee-length versus thigh-length compression stockings and sequential compression devices. *Crit Care Nurs Q* 2007; **30**:255–62.
20. Agu O, Hamilton G, Baker D. Graduated compression stockings in the prevention of venous thromboembolism. *Br J Surg* 1999; **86**:992–1004.
21. Kakkos SK, Griffin M, Geroulakos G,. *et al.* The efficacy of a new portable sequential compression device (SCD Express) in preventing venous stasis. *J Vasc Surg* 2005; **42**:296–303.
22. Blackshear WM Jr, Prescott C, LePain F,. *et al.* Influence of sequential pneumatic compression on postoperative venous function. *J Vasc Surg* 1987; **5**:432–6.
23. Guyton DP, Khayat A, Husni EA,. *et al.* Elevated levels of 6-keto-prostaglandin-F1a from a lower extremity during external pneumatic compression. *Surg Gynecol Obstet* 1988; **166**:338–42.
24. Summaria L, Caprini JA, McMillan R,. *et al.* Relationship between postsurgical fibrinolytic parameters and deep vein thrombosis in surgical patients treated with compression devices. *Am Surg* 1988; **54**:156–60.
25. Comerota AJ, Chouhan V, Harada RN,. *et al.* The fibrinolytic effects of intermittent pneumatic compression: mechanism of enhanced fibrinolysis. *Ann Surg* 1997; **226**:306–13.
26. Kessler CM, Hirsch DR, Jacobs H,. *et al.* Intermittent pneumatic compression in chronic venous insufficiency favorably affects fibrinolytic potential and platelet activation. *Blood Coag Fibrinol* 1996; **7**:437–46.
27. Urbankova J, Quiroz R, Kucher N,. *et al.* Intermittent pneumatic compression and deep vein thrombosis prevention. A meta-analysis in postoperative patients. *Thromb Haemost* 2005; **94**:1181–5.
28. Haddad FS, Kerry RM, McEwen JA,. *et al.* Unanticipated variations between expected and delivered pneumatic compression therapy after elective hip surgery: a possible source of variation in reported patient outcomes. *J Arthroplasty* 2001; **16**:37–46.
29. Comerota AJ, Katz ML, White JV. Why does prophylaxis with external pneumatic compression for deep vein thrombosis fail? *Am J Surg* 1992; **164**:265–8.
30. Geerts WH, Pineo GF, Heit JA,. *et al.* Prevention of venous thromboembolism: the Seventh ACCP Conference on Antithrombotic and Thrombolytic Therapy. *Chest* 2004; **126**:338S–400S.
31. Amaragiri S. Elastic compression stockings for the pevention of DVT. *Cochrane Database Syst Rev* 2004; (1):CD001484.
32. PEP Trialists Group. Prevention of pulmonary embolism and deep vein thrombosis with low dose aspirin: Pulmonary Embolism Prevention (PEP) trial. *Lancet* 2000; **355**:1295–302.
33. Wille-Jorgensen P, Rasmussen M, Andersen B. Heparins and mechanical methods for thromboprophylaxis in colorectal surgery. *Cochrane Database Syst Rev* 2004; **4**:CD001217.

34. Borow M, Goldson HJ. Prevention of postoperative deep venous thrombosis and pulmonary emboli with combined modalities. *Am Surg* 1983; **49**:599–605.
35. Woolson ST, Watt JM. Intermittent pneumatic compression to prevent proximal deep venous thrombosis during and after total hip replacement. A prospective, randomized study of compression alone, compression and aspirin and compression and low-dose warfarin. *J Bone Joint Surg Am Vol* 1991; **73**:507–12.
36. Bradley JG, Krugener GH, Jager HJ. The effectiveness of intermittent plantar venous compression in prevention of deep venous thrombosis after total hip arthroplasty. *J Arthroplasty* 1993; **8**:57–61.
37. Ramos R, Salem BI, De Pawlikowski MP,. *et al.* The efficacy of pneumatic compression stockings in the prevention of pulmonary embolism after cardiac surgery. *Chest* 1996; **109**:82–5.
38. Silbersack Y, Taute BM, Hein W,. *et al.* Prevention of deep-vein thrombosis after total hip and knee replacement. Low-molecular-weight heparin in combination with intermittent pneumatic compression. *J Bone Joint Surg Br Vol* 2004; **86**:809–12.
39. Westrich GH, Bottner F, Windsor RE,. *et al.* VenaFlow plus Lovenox vs VenaFlow plus aspirin for thromboembolic disease prophylaxis in total knee arthroplasty. *J Arthroplasty* 2006; **21**:139–43.
40. Eisele R, Kinzl L, Koelsch T. Rapid-inflation intermittent pneumatic compression for prevention of deep venous thrombosis. *J Bone Joint Surg Am Vol* 2007; **89**:1050–6.
41. Turpie AG, Bauer KA, Caprini JA,. *et al.* Fondaparinux combined with intermittent pneumatic compression vs. intermittent pneumatic compression alone for prevention of venous thromboembolism after abdominal surgery: a randomized, double-blind comparison. *J Thromb Haemost* 2007; **5**:1854–61.
42. Geerts WH, Bergqvist D, Pineo GF,. *et al.* Prevention of venous thromboembolism. American College of Chest Physicians Evidence-based clinical practice guidelines (8th edition). *Chest* 2008; **133**;381s.
43. Nicolaides AN, Fareed J, Kakkar AK,. *et al.* Prevention and treatment of venous thromboembolism: international consensus statement. *Int Angiol* 2006; **25**:101–61.
44. Caprini JA, Arcelus JI, Hoffman K,. *et al.* Prevention of venous thromboembolism in North America: results of a survey among general surgeons. *J Vasc Surg* 1994; **20**:751–8.
45. Caprini JA, Arcelus J, Sehgal LR,. *et al.* The use of low molecular weight heparins for the prevention of postoperative venous thromboembolism in general surgery. A survey of practice in the United States. *Int Angiol* 2002; **21**:78–85.
46. Cohen AT, Tapson VF, Bergmann JF,. *et al.* Venous thromboembolism risk and prophylaxis in the acute care setting (ENDORSE study): a multinational cross-sectional study. *Lancet* 2008; **371**:387–94.
47. Warwick D, Friedman R, Agnelli G,. *et al.* Insufficient duration of venous thromboembolism prophylaxis after total hip or knee replacement when compared with the time course of thromboembolic events: findings from the Global Orthopaedic Registry. *J Bone Joint Surg Br* 2007; **89**:799–807.
48. Amin A, Stemkowski S, Lin J,. *et al.* Thromboprophylaxis rates in US medical centers: success or failure? *J Thromb Haemost* 2007; **5**:1610–6.
49. Allan A, Williams JT, Bolton JP, Le Quesne LP. The use of graduated compression stockings in the prevention of postoperative deep vein thrombosis. *Br J Surg* 1983; **70**:172–4.
50. Barnes RW, Brand RA, Clarke W, Hartley N, Hoak JC. Efficacy of graded-compression antiembolism stockings in patients undergoing total hip arthroplasty. *Clin Orthop* 1978; **132**:61–7.
51. Holford C. Graded compression for preventing deep vein thrombosis. *Br Med J* 1976; **ii**:969–70.
52. Inada K, Shirai N, Hayashi M, Matsumoto K, Hirose M. Postoperative deep venous thrombosis in Japan. Incidence and prophylaxis. *Am J Surg* 1983; **145**:775–9.
53. Rosengarten DS, Laird J, Jeyasingh K, Martin P. The failure of compression stockings (Tubigrip) to prevent deep venous thrombosis after operation. *Br J Surg* 1970; **57**:296–9.
54. Muir KW, Watt A, Baxter G, Grosset DG, Lees KR. Randomized trial of graded compression stockings for prevention of deep-vein thrombosis after acute stroke. *QJM* 2000; **93**:359–64.
55. Shirai N. Study on prophylaxis of postoperative deep vein thrombosis. *Acta Sch Med Univ Gifu* 1985; **33**:1173–83.
56. Turner GM, Cole SE, Brooks JH. The efficacy of graduated compression stockings in the prevention of deep vein thrombosis after major gynaecological surgery. *Br J Obstet Gynaecol* 1984; **91**:588–91.
57. Turpie AG, Hirsh J, Gent M, Julian D, Johnson J. Prevention of deep vein thrombosis in potential neurosurgical patients. A randomized trial comparing graduated compression stockings alone or graduated compression stockings plus intermittent pneumatic compression with control. *Arch Intern Med* 1989; **149**:679–81.
58. Bachman F, McKenna R, Merideth P, Carta S. Intermittent pneumatic compression of the leg and thigh: a new successful method for the prevention of postoperative thrombosis. *Schweiz Med Wochenschr* 1976; **106**:1819–21.

59. Blackshear WM Jr, Prescott C, LePain F, Benoit S, Dickstein R, Seifert KB. Influence of sequential pneumatic compression on postoperative venous function. *J Vasc Surg* 1987; **5**:432–6.
60. Butson AR. Intermittent pneumatic calf compression for prevention of deep venous thrombosis in general abdominal surgery. *Am J Surg* 1981; **142**:525–7.
61. Bynke O, Hillman J, Lassvik C. Does peroperative external pneumatic leg muscle compression prevent post-operative venous thrombosis in neurosurgery? *Acta Neurochir (Wien)* 1987; **88**:46–8.
62. Clark WB, MacGregor AB, Prescott RJ, Ruckley CV. Pneumatic compression of the calf and postoperative deep-vein thrombosis. *Lancet* 1974; **ii**:5–7.
63. Clarke-Pearson DL, Creasman WT, Coleman RE, Synan IS, Hinshaw WM. Perioperative external pneumatic calf compression as thromboembolism prophylaxis in gynecologic oncology: report of a randomized controlled trial. *Gynecol Oncol* 1984; **18**:226–32.
64. Clarke-Pearson DL, Synan IS, Hinshaw WM, Coleman RE, Creasman WT. Prevention of postoperative venous thromboembolism by external pneumatic calf compression in patients with gynecologic malignancy. *Obstet Gynecol* 1984; **63**:92–8.
65. Coe NP, Collins RE, Klein LA,. *et al.* Prevention of deep vein thrombosis in urological patients: a controlled, randomized trial of low-dose heparin and external pneumatic compression boots. *Surgery* 1978; **83**:230–4.
66. Fisher CG, Blachut PA, Salvian AJ, Meek RN, O'Brien PJ. Effectiveness of pneumatic leg compression devices for the prevention of thromboembolic disease in orthopaedic trauma patients: a prospective, randomized study of compression alone versus no prophylaxis. *J Orthop Trauma* 1995; **9**:1–7.
67. Gallus A, Raman K, Darby T. Venous thrombosis after elective hip replacement – the influence of preventive intermittent calf compression and of surgical technique. *Br J Surg* 1983; **70**:17–9.
68. Hills NH, Pflug JJ, Jeyasingh K, Boardman L, Calnan JS. Prevention of deep vein thrombosis by intermittent pneumatic compression of calf. *Br Med J* 1972; **i**:131–5.
69. Hull R, Delmore T, Hirsh J, Gent M. Effectiveness of intermittent pulsitile elastic stockings for the prevention of calf and thigh vein thrombosis in patients undergoing elective knee surgery. *Thromb Res* 1979; **16**:37–45.
70. Hull RD, Raskob GE, Gent M,. *et al.* Effectiveness of intermittent pneumatic leg compression for preventing deep vein thrombosis after total hip replacement. *JAMA* 1990; **263**:2313–7.
71. Knudson MM, Lewis FR, Clinton A, Atkinson K, Megerman J. Prevention of venous thromboembolism in trauma patients. *J Trauma* 1994; **37**:480–7.
72. Kosir M, Kozol R, Perales A,. *et al.* Is DVT prophylaxis overemphasized? A randomized prospective study. *J Surg Res* 1996; **60**:289–92.
73. Skillman JJ, Collins RE, Coe NP,. *et al.* Prevention of deep vein thrombosis in neurosurgical patients: a controlled, randomized trial of external pneumatic compression boots. *Surgery* 1978; **83**:354–8.
74. Turpie AG, Gallus A, Beattie WS, Hirsh J. Prevention of venous thrombosis in patients with intracranial disease by intermittent pneumatic compression of the calf. *Neurology* 1977; **27**:435–8.
75. Turpie AG, Delmore T, Hirsh J,. *et al.* Prevention of venous thrombosis by intermittent sequential calf compression in patients with intracranial disease. *Thromb Res* 1979; **15**:611–6.
76. Weitz J, Michelsen J, Gold K, Owen J, Carpenter D. Effects of intermittent pneumatic calf compression on postoperative thrombin and plasmin activity. *Thromb Haemost* 1986; **56**:198–201.

CHAPTER 20

Pharmacological Prevention of Venous Thromboembolism

Willem M. Lijfering and Jan van der Meer

Division of Haemostasis, Thrombosis and Rheology Department of
Hematology University Medical Center Groningen,
Groningen, The Netherlands

INTRODUCTION

The overall incidence of venous thromboembolism (VTE) is 1–3 per 1000 persons each year and rises exponentially from <0.005% in children to 1% per year at age >80 years (1). Most venous thromboembolic events start in the calf veins, from where they may extend and cause proximal deep vein thrombosis (DVT) and subsequently pulmonary embolism (PE) (2). Patients with DVT or PE remain at risk for recurrent VTE. This risk is most pronounced in the first months after the acute episode and diminishes slowly over subsequent years (3). VTE is now considered a multicausal disease. Gene–gene interactions and acquired or environmental risk factors increase the risk of venous thrombosis (4). Risk factors for VTE are presented in Table 20.1 (5). Despite anticoagulant treatment for 3–6 months, recurrence rate of VTE is 25% within the next 5 years, while the immediate death rate due to pulmonary embolism is 2.6% (6) and the post-thrombotic syndrome occurs in up to 50% of patients (7). Recurrent VTE usually leads to life-long anticoagulant treatment, which increases long term healthcare costs substantially and has serious potential side-effects, particularly major bleeding (8,9). Therefore, it is pivotal to try to decrease the risk of first VTE in addition to recurrence, rather than to apply indefinite anticoagulant treatment after a first episode of VTE. Prevention will probably be more profitable when persons who are at risk of VTE are more precisely identified and, consequently, may have optimal benefit of thromboprophylaxis in high-risk situations. Surveys have shown, however, that many persons who may benefit from thromboprophylaxis do not receive it at all or its dosage and duration are not appropriate (10,11). Therefore, the American College of Chest Physicians (ACCP) has published an evidence-based guideline on the prevention of VTE (12). This guideline addresses a broad range of indications for the prevention of VTE with mechanical thromboprophylaxis (graduated compression stockings and intermittent pneumatic compression devices) and pharmacological thromboprophylaxis. This chapter considers pharmacological thromboprophylaxis in persons at risk of VTE in greater detail and provides updated recommendations; it is, therefore, complementary to the efforts of the ACCP.

Deep Vein Thrombosis and Pulmonary Embolism Edited by Edwin J.R. van Beek, Harry R. Büller and Matthijs Oudkerk
© 2009 John Wiley & Sons, Ltd

Table 20.1   Risk factors for venous thromboembolism

Inherited	Acquired	Transient	Not well established
Antithrombin deficiency	Increasing age	Surgery and major trauma	High factor VIII
Protein C deficiency	Cancer	Pregnancy and puerperium	High factor IX
Protein S deficiency	History of venous thromboembolism	Oral contraceptives	High factor XI
Factor V Leiden	Obesity	Hormone replacement therapy	High TAFI
Prothrombin G20210A	Varicosis	Prolonged immobilization	Hyperhomocysteinaemia
		Hospitalization	Air travel

Types of pharmacological thromboprophylaxis

Currently, there are five types of pharmacological thromboprophylaxis available: low-dose unfractionated heparin (LDUH), low molecular weight heparins (LMWH), fondaparinux, vitamin K antagonists (VKA) and aspirin or other antiplatelet drugs. However, although aspirin is highly effective in reducing major arterial vascular events (13), a number of trials showed no significant benefit of aspirin in the prevention of VTE (14,15) or found that aspirin was inferior to other prophylactic modalities (16,17). Moreover, aspirin use is associated with a small but significant increased risk of major bleeding (18), especially when it is combined with other antithrombotic drugs. For these reasons, aspirin is not recommended to prevent VTE (12,14,16).

Changes in outcome assessment in thromboprophylaxis studies

The main endpoint in most randomized trials on thromboprophylaxis in surgical and also in medical patients was DVT demonstrated by objective techniques, such as the fibrinogen uptake test and venography. These techniques were preferred to the unreliable clinical diagnosis of DVT. They are accurate to detect both proximal and distal DVT, whether or not symptomatic. Although this approach is still appropriate to compare the antithrombotic effect of different anticoagulant drugs, it does not represent the difference in clinical impact of proximal and distal DVT. Proximal DVT is more frequently associated with the post-thrombotic syndrome and (fatal or non-fatal) PE than distal DVT. Because there is no perfect surrogate endpoint (19), most thromboprophylactic anticoagulants have been adopted by health authorities and clinical scientists on the basis of total (proximal plus distal) DVT as assessed by the mentioned objective techniques. In more recent studies, symptomatic or proximal DVT was defined as the primary outcome event. As a consequence, the incidence of DVT was approximately one-fifth of that in previous studies. This is clearly shown in Tables 20.2 and 20.3, which summarize absolute risks of DVT and PE in hospitalized patients not receiving thromboprophylaxis. Although the absolute risk of DVT is high in the presented patient groups (Table 20.2), this risk is mainly related to isolated (asymptomatic) calf vein thrombosis (Table 20.3), of which the clinical relevance remains to be established (20).

Table 20.2   Absolute risk of DVT in hospitalized patients[a]

Patient group	DVT prevalence (%)
Medical patients	10–20
General surgery	20–30
Major gynaecological surgery	20–30
Major urological surgery	20–30
Neurosurgery	20–50
Stroke	20–50
Hip or knee arthroplasty, hip fracture surgery	40–60
Major trauma	40–80
Spinal cord injury	60–100
Critical care patients	10–100

[a]Rates based on objective diagnostic testing for DVT in patients not receiving thromboprophylaxis.

Despite the limitation of the applied screening method and thus the possibility of error in the estimates of the absolute rates of DVT, the relative risk reductions derived from studies comparing two prophylactic regimens are likely to be valid as long as systematic bias has been reduced by concealed randomization of patients, caregivers and outcome adjudicators to the study interventions and by complete follow-up of patients (21). Ultrasonography has been introduced more recently to detect DVT as an alternative for venography. Although it has obvious advantages, ultrasonography is less sensitive in patients with asymptomatic proximal DVT. Thereby, the absolute risk of DVT and the clinical relevance may be underestimated, whereas more patients are required to demonstrate differences in clinical thromboprophylaxis trials. One should be aware of the changes in outcome assessment over time when the results of recent and previous clinical trials are evaluated. Previous trials were designed to demonstrate a difference or non-difference in incidence of all (proximal and distal) DVT and may be underpowered when only proximal DVT is considered.

Bleeding as a serious adverse event outcome due to thromboprophylaxis

Concerns on the side-effects of thromboprophylaxis especially relate to bleeding (22). However, abundant data from meta-analyses and placebo-controlled, blinded, randomized clinical trials on thromboprophylaxis have demonstrated little or no increase in the rates of clinically important bleeding with LDUH, LMWH, fondaparinux or VKA (23–27). In most clinical trials on thromboprophylaxis in surgical patients, major bleeding was defined as bleeding in a critical organ or re-surgery due to bleeding. In recent trials on fondaparinux, the bleeding index was introduced as a measure of surgical blood loss. Although a comparison of this index between groups in a trial is valid, its clinical relevance is uncertain. Moreover, in a comparison between clinical trials, the same criteria for bleeding should be used.

There is convincing evidence that appropriately applied thromboprophylaxis has a favourable risk/benefit ratio and is cost-effective (28–30). Unfortunately, this evidence is inconsistent with current clinical practice. For example, the ENDORSE study showed that more than 50% of hospitalized patients should receive thromboprophylaxis during admission. However, only half of these 50% actually received it (31). Thromboprophylaxis provides an opportunity to improve clinical outcome and also to reduce hospital costs.

RISK STRATIFICATION

Clinical trials on thromboprophylaxis showed a comparable relative risk reduction of VTE when the same dose regimen of anticoagulant drugs was applied in patients at varying levels of VTE risk. It is likely that the aimed for absolute risk reduction can be improved when the dose of anticoagulant drugs is adjusted to the level of VTE risk. To obtain optimal thromboprophylaxis, it should be adjusted to the individual risk of VTE, as well as to the individual risk of bleeding related to anticoagulant thromboprophylaxis. This approach is not feasible in clinical practice. First, we do not know the individual risk, which is determined by numerous risk factors, including unknown genetic variants. Second, most clinical trials were designed to compare the efficacy and safety of anticoagulants at fixed dose and for a standardized treatment time, in a variety of conditions associated with different levels of VTE risk. On the other hand, however, it should be noted that the implementation of thromboprophylaxis will be improved by a simple and uniform regimen, without laboratory monitoring and dose adjustments accordingly, provided that its efficacy and safety have been established. These considerations should be taken into account when evidence-based guidelines are applied in clinical practice.

General surgery

In studies published between 1970 and 1990 (32,33), the observed rates of DVT among general surgical patients not receiving thromboprophylaxis varied between 15 and 40%, and rates of fatal PE between 0.2 and 0.9%. The current absolute risk of thromboembolic events in general surgery is unknown, because studies without thromboprophylaxis are no longer performed in these patients. Advances in surgery and anaesthesiology, improved perioperative care and faster mobilization may have reduced the thromboembolic risk. On the other hand, more extensive surgical procedures in older and sicker patients and preoperative chemotherapy in cancer patients may have increased the risk of VTE.

The type and duration of surgery are clearly related to the risk of DVT (33–35). Individuals undergoing day-care surgery appear to have a low frequency of DVT. For example, only one case of symptomatic VTE occurred in the first month following 2281 day-care hernia repairs (0.04%) (36). Additional factors that affect the risk of VTE in general surgery patients include cancer, previous VTE, obesity, varicose veins, oestrogen use and increasing age (33,35,37).

LDUH and LMWH are the most widely used anticoagulants in the prevention of VTE. Many clinical trials provided convincing evidence of their efficacy and safety when these drugs were used in the perioperative period (12,16). The striking feature of LDUH prophylaxis was the associated reduction in perioperative mortality, with the frequency of PE-associated mortality falling from eight per 1000 to one per 1000 operated patients (38). Concerns about the potential risk of bleeding initiated the development of safer anticoagulant drugs in surgical practice (38,39). As a result, LMWH were introduced, which have been extensively investigated since the first report of its application for thromboprophylaxis in general surgical patients by Kakkar *et al*. in 1982 (40). Additional clinical advantages over LDUH are the once-daily administration and a lower risk of heparin-induced thrombocytopenia (HIT) (41). One meta-analysis showed that LMWH prophylaxis

Table 20.3 Levels of thromboembolism risk in surgical patients without prophylaxis

Level of risk	DVT (%)		PE (%)		Successful prevention strategies
	Calf	Proximal	Clinical	Fatal	
Low risk	2	0.4	0.2	<0.01	No specific prophylaxis; early and 'agressive' mobilization
Minor surgery in patients aged <40 years with no additional risk factors					
Moderate risk	10–20	2–4	1–2	0.1–0.4	LDUH q12h, low dose LMWH oid
Minor surgery in patients with additional risk factors					
Surgery in patients aged 40–60 years with no additional risk factors					
High risk	20–40	4–8	2–4	0.4–1.0	LDUH q8h, adjusted dose LMWH oid
Surgery in patients aged >60 years, or aged 40–60 years with additional risk factors (prior VTE, cancer, thrombophilia)					
Highest risk	40–80	10–20	4–10	0.2–5	Adjusted dose LMWH oid, fondaparinux, oral VKAs (INR, 2–3)
Surgery in patients with multiple risk factors (age >40 years, cancer, prior VTE)					
Hip or knee arthroplasty, hip fracture surgery					
Major trauma; spinal cord injury					

[a] *Source*: Adapted from Geerts *et al.* (12).

reduced the risk of asymptomatic DVT and symptomatic VTE in general surgery patients by >70% compared with no prophylaxis (42). When LDUH and LMWH were directly compared, no single study showed a significant difference in the rates of symptomatic VTE, although LMWH was associated with a significant reduction in the rate of asymptomatic DVT in several trials (43–45). Two meta-analyses that found similar efficacy for LDUH and LMWH reported differences in bleeding rates that were dependent on the dose of LMWH. Low doses of LMWH were associated with less bleeding than LDUH [3.8 vs 5.4%; odds ratio (OR) 0.7], whereas higher doses of LMWH resulted in more bleeding events (7.9 vs 5.3%, respectively; OR 1.5) (42,46).

The selective factor Xa inhibitor fondaparinux has recently been evaluated in patients undergoing abdominal surgery (47). In a double-blind randomized trial, approximately 2000 patients scheduled for major abdominal surgery received once-daily subcutaneous injections of fondaparinux 2.5 mg or dalteparin 5000 IU for 5–9 days postoperatively. There were no significant differences in the rates of all VTE [4.6 vs 6.1%; relative risk reduction (RRR) – 24.6%; 95% confidence interval (CI) – 9.0 to – 47.9%], major bleeding (3.4 vs 2.4%) or death (1.0 vs 1.4%) between the two regimens. A subgroup analysis of patients who underwent cancer surgery, containing 70% of patients, showed similar efficacy of fondaparinux and less efficacy of dalteparin. The risk of all VTE was 4.7 vs 7.7% (RRR – 38.6; 95% CI – 6.7 to – 59.7%).

Although the risk of postoperative DVT is highest within the first 2 weeks after general surgery, VTE, including fatal PE, may occur later (48). Three clinical trials have addressed the use of extended prophylaxis beyond the period of hospitalization after general surgery, but were not sufficiently powered to demonstrate a significant reduction in the risk of VTE, compared with placebo (49–51). To conclude, in patients undergoing major general surgical procedures, routine thromboprophylaxis should in generally be recommended. The modalities that have clearly showed to reduce the risk of DVT and PE include LDUH and LMWH. Fondaparinux may be more effective in patients with an excessively high risk of VTE. Table 20.3 summarizes potential successful strategies, stratified according to the risk of VTE, as recommended by the ACCP (12,16).

Orthopaedic surgery

The natural history of VTE after major orthopaedic surgery has become better defined over the past 30 years. Asymptomatic DVT has been demonstrated in at least half of all patients without thromboprophylaxis (16,52). Symptomatic VTE is the commonest cause of readmission to the hospital following major orthopaedic surgery (53) and the risk of VTE remains higher than expected for at least 2 months after surgery (Figure 20.1) (53–55). In patients undergoing major orthopaedic surgery, routinely performed lung perfusion scans showed defects that were compatible with PE in a proportion as high as 28% (56,57). In another study, approximately 20% of patients undergoing surgery for hip fracture had a negative venogram at hospital discharge, but revealed DVT over the subsequent 3 weeks (58). PE showed to be the cause of death in 14% of patients who died after surgery for hip fracture (59). Unfortunately, there is currently no method to identify orthopaedic patients who will develop symptomatic VTE. Therefore, thromboprophylaxis is recommended in all patients undergoing major orthopaedic surgery of the lower extremities (i.e., hip and knee replacement surgery) (12). Thromboprophylaxis should be continued for 30–42 days after surgery, which significantly reduced the frequency of symptomatic VTE in one meta-analysis

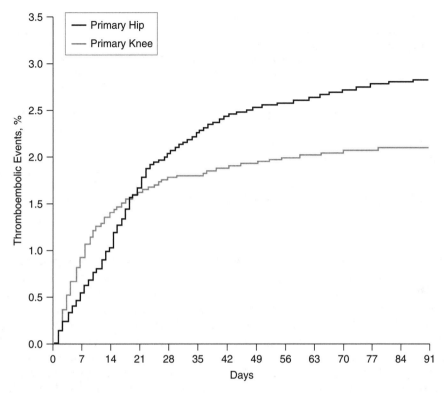

Figure 20.1   Incidence of symptomatic venous thromboembolism in 43 645 patients after primary hip or knee replacement surgery. More than 90% received in-hospital thromboprophylaxis and approximately 30% received warfarin for an average of 4 weeks post-discharge. Reproduced from White RH, Romano PS, Zhou H, Rodrigo J, Bargar W. Incidence and time course of thromboembolic outcomes following total hip or knee arthroplasty. Arch Intern Med 1998; 158:1525–31. Copyright © 1998, American Medical Association

comparing VKA with placebo (1.3 vs 3.3%, OR 0.4) (60), whereas it did not increase the risk of major bleeding due to VKA or LMWH compared with placebo (60,61).

Elective hip replacement surgery

A number of anticoagulant drugs have been evaluated for the prophylaxis of VTE in patients undergoing elective hip replacement (Table 20.4) (62). LDUH has a limited efficacy in this setting. Although it is safe and effective when the dosage of LDUH is adjusted to maintain the activated partial thromboplastin time around the upper range of normal, this approach is impractical in clinical practice (63). VKA have largely been abandoned as prophylaxis of DVT after elective hip replacement surgery because of concerns about their delayed onset of action, variable response within and between patients, need for frequent laboratory monitoring and dose adjustments, interactions with other drugs and lower efficacy compared with LMWH. If VKA are used, they should be administered in doses that are sufficient to prolong the international normalized ratio (INR) to a target of 2.5 (range, 2.0–3.0). The first dose of VKA should be given either the evening before surgery or the evening after surgery. The target range for the INR is usually not reached until at least the third post-operative day (54).

Table 20.4 Prevention of deep vein thrombosis after total hip replacement [a]

Prophylaxis regimen	No. of trials	Combined enrollment	Total DVT Prevalence (%) (95% CI)	RRR (%)	Proximal DVT Prevalence (%) (95% CI)	RRR (%)
Placebo/control	11	598	54.8 (51 to 59)	–	26.6 (23 to 31)	–
LDUH	11	1097	29.2 (26 to 32)	47	18.5 (16 to 21)	31
Warfarin	12	1793	22.3 (20 to 24)	59	5.2 (4 to 6)	81
LMWH	31	8655	15.4 (15 to 16)	72	4.9 (4 to 5)	82
Fondaparinux	2	3411	5.0 (4 to 6)	NA	1.1 (0.7 to 1.8)	NA

[a]Abbreviations: CI, confidence interval; DVT, deep vein thrombosis; LDUH, low-dose unfractionated heparin; LMWH, low molecular wight heparin; RRR, relative risk reduction; NA, no placebo controlled studies available.

LMWH have been studied extensively in patients undergoing elective hip replacement surgery and shown to be effective and safe in the prevention of VTE (12). When the results from five large clinical trials directly comparing VKA with LMWH in elective hip replacement patients are pooled, the respective rates of all DVT were 20.7% (256 of 1238 patients) and 13.7% (238 of 1741 patients; $p = 0.0002$) (64–68). The proximal DVT rates were 4.8 and 3.4%, respectively ($p = 0.08$). The pooled rates of major bleeding were 3.3% in VKA recipients and 5.3% in LMWH recipients. In other randomized clinical trials in elective hip replacement patients, a comparable 4% rate of major bleeding was demonstrated in control patients who received placebo (69,70).

Fondaparinux has been shown to be highly effective in the prevention of DVT among elective hip replacement patients (71–73). In a dose-finding study, fondaparinux showed a statistically significant dose-dependent effect for both efficacy and safety compared with enoxaparin (71). A subcutaneous regimen of 2.5 mg of fondaparinux once daily was selected in further phase III trials starting postoperatively and continued for 5–10 days compared with preoperatively started enoxaparin 40 mg once daily in the EPHESUS trial (conducted in Europe) (72) or postoperatively started enoxaparin 30 mg bid in the PENTHATHLON 2000 trial (conducted in the rest of the world) (73). These studies showed an RRR of all VTE that was – 45.3% (95% CI – 58.9 to -27.4%) in the fondaparinux group compared with the enoxaparin group. The superior efficacy of fondaparinux was also demonstrated for proximal DVT. Both trials showed a non-significant increase in bleeding with fondaparinux. Because of its long half-life (approximately 18 h), patients whose creatinine clearance is <30 mL/min may experience an accumulation of fondaparinux and thus may be at greater risk of bleeding. Furthermore, although the efficacy and safety of extended thromboprophylaxis with fondaparinux were superior in patients after hip fracture surgery compared with placebo (74), its superiority has not been studied yet in elective hip replacement surgery.

Overall, these data indicate that LMWH, and probably fondaparinux by indirect comparison, are more effective than VKA in the prevention of asymptomatic and symptomatic VTE. There is a slight increase in surgical site bleeding and wound haematomas with these more effective forms of prophylaxis. The higher efficacy and bleeding risks are attributable to the earlier onset of the anticoagulant effect of LMWH and fondaparinux compared with VKA.

Elective knee replacement surgery

Elective knee replacement surgery differs from elective hip replacement surgery with respect to the risk of DVT. Without thromboprophylaxis, the rate of venographically detected DVT, particularly distal DVT, is higher after knee replacement surgery than after hip replacement surgery

Table 20.5   Prevention of deep vein thrombosis after total knee replacement [a]

Prophylaxis regimen	No. of trials	Combined enrollment	Total DVT Prevalence (%) (95% CI)	RRR (%)	Proximal DVT Prevalence (%) (95% CI)	RRR (%)
Placebo/control	6	199	64.3 (57 to 71)	–	15.3 (10 to 23)	–
LDUH	2	236	43.2 (37 to 50)	33	11.4 (8 to 16 ')	26
Warfarin	10	1501	44.2 (42 to 47)	31	9.2 (8 to 11)	40
LMWH	18	2776	33.5 (32 to 35)	48	5.3 (4 to 6)	65
Fondaparinux	1	724	12.5 (9 to 16)	NA	2.4 (1.1 to 4.6)	NA

[a]Abbreviations: CI, confidence interval; DVT, deep vein thrombosis; LDUH, low-dose unfractionated heparin; LMWH, low molecular wight heparin; RRR, relative risk reduction; NA, no placebo controlled studies available.

(16). A plausible explanation for this difference is the application of a tourniquet during knee replacement surgery. This also explains why thromboprophylaxis seem to be less effective in patients undergoing elective knee replacement (Tables 20.4 and 20.5) (62).

Extensive data have shown that LMWH prophylaxis is safe and effective after elective knee replacement surgery (Table 20.5) (64,66,6776–78). Two recent meta-analyses confirmed the superior efficacy of LMWH over both LDUH and warfarin, without an increased risk of bleeding (79,80). In a double-blind clinical trial in 1049 patients undergoing elective knee surgery (PEN-TAMAKS), fondaparinux, administered at a dose of 2.5 mg once daily and started about 6 h after surgery, was compared with enoxaparin 30 mg bid started 12–24 h after surgery (81). The rates of all VTE (12.5% vs 27.8%, respectively; p<0.001) and proximal DVT (2.4 vs 5.4%, respectively; $p = 0.06$) were more than halved using fondaparinux (RRR – 63.1%; 95% CI – 75.5 to -44.8%). On the other hand, major bleeding was significantly more common in the fondaparinux group (2.1 vs 0.2%, respectively; $p = 0.006$). This difference was mainly due to more blood loss during surgery in the fondaparinux group, rather than bleeding in critical organs and bleeding leading to re-operation. No trials have been conducted yet comparing the efficacy and safety of extended thromboprophylaxis with either LMWH or fondaparinux as in patients with knee replacement surgery.

Knee arthroscopy

Arthroscopy of the knee, including meniscectomy, synovectomy and reconstruction of the cruciate ligaments, is among the most common orthopaedic procedures, performed in a relatively young age group. Available information about the risk of VTE associated with arthroscopy is controversial, but it is lower than in knee or hip replacement surgery (82,83). The rate of asymptomatic DVT detected by mandatory objective testing ranged from 3 to 18% in patients undergoing knee arthroscopy without prophylaxis (84). In a large series of 8791 knee arthroscopies, the rate of symptomatic VTE was less than 0.15%, and fatal PE was not observed (85). Risk factors for VTE in these patients are unclear. Therapeutic arthroscopy seems to be associated with a higher risk of VTE than diagnostic arthroscopy; the duration of the procedure, probably related to the use of a tourniquet, is a risk factor (86). So far, no sufficiently powered placebo-controlled, randomized clinical trials on thromboprophylaxis have been performed in patients undergoing knee arthroscopy. Therefore, evidence-based recommendations on thromboprophylaxis cannot be made. Patients should be mobilized early after the procedure. Thromboprophylaxis may be considered, however, in patients who are already at high risk of VTE due to additional risk factors.

Laparoscopic surgery

Laparoscopic surgery represents a major advance in surgical practice, as it reduces surgical trauma, patient discomfort and duration of hospital admission. There is considerable controversy, however, regarding the risk of VTE after laparoscopic procedures (87). These often take more time than laparotomy. Both pneumoperitoneum and the reverse Trendelenburg position reduce venous return from the legs, resulting in venous stasis (88). Laparoscopic surgical procedures are associated with a shorter hospital stay and with faster postoperative mobilization. The mobility of patients once discharged from hospital after laparoscopic procedures, compared with patients who remain in hospital, has not been extensively studied (89).

A number of studies have evaluated current practice of thromboprophylaxis after laparoscopic cholecystectomy and reported low rates of thromboembolic complications (90). In a UK study, 91% of 417 surgeons reported that they had never encountered a thromboembolic complication following laparoscopic cholecystectomy, although the majority reported routine use of LDUH in these patients (91). In a Danish study, 80% of surgical departments were not aware of any thromboembolic complication following laparoscopic surgery although, again, thromboprophylaxis was commonly applied (92). In another study, no DVT or PE was reported in the first month after laparoscopic cholecystectomy in 587 cases, of whom only 3% had received thromboprophylaxis (93).

Registries of surgical outcome also indicate a low risk of thromboembolism after laparoscopic procedures. In a review of 50 427 gynaecological laparoscopies, symptomatic VTE was observed in only two per 10 000 patients (94). In a North American analysis of more than 100 000 laparoscopic cholecystectomies, the rate of symptomatic VTE was 0.2% up to 3 months after operation (90), and a Swedish registry reported VTE in only 0.2% of 11 164 patients who underwent laparoscopic cholecystectomy (95).

Considering the reported low rates of VTE, the European Association for Endoscopic Surgery (96) and the ACCP (12) recommend against pharmacological thromboprophylaxis, unless patients have additional thromboembolic risk factors.

Trauma

Among hospitalized patients, those recovering from major trauma have the highest risk of developing VTE. Without prophylaxis, patients with multisystem or major trauma have a DVT risk exceeding 50%, with PE being the third leading cause of death in those who survive beyond the first day (12,16). Factors that are independently associated with an increased risk of VTE include spinal cord injury, lower extremity or pelvic fracture, need for a surgical procedure, increasing age, femoral venous line insertion or major venous repair, prolonged immobility and prolonged hospital stay. Routine thromboprophylaxis in trauma patients has become standard care (12,97). The use of LMWH, started once primary haemostasis has been achieved, is the most effective and simplest option for the majority of moderate- and high-risk trauma patients (16). Current contraindications to early started LMWH prophylaxis include the presence of intracranial bleeding, ongoing and uncontrolled bleeding, an uncorrected major coagulopathy or incomplete spinal cord injury associated with suspected or proven perispinal haematoma. Head injury without haemorrhage, lacerations or contusions of internal organs (such as lungs, liver, spleen or kidneys), a retroperitoneal haematoma associated with pelvic fracture or complete spinal cord injuries are not themselves contraindications to LMWH thromboprophylaxis, provided that there is no evidence of actual bleeding. In most trauma patients, prophylaxis with LMWH can be started within 36 h of injury, although briefly delaying its commencement seems appropriate to ensure that haemostasis has been achieved. Although the optimal duration of prophylaxis in these patients is not known, it should generally be continued until discharge from hospital. If the hospital stay, including the period of rehabilitation, extends beyond 2 weeks and if there is an ongoing risk of VTE, prophylaxis should be continued. Although many trauma patients are not fully mobile at hospital discharge and may be at risk of delayed symptomatic VTE, there are no available data to quantify this risk. Until evidence becomes available, extended prophylaxis of VTE after hospital discharge is not recommended except for patients with hip fracture surgery (see below).

Hip fracture surgery

In the randomized, placebo-controlled double-blind PENTHIFIRA-Plus trial, patients with hip fractures received either fondaparinux 2.5 mg once daily or placebo for 3 weeks after an initial 1 week of treatment with fondaparinux (98). Extended thromboprophylaxis with fondaparinux reduced the incidence of all VTE from 35.0% in the placebo group to 1.4%, with a RRR of − 95.9% (95% CI − 99.7 to -87.2%), while the incidence of symptomatic VTE was reduced from 2.7 to 0.3% (RRR − 89%). Major bleeding was more often observed in the fondaparinux group (2.4%) than in the placebo group (0.6%) ($p = 0.063$), but the incidence of clinically important bleeding was not different.

Spinal cord injury

Without thromboprophylaxis, patients with spinal cord injury are at high risk of DVT (97). Asymptomatic DVT occurs in 60–100% of these patients (16,99). Despite an increased awareness of VTE as a complication of spinal cord injury, PE remains the third leading cause of death (100,101). Although these patients are at highest risk for VTE in the acute care phase, symptomatic DVT or PE may also occur during the rehabilitation phase (99,102). In one study, venographic evidence of DVT was found in 53% of 30 patients who were admitted to a rehabilitation unit, none of whom had received prior thromboprophylaxis (99). Others observed that 10% of all 1649 patients with spinal cord injury undergoing rehabilitation developed symptomatic DVT and that 3% had PE (103). A recent prospective study followed 119 patients with normal duplex ultrasound findings at 2 weeks after acute spinal cord injury for another 6 weeks, when ultrasonography was repeated. Sixty patients received LDUH tid and 59 patients received enoxaparin, 40 mg once daily, in a non-randomized manner. The respective rates of new VTE were 22 and 8%, respectively (102). The very high risk of VTE following spinal cord injury, combined with the currently available results of prevention studies, supports early thromboprophylaxis in all these patients. Its start should be postponed until clinical evidence of primary haemostasis has been obtained. Continued prophylaxis with LMWH or conversion to VKA (target INR, 2.5; range, 2.0–3.0) for the duration of the rehabilitation phase is likely to be beneficial and is recommended (16,99,104). VTE prophylaxis should be continued at least until completion of the in hospital phase of rehabilitation (12,16).

Pregnancy and puerperium

Women who are pregnant or in the postpartum period have a five-fold increased risk of VTE compared with the normal female population of comparable age (105). Its incidence in the general female population, however, is low and ranges from 0.5 to 1 in 1000 deliveries (105,106). Due to this low incidence, thromboprophylaxis is not warranted in pregnant women, with the possible exception of women in whom an additional clinical condition increases the risk of VTE. These conditions may include previous VTE, as one retrospective study found an overall rate of pregnancy-related recurrent VTE of 12 per 100 pregnancies (107). In a cohort study of women with a heritable deficiency of antithrombin, protein C or protein S, the risk of pregnancy related VTE was 59-fold higher than reported in the normal female population of comparable age (108). Another study did not show an increased risk of pregnancy related recurrent VTE in women without evidence of thrombophilia (109). The results of these studies suggest that the risk of VTE during pregnancy or puerperium is strongly increased in women with previous VTE and in asymptomatic women with heritable antithrombin, protein C or protein S deficiency. Thromboprophylaxis should be considered in these women during puerperium and maybe also during pregnancy. These results, however, should be handled with caution as the numbers of women were small.

Air travellers

Since the 1950s, case reports have been published on VTE associated with air travel, which was later called the 'economy class' syndrome (110). The first controlled study on the risk of VTE associated with air travel was conducted in 1986 (111). In this study, death was related to PE in 18% of passengers who suddenly died after air travel. Air travel-related VTE has raised unprecedented interest in the media. A study by Kuipers et al. showed that this information had not unmoved professionals who attended medical conferences (112). A substantial proportion of participants at the 20th International Society of Thrombosis and Haemostasis Congress, the 15th International Society of Developmental Biologists Congress and the 13th Cochrane Colloquium, all of which took place in Australia in 2005, walked around in the airplane or exercised as suggested in in-flight magazines or videos (74%), wore compression stockings (17%) or used aspirin (21%) or LMWH (5%) to prevent VTE during air travel (112). Pathophysiological studies hypothesizing that hypobaric hypoxia or immobilization affected coagulation revealed conflicting results (113). Recently, the first results of large population studies have been published (114–116). A two-fold statistically significant increase in risk of DVT was demonstrated in persons travelling for more than 4 h (115). Interestingly, this risk was not only related to air travel (both in business class and economy class), but also to travelling by train or car. This finding suggests that prolonged immobility contributed to the development of DVT in these persons rather than hypobaric hypoxia.

Figure 20.2 shows the results of a French study group that conducted an epidemiological survey in 135.29 million passengers at Charles de Gaulle airport, Paris (116). The risk of severe PE immediately after air travel increased at increasing distance, up to 4.8 per million passengers arrivals in flights longer than 10 000 km. Extrapolating these results to the Dutch population (in 2006 16.33 million inhabitants, who made 5.39 million vacation trips by airplane, of which 2% were longer than 10 000 km) (117,118), we calculated that only one person per year is seen with severe PE at an emergency department. The risk of symptomatic VTE within 8 weeks after air travel has been estimated to be one per 6500 passengers, which is low, as the risk of VTE in the normal population has been estimated to be approximately two per 6500 persons per 8 weeks (119). Due to these findings, thromboprophylaxis with LMWH during air travel is not recommended. Compression stockings or aspirin are also not recommended, as studies have shown that these precautions do not decrease the risk of VTE during air travel (120). Thromboprophylaxis may be considered, however, in individuals with previous VTE, as these were shown to have an absolute risk of 5% of recurrent (asymptomatic) DVT after long-haul flights, whereas in low-risk subjects no events were recorded (121). Definite conclusions on this issue cannot be drawn yet.

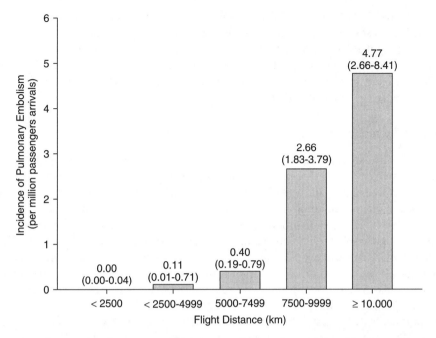

Figure 20.2 Incidence of pulmonary embolism according to distance travelled by air. Values shown above the bars are numbers of cases per million passenger arrivals, with 95% confidence intervals. To convert kilometres to miles, multiply by 0.62. Reproduced from Lapostolle F, Surget V, Borron SW, Desmaizieres M, Sordelet D, Lapandry C, Cupa M, Adnet F. Severe pulmonary embolism associated with air travel. N Engl J Med 2001; 345:779–83. Copyright © 2001, New England Journal of Medicine

Medical patients

Although VTE is still considered to be a risk associated with surgery, it occurs in many groups of hospitalized patients. In the absence of prophylaxis, asymptomatic DVT detected by venography or ultrasonography occurs in 10–20% of medical patients (12). Interestingly, hospitalization for medical illness and hospitalization for surgery account for equal proportions of all VTE cases (22 and 24%, respectively) (3). Several attempts have been made to identify risk factors for VTE in hospitalized medical patients (122–124). Major risk factors include a history of VTE, cancer, increasing age, some thrombophilic defects and prolonged immobility. Additional risk factors include myocardial infarction, stroke, exacerbations of chronic obstructive pulmonary disease and septicaemia.

Three randomized placebo-controlled trials, i.e., the MEDENOX (125), PREVENT (126) and ARTEMIS (127) trials, have evaluated the benefit of thromboprophylaxis in medical patients. Their characteristics and main outcomes are summarized in Table 20.6. All studies showed a decreased risk of proximal or symptomatic VTE as the primary efficacy outcome, and no increased risk of bleeding or death was observed. Although these results seem promising, it should be noted that they were largely driven by asymptomatic VTE. In the MEDENOX trial, only two patients in the placebo group had symptomatic VTE compared with one patient in the 40 mg enoxaparin group after 14 days (125). In the PREVENT study, symptomatic VTE had occurred in 15 patients (0.93%) after 90 days of follow-up and in 21 patients (1.33%) using placebo, a non-significant difference (126). Another issue of concern is the low recruitment rates in these trials. The recruitment rate of patients per centre per month was only 0.97 in the MEDENOX trial, 1.69 in the PREVENT trial and 2.2 in the ARTEMIS trial (128). As none of the trials mentioned the number of screened patients and the reasons for exclusion, it is not possible to assess whether the results of these trials can be extrapolated to the aimed at population of patients. Nevertheless, available evidence supports the benefit of thromboprophylaxis in medical patients who have been admitted to hospital with congestive heart failure, acute respiratory illness or acute infection and who are confined to bed with an additional VTE risk factor.

Acute arterial thromboembolism

Although venous and arterial thromboembolism have long been viewed as separate pathophysiological entities, they share risk factors such as increasing age, obesity, male sex, high factor VIII levels, hypertension and diabetes mellitus (129,130). One potential common pathophysiological substrate for these associations is activation of coagulation (131), a hypothesis which is supported by the efficacy of anticoagulant drugs in prophylaxis of both venous and arterial thromboembolism (132).

Patients hospitalized for acute myocardial infarction (MI) are at high risk of VTE. In a meta-analysis reviewing placebo-controlled studies of antithrombotic drugs, the rate of PE in the placebo group was 3.9% (133). Prevention of recurrent MI rather than prevention of VTE is the primary objective in these patients. Because they receive for this reason combinations of antithrombotic drugs, including aspirin, clopidogrel and glycoprotein IIb/IIIa antagonists and high-dose unfractionated heparin or LMWH, it is likely that the risk of VTE is also reduced.

Patients with acute ischaemic stroke also have an increased risk of VTE. In one study, the incidence of asymptomatic DVT and proximal DVT was 40 and 18%, respectively, after 21 days, while clinical DVT and PE occurred in 3 and 5% of these patients (134). In meta-analyses, treatment with LMWH compared with placebo was associated with a significant decrease in the incidence of DVT (from 5.6 to 2.9%) and symptomatic PE (from 1.9 to 0.7%) (135,136). On the other hand, these meta-analyses also showed that LMWH significantly increased the risk of major bleeding (1.1 to 2.3%), while end-of-trial death and disability were non-significantly reduced (OR 0.87). Therefore, whether LMWH should be used in the routine management of patients with ischemic stroke remains a matter of debate (12).

Cancer

In cancer patients, VTE is common and the second cause of death (137–139). Compared with non-cancer patients, the risk of symptomatic VTE is 6–7 times higher in cancer patients, with similar risks for DVT and PE separately (3,140). In addition, VTE recurs three times more frequently in cancer patients than in patients who do not have cancer, whereas required long-term oral anticoagulation is associated with a two-fold higher risk of bleeding compared with patients who do not have cancer (141). Cancer is also an independent predictor of failure of thromboprophylaxis (i.e., the development of VTE despite anticoagulant treatment) (35,42). Cancer patients at particularly high risk for VTE include older patients, patients with cancers of the brain, pancreas, gastrointestinal tract, ovary, kidney, urinary bladder or lung, haematological malignancies and patients with metastatic disease (140,142).

Evidence-based information about the benefits of thromboprophylaxis in hospitalized patients with cancer is scarce. Three double-blind, placebo-controlled, multicentre trials of thromboprophylaxis with either LMWH (enoxaparin 40 mg or dalteparin 5000 IU once daily) or fondaparinux (2.5 mg once daily) in acutely ill hospitalized patients have been reported (125–127). Only one study provided outcome data for cancer patients who had a 1.6-fold increased risk of (a) symptomatic VTE compared with medical patients without cancer ($p = 0.08$) (143,144). On the other hand, analysis of the PREVENT trial data showed that proximal DVT was associated with an

Table 20.6 Main design of MEDENOX, PREVENT and ARTEMIS trials [a]

MEDENOX [125] [b]	PREVENT [126]	ARTEMIS [127]
Treatments	*Treatments*	*Treatments*
Enoxaparin 40 mg, placebo once daily for 14 days	Dalteparin 5000 IU, placebo once daily for 14 days	Fondaparinux 2.5 mg, placebo once daily for 6 to 14 days
Eligibility criteria	*Eligibility criteria*	*Eligibility criteria*
Age $\geq$ 40 years	Age $\geq$40 years	Age $\geq$60 years
Expected hospital stay $\geq$16 days	Expected hospital stay $\geq$ 4 days	Expected bed rest $\geq$4 days and CHF (NYHA III/IV) or acute or chronic lungdisease or acute infections; no other risk factor analysis required
Recent immobilization ($\leq$3 days) and CHF (NYHA III/IV) or acute respiratory illness or infection or bone/joint or inflamed bowel if $\geq$1 added risk for VTE (i.e., aged >75 years, cancer, previous VTE, obesity, varicose veins, hormones, or chronic heart or lung failure)	Recent immobilization ($\leq$ 3 days) and CHF (NYHA III/IV) or acute respiratory illness or infection or bone/joint or inflamed bowel if $\geq$1 added risk for VTE (i.e., aged >75 years, cancer, previous VTE, obesity, varicose veins, hormones, or chronic heart or lung failure)	
Primary efficacy/safety	*Primary efficacy/safety*	*Primary efficacy/safety*
At day 14/at day 110	At day 21/at day 21	At day 6–15/at day 8–17
Total No. of patients	Total No. of patients	Total No. of patients
579	3706	849
Proximal DVT or symptomatic VTE	Proximal DVT or symptomatic VTE	Proximal DVT or symptomatic VTE
Enoxaparin 2.1%	Dalteparin 2.6%	Fondaparinux 1.5%
Placebo 6.6%	Placebo 5.0%	Placebo 3.4%
$p = 0.037$	$p = 0.002$	$p = 0.085$
Major bleeding	*Major bleeding*	*Major bleeding*
Enoxaparin 3.4%	Dalteparin 0.49%	Fondaparinux 0.2%
Placebo 2.0%	Placebo 0.16%	Placebo 0.2%
$p =$ not significant	$p = 0.15$	$p =$ not significant
Death	*Death*	*Death*
Enoxaparin 11.4%	Dalteparin 2.35%	Fondaparinux 3%
Placebo 13.9%	Placebo 2.32%	Placebo (6%)
$p = 0.31$	$p =$ not significant	$p = 0.06$

[a]Abbreviations: VTE, venous thromboembolism; DVT, deep vein thrombosis; PE, pulmonary embolism; CHF, congestive heart failure; NYHA, New York Heart Association.
[b]MEDENOX included a 20 mg enoxaparin arm of 287 patients with event rates equivalent to placebo. Number includes only placebo and patients receiving 40 mg treatment.

increased mortality rate (126). Although none of the deaths was considered related to VTE, one-third of the deaths were due to cancer, suggesting that asymptomatic VTE in patients with cancer in this study most likely was associated with advanced malignancy (145). In spite of the absence of data from appropriate studies on the efficacy of thromboprophylaxis in hospitalized patients with cancer, while none of the three randomized trials have reported bleeding data specifically in the subgroup of patients with cancer (125–127), the low overall complication rates of prophylaxis in these trials appear to justify the application of LMWH or fondaparinux in hospitalized patients with cancer, according to the ACCP and the American Society of Clinical Oncology (ASCO) guidelines (12,142).

Cancer patients receiving chemotherapy account for 13% of the overall burden of VTE in the cancer population (48). Still, the ASCO and ACCP guidelines do not recommend routine use of thromboprophylaxis in outpatients with cancer receiving chemotherapy, because of conflicting data from clinical trials, concern about bleeding and the need for laboratory monitoring and dose adjustment in patients with renal insufficiency (12,142). The ASCO guideline makes one exception for cancer patients receiving thalidomide or lenalidomide (an analogue of thalidomide) in combination with dexamethasone or other chemotherapy (142), because the incidence of VTE was 15–24% in patients who received thalidomide in combination with dexamethasone or other chemotherapeutic agents (146–149). Recent non-randomized studies of thalidomide-containing regimens in patients with multiple myeloma have suggested efficacy of thromboprophylaxis with LMWH (149,150) or low-dose warfarin (149). This recommendation should be treated with some caution, as it is based on extrapolation of results from studies on postoperative thromboprophylaxis in orthopaedic surgery.

Hormonal manipulation also affects the thrombotic risk (151,152). The rate of VTE increased by 2–5-fold among women whose breast cancer had been treated with the selective oestrogen receptor modulator tamoxifen (151,153). In a double-blind clinical trial on the primary prevention with tamoxifen in women at increased risk of breast cancer, 13 000 women were randomized to receive tamoxifen or placebo for 5 years. The risk of DVT was increased in the tamoxifen group compared with women who received placebo (0.13 vs 0.08% per year), as was the risk of PE (0.07 vs 0.02% per year) (153). Among 9000 postmenopausal women with early breast cancer who were followed for a median period of 33 months, VTE occurred in 5.3% of those treated with tamoxifen and in 3.1% of those treated with anastrozole (154). No clinical trials have studied the effects of thromboprophylaxis in cancer patients receiving hormonal manipulation chemotherapy. Although these findings are interesting, there is need for additional studies before recommendations can be made regarding thromboprophylaxis in these patients.

There is strong evidence that LDUH reduces the risk of DVT and fatal PE following cancer surgery (32), while LMWH is at least as effective as LDUH (42,155). In cancer surgery, the effect of prophylaxis depends on the dose of anticoagulants. Among general surgical patients with underlying malignancy, prophylaxis with dalteparin 5000 IU once daily was more effective than 2500 IU once daily (156). Two placebo-controlled clinical trials in cancer surgery patients showed that extended LMWH prophylaxis (enoxaparin 40 mg once daily or dalteparin 5000 IU once daily) for 3 weeks after hospital discharge reduced the risk of late asymptomatic DVT by 60%, whereas there were no significant differences in the rate of bleeding or other complications (50,51). Therefore, thromboprophylaxis is recommended for at least 7–10 days after cancer surgery, and prolonged prophylaxis for another 3 weeks may be considered.

Previous VTE

Patients with previous VTE are at high risk of recurrence, ranging from 8.6% after 6 months to 30.3% after 8 years (157). In an observational study of 1231 consecutive patients with VTE, 19% had at least one recurrence associated with environmental risk factors (i.e., major surgery, prolonged immobility or serious illness) (158). In a case–control study, patients with a history of VTE were approximately eight times more likely to develop a recurrence when exposed to environmental risk factors than patients without a history of DVT or PE (159). Therefore, thromboprophylaxis should be considered in all persons with prior VTE after anticoagulant treatment has been stopped when they are exposed to environmental risk factors. For the same reason, use of oral contraception should be discouraged (160).

Thrombophilic defects

Since 1965, an increasing number of thrombophilic defects have been identified as risk factors for VTE. These include hereditary deficiencies of antithrombin, protein C and protein S, factor V Leiden, prothrombin G20210A, high levels of factors VIII, IX, XI and thrombin activatable fibrinolysis inhibitor (TAFI) (161–167). In addition, hyperhomocysteinaemia was shown to be a metabolic thrombophilic defect (168). Together, their prevalence is approximately 25% in the normal population and more than 60% in subjects with venous thrombosis (4). Although these thrombophilic defects are often summarized under the same denominator, i.e., 'thrombophilia', this approach may be inappropriate to assess the associated absolute risk of VTE because it varies for different thrombophilic defects. While high levels of factors IX, FXI, TAFI and hyperhomocysteinaemia were previously identified as risk factors for VTE, a recent study showed that the associated risk was actually due to concomitance of high factor VIII levels (169). The same study showed that annual incidences of VTE in subjects with factor V Leiden, prothrombin G20210A or high factor VIII levels were increased 3–5-fold compared with the normal population. However, these were 15–19-fold higher in subjects with heritable antithrombin, protein C or protein S deficiency. The authors stated that thromboprophylaxis is justified in high-risk situations in still asymptomatic subjects with one of these deficiencies (169). It should be noted, however, that antithrombin, protein C or protein S deficiencies are rare, even in patients with venous thrombosis (4). Considering the cost–benefit ratio and the possible psychological burden of the knowledge of a heritable deficiency, it is not justified to screen all patients with a first episode of VTE for one of these deficiencies. However, a clinician should be aware of these thrombophilic deficiencies when a patient reveals VTE at age below 40 years and/or notes a history of VTE in more than 20% of first-degree relatives (169).

SOME REMAINING ISSUES

Timing of thromboprophylaxis initiation in surgery

In Europe, LMWH prophylaxis is generally started 10–12 h before surgery, in practice usually the evening before. In North America, prophylaxis with LMWH is usually started 12–24 h after surgery, to both minimize the risk of bleeding and to simplify same-day hospital admission for elective surgery. One review suggested that any difference in efficacy between a preoperative and a postoperative start of LMWH is likely to be small (170), although a subsequent meta-analysis concluded that preoperative initiation of LMWH was significantly more effective than a postoperative start (171). A systematic review concluded that LMWH administered close to the time of surgery reduced the risk of VTE, but this benefit was offset by an increased risk of major bleeding (172). Studies on thromboprophylaxis with fondaparinux also support the statement that dosing in close proximity to surgery enhances the prophylactic efficacy of the drug, while on the other hand major bleeding in patients who received a first dose within 6 h of skin closure had significantly more major bleeds (3.2%) compared with waiting for 6 h or longer (2.1%, P = 0.045) (173). Moreover, these studies strongly suggested that fondaparinux started after surgery was more effective than enoxaparin, whether the first dose of enoxaparin was given prior to or after surgery. Although there are no data available from a head-to-head comparison of LMWH started preoperatively versus LMWH started after surgery, it is the current opinion that a postoperative start of LMWH may also be preferred.

Duration of thromboprophylaxis in medical patients

The optimal duration of thromboprophylaxis in medical patients is unknown. In recent clinical trials with LMWH or fondaparinux, the maximum treatment time was 14 days (125–127). One review showed that it is likely that thrombosis has already started in some patients before they are admitted to the hospital and that patients may remain at risk of VTE after discharge (174). To date, however, clinical trials to assess the benefits of extended thromboprophylaxis in acutely ill medical patients have not been performed.

Critical care patients

There is a paucity of critical care-specific data about thromboprophylaxis (12). The risk of VTE in critically ill patients ranges from 10 to 100%, reflecting the heterogeneity of these patients. A standardized approach to thromboprophylaxis is recommended, but it should be adjusted to variations in risk of VTE and risk of bleeding, both of which may change over time in the same patient. Mechanical thromboprophylaxis should be preferred when the risk of bleeding is high or when there is an overt major bleeding. Dose adjustments of anticoagulant drugs are required in patients with renal insufficiency.

Under-use of thromboprophylaxis

Despite the ACCP guideline and other evidence-based guidelines, there is a widespread under-use of thromboprophylaxis in medical and surgical patients. Previous studies conducted in different countries have shown that only 35–42% of patients in the highest risk groups receive adequate thromboprophylaxis (175–177), with a lowest score of 16% for hospitalized medical patients in Canada (178). This may be explained by the complexity of available guidelines. The latest ACCP guideline on VTE thromboprophylaxis supports educational initiatives to increase the awareness and understanding of management guidelines (12). Another contributory factor is the absence of formal protocols for the prevention of VTE in medical patients in many hospitals. The ACCP emphasizes the implementation of such protocols and suggests the application of computer-generated reminders to improve appropriate thromboprophylaxis in patients at risk (12).

REFERENCES

1. White RH. The epidemiology of venous thromboembolism. *Circulation* 2003; **107**(Suppl):I4–I8.
2. Cogo A, Lensing AW, Prandoni P, Hirsh J. Distribution of thrombosis in patients with symptomatic deep vein thrombosis. Implications for simplifying the diagnostic process with compression ultrasound. *Arch Intern Med* 1993; **153**:2777–80.
3. Heit JA, Mohr DN, Silverstein MD, Petterson TM, O'Fallon WM, Melton LJ III. Predictors of recurrence after deep vein thrombosis and pulmonary embolism: a population-based cohort study. *Arch Intern Med* 2000; **160**:761–8.
4. Rosendaal FR. Venous thrombosis: a multicausal disease. *Lancet* 1999; **353**:1167–73.
5. Martinelli I. Risk factors in venous thromboembolism. *Thromb Haemost* 2001; **86**:395–403.
6. Hansson PO, Sörbo J, Eriksson H. Recurrent venous thromboembolism after deep vein thrombosis: incidence and risk factors. *Arch Intern Med* 2000; **160**:769–74.
7. Prandoni P, Lensing AW, Prins MH, Frulla M, Marchiori A, Bernardi E, Tormene D, Mosena L, Pagnan A, Girolami A. Below-knee elastic compression stockings to prevent the post-thrombotic syndrome: a randomized, controlled trial. *Ann Intern Med* 2004; **141**:249–56.
8. Palareti G, Leali N, Coccheri S, Poggi M, Manotti C, D'Angelo A, Pengo V, Erba N, Moia M, Ciavarella N, Devoto G, Berrettini M, Musolesi S. Bleeding complications of oral anticoagulant treatment: an inception-cohort, prospective collaborative study (ISCOAT). Italian Study on Complications of Oral Anticoagulant Therapy. *Lancet* 1996; **348**:423–8.
9. Schulman S, Granqvist S, Holmström M, Carlsson A, Lindmarker P, Nicol P, et al. The duration of oral anticoagulant therapy after a second episode of venous thromboembolism. The Duration of Anticoagulation Trial Study Group. *N Engl J Med* 1997; **336**:393–8.
10. Arnold DM, Kahn SR, Shrier I. Missed opportunities for prevention of venous thromboembolism: an evaluation of the use of thromboprophylaxis guidelines. *Chest* 2001; **120**:1964–71.
11. Goldhaber SZ, Tapson VF, DVT FREE Steering Committee. A prospective registry of 5,451 patients with ultrasound-confirmed deep vein thrombosis. *Am J Cardiol* 2004; **93**:259–62.
12. Geerts WH, Pineo GF, Heit JA, Bergqvist D, Lassen MR, Colwell CW, Ray JG. Prevention of venous thromboembolism: the Seventh ACCP Conference on Antithrombotic and Thrombolytic Therapy. *Chest* 2004; **126**(3 Suppl):338S–400S.
13. Patrono C, Coller B, Dalen JE, FitzGerald GA, Fuster V, Gent M, Hirsh J, Roth G. Platelet-active drugs: the relationships among dose, effectiveness and side-effects. *Chest* 2001; **119**(1 Suppl):39S–63S.
14. Pulmonary Embolism Prevention (PEP) Trial Collaborative Group. Prevention of pulmonary embolism and deep vein thrombosis with low dose aspirin: Pulmonary Embolism Prevention (PEP) Trial. *Lancet* 2000; **355**:1295–302.
15. Powers PJ, Gent M, Jay RM, Julian DH, Turpie AG, Levine M, Hirsh J. A randomized trial of less intense postoperative warfarin or aspirin therapy in the prevention of venous thromboembolism after surgery for fractured hip. *Arch Intern Med* 1989; **149**:771–4.
16. Geerts WH, Heit JA, Clagett GP, Pineo GF, Colwell CW, Anderson FA Jr, Wheeler HB. Prevention of venous thromboembolism. *Chest* 2001; **119**(1 Suppl):132S–175S.
17. Gent M, Hirsh J, Ginsberg JS, Powers PJ, Levine MN, Geerts WH, Jay RM, Leclerc J, Neemeh JA, Turpie AG. Low-molecular-weight heparinoid orgaran is more effective than aspirin in the prevention of venous thromboembolism after surgery for hip fracture. *Circulation* 1996; **93**:80–4.
18. Antiplatelet Trialists' Collaboration. Collaborative overview of randomised trials of antiplatelet therapy – III. Reduction in venous thrombosis and pulmonary embolism by antiplatelet prophylaxis among surgical and medical patients. Antiplatelet Trialists' Collaboration. *BMJ* 1994; **308**:235–46.
19. Fleming TR, DeMets DL. Surrogate end points in clinical trials: are we being misled? *Ann Intern Med* 1996; **125**:605–13.
20. Di Nisio M, Wichers IM, Middeldorp S. Treatment for superficial thrombophlebitis of the leg. *Cochrane Database Syst Rev* 2007; CD004982.
21. Rodgers A, MacMahon S. Systematic underestimation of treatment effects as a result of diagnostic test inaccuracy: implications for the interpretation and design of thromboprophylaxis trials. *Thromb Haemost* 1995; **73**:167–71.
22. van Ooijen B. Subcutaneous heparin and postoperative wound hematomas. A prospective, double-blind, randomized study. *Arch Surg* 1986; **121**:937–40.
23. Nurmohamed MT, Rosendaal FR, Büller HR, Dekker E, Hommes DW, Vandenbroucke JP, Briët E. Low-molecular-weight heparin versus standard heparin in general and orthopaedic surgery: a meta-analysis. *Lancet* 1992; **340**:152–6.

24. Koch A, Ziegler S, Breitschwerdt H, Victor N. Low molecular weight heparin and unfractionated heparin in thrombosis prophylaxis: meta-analysis based on original patient data. *Thromb Res* 2001; **102**:295–309.

25. Kakkar VV, Cohen AT, Edmonson RA, Phillips MJ, Cooper DJ, Das SK, Maher KT, Sanderson RM, Ward VP, Kakkar S. Low molecular weight versus standard heparin for prevention of venous thromboembolism after major abdominal surgery. The Thromboprophylaxis Collaborative Group. *Lancet* 1993; **341**:259–65.

26. Koopman MM, Prandoni P, Piovella F, Ockelford PA, Brandjes DP, van der Meer J, Gallus AS, Simonneau G, Chesterman CH, Prins MH. Treatment of venous thrombosis with intravenous unfractionated heparin administered in the hospital as compared with subcutaneous low-molecular-weight heparin administered at home. The Tasman Study Group. *N Engl J Med* 1996; **334**:682–7.

27. Turpie AG, Eriksson BI, Bauer KA, Lassen MR. New pentasaccharides for the prophylaxis of venous thromboembolism: clinical studies. *Chest* 2003; **124**(6 Suppl):371S–378S.

28. Sullivan SD, Kahn SR, Davidson BL, Borris L, Bossuyt P, Raskob G. Measuring the outcomes and pharmacoeconomic consequences of venous thromboembolism prophylaxis in major orthopaedic surgery. *Pharmacoeconomics* 2003; **21**:477–96.

29. Mamdani MM, Weingarten CM, Stevenson JG. Thromboembolic prophylaxis in moderate-risk patients undergoing elective abdominal surgery: decision and cost-effectiveness analyses. *Pharmacotherapy* 1996; **16**:1111–27.

30. Etchells E, McLeod RS, Geerts W, Barton P, Detsky AS. Economic analysis of low-dose heparin vs the low-molecular-weight heparin enoxaparin for prevention of venous thromboembolism after colorectal surgery. *Arch Intern Med* 1999; **159**:1221–8.

31. Cohen AT, Tapson VF, Bergmann JF, Goldhaber SZ, Kakkar AK, Deslandes B, Huang W, Zayaruzny M, Emery L, Anderson FA Jr, ENDORSE Investigators. Venous thromboembolism risk and prophylaxis in the acute hospital care setting (ENDORSE study): a multinational cross-sectional study. *Lancet* 2008; **371**:387–94.

32. Clagett GP, Reisch JS. Prevention of venous thromboembolism in general surgical patients. Results of meta-analysis. *Ann Surg* 1988; **208**:227–40.

33. Pezzuoli G, Neri Serneri GG, Settembrini P, Coggi G, Olivari N, Buzzetti G, Chierichetti S, Scotti A, Scatigna M, Carnovali M. Prophylaxis of fatal pulmonary embolism in general surgery using low-molecular weight heparin Cy 216: a multicentre, double-blind, randomized, controlled, clinical trial versus placebo (STEP). STEP Study Group. *Int Surg* 1989; **74**:205–10.

34. Ageno W. Applying risk assessment models in general surgery: overview of our clinical experience. *Blood Coagul Fibrinol* 1999; **10** (Suppl):S71–S78.

35. Flordal PA, Berggvist D, Burmark US, Ljungström KG, Törngren S. Risk factors for major thromboembolism and bleeding tendency after elective general surgical operations. The Fragmin Multicentre Study Group. *Eur J Surg* 1996; **162**:783–9.

36. Riber C, Alstrup N, Nymann T, Bogstad JW, Wille-Jørgensen P, Tønnesen H. Postoperative thromboembolism after day-case herniorrhaphy. *Br J Surg* 1996; **83**:420–21.

37. Wille-Jørgensen P, Ott P. Predicting failure of low-dose prophylactic heparin in general surgical procedures. *Surg Gynecol Obstet* 1990; **171**:126–30.

38. Prevention of fatal postoperative pulmonary embolism by low doses of heparin. An international multicentre trial. *Lancet* 1975; **ii**:45–51.

39. Collins R, Scrimgeour A, Yusuf S, Peto R. Reduction in fatal pulmonary embolism and venous thrombosis by perioperative administration of subcutaneous heparin. Overview of results of randomized trials in general, orthopedic and urologic surgery. *N Engl J Med* 1988; **318**:1162–73.

40. Kakkar VV, Djazaeri B, Fok J, Fletcher M, Scully MF, Westwick J. Low-molecular-weight heparin and prevention of postoperative deep vein thrombosis. *Br Med J* 1982; **284**:375–9.

41. Warkentin TE, Levine MN, Hirsh J, Horsewood P, Roberts RS, Gent M, Kelton JG. Heparin-induced thrombocytopenia in patients treated with low-molecular-weight heparin or unfractionated heparin. *N Engl J Med* 1995; **332**:1330–5.

42. Mismetti P, Laporte S, Darmon JY, Buchmüller A, Decousus H. Meta-analysis of low molecular weight heparin in the prevention of venous thromboembolism in general surgery. *Br J Surg* 2001; **88**:913–30.

43. Kakkar VV, Murray WJ. Efficacy and safety of low-molecular-weight heparin (CY216) in preventing postoperative venous thrombo-embolism: a co-operative study. *Br J Surg* 1985; **72**:786–91.

44. Bergqvist D, Mätzsch T, Burmark US, Frisell J, Guilbaud O, Hallböök T, Horn A, Lindhagen A, Ljungnér H, Ljungström KG, et al. Low molecular weight heparin given the evening before surgery compared with conventional low-dose heparin in prevention of thrombosis. *Br J Surg* 1988; **75**:888–91.

45. European Fraxiparin Study (EFS) Group. Comparison of a low molecular weight heparin and unfractionated heparin for the prevention of deep vein thrombosis in patients undergoing abdominal surgery. The European Fraxiparin Study (EFS) Group. *Br J Surg* 1988; **75**:1058–63.

46. Koch A, Bouges S, Ziegler S, Dinkel H, Daures JP, Victor N. Low molecular weight heparin and unfractionated heparin in thrombosis prophylaxis after major surgical intervention: update of previous meta-analyses. *Br J Surg* 1997; **84**:750–9.

47. Agnelli G, Bergqvist D, Cohen AT, Gallus AS, Gent M, PEGASUS investigators. Randomized clinical trial of postoperative fondaparinux versus perioperative dalteparin for prevention of venous thromboembolism in high-risk abdominal surgery. *Br J Surg* 2005; **92**:1212–20.

48. Heit JA, O'Fallon WM, Petterson TM, Lohse CM, Silverstein MD, Mohr DN, Melton LJ III. Relative impact of risk factors for deep vein thrombosis and pulmonary embolism: a population-based study. *Arch Intern Med* 2002; **162**:1245–8.

49. Lausen I, Jensen R, Jorgensen LN, Rasmussen MS, Lyng KM, Andersen M, Raaschou HO, Wille-Jørgensen P. Incidence and prevention of deep venous thrombosis occurring late after general surgery: randomised controlled study of prolonged thromboprophylaxis. *Eur J Surg* 1998; **164**: 657–63.

50. Bergqvist D, Agnelli G, Cohen AT, Eldor A, Nilsson PE, Le Moigne-Amrani A, Dietrich-Neto F, ENOXACAN II Investigators. Duration of prophylaxis against venous thromboembolism with enoxaparin after surgery for cancer. *N Engl J Med* 2002; **346**:975–80.

51. Rasmussen MS. Preventing thromboembolic complications in cancer patients after surgery: a role for prolonged thromboprophylaxis. *Cancer Treat Rev* 2002; **28**:141–4.

52. Prevention of venous thrombosis and pulmonary embolism. NIH Consensus Development. *JAMA* 1986; **256**:744–9.

53. White RH, Romano PS, Zhou H, Rodrigo J, Bargar W. Incidence and time course of thromboembolic outcomes following total hip or knee arthroplasty. *Arch Intern Med* 1998; **158**:1525–31.

54. Caprini JA, Arcelus JI, Motykie G, Kudrna JC, Mokhtee D, Reyna JJ. The influence of oral anticoagulation therapy on deep vein thrombosis rates four weeks after total hip replacement. *J Vasc Surg* 1999; **30**:813–20.

55. Douketis JD, Eikelboom JW, Quinlan DJ, Willan AR, Crowther MA. Short-duration prophylaxis against venous thromboembolism after total hip or knee replacement: a meta-analysis of prospective studies investigating symptomatic outcomes. *Arch Intern Med* 2002; **162**:1465–71.

56. Eriksson BI, Kälebo P, Anthymyr BA, Wadenvik H, Tengborn L, Risberg B. Prevention of deep-vein thrombosis and pulmonary embolism after total hip replacement. Comparison of low-molecular-weight heparin and unfractionated heparin. *J Bone Joint Surg Am* 1991; **73**:484–93.

57. Stulberg BN, Insall JN, Williams GW, Ghelman B. Deep-vein thrombosis following total knee replacement. An analysis of six hundred and thirty-eight arthroplasties. *J Bone Joint Surg Am* 1984; **66**:194–201.

58. Planes A, Vochelle N, Darmon JY, Fagola M, Bellaud M, Huet Y. Risk of deep-venous thrombosis after hospital discharge in patients having undergone total hip replacement: double-blind randomised comparison of enoxaparin versus placebo. *Lancet* 1996; **348**:224–8.

59. Perez JV, Warwick DJ, Case CP, Bannister GC. Death after proximal femoral fracture – an autopsy study. *Injury* 1995; **26**:237–40.

60. Eikelboom JW, Quinlan DJ, Douketis JD. Extended-duration prophylaxis against venous thromboembolism after total hip or knee replacement: a meta-analysis of the randomised trials. *Lancet* 2001; **358**:9–15.

61. Hull RD, Pineo GF, Stein PD, Mah AF, MacIsaac SM, Dahl OE, Butcher M, Brant RF, Ghali WA, Bergqvist D, Raskob GE. Extended out-of-hospital low-molecular-weight heparin prophylaxis against deep venous thrombosis in patients after elective hip arthroplasty: a systematic review. *Ann Intern Med* 2001; **135**:858–69.

62. Agnelli G. Prevention of venous thromboembolism in orthopedic surgery. In Colman RW, Marder VJ, Clowes AW, George JN, Goldhaber SZ (eds), *Hemostasis and Thrombosis*, 5th edn. Lippincott Williams & Wilkins, Philedelphia, PA, 2006, pp. 1369–81.

63. Leyvraz PF, Richard J, Bachmann F, Van Melle G, Treyvaud JM, Livio JJ, Candardjis G. Adjusted versus fixed-dose subcutaneous heparin in the prevention of deep-vein thrombosis after total hip replacement. *N Engl J Med* 1983; **309**:954–8.

64. RD Heparin Arthroplasty Group. RD heparin compared with warfarin for prevention of venous thromboembolic disease following total hip or knee arthroplasty. RD Heparin Arthroplasty Group. *J Bone Joint Surg Am* 1994; **76**:1174–85.

65. Francis CW, Pellegrini VD Jr, Totterman S, Boyd AD Jr, Marder VJ, Liebert KM, Stulberg BN, Ayers DC, Rosenberg A, Kessler C, Johanson NA. Prevention of deep-vein thrombosis after total hip arthroplasty. Comparison of warfarin and dalteparin. *J Bone Joint Surg Am* 1997; **79**:1365–72.

66. Hull R, Raskob G, Pineo G, Rosenbloom D, Evans W, Mallory T, Anquist K, Smith F, Hughes G, Green D, et al. A comparison of subcutaneous low-molecular-weight heparin with warfarin sodium for prophylaxis against deep-vein thrombosis after hip or knee implantation. *N Engl J Med* 1993; **329**:1370–6.

67. Hamulyák K, Lensing AW, van der Meer J, Smid WM, van Ooy A, Hoek JA. Subcutaneous low-molecular weight heparin or oral anticoagulants for the prevention of deep-vein thrombosis in elective hip and knee replacement? Fraxiparine Oral Anticoagulant Study Group. *Thromb Haemost* 1995; **74**:1428–31.

68. Hull RD, Pineo GF, Francis C, Bergqvist D, Fellenius C, Soderberg K, Holmqvist A, Mant M, Dear R, Baylis B, Mah A, Brant R. Low-molecular-weight heparin prophylaxis using dalteparin extended out-of-hospital vs in-hospital warfarin/out-of-hospital placebo in hip arthroplasty patients: a double-blind, randomized comparison. North American Fragmin Trial Investigators. *Arch Intern Med* 2000; **160**:2208–15.

69. Colwell CW Jr, Spiro TE, Trowbridge AA, Stephens JW, Gardiner GA Jr, Ritter MA. Efficacy and safety of enoxaparin versus unfractionated heparin for prevention of deep venous thrombosis after elective knee arthroplasty. Enoxaparin Clinical Trial Group. *Clin Orthop Relat Res* 1995; **321**:19–27.

70. Turpie AG, Levine MN, Hirsh J, Carter CJ, Jay RM, Powers PJ, Andrew M, Hull RD, Gent M. A randomized controlled trial of a low-molecular-weight heparin (enoxaparin) to prevent deep-vein thrombosis in patients undergoing elective hip surgery. *N Engl J Med* 1986; **315**:925–9.

71. Turpie AG, Gallus AS, Hoek JA; Pentasaccharide Investigators. A synthetic pentasaccharide for the prevention of deep-vein thrombosis after total hip replacement. *N Engl J Med* 2001; **344**:619–25.

72. Lassen MR, Bauer KA, Eriksson BI, Turpie AG, European Pentasaccharide Elective Surgery Study (EPHESUS) Steering Committee. Postoperative fondaparinux versus preoperative enoxaparin for prevention of venous thromboembolism in elective hip-replacement surgery: a randomised double-blind comparison. *Lancet* 2002; **359**:1715–20.

73. Turpie AG, Bauer KA, Eriksson BI, Lassen MR, PENTATHALON 2000 Study Steering Committee. Postoperative fondaparinux versus postoperative enoxaparin for prevention of venous thromboembolism after elective hip-replacement surgery: a randomised double-blind trial. *Lancet* 2002; **359**:1721–6.

74. Turpie AG, Eriksson BI, Bauer KA, Lassen MR. New pentasaccharides for the prophylaxis of venous thromboembolism: clinical studies. *Chest* 2003; **124**(Suppl):371S–378S.

75. Eriksson BI, Bauer KA, Lassen MR, Turpie AG, Steering Committee of the Pentasaccharide in Hip-Fracture Surgery Study. Fondaparinux compared with enoxaparin for the prevention of venous thromboembolism after hip-fracture surgery. *N Engl J Med* 2001; **345**:1298–304.

76. Leclerc JR, Geerts WH, Desjardins L, Laflamme GH, L'Espérance B, Demers C, Kassis J, Cruickshank M, Whitman L, Delorme F. Prevention of venous thromboembolism after knee arthroplasty. A randomized, double-blind trial comparing enoxaparin with warfarin. *Ann Intern Med* 1996; **124**:619–26.

77. Heit JA, Berkowitz SD, Bona R, Cabanas V, Corson JD, Elliott CG, Lyons R. Efficacy and safety of low molecular weight heparin (ardeparin sodium) compared to warfarin for the prevention of venous thromboembolism after total knee replacement surgery: a double-blind, dose-ranging study. Ardeparin Arthroplasty Study Group. *Thromb Haemost* 1997; **77**:32–8.

78. Fitzgerald RH Jr, Spiro TE, Trowbridge AA, Gardiner GA Jr, Whitsett TL, O'Connell MB, Ohar JA, Young TR, Enoxaparin Clinical Trial Group. Prevention of venous thromboembolic disease following primary total knee arthroplasty. A randomized, multicenter, open-label, parallel-group comparison of enoxaparin and warfarin. *J Bone Joint Surg Am* 2001; **83-A**:900–6.

79. Howard AW, Aaron SD. Low molecular weight heparin decreases proximal and distal deep venous thrombosis following total knee arthroplasty. A meta-analysis of randomized trials. *Thromb Haemost* 1998; **79**:902–6.

80. Brookenthal KR, Freedman KB, Lotke PA, Fitzgerald RH, Lonner JH. A meta-analysis of thromboembolic prophylaxis in total knee arthroplasty. *J Arthroplasty* 2001; **16**:293–300.

81. Bauer KA, Eriksson BI, Lassen MR, Turpie AG, Steering Committee of the Pentasaccharide in Major Knee Surgery Study. Fondaparinux compared with enoxaparin for the prevention of venous thromboembolism after elective major knee surgery. *N Engl J Med* 2001; **345**:1305–10.

82. Bergqvist D, Lowe G. Venous thromboembolism in patients undergoing laparoscopic and arthroscopic surgery and in leg casts. *Arch Intern Med* 2002; **162**:2173–6.

83. Ettema HB, Hoppener MR, Veeger NJ, Büller HR, van der Meer J. Low incidence of venographically detected deep vein thrombosis after knee arthroscopy without thromboprophylaxis: a prospective cohort study. *J Thromb Haemost* 2006; **4**:1411–3.

84. Stringer MD, Steadman CA, Hedges AR, Thomas EM, Morley TR, Kakkar VV. Deep vein thrombosis after elective knee surgery. An incidence study in 312 patients. *J Bone Joint Surg Br* 1989; **71**: 492–7.

85. Small NC. Complications in arthroscopic surgery performed by experienced arthroscopists. *Arthroscopy* 1988; **4**:215–21.

86. Demers C, Marcoux S, Ginsberg JS, Laroche F, Cloutier R, Poulin J. Incidence of venographically proved deep vein thrombosis after knee arthroscopy. *Arch Intern Med* 1998; **158**:47–50.

87. Zacharoulis D, Kakkar AK. Venous thromboembolism in laparoscopic surgery. *Curr Opin Pulm Med* 2003; **9**:356–61.

88. Wilson YG, Allen PE, Skidmore R, Baker AR. Influence of compression stockings on lower-limb venous haemodynamics during laparoscopic cholecystectomy. *Br J Surg* 1994; **81**:841–4.

89. Zacharoulis D, Kakkar AK. Venous thromboembolism in laparoscopic surgery. *Curr Opin Pulm Med* 2003; **9**:356–61.

90. White RH, Zhou H, Romano PS. Incidence of symptomatic venous thromboembolism after different elective or urgent surgical procedures. *Thromb Haemost* 2003; **90**:446–55.

91. Bradbury AW, Chan YC, Darzi A, Stansby G. Thromboembolism prophylaxis during laparoscopic cholecystectomy. *Br J Surg* 1997; **84**:962–4.

92. Filtenborg Tvedskov T, Rasmussen MS, Wille-Jørgensen P. Survey of the use of thromboprophylaxis in laparoscopic surgery in Denmark. *Br J Surg* 2001; **88**:1413–6.

93. Blake AM, Toker SI, Dunn E. Deep venous thrombosis prophylaxis is not indicated for laparoscopic cholecystectomy. *J Soc Laparosc Surg* 2001; **5**:215–9.

94. Chamberlain G, Brown JC. *Gynecologic Laparoscopy: the Report of a Working Party in a Confidential Enquiry of Gynaecological Laparoscopy*. Royal College of Obstetricians and Gynecologists, London, 1978.

95. Lindberg F, Bergqvist D, Rasmussen I. Incidence of thromboembolic complications after laparoscopic cholecystectomy: review of the literature. *Surg Laparosc Endosc* 1997; **7**:324–31.

96. Neudecker J, Sauerland S, Neugebauer E, Bergamaschi R, Bonjer HJ, Cuschieri A, Fuchs KH, Jacobi Ch, Jansen FW, Koivusalo AM, Lacy A, McMahon MJ, Millat B, Schwenk W. The European Association for Endoscopic Surgery clinical practice guideline on the pneumoperitoneum for laparoscopic surgery. *Surg Endosc* 2002; **16**:1121–43.

97. Rogers FB, Cipolle MD, Velmahos G, Rozycki G, Luchette FA. Practice management guidelines for the prevention of venous thromboembolism in trauma patients: the EAST practice management guidelines work group. *J Trauma* 2002; **53**:142–64.

98. Eriksson BI, Lassen MR, PENTasaccharide in HIp-FRActure Surgery Plus Investigators. Duration of prophylaxis against venous thromboembolism with fondaparinux after hip fracture surgery: a multicenter, randomized, placebo-controlled, double-blind study. *Arch Intern Med* 2003; **163**:1337–42.

99. Spinal Cord Injury Thromboprophylaxis Investigators. Prevention of venous thromboembolism in the acute treatment phase after spinal cord injury: a randomized, multicenter trial comparing low-dose heparin plus intermittent pneumatic compression with enoxaparin. *J Trauma* 2003; **54**:1116–24.

100. Waring WP, Karunas RS. Acute spinal cord injuries and the incidence of clinically occurring thromboembolic disease. *Paraplegia* 1991; **29**:8–16.

101. DeVivo MJ, Krause JS, Lammertse DP. Recent trends in mortality and causes of death among persons with spinal cord injury. *Arch Phys Med Rehabil* 1999; **80**:1411–9.

102. Powell M, Kirshblum S, O'Connor KC. Duplex ultrasound screening for deep vein thrombosis in spinal cord injured patients at rehabilitation admission. *Arch Phys Med Rehabil* 1999; **80**:1044–6.

103. Chen D, Apple DF Jr, Hudson LM, Bode R. Medical complications during acute rehabilitation following spinal cord injury – current experience of the model systems. *Arch Phys Med Rehabil* 1999; **80**:1397–401.

104. Hadley, MN Deep venous thrombosis and thromoembolism inpatients with cervical spinal cord injuries. *Neurosurgery* 2002; **50**(Suppl), S73–S80.

105. Heit JA, Kobbervig CE, James AH, Petterson TM, Bailey KR, Melton LJ III. Trends in the incidence of venous thromboembolism during pregnancy or postpartum: a 30-year population-based study. *Ann Intern Med* 2005; **143**:697–706.

106. Toglia MR, Weg JG. Venous thromboembolism during pregnancy. *N Engl J Med* 1996; **335**:108–14.

107. De Stefano V, Martinelli I, Rossi E, Battaglioli T, Za T, Mannuccio Mannucci P, Leone G. The risk of recurrent venous thromboembolism in pregnancy and puerperium without antithrombotic prophylaxis. *Br J Haematol* 2006; **135**:386–91.

108. Folkeringa N, Brouwer JL, Korteweg FJ, Veeger NJ, Erwich JJ, van der Meer J. High risk of pregnancy-related venous thromboembolism in women with multiple thrombophilic defects. *Br J Haematol* 2007; **138**:110–6.

109. Brill-Edwards P, Ginsberg JS, Gent M, Hirsh J, Burrows R, Kearon C, Geerts W, Kovacs M, Weitz JI, Robinson KS, Whittom R, Couture G, Recurrence of Clot in This Pregnancy Study Group. Safety of withholding heparin in pregnant women with a history of venous thromboembolism. Recurrence of Clot in This Pregnancy Study Group. *N Engl J Med* 2000; **343**:1439–44.

110. Symington IS, Stack BH. Pulmonary thromboembolism after travel. *Br J Dis Chest* 1977; **71**:138–40.

111. Sarvesvaran R. Sudden natural deaths associated with commercial air travel. *Med Sci Law* 1986; **26**:35–8.

112. Kuipers S, Cannegieter SC, Middeldorp S, Rosendaal FR, Buller HR. Use of preventive measures for air travel-related venous thrombosis in professionals who attend medical conferences. *J Thromb Haemost* 2006; **4**:2373–6.

113. Kuipers S, Schreijer AJ, Cannegieter SC, Büller HR, Rosendaal FR, Middeldorp S. Travel and venous thrombosis: a systematic review. *J Intern Med* 2007; **262**:615–34.

114. Schreijer AJ, Cannegieter SC, Meijers JC, Middeldorp S, Buller HR, Rosendaal FR. Activation of coagulation system during air travel: a crossover study. *Lancet* 2006; **367**:832–8.

115. Cannegieter SC, Doggen CJ, van Houwelingen HC, Rosendaal FR. Travel-related venous thrombosis: results from a large population-based case control study (MEGA Study). *PLoS Med* 2006; **3**(8):1258–65.

116. Lapostolle F, Surget V, Borron SW, Desmaizieres M, Sordelet D, Lapandry C, Cupa M, Adnet F. Severe pulmonary embolism associated with air travel. *N Engl J Med* 2001; **345**:779–83.

117. Central Bureau of Statistics (CBS), The Netherlands. URL: http://statline.cbs.nl/StatWeb/Table.asp?STB = T&LA = nl&DM = SLNL&PA = 37296ned&D1 = a&D2 = 0,10,20,30,40,50,(1–1)-l&HDR = G1. Accessed 23 January 2008.

118. Central Bureau of Statistics (CBS), the Netherlands. URL: http://www.cbs.nl/NR/rdonlyres /C3619414–3E5B–431A–8554-A79B2E730477/0/2007g82pub.pdf. Accessed 23 January 2008.

119. Rosendaal FR. Interventions to prevent venous thrombosis after air travel: are they necessary? No. *J Thromb Haemost* 2006; **4**:2306–7.

120. Chee YL, Watson HG. Air travel and thrombosis. *Br J Haematol* 2005; **130**:671–80.

121. Belcaro G, Geroulakos G, Nicolaides AN, Myers KA, Winford M. Venous thromboembolism from air travel: the LONFLIT study. *Angiology* 2001; **52**:369–74.

122. Cohen, AT. Venous thromboembolic disease management of the nonsurgical moderate-and high-risk patient. *Semin Hematol* 2000; **37**(Suppl):19–22.

123. Bergmann, JF, Mouly, S. Thromboprophylaxis in medical patients: focus on France. *Semin Thromb Hemost* 2002; **28**(Suppl):51–55.

124. Samama MM. An epidemiologic study of risk factors for deep vein thrombosis in medical outpatients: the Sirius study. *Arch Intern Med* 2000; **160**:3415–20.

125. Samama MM, Cohen AT, Darmon JY, Desjardins L, Eldor A, Janbon C, Leizorovicz A, Nguyen H, Olsson CG, Turpie AG, Weisslinger N. A comparison of enoxaparin with placebo for the prevention of venous thromboembolism in acutely ill medical patients: Prophylaxis in Medical Patients with Enoxaparin Study Group. *N Engl J Med* 1999; **341**:793–800.

126. Leizorovicz A, Cohen AT, Turpie AG, Olsson CG, Vaitkus PT, Goldhaber SZ; PREVENT Medical Thromboprophylaxis Study Group. Randomized, placebo-controlled trial of dalteparin for the prevention of venous thromboembolism in acutely ill medical patients. *Circulation* 2004; **110**:874–9.

127. Cohen AT, Davidson BL, Gallus AS, Lassen MR, Prins MH, Tomkowski W, Turpie AG, Egberts JF, Lensing AW; ARTEMIS Investigators. Efficacy and safety of fondaparinux for the prevention of venous thromboembolism in older acute medical patients: randomised placebo controlled trial. *BMJ* 2006; **332**:325–9.

128. Schulman S. Thromboprophylaxis in medical patients – why not for all? *Pathophysiol Haemost Thromb* 2006; **35**:141–5.

129. Lowe GD. Arterial disease and venous thrombosis: are they related and if so, what should we do about it? *J Thromb Haemost* 2006; **4**:1882–5.

130. Prandoni P. Venous thromboembolism and atherosclerosis: is there a link? *J Thromb Haemost* 2007; **5**(Suppl):270–5.

131. Lowe GD. Can haematological tests predict cardiovascular risk? The 2005 Kettle Lecture. *Br J Haematol* 2006; **133**:232–50.

132. Hirsh J, Guyatt G, Albers G, Schunemann H (eds). The Seventh ACCP Conference on Antithrombotic and Thrombolytic Therapy: Evidence Based Guidelines. *Chest* 2004; **126**(Suppl):1S–703S.

133. Collins R, MacMahon S, Flather M, Baigent C, Remvig L, Mortensen S, Appleby P, Godwin J, Yusuf S, Peto R. Clinical effects of anticoagulant therapy in suspected acute myocardial infarction: systematic overview of randomised trials. *BMJ* 1996; **313**:652–9.

134. Kelly J, Rudd A, Lewis RR, Coshall C, Moody A, Hunt BJ. Venous thromboembolism after acute ischemic stroke: a prospective study using magnetic resonance direct thrombus imaging. *Stroke* 2004; **35**:2320–5.

135. Bath PM, Iddenden R, Bath FJ. Low-molecular-weight heparins and heparinoids in acute ischemic stroke: a meta-analysis of randomized controlled trials. *Stroke* 2000; **31**:1770–8.

136. Sandercock P, Counsell C, Stobbs SL. Low-molecular-weight heparins or heparinoids versus standard unfractionated heparin for acute ischaemic stroke. *Cochrane Database Syst Rev* 2005; **2**:CD000119.

137. Prandoni P, Falanga A, Piccioli A. Cancer and venous thromboembolism. *Lancet Oncol* 2005; **6**:401–10.

138. Rickles FR, Edwards RL. Activation of blood coagulation in cancer: Trousseau's syndrome revisited. *Blood* 1983; **62**:14–31.

139. Shen VS, Pollak EW. Fatal pulmonary embolism in cancer patients: is heparin prophylaxis justified? *South Med J* 1980; **73**:841–3.

140. Blom JW, Doggen CJ, Osanto S, Rosendaal FR. Malignancies, prothrombotic mutations and the risk of venous thrombosis. *JAMA* 2005; **293**:715–22.

141. Prandoni P, Lensing AW, Piccioli A, Bernardi E, Simioni P, Girolami B, Marchiori A, Sabbion P, Prins MH, Noventa F, Girolami A. Recurrent venous thromboembolism and bleeding complications during anticoagulant treatment in patients with cancer and venous thrombosis. *Blood* 2002; **100**:3484–8.

142. Lyman GH, Khorana AA, Falanga A, Clarke-Pearson D, Flowers C, Jahanzeb M, Kakkar A, Kuderer NM, Levine MN, Liebman H, Mendelson D, Raskob G, Somerfield MR, Thodiyil P, Trent D, Francis CW, American Society of Clinical Oncology. American Society of Clinical Oncology guideline: recommendations for venous thromboembolism prophylaxis and treatment in patients with cancer. *J Clin Oncol* 2007; **25**:5490–505.

143. Alikhan R, Cohen AT, Combe S, Samama MM, Desjardins L, Eldor A, Janbon C, Leizorovicz A, Olsson CG, Turpie AG; MEDENOX Study. Risk factors for venous thromboembolism in hospitalized patients with acute medical illness: analysis of the MEDENOX Study. *Arch Intern Med* 2004; **164**:963–8.

144. Alikhan R, Cohen AT, Combe S, Samama MM, Desjardins L, Eldor A, Janbon C, Leizorovicz A, Olsson CG, Turpie AG. Prevention of venous thromboembolism in medical patients with enoxaparin: a subgroup analysis of the MEDENOX study. *Blood Coagul Fibrinol* 2003; **14**:341–6.

145. Vaitkus PT, Leizorovicz A, Cohen AT, Turpie AG, Olsson CG, Goldhaber SZ; PREVENT Medical Thromboprophylaxis Study Group. Mortality rates and risk factors for asymptomatic deep vein thrombosis in medical patients. *Thromb Haemost* 2005; **93**:76–9.

146. Cavo M, Zamagni E, Cellini C, Tosi P, Cangini D, Cini M, Valdrè L, Palareti G, Masini L, Tura S, Baccarani M. Deep-vein thrombosis in patients with multiple myeloma receiving first-line thalidomide-dexamethasone therapy. *Blood* 2002; **100**:2272–3.

147. Zangari M, Anaissie E, Barlogie B, Badros A, Desikan R, Gopal AV, Morris C, Toor A, Siegel E, Fink L, Tricot G. Increased risk of deep-vein thrombosis in patients with multiple myeloma receiving thalidomide and chemotherapy. *Blood* 2001; **98**:1614–5.

148. Bennett CL, Angelotta C, Yarnold PR, Evens AM, Zonder JA, Raisch DW, Richardson P. Thalidomide- and lenalidomide-associated thromboembolism among patients with cancer. *JAMA* 2006; **296**:2558–60.

149. Kakkar AK, Haas S, Wolf H, Encke A. Evaluation of perioperative fatal pulmonary embolism and death in cancer surgical patients: the MC-4 cancer substudy. *Thromb Haemost* 2005; **94**:867–71.

150. Kearon C, Hirsh J. Management of anticoagulation before and after elective surgery. *N Engl J Med* 1997; **336**:1506–11.

151. Fisher B, Costantino J, Redmond C, Poisson R, Bowman D, Couture J, Dimitrov NV, Wolmark N, Wickerham DL, Fisher ER, et al. A randomized clinical trial evaluating tamoxifen in the treatment of patients with node-negative breast cancer who have oestrogen-receptor-positive tumors. *N Engl J Med* 1989; **320**:479–84.

152. Saphner T, Tormey DC, Gray R. Venous and arterial thrombosis in patients who received adjuvant therapy for breast cancer. *J Clin Oncol* 1991; **9**:286–94.

153. Fisher B, Costantino JP, Wickerham DL, Redmond CK, Kavanah M, Cronin WM, Vogel V, Robidoux A, Dimitrov N, Atkins J, Daly M, Wieand S, Tan-Chiu E, Ford L, Wolmark N. Tamoxifen for prevention

of breast cancer: report of the National Surgical Adjuvant Breast and Bowel Project P-1 Study. *J Natl Cancer Inst* 1998; **90**:1371–88.

154. Baum M, Budzar AU, Cuzick J, Forbes J, Houghton JH, Klijn JG, Sahmoud T, ATAC Trialists' Group. Anastrozole alone or in combination with tamoxifen versus tamoxifen alone for adjuvant treatment of postmenopausal women with early breast cancer: first results of the ATAC randomised trial. *Lancet* 2002; **359**:2131–9.

155. Efficacy and safety of enoxaparin versus unfractionated heparin for prevention of deep vein thrombosis in elective cancer surgery: a double-blind randomized multicentre trial with venographic assessment. ENOXACAN Study Group. *Br J Surg* 1997; **84**:1099–103.

156. Bergqvist D, Burmark US, Flordal PA, Frisell J, Hallböök T, Hedberg M, Horn A, Kelty E, Kvitting P, Lindhagen A, et al. Low molecular weight heparin started before surgery as prophylaxis against deep vein thrombosis: 2500 versus 5000 XaI units in 2070 patients. *Br J Surg* 1995; **82**:496–501.

157. Prandoni P, Lensing AW, Cogo A, Cuppini S, Villalta S, Carta M, Cattelan AM, Polistena P, Bernardi E, Prins MH. The long-term clinical course of acute deep venous thrombosis. *Ann Intern Med* 1996; **125**:1–7.

158. Anderson FA Jr, Wheeler HB. Physician practices in the management of venous thromboembolism: a community-wide survey. *J Vasc Surg* 1992; **16**:707–14.

159. Sevitt S, Gallagher NG. Prevention of venous thrombosis and pulmonary embolism in injured patients. A trial of anticoagulant prophylaxis with phenindione in middle-aged and elderly patients with fractured necks of femur. *Lancet* 1959; **ii**:981–9.

160. Christiansen SC, Cannegieter SC, Koster T, Vandenbroucke JP, Rosendaal FR. Thrombophilia, clinical factors and recurrent venous thrombotic events. *JAMA* 2005; **293**:2352–61.

161. Brouwer JL, Veeger NJ, Kluin-Nelemans HC, van der Meer J. The pathogenesis of venous thromboembolism: evidence for multiple interrelated causes. *Ann Intern Med* 2006; **145**:807–15.

162. Middeldorp S, Henkens CM, Koopman MM, van Pampus EC, Hamulyák K, van der Meer J, Prins MH, Büller HR. The incidence of venous thromboembolism in family members of patients with factor V Leiden mutation and venous thrombosis. *Ann Intern Med* 1998; **128**:15–20.

163. Bank I, Libourel EJ, Middeldorp S, Hamulyák K, van Pampus EC, Koopman MM, Prins MH, van der Meer J, Büller HR. Prothrombin 20210A mutation: a mild risk factor for venous thromboembolism but not for arterial thrombotic disease and pregnancy-related complications in a family study. *Arch Intern Med* 2004; **164**:1932–7.

164. Bank I, Libourel EJ, Middeldorp S, Hamulyák K, van Pampus EC, Koopman MM, Prins MH, van der Meer J, Büller HR. Elevated levels of FVIII:C within families are associated with an increased risk for venous and arterial thrombosis. *J Thromb Haemost* 2005; **3**:79–84.

165. van Hylckama Vlieg A, van der Linden IK, Bertina RM, Rosendaal FR. High levels of factor IX increase the risk of venous thrombosis. *Blood* 2000; **95**:3678–82.

166. Meijers JC, Tekelenburg WL, Bouma BN, Bertina RM, Rosendaal FR. High levels of coagulation factor XI as a risk factor for venous thrombosis. *N Engl J Med* 2000; **342**:696–701.

167. van Tilburg NH, Rosendaal FR, Bertina RM. Thrombin activatable fibrinolysis inhibitor and the risk for deep vein thrombosis. *Blood* 2000; 2855–9.

168. den Heijer M, Koster T, Blom HJ, Bos GM, Briet E, Reitsma PH, Vandenbroucke JP, Rosendaal FR. Hyperhomocysteinemia as a risk factor for deep-vein thrombosis. *N Engl J Med* 1996; **334**:759–761.

169. Lijfering WM, Coppens M, Veeger NJ, Middeldorp S, Hamulyák K, Prins MH, Büller HR, van der Meer J. Thrombophilic risk factors for first venous thrombosis, recurrence and its implications (abstract). *J Thromb Hamemost* 2007; **5**(1 Suppl):O–T-007.

170. Hull RD, Brant RF, Pineo GF, Stein PD, Raskob GE, Valentine KA. Preoperative vs postoperative initiation of low-molecular-weight heparin prophylaxis against venous thromboembolism in patients undergoing elective hip replacement. *Arch Intern Med* 1999; **159**:137–41.

171. Hull RD, Pineo GF, Francis C, Bergqvist D, Fellenius C, Soderberg K, Holmqvist A, Mant M, Dear R, Baylis B, Mah A, Brant R. Low-molecular-weight heparin prophylaxis using dalteparin extended out-of-hospital vs in-hospital warfarin/out-of-hospital placebo in hip arthroplasty patients: a double-blind, randomized comparison. North American Fragmin Trial Investigators. *Arch Intern Med* 2000; **160**:2208–15.

172. Strebel N, Prins M, Agnelli G, Büller HR. Preoperative or postoperative start of prophylaxis for venous thromboembolism with low-molecular-weight heparin in elective hip surgery? *Arch Intern Med* 2002; **162**:1451–6.

173. Turpie A, Bauer K, Eriksson B, Lassen M, Steering Committees of the Pentasaccharide Orthopedic Prophylaxis Studies. Efficacy and safety of fondaparinux in major orthopedic surgery according to the timing of its first administration. *Thromb Haemost* 2003; **90**:364–6.

174. Turpie AG. Extended duration of thromboprophylaxis in acutely ill medical patients: optimizing therapy? *J Thromb Haemost* 2007; **5**:5–11.

175. Deheinzelin D, Braga AL, Martins LC, Martins MA, Hernandez A, Yoshida WB, Maffei F, Monachini M, Calderaro D, Campos W Jr, Sguizzatto GT, Caramelli B, Trombo Risc Investigators. Incorrect use of thromboprophylaxis for venous thromboembolism in medical and surgical patients: results of a multicentric, observational and cross-sectional study in Brazil. *J Thromb Haemost* 2006; **4**:1266–70.

176. Ahmad HA, Geissler A, MacLellan DG. Deep venous thrombosis prophylaxis: are guidelines being followed? *ANZ J Surg* 2002; **72**:331–4.

177. Learhinan ER, Alderman CP. Venous thromboembolism prophylaxis in a South Australian teaching hospital. *Ann Pharmacother* 2003; **37**:1398–402.

178. Kahn SR, Panju A, Geerts W, Pineo GF, Desjardins L, Turpie AG, Glezer S, Thabane L, Sebaldt RJ; CURVE study investigators. Multicenter evaluation of the use of venous thromboembolism prophylaxis in acutely ill medical patients in Canada. *Thromb Res* 2007; **119**:145–55.

CHAPTER 21

Vena Cava Filters and Venous Thromboembolism

Patrick Mismetti, Silvy Laporte, Fabrice Guy Barral and Hervé Decousus

Thrombosis Research Group: EA 3065 - CIE3, University Hospital of Saint-Etienne, University Jean Monnet Saint-Etienne, France

INTRODUCTION

John Hunter is credited with the first femoral vein ligation in managing a patient with deep vein thrombosis (DVT) and to prevent pulmonary embolism (PE) as early as 1784 (1). Subsequently, with the observation that venous interruption led to chronic venous insufficiency, the technique was amended and inferior vena cava placation became the preferred technique, initially through surgery and later through external clip placement (2,3). In spite of these attempts, complication rates were high with 1.7% fatal PE, 2.3% non-fatal PE, an operative mortality rate of up to 12% and chronic venous insufficiency in nearly two-thirds of patients (3). Given the high operative mortality and morbidity rates, surgical interruption was gradually replaced by intraluminal devices, which were much safer to introduce and did not require general anaesthesia.

The first inferior cava filters were developed in the 1970s and although these initially could show migration, with expertise and redesign they progressively became more efficient and safe (4,5). Although there is no doubt that these devices have significantly improved in terms of effectiveness and safety, there are a number of complications that one can ascribe to the procedure, including femoral vein thrombosis at the insertion site, bleeding, caval perforation, filter misplacement (and resultant renal vein thrombosis or inferior vena cava obstruction) and filter migration (Figure 21.1). Indeed, for a long time the surgical introduction of filters was safer than the percutaneous method as large introducer sheaths were required (6,7). However, with the development of smaller introducer sheaths and the progressive experience of interventional radiologists, the technique became firmly established and complication rates decreased (8,9).

DIFFERENT TYPES OF FILTERS

Currently, at least 10 types of vena cava filter are in use in North America and Europe. These are either permanent, with no possibility of removal, such as the Greenfield (Boston Scientific,

Deep Vein Thrombosis and Pulmonary Embolism   Edited by Edwin J.R. van Beek, Harry R. Büller and Matthijs Oudkerk
© 2009 John Wiley & Sons, Ltd

Boston, MA, USA), Bird's Nest (Cook, Bloomington, IN, USA), Venatech (B. Braun, Boulogne, France) and Simon Nitinol (Bard, Tempe, AZ, USA) filters, or optionally retrievable, such as the Günther Tulip (Cook), Recovery (Bard), OptEase (Johnson and Johnson, Cordis Endovascular, Miami, FL, USA), Tempofilter II (B. Braun) and ALN (ALN Implants Chirurgicaux, Ghisonaccia, France) filters.

The effectiveness of these filters has been shown in mostly small studies. In a meta-analysis of 13 series of consecutive patients with stainless-steel Greenfield filters, a 2.4% non-fatal recurrence rate and a 0.7% fatal recurrence rate were shown in 1094 patients (10). In another review paper, aimed at the evaluation of newer filters, a recurrent PE rate of 2.9% and a fatal PE incidence of 0.8% were observed (11).

RECOMMENDATIONS FOR USE

As with all invasive procedures, insertion of a vena cava filter may be associated with a risk of serious adverse events, justifying consideration of the benefit-to-risk ratio in all indications (12). On this basis, IVC filters should be recommended mainly in the following situations:

1. When the risk of death due to PE is high (> 5% at 3 months) even under anticoagulation (13), for instance:
   - in patients with haemodynamically unstable PE
   - in patients at risk of recurrence of life-threatening PE, such as those with chronic pulmonary heart disease and chronic thromboembolic pulmonary hypertension, especially if a surgical treatment if proposed (see also Chapter 25).

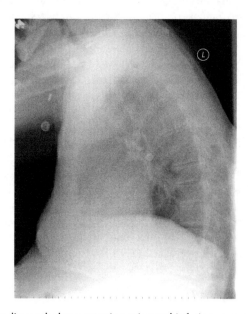

Figure 21.1   Lateral chest radiograph demonstrating migrated inferior vena cava filter located in the right heart

2. In patients experiencing recurrent PE despite optimal and well-conducted anticoagulation.
3. In patients with a contraindication to anticoagulant therapy for VTE, mainly due to bleeding or the risk of fatal bleeding, because the risk of PE recurrence or PE-related death may then reach 20% (14,15).

In these specific situations, indications for IVC filter placement are very widely accepted and intuitive and a randomized clinical trial is no longer realistic or feasible. In the absence of more convincing data, the most recent guidelines for the treatment of VTE only include a low-grade recommendation (grade 2C) for the use of vena cava filters (13,16).

POTENTIAL INDICATIONS WITHOUT RECOMMENDATIONS

The frequency of the specific situations described below is low and cannot in itself explain the impressive increase in the use of vena cava filters, especially in the USA, with about 30 000–40 000 filters inserted in 2004 (10). However, the frequency of use of these filters seems to differ on the two sides of the Atlantic Ocean, as shown by two prospective registries in North America, including 5541 patients (17) and 1691 patients (18), and one European registry including 14 314 patients at the time of publication (19). These registries indicate the use of IVC filters in 15 and 12% of VTE patients in the USA, compared with a mere 2% in Europe. Although their use was prompted by a contraindication to anticoagulant treatment in one-third of the patients, both the discrepancy between the USA and Europe and the high utilization rate of vena cava filters in the USA were mainly due to their employment in indications other than those described above as intuitive (20).

These potential indications, not as widely accepted, include:

1. episodes of VTE in patients at high risk of recurrence without any contraindication to or failure of anticoagulant therapy
2. primary prevention of PE in high-risk situations such as trauma, major orthopaedic surgery, neurosurgery or bariatric surgery [about 30–50% of patients in published cohorts (21)].

With respect to the first indication, the risk of fatal PE is now relatively low in patients treated with conventional anticoagulants, with 0.5% of fatal PE in DVT patients(22) and 1.5% in PE patients(23) in recent randomized clinical trials and 1.7% in VTE patients in a recent prospective cohort (24). This low incidence may counterbalance the value of filters in this context. In primary prevention, the considerations are the same, with an even lower risk of fatal PE, less than 0.5%, even after trauma, hip fracture or bariatric surgery (25–27). Furthermore, full efficacy of vena cava filters is not guaranteed, the estimated incidence of PE ranging from 0.5 to 6% despite filter insertion (10,11,28). Finally, in addition to the low risk of fatal PE and the only partial efficacy of vena cava filters in preventing PE, the occurrence of adverse events after filter implantation is not negligible, as shown in several cohorts (28), with:

- a 4–10% rate of adverse events related to filter insertion (haematoma, infection, etc.)
- a 5–70% rate of migration
- a 3–25% rate of acute vena caval perforation

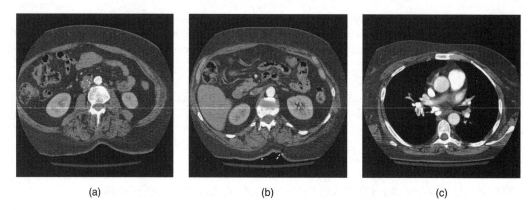

(a)   (b)   (c)

Figure 21.2 Patient with inferior vena cava thrombosis (a), with contrast from the renal vein entering above the filter (b) and a new filling defect in the right lower lobe indicating PE (c)

- a 5–30% rate of filter thrombosis (Figure 21.2)
- an approximately 0.1% mortality rate related to the filter insertion procedure.

Ultimately, the placement of a vena cava filter needs to be considered like a surgical procedure and the consenting process must include a balanced consideration of the possible benefits and adverse events.

A review of the literature revealed only one randomized controlled trial with 400 participants (29,30). The main results of this trial, PREPIC (Prévention du Risque d'Embolie Pulmonaire par Interruption Cave), are shown in Figure 21.3. This trial compared the effectiveness of vena cava filter insertion with no vena cava filter insertion in patients with documented proximal DVT or PE who received concurrent anticoagulation for at least 3 months. Permanent vena cava filters prevented PE at 8 years [hazard ratio (HR) 0.37, 95% confidence interval (CI) 0.17 to 0.79 in favour of filter insertion], but this benefit was counterbalanced by an excess of DVT in the filter group (HR 1.52, 95% CI 1.02 to 2.27), mainly due to filter-related thrombosis (30). This study did not demonstrate any difference in death rates between the two groups.

These results warrant several comments:

1. This trial evaluated the efficacy of permanent vena cava filters. The increased incidence of DVT in the filter group mainly appeared at least 6 months after insertion, as recently confirmed by a comparative, but not randomized study (31). The necessity for continuing anticoagulation in patients having received a vena cava filter is now supported by the recommendations of the 8th Conference of the ACCP (13).
2. The steering committee strongly recommended the predominant inclusion of patients at high risk of PE (29). This explains the advanced age of this population, close to 75 years compared with 65 years in the majority of randomized clinical trials in standard VTE patients. However, less than 40% of the patients presented with symptomatic concomitant PE, while 10% had undergone surgery within the previous 3 months and should therefore be considered as patients with provoked DVT.

One of the most important risk factors for VTE recurrence in anticoagulated patients is the presence of active cancer (19,32). Some studies have reported a high incidence of filter-related

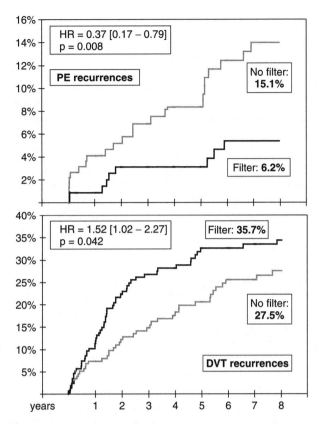

Figure 21.3 Results of comparison between patients with proximal DVT treated with anticoagulants plus a permanent vena cava filter (filter) and patients treated with anticoagulants alone (no filter) at 8 years: PREPIC study (30)

adverse events, ranging from 7 to 13% (33–35). However, these results should be interpreted cautiously since they were observed in a non-comparative trial. The subgroup of cancer patients in the randomized clinical trial PREPIC (13% of patients) does not allow more robust conclusions (36). It is not surprising to read that the latest ACCP recommendations advise against the systematic use of vena cava filters in patients presenting with VTE who have no contraindication to anticoagulant therapy (grade 1A) (13).Data on the use of vena cava filters as primary prevention in patients at high risk of VTE are only available for patient cohorts and do not allow any conclusions to be drawn regarding their effectiveness in the context of orthopaedic or trauma surgery (37,38), cancer surgery (39), bariatric surgery(40) or neurosurgery. Trials are needed to confirm their benefit and assess their safety accurately. The latest ACCP recommendations therefore advise against the routine use of vena cava filters in these situations (25).

OPTIMIZATION OF THE BENEFIT-TO-RISK RATIO OF VENA CAVA FILTERS: RETRIEVABLE FILTERS AND SPECIFIC POPULATIONS

Two avenues could be explored to optimize the benefit-to-risk ratio of vena cava filters: temporary filter placement and better selection of the population likely to benefit from such treatment.

Retrievable filters

The majority of the data have been derived from studies assessing permanent vena cava filters. In the PREPIC trial, the benefit of filters compared with no filters, with regard to preventing PE, appeared early after filter insertion, whereas the negative effect on DVT appeared long after filter insertion, becoming significant at 2 years (29,30). This suggests that such treatment could be optimized by judiciously defining the duration of filter placement and one could envisage implantation of the filter during the period when there is a risk of PE and its removal before the period corresponding to a risk of filter-related thrombosis occurs. The same scenario may be suggested for patients with a transient contraindication to anticoagulant therapy (e.g., a bleeding gastrointestinal ulcer), which is no longer applicable once the risk of haemorrhage has been controlled. Removal of the filter would avoid the necessity for an extended duration of anticoagulation as currently recommended for patients receiving vena cava filters (41). Similarly, in primary prevention, both the risk of thromboembolism and the risk of bleeding after surgery or trauma are transient. Once these risks are close to zero, filter removal could diminish the incidence of filter-related adverse events over time.

The first retrievable filters were developed around 20 years ago (the Amplatz filter) and several models are now available. Figure 21.4 shows an example of a procedure where a filter is removed at a time that the risk for recurrent PE has passed. Moreover, the permitted interval between implantation and removal, initially highly restrictive (<2 weeks), has now increased to several weeks or months in published observational patient cohorts (28). The potential value of retrievable filters is illustrated by the number of publications over the last 3 years, with more than 100 papers referenced in PubMed.

Even though the majority of cohorts were retrospective, it is important to note that the rate of filter-related adverse events remain high. In a recent prospective cohort of consecutive patients in whom a retrievable filter (ALN) was inserted, the rate of filter related-complications was about 12%, including filter tilt (6%), insertion site haematoma (4%) and filter migration (1%) (42). In addition, in some cases, filter removal was reported to be impossible and successful removal was not guaranteed. Failures of filter removal can reach 12% in observational studies (28). Such failures may outweigh the potential value of these types of filter since their benefit is directly linked to the possibility of removal.

Prospective randomized clinical trials are needed to assess the efficacy and safety of retrievable filters and the rate of successful removal when planned. Furthermore, as for all surgical implants, in addition to the overall feasibility of the procedure, transfer of the technique to other less

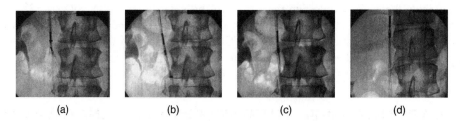

(a) (b) (c) (d)

Figure 21.4 Different steps of the retrieval of the ALN filter. (a) The olive is caught in a wire loop, inserted through the internal jugular vein. (b) The top of the filter is stabilized between the pincers and the outer sheath is advanced over the filter. (c) The entire filter is within the retrieval sheath. (d) The filter is pulled back in the retrieval sheath and removed through the jugular vein

experienced centres and/or investigators warrants evaluation in clinical practice and careful audit is essential in these situations.

Specific populations

In order to optimize the benefit-to-risk ratio, retrievable filters should be assessed in patients at high risk of PE, especially fatal PE. Clinical prognostic factors for fatal PE were identified in 15 520 patients presenting with an acute VTE (Table 21.1) (24). Symptomatic PE, especially massive PE, is significantly associated with an increased risk of fatal PE within 3 months, as are immobilization for neurological disease, advanced age, cancer and cardiac or respiratory disease, even if the trial was insufficiently powered to confirm definitively the statistical significance of the last predictor.

On the basis of the data from this prospective cohort and the single randomized clinical trial (PREPIC 1), a new randomized clinical trial, PREPIC 2, was recently started to assess the effectiveness of a retrievable filter (ALN) in patients with acute symptomatic PE anticoagulated with conventional therapy. To be included, patients also have to suffer from a DVT or a superficial vein thrombosis of the lower limb and at least one other risk factor for fatal PE, as previously identified (ClinicalTrials.gov identifier: NCT 00457158).

The same approach could be used for primary prevention in patients at high risk of VTE. Most of the multivariate studies show that cancer, advanced age, high body mass index ($>55 \text{ kg/m}^2$ in the context of bariatric surgery) and, above all, a history of VTE, are associated with an increased risk of VTE. These demographic and clinical characteristics of patients could be used to define the population likely to benefit from filter implantation (26,27,43). Once again, in view of the lack of reliable data and the current recommendations, the use of vena cava filters should be strictly

Table 21.1   Independent significant clinical predictors for fatal PE within 3 months in the RIETE study (24)

	OR	95% CI	*p*	Significant in the validation dataset
Venous thromboembolism at inclusion				
Distal/proximal DVT	1.00		<0.0001	Yes
Symptomatic non-massive PE	5.95	3.70 to 5.44		
Massive PE	16.3	8.50 to 31.4		
Immobilization>4 days for neurological disease	2.90	1.61 to 4.86	0.0001	Yes
Age>75 years	2.31	1.67 to 3.21	<0.0001	Yes
Cancer	2.40	1.72 to 3.25	<0.0001	Yes
Cardiac or respiratory disease	1.90	1.35 to 2.65	0.0001	No
Recent surgery	0.53	0.20 to 0.95	0.034	No

reserved for patients at high risk of PE, especially those with a history of VTE and discussed on a case-by-case basis.

CONCLUSION

Permanent vena cava filters, and also retrievable filters, may be considered valuable aids to the management of patients at high risk of VTE recurrence and/or patients with a contraindication to anticoagulant treatment. Fortunately, the majority of patients may warrant less invasive methods of VTE prophylaxis or treatment. The use of vena cava filters is increasing, probably due to the availability of more easy-to-insert implants, but more trials are definitely needed to confirm their benefit and assess accurately their safety and feasibility of removal in clinical practice.

REFERENCES

1. Hunter J. Observations on inflammation of internal coat of veins. *Trans Soc Improvement Med Chir Knowledge* 1793; **1**:18.
2. Piccone VA, Vida E, Yarnoz M, Glass BS, LeVeen HH. The late results of caval ligation. *Surgery* 1970; **68**:980–98.
3. Greenfield LJ. Evolution of venous interruption for pulmonary thromboembolism. *Arch Surg* 1992; **127**:622–26.
4. Mobin-Uddin K, Utley JR, Bryant LR. The inferior vena cava umbrella filter. *Prog Cardiovasc Dis* 1975; **17**:391–99.
5. Rectenwald JE. Vena cava filters: uses and abuses. *Sem Vasc Surg* 2005; **18**:166–175.
6. Alexander JJ, Yuhas JP, Piotrowski JJ. Is the increasing use of prophylactic percutaneous IVC filters justified? *Am J Surg* 1994; **168**:102–106.
7. Mewissen MW, Erickson SJ, Foley WD, Lipchik EO, Olson DL, McCann KM. Thrombosis of venous insertion sites after inferior vena caval filter placement. *Radiology* 1989; **173**:155–57.
8. Greenfield LJ, Cho KJ, Tauscher JR. Limitations of percutaneous insertion of Greenfield filters. *J Cardiovasc Surg* 1990; **31**:344–350.
9. Ammann ME, Eibenberger K, Winkelbauer F,. *et al.* Thromboserate nach Kavafilterimplantation. Langzeitergebnisse. *Untraschall Med* 1994; **15**:95–8.
10. Becker DM, Philbrick JT, Selby JB. Inferior vena cava filters. Indications, safety, effectiveness [review]. *Arch Intern Med* 1992; **152**:1985–94.
11. Ballew KA, Philbrick JT, Becker DM, Vena cava filter devices. *Clin Chest Med* 1995; **16**:295–305.
12. Stein PD, Kayali F, Olson RE. Twenty-one-year trends in the use of inferior vena cava filters. *Arch Intern Med* 2004; **164**:1541–45.
13. Kearon C, Kahn SR, Agnelli G,. *et al.* Antithrombotic therapy for venous thrombembolic disease. American College of Chest Physicians evidence-based clinical practice guidelines (8th edition). *Chest* 2008; **133**:454S–545S.
14. Barrit DW, Jordan SC. Anticoagulant drugs in the treatment of pulmonary embolism: a controlled trial. *Lancet* 1960; 1309–1312.
15. Brandjes DP, Heijboer H, Büller HR,. *et al.* Acenocoumarol and heparin compared with acenocoumarol alone in the initial treatment of proximal thrombosis. *N Engl J Med* 1992; **327**:1485–89.
16. Debourdeau P, Farge-Bancel D, Bosquet L,. *et al.* 2008 standards, options: recommendations for venous thrombembolic events treatment and central venous catheter thrombosis management in cancer patients. *Bull Cancer* 2008; **95**:750–761.
17. Seddighzadeh A, Shetty R, Goldhaber SZ. Venous thrombembolism in patients with active cancer. *Thromb Haemost* 2007; **98**:656–661.
18. Spencer FA, Gore JM, Lessard D,. *et al.* Patient outcomes after deep vein thrombosis and pulmonary embolism. The Worcester venous thrombembolism study. *Arch Intern Med* 2008; **168**:425–30.
19. Monreal M, Falga C, Valdés M,. *et al.* Fatal pulmonary embolism and fatal bleeding in cancer patients with venous thromboembolism. *J Thromb Haemost* 2006; **4**:1950–56.
20. Jaff MR, Goldhaber SZ, Tapson VF, on behalf of the DVT-FREE Registry. High utilization rate of vena cava filters in deep vein thrombosis. *Thromb Haemost* 2005; **93**:1117–19.

21. Rutherford RB. Prophylactic indications for vena cava filters: critical appraisal. *Semin Vasc Surg* 2005; **18**:158–165.
22. Büller HR, Davidson BL, Decousus H, *et al.*, for the Matisse DVT investigators. Fondaparinux or enoxaparin for the initial treatment of symptomatic deep vein thrombosis: a randomised trial. *Ann Intern Med* 2004; **140**:867–73.
23. Büller HR, Davidson BL, Decousus H, *et al.*, for the Matisse PE investigators. Subcutaneous fondaparinux versus intravenous unfractionated heparin in the initial treatment of pulmonary embolism. *N Engl J Med* 2003; **349**:1695–1702.
24. Laporte S, Mismetti P, Décousus H, Uresandi F, Otero R, Lobo JL, Monreal M, RIETE Investigators. Clinical predictors for fatal pulmonary embolism in 15,520 patients with venous thromboembolism: findings from the Registro Informatizado de la Enfermedad TromboEmbolica venosa (RIETE) Registry. *Circulation* 2008; **117**:1711–16.
25. Geerts WH, Bergqvist D, Pineo GF,. *et al*. Prevention of venous thromboembolism. American College of Chest Physicians evidence-based clinical practice guidelines (8th edition). *Chest* 2008; **133**:381S–453S.
26. Rosencher N, Vielpeau C, Emmerich J,. *et al*. Venous thromboembolism and mortality after hip fracture surgery. *J Thromb Haemost* 2005; **3**:1–9.
27. Hamad GG, Bergqvist D. Venous thromboembolism in bariatric surgery surgery patients: an update of risk and prevention. *Surg Obesity Related Dis* 2007; **3**:97–102.
28. Imberti D, Prisco D. Retrievable vena cava filters: key considerations. *Thromb Res* 2008; **122**:442–49.
29. Decousus H, Leizorovicz A, Parent F,. *et al*. A clinical trial of vena caval filters in the prevention of pulmonary embolism in patients with proximal deep-vein thrombosis. Prévention du Risque d'Embolie Pulmonaire par Interruption Cave Study Group. *N Engl J Med* 1998; **338**:409–15.
30. The PREPIC Study Group. Eight-year follow-up of patients with permanent vena cava filters in the prevention of pulmonary embolism: the PREPIC randomized study. *Circulation* 2005; **112**:416–22.
31. Billett HH, Jacobs LG, Madsen EM, Giannattasio ER, Mahesh S, Cohen HW. Efficacy of inferior vena cava filters in anticoagulated patients. *J Thromb Haemost* 2007; **5**:1848–53.
32. Prandoni P, Lensing AW, Piccioli A, Bernardi E, Simioni P, Girolami B, Marchiori A, Sabbion P, Prins MH, Noventa F, Girolami A. Recurrent venous thromboembolism and bleeding complications during anticoagulant treatment in patients with cancer and venous thrombosis. *Blood* 2002; **100**:3484–88.
33. Jarrett BP, Dougherty MJ, Calligaro KD. Inferior vena cava filters in malignant disease. *J Vasc Surg* 2002; **36**:704–707.
34. Schunn C, Schunn G, Hobbs G,. *et al*. Inferior vena cava filter placement in late-stage cancer. *Vasc Endovasc Surg* 2006; **40**:287–94.
35. Wallace MJ, Jean JL, Gupta S,. *et al*. Use of inferior vena caval filters and survival in patients with malignancy. *Cancer* 2004; **101**:1902–1907.
36. Mismetti P, Rivron-Guillot K, Moulin N. Vena cava filters and treatment of venous thromboembolism in cancer patients. *Pathol Biol* 2008; **56**:229–32.
37. Strauss EJ, Egol KA, Alaia M,. *et al*. The use of retrievable inferior cava filters in orthopedic patients. *J Bone Joint Surg Br* 2008; **90**:662–67.
38. Giannoudis PV, Pountos I, Pape HC,. *et al*. Safety and efficacy of vena cava filters in trauma patients. *Injury Int J Care Injured* 2007; **38**:7–18.
39. Adib T, Belli A, McCall, *et al*.. The use of inferior vena cava filters prior to major surgery in women with gynaecological cancer. *BJOG* 2008; **115**:902–907.
40. Piano G, Ketteler ER, Prachand V,. *et al*. Safety, feasibility and outcome of retrievable vena cava filters in high-risk surgical patients. *J Vasc Surg* 2007; **45**:784–88.
41. Kearon C. Long-term management of patients after venous thromboembolism. *Circulation* 2004; **110**:I10–I18.
42. Mismetti P, Rivron-Guillot K, Quenet S,. *et al*. A prospective long-term study of 220 patients with a retrievable vena cava filters for secondary prevention of venous thromboembolism. *Chest* 2007; **131**:223–29.
43. Schiff RL, Kahn SR, Shrier I,. *et al*. Identifying orthopedic patients at high risk for venous thromboembolism despite thromboprophylaxis. *Chest* 2005; **128**:3364–71.

PART VI

Conservative and Surgical Treatment

CHAPTER 22

Initial and Long-Term Treatment of Deep Vein Thrombosis

Gary Raskob

College of Public Health University of Oklahoma Health Sciences Center, Oklahoma, USA

OBJECTIVES OF TREATMENT AND OVERVIEW OF APPROACHES

The objectives of treatment in patients with established deep vein thrombosis (DVT) are to (1) prevent death from pulmonary embolism (PE), (2) alleviate the acute leg symptoms such as pain and swelling, (3) prevent morbidity from recurrent DVT and/or PE and (4) prevent the post-thrombotic syndrome and minimize post-thrombotic symptoms.

Symptomatic thrombosis of the popliteal or more proximal deep veins of the leg, known as 'proximal vein thrombosis', is a serious and potentially lethal condition. Inadequately treated proximal vein thrombosis results in a 20–50% incidence of symptomatic recurrent venous thromboembolic events (1–3), which may include fatal PE.

Symptomatic DVT that remains limited to the calf veins is associated with low risk (1%) of clinically important PE. Symptomatic extension of calf vein thrombosis into the popliteal vein or more proximally occurs in 15–25% of patients with untreated calf vein thrombosis (4,5).

Thrombosis may also occur in the deep veins of the upper extremity and these thrombi may cause symptoms or result in PE, including fatal embolism (6). Much less high-quality evidence from clinical research is available to guide clinical recommendations for the treatment of upper extremity DVT. In general, patients with upper extremity DVT should receive similar treatment to that for patients with DVT of the legs (7). The remainder of this chapter will focus on the treatment of DVT of the legs.

The post-thrombotic syndrome is a frequent complication of DVT (8). A prospective study documented a 25% incidence of moderate-to-severe post-thrombotic symptoms within 2 years after the initial diagnosis of proximal vein thrombosis in patients who were treated with initial heparin and oral anticoagulants for 3 months (9). This study also demonstrated that ipsilateral recurrent venous thrombosis is strongly associated with the subsequent development of moderate or severe post-thrombotic symptoms. Thus, prevention of ipsilateral recurrent DVT probably reduces the incidence of the post-thrombotic syndrome.

For most patients, the objectives of treatment as listed above are achieved by providing adequate anticoagulant treatment, both as initial therapy and continued long term for 3 months or

Deep Vein Thrombosis and Pulmonary Embolism Edited by Edwin J.R. van Beek, Harry R. Büller and Matthijs Oudkerk
© 2009 John Wiley & Sons, Ltd

longer. Adequate anticoagulant treatment reduces the incidence of symptomatic extension and/or recurrence of thromboembolism during the first 3 months after diagnosis from 25% or more to 4% or less (1–3,5,10). Use of a properly fitted graded compression stocking, with an ankle pressure gradient of 30–40 mmHg, applied as soon after diagnosis as the patient's symptoms will allow and continued for at least 2 years, is effective in reducing the incidence of post-thrombotic symptoms, including moderate-to-severe symptoms (11).

Thrombolytic therapy, either by systemic infusion or catheter-directed infusion, is currently indicated only for selected patients with DVT (7) (see the section 'Thrombolytic therapy' below). The main rationale for using thrombolytic therapy for DVT is to prevent post-thrombotic symptoms, but the evidence that it is effective for this purpose is not definitive. In selected patients with extensive iliofemoral thrombosis, thrombolytic therapy may also be indicated or required to relieve the acute symptoms caused by venous outflow obstruction. A more complete overview of thrombolytic therapy is provided in Chapter 24. Catheter-directed thrombolytic therapy may also be combined with interventional procedures such as angioplasty or stent placement to correct the underlying venous lesion(s), as is more fully described in Chapter 26. Regardless of whether it is given by systemic or catheter-directed infusion, thrombolytic therapy must be followed by adequate anticoagulant therapy to prevent recurrent venous thromboembolism.

The use of an inferior vena cava filter is indicated to prevent death from PE in patients with proximal vein thrombosis in whom anticoagulant treatment is contraindicated and in the rare patient in whom adequate anticoagulant treatment is ineffective (see also Chapter 21). The insertion of a vena cava filter increases the risk of subsequent recurrent DVT (12), and this has led to the development of retrievable filters. Therefore, if the contraindication to anticoagulant therapy is transient, anticoagulant therapy should be given to these patients when it is safe to do so and continued long term to prevent recurrent venous thrombosis of the legs (7).The use of removable filters has the potential to avoid the increased risk of recurrent DVT associated with placement of a permanent vena cava filter. However, the benefits (reduced DVT) and risks (subsequent PE) of removable filters compared with conventional permanent filters, such as the Greenfield filter, should be evaluated by definitive randomized trials before firm recommendations are made to remove vena cava filters routinely. In patients with DVT confined to the calf veins, in whom a contraindication to anticoagulant therapy is present, monitoring for proximal extension of thrombosis using serial ultrasound imaging may be used as an alternative to insertion of a vena cava filter.

EVIDENCE-BASED RECOMMENDATIONS

In this section, the recommendations for treatment are linked to the strength of the evidence from clinical trials using the approach for grading evidence of the American College of Chest Physicians Evidence-based Clinical Practice Guidelines (13). This approach grades treatment recommendations based on both the clinical benefits and risks of the treatment (grade 1 or 2) and on the methodological quality of the underlying clinical research evidence for a particular treatment (grade A, B or C) (13). Recommendations classified as 1A are the strongest. These recommendations indicate a clear risk-to-benefit conclusion (grade 1) and are supported by evidence from scientifically valid randomized clinical trials (grade A evidence). Grade 1A recommendations should be implemented for most patients (13). Grade 2A recommendations also are supported by definitive clinical trial evidence (grade A), but the results indicate a less clear risk-to-benefit conclusion (grade 2); such recommendations may or may not be appropriate for the individual patient, depending on the clinical circumstances and on patient values and preferences. Grade 1B or 1C recommendations, which are based on weaker quality evidence (grade B or C), but apparently clear risk–benefit conclusions (grade 1), can apply to most patients in most circumstances, although these recommendations may change in the future as higher quality research evidence becomes available. Grade 2B and 2C recommendations are the weakest and, in these cases, other alternative treatments may be equally appropriate (13), depending on the clinical circumstances and on patient values and preferences.

INITIAL TREATMENT OF DEEP VEIN THROMBOSIS

Anticoagulant therapy

Anticoagulant therapy is the initial treatment of choice for most patients with symptomatic DVT (grade 1A) (7). The absolute contraindications to anticoagulant treatment include intracranial bleeding, severe active bleeding, recent brain, eye or spinal cord surgery and malignant hypertension. Relative contraindications include recent major surgery, recent large thromboembolic stroke, active gastrointestinal tract bleeding, severe hypertension, severe renal or hepatic failure and severe thrombocytopenia (platelets <50 000/L).

Initial therapy with continuous intravenous heparin was the standard approach for the treatment of DVT from the 1960s through the 1980s. During the 1990s, low molecular weight heparin (LMWH) given by subcutaneous injection once or twice daily was evaluated in clinical trials and shown to be as effective and safe as continuous intravenous heparin for the initial treatment of patients with proximal DVT.

The synthetic pentasaccharide fondaparinux, which selectively inhibits factor Xa, has been evaluated by large randomized clinical trials (14,15). Fondaparinux is as effective and safe as LMWH for treatment of established DVT (7,14).

The advantage of LMWH and fondaparinux is that these drugs do not require anticoagulant monitoring (grade 1A) (7) and can be given in fixed doses by subcutaneous injection. LMWH given once or twice daily or fondaparinux given once daily are preferred over intravenous unfractionated heparin for the initial treatment of most patients with DVT (grade 1A) (7). Treatment with LMWH or fondaparinux allows outpatient therapy for many patients with DVT. Table 22.1 lists the specific drug regimens that are effective for the initial treatment of DVT as shown by high-quality randomized clinical trials. Intravenous unfractionated heparin is suggested in place of LMWH or fondaparinux for initial anticoagulant therapy in patients with severe renal failure (grade 2C) (7).

If unfractionated heparin is used for initial therapy, it is important to achieve an adequate anticoagulant effect, defined as an activated partial thromboplastin time (aPTT) above the lower limit of therapeutic range within the first 24 h (16,17). Failure to achieve an adequate aPTT effect early during therapy is associated with a high incidence (25%) of recurrent venous thromboembolism (16). Two-thirds of the recurrent events occur between 2 and 12 weeks after the initial diagnosis, despite treatment with oral anticoagulants (17). The clinical trial data indicate that initial management with either adequate unfractionated heparin or with LMWH or fondaparinux is critical to reducing the long-term risk of recurrent venous thromboembolism (3,16,17).

Initial treatment with LMWH, fondaparinux or unfractionated heparin should be continued for at least 5 days (grade 1C) (7).

Table 22.1   Regimens of LMWH and fondaparinux for treatment of deep vein thrombosis

Drug	Regimen
Enoxaparin	1.0 mg/kg bid[a]
Dalteparin	200 IU/kg once daily[b]
Tinzaparin	175 IU/kg once daily[c]
Nadroparin	6150 IU bid for 50–70 kg[d]
Reviparin	4200 IU bid for 46–60 kg[e]
Fondaparinux	7.5 mg once daily for 50–100 kg[f]

[a]A once-daily regimen of 1.5 mg/kg can be used but probably is less effective in patients at high risk of recurrence, such as those with cancer and in obese patients.
[b]After 1 month, can be followed by 150 IU/kg once daily as an alternative to an oral vitamin K antagonist for long-term treatment in patients with cancer.
[c]This regimen can also be used for long-term treatment as an alternative to an oral vitamin K antagonist.
[d]4100 IU bid if patient weighs <50 kg or 9200 IU bid if patient weighs >70 kg.
[e]3500 IU bid if patient weighs 35–45 kg or 6300 IU bid if patient weighs >60 kg.
[f]5 mg once daily if patient weighs <50 kg or 10 mg once daily if patient weighs >100 kg.

Thrombolytic therapy

The role of thrombolytic therapy in patients with DVT is limited. Thrombolytic therapy may be indicated in patients with acute massive proximal vein thrombosis (e.g., phlegmasia cerulea dolens with impending venous gangrene) or in selected patients with acute extensive proximal vein thrombosis (e.g., extensive iliofemoral thrombosis), symptoms for <14 days, good functional status, life expectancy for >1 year, who have a low risk of bleeding, with the goal of reducing acute symptoms and post-thrombotic morbidity. Thrombolytic therapy can be given by catheter-directed infusion (grade 2B) or by systemic infusion (grade 2C) (7). The catheter-directed approach may be associated with a lower risk of major bleeding, particularly intracranial bleeding, than systemic injection and is probably preferred if the appropriate expertise and facilities are available. After successful catheter-directed thrombolysis, correction of the underlying venous lesion with angioplasty and/or stenting may be indicated (grade 2C) (7). Further randomized clinical trials of sufficient size and follow-up are required to determine the relative benefits, risks and cost-effectiveness of catheter-directed thrombolysis, with or without mechanical adjuncts such as thrombus fragmentation, aspiration, angioplasty or stent placement, compared with standard anticoagulant therapy alone.

Inferior vena cava filter

Insertion of an inferior vena cava filter is indicated for patients with acute DVT who have a contraindication to anticoagulant therapy (grade 1C), (7) and for the rare patient who has recurrent venous thromboembolism during adequate anticoagulant therapy.

Insertion of a vena cava filter is effective for preventing clinically important PE. However, use of a filter results in an increased incidence of recurrent DVT 1–2 years after insertion (increase in cumulative incidence at 2 years from 12 to 21%) (12). If the contraindication to anticoagulant therapy is transient, long-term anticoagulant treatment should be started as soon as safely possible after placement of a vena cava filter to prevent morbidity from recurrent DVT (grade 1C) (7).

LONG-TERM TREATMENT OF DEEP VEIN THROMBOSIS

Long-term anticoagulant therapy is required to prevent a high frequency (15–25%) of symptomatic extension of thrombosis and/or recurrent venous thromboembolic events (1,5,7). Oral anticoagulant treatment using a vitamin K antagonist (e.g., warfarin) is currently the preferred approach for long-term treatment in most patients. Treatment with adjusted doses of unfractionated heparin or LMWH is indicated for selected patients in whom vitamin K antagonists are contraindicated (e.g., pregnant women) or impractical or in patients with concurrent cancer for whom LMWH regimens have been shown to be more effective (7,18,19).

Vitamin K antagonist therapy

Treatment with a vitamin K antagonist is started together with initial LMWH, fondaparinux or unfractionated heparin on the first treatment day rather than delayed (grade 1A) and overlapped for at least 4–5 days; the heparin or fondaparinux is then discontinued provided that the international normalized ratio (INR) is 2.0 or more for 24 h (grade 1C) (7).

The preferred intensity of the anticoagulant effect of treatment using a vitamin K antagonist has been established by clinical trials (7,20–23). The dose of the vitamin K antagonist should be adjusted to maintain a target INR of 2.5 (range, 2.0–3.0), for all treatment durations (grade 1A) (7). For patients with unprovoked DVT who have a strong preference for less frequent INR testing, after the 3 months of vitamin K antagonist therapy at conventional intensity (INR 2.0–3.0), low-intensity therapy (target INR 1.75, range 1.5–1.9) is preferable to stopping anticoagulant therapy (grade 1A), but less effective than conventional intensity therapy (21). Importantly, low-intensity vitamin K antagonist therapy did not reduce bleeding in the single randomized trial that directly compared these regimens, (21) and therefore, the reason to select low-intensity therapy would be based on patient preference for somewhat less frequent monitoring. High-intensity vitamin K antagonist treatment (INR 3.1 to 4.0) should not be used (grade 1A) (7) because it does not improve effectiveness in patients with the antiphospholipid syndrome and recurrent thrombosis (22) and results in more bleeding (23).

The appropriate duration of oral anticoagulant treatment for venous thromboembolism using a vitamin K antagonist has been evaluated by multiple randomized clinical trials (7,20,24–29). Treatment should be continued for at least 3 months in patients with a first episode of proximal-vein thrombosis secondary to a transient (reversible) risk factor (grade 1A) (7). Stopping treatment at 4 to 6 weeks resulted in an increased incidence of recurrent venous thromboembolism during the following 6–12 months (absolute risk increase 8%). In contrast, treatment for 3–6 months resulted in a low rate of recurrent venous thromboembolism during the following 1–2 years (annual incidence 3%). For patients with a first episode of unprovoked DVT, anticoagulant therapy with a vitamin K antagonist should be continued for at least 3 months (grade 1A) (7). The term 'unprovoked' refers to the clinical presentation of symptomatic DVT in the absence of a provoking risk factor, such as surgery or hospitalization for medical illness, and has also been called 'idiopathic' thrombosis. After 3 months of therapy, patients with unprovoked (idiopathic) DVT should be evaluated for the benefits and risks of extended long-term therapy (grade 1C) (7). For patients with a first unprovoked proximal vein thrombosis, in whom risk factors for bleeding are absent and for whom good anticoagulant (INR) monitoring is achievable, continued long-term treatment is recommended (grade 1A) (7). This recommendation places a higher value on avoiding recurrent venous thromboembolism and a lower value on the risks and burden of continued long-term anticoagulant treatment. Such treatment should be continued indefinitely. The term 'indefinite' means that the therapy does not have a scheduled stop date, but may be stopped if the patient's risk of bleeding subsequently increases or if there is a change in the patient's preference. The need for an 'indefinite' duration of therapy is based on the results of a randomized trial which found a loss of benefit upon withdrawal of anticoagulant treatment at 12 months, with similar rates of recurrent venous thromboembolism at 2 years among patients who were treated for only 6 months or for 1 year (29). If indefinite anticoagulant treatment is prescribed, the risks and benefits of continuing such treatment and the patient's preference, should be reassessed at periodic intervals (grade 1C) (7).

Oral vitamin K antagonist treatment should be given indefinitely for most patients with a second episode of unprovoked venous thromboembolism (grade 1A) (7). Stopping treatment at 3–6 months in these patients results in a high incidence (21%) of recurrent venous thromboembolism during the following 4 years. The risk of recurrent thromboembolism was reduced by 87% (from 21 to 3%) by continuing anticoagulant treatment (27). This benefit was partially offset by an increase in the cumulative incidence of major bleeding (from 3 to 9%). More recent clinical trials of indefinite duration vitamin K antagonist therapy (21) and a meta-analysis of seven trials (30) suggest the rate of major bleeding to be 1.1% per patient-year, compared with 0.6% per patient-year without anticoagulation. However, the risk of major bleeding in an individual patient may differ from these estimates and should be considered carefully in weighing the risks and benefits of indefinite therapy. On the other hand, all of the available evidence indicates that patients with unprovoked venous thromboembolism lose the benefit of protection against recurrent thromboembolism when anticoagulants are withdrawn (7), even after one or more years of therapy. Therefore, the patient's values and preferences regarding preventing recurrent thromboembolism, avoiding bleeding and the inconvenience of continued anticoagulant treatment weigh significantly on the decision and should be discussed in detail with patients.

A variety of prothrombotic conditions or markers reportedly are associated with an increased risk of recurrent venous thromboembolism, as described in more detail in Chapter 1. These conditions include deficiencies of the naturally occurring inhibitors of coagulation such as antithrombin, protein C and protein S, specific gene mutations including factor V Leiden and prothrombin 20210A, elevated levels of coagulation factor VIII, elevated levels of homocysteine and the presence of antiphospholipid antibodies. The presence of residual DVT assessed by compression ultrasonography (31), elevated levels of plasma D-dimer after discontinuation of anticoagulant treatment (32) and male gender (33) have been associated with an increased incidence of recurrent thromboembolism. However, the available data are limited to subgroup analyses of randomized trials and data from observational studies. No randomized trials have been performed, a priori, in these subgroups of patients with thrombophilic conditions to evaluate the risk–benefit of different durations of anticoagulant treatment. The role of these parameters in guiding clinical decision making about the duration of treatment remains uncertain and further well-designed randomized trials are needed.

For patients with a first episode of DVT and documented antiphospholipid antibodies or two or more hereditary thrombophilic conditions (e.g., combined factor V Leiden and prothrombin 20210A gene mutations), the risk of recurrent venous thromboembolism is particularly high and many of these patients may be considered for indefinite anticoagulant treatment. For patients with a first episode of DVT who have documented deficiency of antithrombin, protein C or protein S or the factor V Leiden or prothrombin 20210A gene mutation, hyper-homocysteinaemia or high factor VIII levels (>90th percentile), the duration of treatment should be individualized after the patients have completed at least 3 months of anticoagulant therapy. Some of these patients also may be candidates for indefinite therapy.

Low molecular weight heparin

The use of LMWH for long-term treatment of venous thromboembolism has been evaluated in clinical trials. The studies indicate that long-term treatment with subcutaneous LMWH for 3–6 months is at least as effective and in cancer patients, more effective than, an oral vitamin K antagonist adjusted to maintain the INR between 2.0 and 3.0 (18,19,34). LMWH also was associated with less bleeding complications because of a reduction in minor bleeding (34).

For patients with DVT and concurrent cancer, LMWH is recommended for the first 3–6 months of long-term treatment (grade 1A) (7). The patients should receive subsequent anticoagulant therapy with either LMWH or a vitamin K antagonist indefinitely or until the cancer resolves (grade 1C). The regimens of LMWH that are established as effective for long-term treatment are dalteparin 200 U/kg once daily for 1 month, followed by 150 U/kg daily thereafter (18), or tinzaparin 175 U/kg once daily (19,34).

Long-acting pentasaccharides: idraparinux and idrabiotaparinux

Idraparinux is a hypermethylated derivative of fondaparinux that inhibits factor Xa indirectly through its action on antithrombin. The very high affinity for antithrombin influences the idraparinux pharmacokinetics, such that the elimination half-life from the plasma of idraparinux is approximately 80 h (35). This long elimination half-life enables idraparinux to be given once weekly by subcutaneous injection, instead of once daily as for fondaparinux. Following promising results in a phase II study of patients with DVT (36), idraparinux 2.5 mg given once weekly was evaluated as an alternative to standard therapy with a heparin and vitamin K antagonist for the treatment of patients with either DVT or PE (37) and for extended anticoagulant therapy in patients with venous thromboembolism who had completed an initial 6 months of anticoagulant therapy (38).

In the study of 2904 patients with DVT, the incidence of symptomatic recurrent venous thromboembolism at 3 months was 2.9% in the idraprinux group compared with 3.0% for standard therapy, indicating non-inferiority of idraparinux (37). The rates of clinically relevant bleeding during 3 months of treatment were 4.5% for idraparinux and 7.0% for standard therapy ($p < 0.01$); at 6 months, bleeding rates were similar (8.3 and 8.1% respectively). In the study of 2215 patients with PE, however, the rate of recurrent thromboembolism was 3.4% for idraparinux and 1.6% for standard therapy ($p < 0.05$), indicating that idraparinux was less efficacious in this patient group (37). The difference in efficacy was due to an excess of fatal and non-fatal recurrent PE within the first 1–2 weeks of treatment.

These results establish the concept that patients with DVT can be treated with a single long-acting anticoagulant given once weekly, without anticoagulant monitoring, and achieve similar effectiveness and safety to current standard therapy with LMWH overlapped with, and followed by, a vitamin K antagonist, when used for 3–6 months of treatment. For patients with PE, either larger doses of idraparinux are needed or an alternate anticoagulant will need to be given for initial therapy.

In the study of extended anticoagulant therapy, 1215 patients who had received 6 months of anticoagulant therapy were randomly assigned to continue anticoagulant therapy using 2.5 mg idraparinux subcutaneously given once weekly, without anticoagulant monitoring or to subcutaneous placebo, for a further 6 months (38). Among the 1215 patients, recurrent venous thromboembolism occurred in 1.0% given idraparinux and in 3.7% given placebo ($p < 0.01$). Major bleeding occurred in 11 patients (1.9%) given idraparinux, including three intracranial bleeds, compared with none who received placebo ($p < 0.01$). Hence idraparinux was effective for preventing recurrent venous thromboembolism but, associated with an increased risk of major bleeding (38).

Collectively, the phase III studies with idraparinux suggest that an approach using subcutaneous injection once weekly, without anticoagulant monitoring, is a feasible strategy for long-term anticoagulant therapy of patients with DVT. However, further understanding of the pharmacokinetics of idraparinux, including the time to achieve a steady state and the distribution kinetics of the drug, are needed. The regimen will need to be modified to ensure that the drug does not accumulate once a steady state is achieved and contribute to an increased bleeding incidence. Such studies are required before this approach can be implemented in clinical practice and are in progress with a modified form of idraparinux, known as idrabiotaparinux.

Idrabiotaparinux, formerly known as SSR12517E, is a biotinylated form of idraparinux which exhibits essentially the same pharmacokinetic profile as idraprinux, but which has the advantage that its anticoagulant effect can be rapidly neutralized by the intravenous infusion of avidin (35). Avidin is a large protein derived from egg white, which binds to the biotin moiety of idrabiotaparinux, and the complex is then cleared by the kidneys. Idrabiotaprinux is undergoing phase III evaluation in an equipotency study of patients with DVT and in patients with PE following an initial course of LMWH.

New oral anticoagulants

Several new oral anticoagulants which bind directly to the target coagulation enzyme of either thrombin or factor Xa are currently undergoing evaluation in phase III clinical trials for the treatment of patients with DVT (35). The potential advantages of these drugs are (1) they can be administered orally once or twice daily without the need for anticoagulant monitoring and dose titration, (2) there are fewer clinically relevant drug interactions and (3) because of a fast onset of anticoagulant action, similar to that of LMWH, they have the potential to simplify treatment by replacing the current approach of a parenteral drug (LMWH or fondaparinux) followed by an oral vitamin K antagonist with a single drug given for both initial and long-term therapy.

The first such drug to undergo phase III studies was ximelagatran, an oral direct thrombin inhibitor. Ximelagatran was shown to be of similar effectiveness to standard therapy with LMWH followed by a vitamin K antagonist(39), and was also effective for preventing recurrent venous thromboembolism during extended long-term therapy, with a rate of major bleeding similar to that with placebo (40). However, the drug was associated with hepatotoxicity (35). The studies with ximelagatran were nevertheless important conceptually by establishing the feasibility of effectively treating DVT using a single drug given orally without anticoagulant monitoring.

The new oral anticoagulant drugs currently undergoing evaluation in phase III trials for the treatment of DVTs are the direct thrombin inhibitor dabigatran and the direct factor Xa inhibitors rivaroxaban and apixaban (35). Several other oral direct factor Xa inhibitors are also potential candidates for clinical evaluation for the treatment of DVT (35).

SIDE-EFFECTS OF ANTICOAGULANT THERAPY

Bleeding

Bleeding is the most common side effect of anticoagulant therapy. Bleeding can be classified as major or minor according to standardized international criteria. Major bleeding is defined as clinically overt bleeding resulting in a decline of haemoglobin of at least 2 g/dL, transfusion of at least 2 U of packed red cells or bleeding that is retroperitoneal or intracranial. The rates of major bleeding in clinical trials of initial therapy with intravenous heparin, LMWH or fondaparinux are

1–2% (14,15,41). Patients at increased risk of major bleeding are those who underwent surgery or experienced trauma within the previous 14 days, those with a history of gastrointestinal bleeding, peptic ulcer disease or genitourinary bleeding and those with miscellaneous conditions predisposing to bleeding, such as thrombocytopenia, liver disease and multiple invasive lines.

Major bleeding occurs in approximately 2% of patients during the first 3 months of oral anti-coagulant treatment using a vitamin K antagonist and in approximately 1% per year of treatment thereafter (42). A meta-analysis suggests the clinical impact of major bleeding during long-term oral vitamin K antagonist treatment is greater than widely appreciated. The estimated case fatality rate for major bleeding is 13% and the rate of intracranial bleeding was 1.15 per 100 patient-years (42). These risks are important considerations in the decision about extended or indefinite antico-agulant therapy in patients with DVT.

Heparin-induced thrombocytopenia

Heparin or LMWH may cause thrombocytopenia. In large clinical studies of acute venous throm-boembolism treatment, thrombocytopenia occurred in fewer than 1% of more than 2000 patients treated with unfractionated heparin or LMWH (14,15). Nevertheless, heparin-induced thrombo-cytopenia (HIT) can be a serious complication when accompanied by extension or recurrence of venous thromboembolism or the development of arterial thrombosis. Such complications may pre-cede or coincide with the fall in platelet count and have been associated with a high rate of limb loss and a high mortality. Heparin in all forms should be discontinued when the diagnosis of HIT is made on clinical grounds and treatment with an alternative anticoagulant such as danaparoid, lepirudin or argatroban should be initiated. Treatment with an oral vitamin K antagonist should be started or resumed once the thrombocytopenia resolves. It is given in low daily doses overlapping for at least 5 days with the alternative anticoagulant that is discontinued once a stable INR is achieved.

Heparin-induced osteoporosis

Osteoporosis may occur as a result of long-term treatment with heparin or LMWH (usually after more than 6 months). The earliest clinical manifestation of heparin-associated osteoporosis usually consists of non-specific low back pain primarily involving the vertebrae or the ribs. Patients may also present with spontaneous fractures. Up to one-third of patients treated with long-term heparin may have a subclinical reduction in bone density. Whether these patients are predisposed to future fractures is not known. The incidence of symptomatic osteoporosis in clinical trials of LMWH treatment for 3–6 months was very low and not increased compared with warfarin treatment (18,34). Patients with osteoporosis or fractures often had other risk factors such as bone metastases.

Hepatotoxicity

Heparin or LMWH may cause elevated liver transaminase levels. These elevations are of unknown clinical significance and usually return to normal after the heparin or LMWH is discontinued. Awareness of this biochemical effect is important so as to avoid unnecessary interruption of heparin therapy and unnecessary liver biopsies in patients who may develop elevated transaminase levels during heparin or LMWH therapy.

The oral direct thrombin inhibitor ximelagatran was denied approval by the FDA and withdrawn from the world market due to associated hepatotoxicity(35), manifest by elevated liver transaminase enzymes, combined elevation of transaminases and bilirubin (Hy's rule) and, in three cases, clinical features of liver failure and death. This has led to increased sensitivity on the part of regulatory authorities to safety monitoring for hepatotoxicity in the ongoing clinical development of new oral anticoagulants and their evaluation for the treatment of venous thromboembolism. If these new drugs are successful, periodic monitoring of liver transaminase enzymes will probably be required.

REFERENCES

1. Hull R, Delmore T, Genton E, *et al.* Warfarin sodium versus low-dose heparin in the long-term treatment of venous thrombosis. *N Engl J Med* 1979; **301**:855–58.
2. Hull R, Raskob G, Hirsh J, *et al.* Continuous intravenous heparin compared with intermittent subcutaneous heparin in the initial treatment of proximal vein thrombosis. *N Engl J Med* 1986; **315**:1109–14.
3. Brandjes D, Heijboer H, Büller H, *et al.* Acenocoumarol and heparin compared with acenocoumarol alone in the initial treatment of proximal vein thrombosis. *N Engl J Med* 1992; **327**:1485–89.
4. Moser KM, Lemoine JR. Is embolic risk conditioned by localization of deep venous thrombosis? *Ann Intern Med* 1981; **94**:439–44.
5. Lagerstedt C, Olsson C, Fagher B, *et al.* Need for long-term anticoagulant treatment in symptomatic calf-vein thrombosis. *Lancet* 1986; **ii**:515–18.
6. Prandoni P, Polistena P, Bernardi E, *et al.* Upper-extremity deep vein thrombosis. Risk factors, diagnosis and complications. *Arch Intern Med* 1997; **157**:57–62.
7. Kearon C, Kahn S, Agnelli G, Goldhaber S, Raskob G, Comerota A. Antithrombotic therapy for venous thromboembolic disease: American College of Chest Physicians Evidence-based Clinical Practice Guidelines (8th edition). *Chest* 2008; **133**(Suppl):454S–545S.
8. Kahn S, Ginsberg J. Relationship between deep venous thrombosis and the postthrombotic syndrome. *Arch Intern Med* 2004; **164**:17–26.
9. Prandoni P, Lensing AWA, Cogo A, *et al.* The long-term clinical course of acute deep venous thrombosis. *Ann Intern Med* 1996; **125**:1–7.
10. van Dongen CJJ, van der Belt AGG, Prins MH, *et al.* Fixed dose subcutaneous low-molecular weight heparins versus adjusted dose unfractionated heparin for venous thromboembolism. *Cochrane Database Syst Rev* 2004; **(4)**: CD001100.
11. Brandjes D, Büller H, Heijboer H, *et al.* Randomized trial of the effect of compression stockings in patients with symptomatic proximal-vein thrombosis. *Lancet* 1997; **349**:759–62.
12. Decousus H, Leizorovicz A, Parent F, *et al.* A clinical trial of vena caval filters in the prevention of pulmonary embolism in patients with proximal deep-vein thrombosis. *N Engl J Med* 1998; **338**:409–16.
13. Guyatt G, Cook D, Jaeschke R, Pauker S, Schunemann H. Grades of recommendation for antithrombotic agents: American College of Chest Physicians Clinical Practice Guidelines (8th edition). *Chest* 2008; **133**(Suppl):123S–131S.
14. Büller H, Davidson B, Decousus H, *et al.* Fondaparinux or enoxaparin for the initial treatment of symptomatic deep venous thrombosis. A randomized trial. *Ann Intern Med* 2004; **140**:867–73.
15. Matisse Investigators. Subcutaneous fondaparinux versus intravenous unfractionated heparin in the initial treatment of pulmonary embolism. *N Engl J Med* 2003; **349**:1695–1702.
16. Hull RD, Raskob GE, Brant RF, *et al.* Relation between the time to achieve the lower limit of the APTT therapeutic range and recurrent venous thromboembolism during heparin treatment for deep vein thrombosis. *Arch Intern Med* 1997; **157**:2562–68.
17. Hull RD, Raskob GE, Brant RF, *et al.* The importance of initial heparin treatment on long-term clinical outcomes of antithrombotic therapy: The emerging theme of delayed recurrence. *Arch Intern Med* 1997; **157**:2317–21.
18. Lee A, Levine M, Baker R, *et al.* Low-molecular-weight heparin versus a coumarin for the prevention of recurrent venous thromboembolism in patients with cancer. *N Engl J Med* 2003; **349**:146–153.
19. Hull R, Pineo G, Brant R, *et al.* Long-term low-molecular weight heparin versus usual care in proximal vein thrombosis patients with cancer. *Am J Med* 2006; **119**:1062–72.

20. Ridker P, Goldhaber S, Danielson E, *et al.* Long-term low-intensity warfarin therapy for the prevention of recurrent venous thromboembolism. *N Engl J Med* 2003; **348**:1425–34.
21. Kearon C, Ginsberg J, Kovacs M, *et al.* Comparison of low-intensity warfarin therapy with conventional intensity warfarin therapy for long-term prevention of recurrent venous thromboembolism. *N Engl J Med* 2003; **349**:631–39.
22. Crowther M, Ginsberg J, Julian J, *et al.* A comparison of two intensities of warfarin for the prevention of recurrent thrombosis in patients with the antiphospholipid antibody syndrome. *N Engl J Med* 2003; **349**:1133–38.
23. Hull R, Hirsh J, Jay R, *et al.* Different intensities of oral anticoagulant therapy in the treatment of proximal vein thrombosis. *N Engl J Med* 1982; **307**:1676–81.
24. Optimum duration of anticoagulation for deep-vein thrombosis and pulmonary embolism. Research Committee of the British Thoracic Society. *Lancet* 1992; **340**:873–76.
25. Schulman S, Rhedin A-S, Lindmarker P, *et al.* A comparison of six weeks with six months of oral anti-coagulant therapy after a first episode of venous thromboembolism. *N Engl J Med* 1995; **332**:1661–65.
26. Levine M, Hirsh J, Gent M, *et al.* Optimal duration of oral anticoagulant therapy: a randomized trial comparing four weeks with three months of warfarin in patients with proximal deep-vein thrombosis. *Thromb Haemost* 1995; **74**:606–611.
27. Schulman S, Granqvist S, Holmström M, *et al.* The duration of oral anticoagulant therapy after a second episode of venous thromboembolism. *N Engl J Med* 1997; **336**:393–398.
28. Kearon C, Gent M, Hirsh J, *et al.* A comparison of three months of anticoagulation with extended anticoagulation for a first-episode of idiopathic venous thromboembolism. *N Engl J Med* 1999; **340**:901–907.
29. Agnelli G, Prandoni P, Santamaria M, *et al.* Three months versus one year of oral anticoagulant therapy for idiopathic deep-venous thrombosis. *N Engl J Med* 2001; **345**:165–169.
30. Ost D, Tepper J, Mihara H *et al.* Duration of anticoagulation following venous thromboembolism: a meta-analysis. *JAMA* 2005; **294**:706–15.
31. Prandoni P, Lensing A, Prins M, *et al.* Residual venous thrombosis as a predictive factor of recurrent venous thromboembolism. *Ann Intern Med* 2002; **137**:955–60.
32. Eichinger S, Minar E, Bialonczyk C, *et al.* D-dimer levels and risk of recurrent venous thromboembolism. *JAMA* 2003; **290**:1071–74.
33. Kyrle P, Minar E, Bialonczyk, *et al.* The risk of recurrent venous thromboembolism in men and women. *N Engl J Med* 2004; **350**:2558–63.
34. Hull R, Pineo G, Brant R, *et al.* Self-managed long-term low-molecular weight heparin therapy: the balance of benefits and harms. *Am J Med* 2007; **120**:72–82.
35. Weitz J, Hirsh J, Samama M. New antithrombotic drugs: American College of Chest Physicians Clinical Practice Guidelines (8th edition). *Chest* 2008; **133**(Suppl):234S–256S.
36. Persist Investigators. A novel long-acting synthetic factor Xa inhibitor (SanOrg 34006) to replace warfarin for secondary prevention in deep-vein thrombosis: a phase II evaluation. *J Thromb Haemost* 2004; **2**:47–53.
37. The van Gogh Investigators. Idraparinux versus standard therapy for venous thromboembolic disease. *N Engl J Med* 2007; **357**:1094–1104.
38. The van Gogh Investigators. Extended prophylaxis of venous thromboembolism with idraparinux. *N Engl J Med* 2007; **357**:1105–12.
39. Fiessinger J, Huisman M, Davidson B, *et al.* Ximelagatran versus low-molecular-weight heparin and warfarin for the treatment of deep-vein thrombosis. *JAMA* 2005; **293**:681–689.
40. Schulman S, Wahlander K, Lundstrom T, *et al.* Secondary prevention of venous thromboembolism with the oral direct thrombin inhibitor ximelagatran. The THRIVE III Study. *N Engl J Med* 2003; **349**:1713–21.
41. Quinlan D, McQuillan A, Eikelboom J. Low-molecular-weight heparin compared with intravenous unfractionated heparin for treatment of pulmonary embolism. *Ann Intern Med* 2004; **140**:175–183.
42. Linkins L, Choi P, Douketis J. Clinical impact of bleeding in patients taking oral anticoagulant therapy for venous thromboembolism. A meta-analysis. *Ann Intern Med* 2003; **139**:893–900.

CHAPTER 23

Initial and Long-term Treatment of Patients with Pulmonary Embolism

Guy Meyer[1] and Victor Tapson[2]

[1]Division of Pulmonary and Intensive Care Medicine, Assistance Publique Hopitaux de Paris, Faculté de Medecine, Université Paris Descartes, Hôpital Européen Georges Pompidou, Paris, France
[2]Division of Pulmonary and Critical Care Medicine, Duke University Medical Center, Durham, USA

INTRODUCTION

Deep vein thrombosis (DVT) and pulmonary embolism (PE) are considered to be different manifestations of the same disease – venous thromboembolism – and there is little difference in the anticoagulant treatment of these two manifestations. However, the treatment of PE differs from that of DVT in several respects, which will be described here. Patients with massive PE generally suffer respiratory failure and circulatory collapse, requiring specific symptomatic treatment. Thrombolytic treatment and pulmonary embolectomy may also be considered in these patients. There are generally two phases of PE treatment: initial parenteral anticoagulation treatment with heparin, low molecular weight heparin or fondaparinux and long-term treatment with oral anticoagulants. However, the development of new oral compounds for both initial and long-term treatment may eliminate this distinction in the near future.

INITIAL TREATMENT OF PULMONARY EMBOLISM

Risk stratification for patients with pulmonary embolism

The definition of massive PE has long been based on the extent of pulmonary vascular obstruction, as assessed by pulmonary angiography. Pulmonary vascular resistance increases sharply when vascular obstruction exceeds 50–60% (1). This level of pulmonary vascular obstruction has therefore been used in the past to define massive PE. However, recent data strongly suggest that PE-related mortality is linked to clinical findings at the time of diagnosis rather than to the degree

Deep Vein Thrombosis and Pulmonary Embolism   Edited by Edwin J.R. van Beek, Harry R. Büller and Matthijs Oudkerk
© 2009 John Wiley & Sons, Ltd

of vascular obstruction itself. In the ICOPER registry, the mortality rate was 58% in patients with haemodynamic instability but only 15% in clinically stable patients (2). In the same study, a systolic blood pressure below 90 mmHg was independently associated with a greater risk of death [odds ratio (OR), 2.9; 95% confidence interval (CI), 1.7 to 5.0]. Another large, multicentre registry included 1001 patients with major PE, defined as right heart failure or pulmonary hypertension (3). Four patient groups were defined prospectively: (1) patients with evidence of right ventricular pressure overload or pulmonary hypertension, but with normal blood pressure; (2) patients with arterial hypotension (systolic blood pressure <90 mmHg or a drop of at least 40 mmHg for more than 15 min), but without cardiogenic shock or need for catecholamine support; (3) patients with arterial hypotension and cardiogenic shock and/or need for catecholamine administration to maintain adequate tissue perfusion; (4) patients with circulatory collapse who underwent cardiopulmonary resuscitation. The hospital mortality rate was 8.1% in group 1, 15.2% in group 2, 25% in group 3 and 62.5% in group 4 (3). Other studies have confirmed these findings, suggesting that the early mortality rate in patients with shock exceeds 25% (4–6). Based on these data, the definition of massive PE is now based on clinical rather than angiographic parameters and, more specifically, on the presence of haemodynamic instability (persistent arterial hypotension and/or cardiogenic shock) at presentation (7).

PE patients in a stable haemodynamic condition at presentation have a low death rate on anticoagulant treatment, provided that they have no major underlying disease. A meta-analysis comparing unfractionated heparin with low molecular weight heparin for the initial treatment of PE found in-hospital mortality rates of 1.4% for unfractionated heparin and 1.2% for low molecular weight heparin, but most patients had asymptomatic PE with symptomatic deep venous thrombosis (8). More recently, the overall mortality rate of 1017 clinically stable patients with symptomatic PE included in a multicentre randomized clinical trial and receiving low molecular weight heparin followed by a course of 6 months of oral anticoagulant treatment was reported to be 4.4% (9).

Several studies have tried to identify a subgroup of patients with 'submassive PE' who may have a higher mortality rate than other patients with normal blood pressure. Ribeiro *et al.* showed that the mortality rate was higher in patients with right ventricular dysfunction (10 deaths among 70 patients; 14%) than in those with normal findings on echocardiography (no death among 56 patients; $p = 0.002$), although patients with haemodynamic instability were not assessed separately (10). In the ICOPER study, the in-hospital death rate of patients with right ventricular dysfunction on echocardiography was 18% although, again, patients with shock were not analysed separately (11). Several more recent studies have investigated the outcome of patients with normal blood pressure and right ventricular dysfunction on echocardiography (5,6,12–14). The mortality rate in these studies varied between 3 and 16% in patients with right ventricular dysfunction and between 0 and 8% in patients with normal echocardiography results. Although most studies have reported higher mortality rates in patients with right ventricular dysfunction (11,15,16), this has not been found in all studies (6,17). Right ventricular dysfunction on echocardiography was not defined in the same way in all studies and treatment was not controlled, with some patients receiving thrombolytic treatment. These limitations may account for the discrepancies observed.

High levels of brain natriuretic peptide, pro-brain natriuretic peptide and cardiac troponins T and I have all been associated with a greater risk of death in patients with PE. In one series, the in-hospital mortality of patients with normal blood pressure, high troponin levels and an enlarged right ventricle was 25% (18). Another study by the same group showed that clinically stable patients with high pro-brain natriuretic peptide levels had a mortality rate of 17% (19). Scridon *et al.* observed an overall 30 day mortality rate of 19.9% in another series of 141 patients with PE. Troponin I concentrations were high in 52% of the patients and the combination of right ventricular enlargement and high troponin I concentration found in 32% of the subjects was associated with a mortality rate of 38% (16). However, in most studies, patients in a stable haemodynamic condition and patients with shock were not analysed separately and different threshold values were used to define high levels of biomarkers. In addition, these findings were obtained in small numbers of patients recruited in single-centre studies and require confirmation in larger studies.

Aujesky *et al.* recently described a clinical score for predicting early mortality in patients with PE. This score was derived from a large hospital database and has been successively validated in several independent cohorts (20,21). Higher scores are associated with advanced age, being male, the number of associated co-morbid conditions and several clinical abnormalities. Patients can be assigned to five groups based on this score. Mortality rates 3 months after diagnosis are as follows: 2.5% for groups I and II, 7% for group III, 11% for group IV and 24% for group V (20–23).

Anticoagulant treatment

DVT and PE are considered to be different manifestations of the same disease process. Thus, most studies on the initial anticoagulant treatment of venous thromboembolism have included principally patients with DVT. Patients with PE comprise only a minority of the patients studied and their outcome is generally not given separately. However, patients treated for PE are more likely to die of recurrent PE than patients with DVT. The risk of fatal recurrent PE is four times higher in patients with PE than in patients with DVT during 3 months of anticoagulant treatment (1.5 versus 0.4%) (24). As a result, recent studies have specifically evaluated patients with PE (9,25). In the most recent large randomized trial, strikingly different results were obtained with idraparinux in patients with deep venous thrombosis and patients with PE (9).

Unfractionated heparin

Barritt and Jordan carried out the only randomized controlled trial comparing unfractionated heparin with no treatment in a small group of patients with PE diagnosed on clinical grounds (26). In this study, unfractionated heparin treatment was associated with a significantly lower rate of recurrent PE and death due to PE. Based on these data and the results of additional studies in patients with DVT, the experts of the last consensus conference of the American College of Chest Physicians (ACCP) strongly recommended the use of unfractionated heparin (or low molecular weight heparin) for the initial treatment of PE (27). No specific comparative trials have addressed the issues of the initiation of unfractionated heparin treatment, the overlap with oral anticoagulant treatment and monitoring of the anticoagulant effect of unfractionated heparin in patients with PE. The mode of administration of unfractionated heparin in patients with PE is therefore largely based on studies in patients with DVT. Most patients dying from PE do so within the first few hours of admission to hospital (28). This finding and the high mortality rate observed in untreated patients justify the early initiation of anticoagulant treatment while awaiting objective confirmation if PE is strongly suspected on clinical grounds.

The largest study of the use of unfractionated heparin in patients with PE reported to date is the Matisse PE trial, a randomized controlled trial comparing fondaparinux with unfractionated heparin for the initial treatment of PE (25). In this trial, 1110 patients with PE received unfractionated heparin as an initial intravenous bolus of at least 5000 IU, followed by at least 1250 IU per hour administered as a continuous intravenous infusion. The dose was subsequently adjusted to obtain an APTT value between 1.5 and 2.5 times the control value. Warfarin treatment was initiated in all patients within 72 h of the start of anticoagulant treatment. After 3 months of follow-up, 56 patients had experienced symptomatic and objectively confirmed recurrent venous thromboembolism (5.0%), 12 patients had experienced a major bleeding episode (1.1%) and 48 patients had died (4.4%) (25). These results confirm, in a large group of patients, that treatment with unfractionated heparin followed by warfarin is a safe and effective therapeutic option for patients with PE.

The use of unfractionated heparin is hampered by the need for an intravenous line, frequent dose adjustment and APTT monitoring. However, the results of the recent FIDO study suggest that this approach may be simplified in a significant number of patients (29). In this study, patients with venous thromboembolism, including 134 patients with PE, were allocated to groups given subcutaneous low molecular weight heparin twice daily or subcutaneous unfractionated heparin at an initial dose of 330 IU followed by 250 IU, twice daily, without APTT monitoring and dose adjustment. Both treatments overlapped with warfarin, which was continued for 3 months. The 139 patients with PE were not analysed separately, but recurrence and bleeding rates were low in both groups and did not differ significantly, allowing the authors to conclude that fixed-dose, unmonitored subcutaneous unfractionated heparin treatment is not inferior to a fixed dose of low molecular weight heparin for the initial treatment of venous thromboembolism (29). There is some evidence to suggest that the use of unfractionated heparin is associated with a higher risk of heparin-induced thrombocytopenia in patients receiving thromboprophylaxis after surgery, but there is little to suggest that this risk is increased during the short period of initial treatment for established venous thromboembolism (30). Indeed, no episode of heparin-induced thrombocytopenia was reported in patients receiving unfractionated heparin in the FIDO and Matisse PE studies, although platelet count was not routinely monitored in the FIDO study (25,29).

Unfractionated heparin is the only available option for the initial treatment of patients with PE and severe renal dysfunction. Due to its short half-life, unfractionated heparin is also a safe option for patients with a high risk of bleeding, such as patients who have recently suffered bleeding or undergone surgery. The use of low molecular weight heparin together with thrombolytic treatment has not been evaluated in PE. Thus, unfractionated heparin should be used in patients with massive PE receiving thrombolytic therapy.

Low molecular weight heparin

The THESEE study is the largest randomized study to have compared low molecular weight heparin and unfractionated heparin for the initial treatment of PE (31). In total, 612 patients with symptomatic PE were randomized to groups receiving tinzaparin at a fixed dose of 175 IU/kg subcutaneously once daily or intravenous heparin with dose adjustment to maintain APTT between two and three times the control value. In both treatment groups, warfarin was introduced between the first and third days of treatment and was continued for at least 3 months, with the international normalized ratio (INR) maintained at 2–3. By day 8, three of the 304 patients given tinzaparin had experienced a recurrent venous thromboembolic event, three had suffered major bleeding and four had died. Two of the 308 patients given unfractionated heparin had experienced recurrent disease, five had suffered major bleeding and three had died. The combined endpoint of recurrent thromboembolism, major haemorrhage or death was reached by nine patients (3%) in the tinzaparin group and nine patients in the heparin group (2.9%). At the end of the 3 month follow-up period, no difference was observed between the groups (31). Quinlan *et al*. carried out a meta-analysis of 12 trials comparing low molecular weight heparin and unfractionated heparin as initial treatments in 1951 patients with either symptomatic PE or asymptomatic PE and symptomatic DVT (8). They found a non-significant trend in favour of low molecular weight heparin for recurrent venous thromboembolism [relative risk (RR), 0.68; 95% CI, 0.42 to 1.09), major bleeding (RR, 0.67; 95%CI, 0.36 to 1.27) and death (RR, 0.77; 95% CI, 0.52 to 1.55) (8). The largest group of patients with pulmonary embolism receiving low molecular weight heparin followed by oral anticoagulant treatment reported to date is that studied in the recent van Gogh trial (9). In this study, 1120 clinically stable patients with symptomatic PE received standard treatment with unfractionated heparin ($n = 119$; 10.9%), low molecular weight heparin (tinzaparin or enoxaparin) ($n = 914$; 83.7%) or both low molecular weight heparin and unfractionated heparin ($n = 59$; 5.4%), followed by oral anticoagulant treatment for 3 or 6 months. After 3 months of treatment, 18 patients (1.6%) had experienced recurrent venous thromboembolism, 24 (2.1%) had suffered major bleeding and 32 (2.9%) had died. In the group of 1017 patients given 6 months of anticoagulant treatment, 20 patients (2%) had recurrent venous thromboembolism, 28 (2.6%) presented with major bleeding and 45 (4.4%) had died (9). A few patients received unfractionated heparin as the initial treatment, but these results mostly reflect the use of low molecular weight heparin and confirm, in a large group of patients, that the use of a fixed dose of low molecular weight heparin is a safe and effective treatment for patients with symptomatic PE.

Studies assessing low molecular weight heparin for the initial treatment of PE used a fixed dose of the drug adjusted for body weight, without anti-Xa monitoring. There is no convincing evidence to suggest that the risk of recurrent venous thromboembolism or bleeding depends on anti-Xa level in patients receiving low molecular weight heparin for the treatment of venous thromboembolism. Low molecular weight heparin may accumulate, increasing the risk of bleeding, in patients with renal failure (32). In such patients, it is generally recommended to use unfractionated heparin with dose adjusted to the APTT rather than low molecular weight heparin with anti-Xa measurement (27). Heparin-induced thrombocytopenia is a rare complication in medical patients treated with therapeutic doses of low molecular weight heparin. In a series of 728 patients receiving therapeutic doses of low molecular weight heparin for various indications, heparin-induced thrombocytopenia was observed in 0.8% of patients and was more frequent in patients who had (1.7%) previously been exposed to unfractionated heparin or low molecular weight heparin than in those who had not (0.3%) (33). Medical patients treated with therapeutic doses of low molecular weight heparin for periods of only 5–7 days are thought to have a low risk of heparin-induced thrombocytopenia and routine platelet count monitoring is therefore not required in these patients (34).

Fondaparinux

The use of fondaparinux for the initial treatment of PE was evaluated in the Matisse PE study (25). In this study, 2213 patients with PE were randomized to groups receiving fondaparinux subcutaneously once daily at a fixed dose adapted to body weight (5.0, 7.5 and 10.0 mg in patients weighing less than 50 kg, 50–100 kg and more than 100 kg, respectively) or heparin, given as a constant intravenous infusion, adapted to maintain APTT value between 1.5 and 2.5 times the control value. Oral anticoagulant treatment was started after 1–3 days of treatment in both groups and was continued for at least 3 months, with dose adaptation to maintain INR between 2 and 3. The study was designed as a non inferiority trial and the main end-point was the rate of objectively confirmed recurrent venous thromboembolism during the 3 month study period. Forty-two of the 1103 patients assigned to the fondaparinux group (3.8%) experienced symptomatic and objectively confirmed recurrent venous thromboembolism, versus 56 of the 1110 patients assigned to the unfractionated heparin group (5.0%), giving an absolute difference of – 1.2% in favour of fondaparinux (95% CI, – 3.0 to 0.5). This result indicates that a true difference of more than 0.5% in favour of heparin was unlikely, allowing the authors to conclude that fondaparinux was not inferior to heparin (25). Major bleeding was observed during initial treatment in 14 patients (1.2%) on fondaparinux and 12 patients (1.1%) on heparin. At the end of the 3 month period of treatment, 57 deaths (5.2%) were recorded in patients initially treated with fondaparinux and 48 (4.4%) deaths were recorded in patients initially treated with heparin (25).

Idraparinux

Idraparinux is a long-acting synthetic antithrombin inhibitor administered subcutaneously once per week. This compound was developed for both the initial and long-term treatment of venous thromboembolism. In the van Gogh PE study, 2215 patients with symptomatic and objectively confirmed PE were allocated to either idraparinux or standard treatment (9). Patients in the idraparinux received 2.5 mg of this drug in the form of a once weekly subcutaneous injection. For patients with a creatinine clearance of less than 30 mL/min, the second and subsequent doses were reduced to 1.5 mg. Patients in the standard treatment group received either unfractionated heparin (about 15% of the patients) or low molecular weight heparin (about 85% of the patients) followed by warfarin or acenocoumarol, initiated within 24 h of randomization with subsequent dose adjustments to keep the INR value between 2 and 3. Treatment was administered for 3 or 6 months in the two groups, as decided by the local investigator. The primary outcome was symptomatic recurrent venous thromboembolism, including deaths attributed to PE. The incidence of the primary outcome was expected to be 4% for the standard treatment group at 3 months and the study was designed to demonstrate the non inferiority of idraparinux with respect to standard treatment. The standard treatment was given to 1120 patients and 1095 patients received idraparinux. After 3 months of treatment, recurrent venous thromboembolism had occurred in 37 patients on idraparinux (3.4%) and 18 patients (1.6%) on standard treatment (OR, 2.14; 95% CI, 1.21 to 3.78). In total, 2010 patients were given 6 months of anticoagulant treatment: 993 were allocated to the idraparinux group and 1017 to the standard therapy group. Recurrent venous thromboembolism occurred in 40 patients (4%) allocated to the idraparinux group and 20 patients (2%) allocated to the standard therapy group (hazard ratio, 2.09; 95% CI, 1.22 to 3.57). The difference in the incidence of recurrent events between the groups originated mostly during the first 2 weeks of treatment and was related to objectively confirmed recurrent events and PE-related deaths. It should be noted, however, that the rate of recurrent venous thromboembolism in the standard treatment group was lower than expected in PE patients and was even lower in patients with PE than in patients with DVT receiving the same standard treatment. More patients receiving idraparinux in the PE study died during the 6 month treatment period [64 patients (6.4%) versus 45 patients (4.4%) on standard treatment, $p = 0.04$]. In patients treated for 6 months, clinically relevant bleeding occurred in 76 patients allocated to the idraparinux group (7.7%) and 99 patients (9.7%) allocated to the standard treatment group ($p = 0.10$). Significantly less bleeding was observed with idraparinux than with the standard treatment after 3 and 6 months of treatment (9).

Treatment of circulatory collapse and respiratory failure

Occasionally, patients with PE present with circulatory collapse or respiratory failure. In large registries, these patients account for less than 5% of all patients admitted with PE (2). The treatment of these patients combines symptomatic interventions to reverse haemodynamic instability and respiratory failure and treatments aiming to decrease pulmonary vascular obstruction rapidly. Thrombolytic treatment and mechanical interventions are discussed in other chapters of this book and will not be detailed here.

Oxygen

Oxygen is usually administered through a face mask or nasal prongs in cases of moderate hypoxaemia; mechanical ventilation is rarely indicated in the absence of profound hypotension. When mechanical ventilation is required, oral intubation is the preferred option, to minimize the risk of bleeding in patients receiving thrombolytic treatment. Positive expiratory pressure and high tidal volumes should be avoided to limit the detrimental effects of mechanical ventilation on right heart function.

Fluid loading

The traditional first-line treatment for hypotension is volume expansion. However, evidence from animal experiments suggests that, in cases of pulmonary hypertension, this approach may increase myocardial oxygen consumption, resulting in right ventricular ischaemia and a deterioration of right ventricular function. However, some clinical data suggest that fluid loading may improve the haemodynamic status of patients with massive PE (35). In an uncontrolled series of 13 normotensive patients with acute PE and a low cardiac index, a 500 mL infusion of dextran over 20 min was found to be associated with a significant increase in cardiac index, from 1.6 ± 0.1 to 2.0 ± 0.1 L/min/m^2 (36). The effect of fluid loading on cardiac index was inversely correlated with baseline right ventricular end-diastolic volume index.

Inotropes and vasopressors

In animals with experimental massive PE and profound hypotension, isoproterenol treatment was associated with deleterious effects on systemic arterial pressure, the positive inotropic and pulmonary vasodilatory effects of isoproterenol being outweighed by the damaging effects of peripheral vasodilation (35,37). In a small series of nine normotensive patients with PE, isoproterenol was associated with an increase in cardiac output, a slight decrease in systemic arterial pressure and no significant change in pulmonary arterial pressure (37). In animal experiments, norepinephrine improved right ventricular function and increased systemic arterial pressure over a wide range of blood pressure and right ventricular afterload, suggesting that its effects were not limited to the subset of animals with profound hypotension (35). Evidence relating to the effects of norepinephrine in patients with massive PE and shock is anecdotal, coming from small case series or single case reports. All the patients also received thrombolytic treatment and other vasopressors, making it difficult to determine treatment outcome (38–40). Epinephrine combines the beneficial vasoconstrictive effects of norepinephrine with the positive inotropic effects of dobutamine and appears to be the drug of choice in PE patients with marked hypotension. However, our knowledge of the effects of epinephrine in patients with PE has been gleaned from only a few case reports and is therefore not necessarily reliable (38,41). Both dopamine and dobutamine have been shown to increase cardiac output in experimental PE. The effects of dopamine on cardiac output appear to be limited by concurrent tachycardia (42). The effects of dobutamine on haemodynamics and gas exchange in patients with PE have been described in two small case series (43,44). In these studies, dobutamine raised cardiac output and improved oxygen transport, although arterial PO_2 fell in some patients (44).

Nitric oxide

Inhaled nitric oxide induces selective pulmonary arterial vasodilation, inducing an increase in cardiac output in patients with increased right ventricular afterload. Clinical experience with inhaled nitric oxide in patients with PE is limited to a small case series and a few case reports. Capellier *et al.* reported the use of nitric oxide in four patients with massive PE, one of whom was on mechanical ventilation (45). The other three patients were breathing spontaneously and received nitric oxide through a face mask, along with oxygen. Inhaled nitric oxide, at concentrations of 5–20 ppm, induced a dose-dependent decrease in pulmonary artery pressure and an increase in cardiac output and blood oxygen saturation in all patients (45). One of the four patients also underwent thrombolysis and haemodynamic support. All patients improved initially, but the clinical condition of two patients subsequently deteriorated and these patients ultimately died as a consequence of PE (45). It has also been shown that inhaled nitric oxide can correct the profound hypoxaemia associated with right to left shunt through a patent foramen ovale in patients with massive PE (46).

In clinical practice, moderate fluid loading may improve the haemodynamic status of patients with massive PE. If shock persists after a 500 mL fluid challenge, inotropic support is indicated, using dobutamine in cases of moderate systemic hypotension or norepinephrine in cases of profound systemic hypotension. In such cases, inhaled nitric oxide may also help to stabilize the haemodynamic condition of the patient.

Is it possible to treat some patients with PE at home?

Randomized controlled trials have shown that the treatment of DVT with low molecular weight heparin administered primarily at home is as safe as treatment with unfractionated heparin in hospital (47,48). The evidence is less clear for patients with PE, but at least some of these patients may be treated at home. A total of 158 patients with PE were included in a multicentre prospective cohort study. All patients were treated with dalteparin (200 U/kg sc daily) for a minimum of 5 days and warfarin for 3 months. Patients with haemodynamic instability, hypoxaemia requiring oxygen therapy, admission for another medical condition, severe pain requiring parenteral analgesia or with a high risk of major bleeding were initially treated in the hospital, whereas other patients were managed primarily as outpatients. Fifty patients were managed as inpatients and 108 as outpatients. Twenty-seven patients were managed for an average of 2.5 days as inpatients and then completed dalteparin treatment as outpatients. The remaining 81 patients were managed exclusively as outpatients. For all outpatients, the overall rate of recurrence of symptomatic venous thromboembolism was 5.6%, with major bleeding occurring in only 1.9% of cases. Of the four deaths, none was due to PE or major bleeding (49). These results suggest that outpatient management of PE is feasible and safe for most patients. In a second study, the same group was able to treat 80% of the patients as outpatients, but this study included both patients with DVT and patients with PE (50). In the Matisse PE study, 14% of the patients assigned to the fondaparinux group received at least some of their treatment as outpatients (25). A randomized controlled trial is under way to compare treatment administered on an outpatient basis with initial treatment administered at hospital in patients with PE and a low risk of death.

LONG-TERM TREATMENT

Data on the long-term treatment of patients with PE are scarce and only one study has compared different durations of anticoagulant treatment in these patients (51). Several large randomized trials have compared different durations of anticoagulant treatment in patients with venous thromboembolism, but the outcome of patients with PE included in these studies is generally not given separately. Recommendations on the optimal duration of anticoagulant treatment for patients with PE are based principally on data from venous thromboembolism studies, in which most patients have symptomatic DVT and either asymptomatic PE or no PE at all. Should the duration of anticoagulant treatment be the same for patients with PE and patients with DVT? To answer this question, studies comparing the long-term outcome of patients with these two conditions are required. However, far less is known about the long-term outcome of patients with PE than about the long-term follow-up of patients with DVT.

Recurrent venous thromboembolism during anticoagulant treatment in patients with PE and in patients with DVT

Using the California Patient Discharge Data Set, Murin *et al.* reported the outcome of 71 250 patients hospitalized with a principal diagnosis of venous thrombosis alone and 21 625 patients diagnosed with PE. In the venous thrombosis cohort, the rate of rehospitalization for recurrent venous thromboembolism after 6 months of follow-up was 6.4% in patients who had initially had a DVT and 5.8% in patients who had initially had a PE (52). Patients who had initially had a PE tended to have recurrences in the form of another PE (RR, 4.2; 95% CI, 3.8 to 4.7), whereas patients who had initially had DVT tended to have recurrences in the form of DVT (RR, 2.7; 95% CI, 2.3 to 3.1) (Table 23.1). In an analysis of 25 prospective studies in which patients with symptomatic DVT or PE were treated with 5–10 days of heparin followed by 3 months of oral anticoagulants, the rate of fatal PE during anticoagulant treatment was 0.4% (95% CI, 3.2 to 4.4) in patients who had initially had DVT and 1.5% (95% CI, 0.9 to 2.2) in those who had initially had PE (24).

In the Matisse PE study, the rate of recurrent venous thromboembolism after 6 months of treatment with heparin or fondaparinux followed by warfarin was 4.4% in 2213 patients with PE. Among the 98 patients who had a recurrent thromboembolic event during 3 months of anticoagulant treatment, the recurrence took the form of a new PE in 69 patients (70.4%) and DVT in 29 patients (29.6%) (25). In the Matisse DVT study, a recurrent venous thromboembolism was observed in 88 (4%) of the 2205 patients with DVT receiving fondaparinux or low molecular weight heparin followed by warfarin for 3 months. The recurrence took the form of a new DVT in 46 patients (52.3%) and PE in 42 patients (47.7%) (Table 23.1) (53).

In the van Gogh studies, the rate of recurrent venous thromboembolism after 6 months of anticoagulant treatment with conventional treatment or idraparinux was 3.7% in the 2267 patients who had had DVT and 3.0% in the 2010 patients who had had PE at inclusion. Among the 60 patients with PE who had a recurrent thromboembolic event during 6 months of anticoagulant treatment, the recurrence took the form of a new PE in 35 patients (58.3%) and DVT in 25 patients (41.7%). Among the 84 recurrences occurring in patients with an initial DVT, the recurrence took the form of a new DVT in 36 patients (42.9%) and PE in 48 patients (57.1%) (9). Hence, in this large study, no difference was observed in the rate or clinical manifestation of recurrence between patients who had initially had DVT and those who had initially had PE (Table 23.1). These results suggest that the rate of recurrences during anticoagulant treatment, is not higher in patients with PE than in patients with DVT. The recurrence was most often a new DVT in patients who had had a DVT and a new PE in patients who had had a PE in earlier studies, but this was not the case in the most recent van Gogh trial.

Table 23.1 Recurrences during anticoagulant treatment in patients with PE and patients with DVT

Study	DVT (*n*)	PE (*n*)	Overall VTE recurrence rate (%)		Type of recurrence, DVT/PE (%)[a]	
			Patients with initial DVT	Patients with with initial PE	Patients with initial DVT	Patients with initial PE
Douketis (24)	2429	949	5.3	4.7	79/21	19/81
Murin (52)	71250	21625	6.4	5.8	86/14	34/66
Matisse (25,53)	2205	2213	4.0	4.4	52/48	30/70
van Gogh (9)	2267	2010	3.7	3.0	43/57	42/58

[a]The percentages refer to the rate of DVT/PE in the recurrent events.

Recurrent venous thromboembolism in patients with PE after the cessation of anticoagulant treatment (cohort studies)

Eichinger *et al*. reported data for a cohort of 464 patients with a first episode of unexplained venous thromboembolism who had been treated with oral anticoagulants for at least 3 months (54). The patients entered the study at the end of their oral anticoagulant treatment. After an average follow-up period of 30 months, 54 patients (12.4%) had experienced recurrent venous thromboembolism. Recurrent venous thromboembolism occurred in 28 (17.3%) of the 162 patients with symptomatic PE and in 26 (9.5%) of the 274 patients with DVT without symptoms of PE. A first symptomatic PE conferred a relative risk of recurrence of 2.2 (95% CI, 1.3 to 3.7; $p = 0.005$) and remained an independent risk factor for recurrence after adjustment for other risk factors. In addition, patients who had initially had PE had a higher risk of subsequent PE than patients who had initially had DVT (RR, 4.0; 95% CI, 1.3 to 12.3) (54). The 10 year incidence of recurrent venous thromboembolism in patients with an initial PE is known from two long-term studies. In the report by Pengo *et al*., the cumulative incidence of recurrent venous thromboembolism was 4.9% after 3 months, 8.0% after 1 year, 22.1% after 5 years and 29.1% (95% CI, 16.9 to 41.3) after 10 years of follow-up (55). In the study by Schulman *et al*., the cumulative 10 year recurrence rate after 6 weeks or 6 months of anticoagulant therapy for a first episode of venous thromboembolism was 34.5% for the 107 patients who had had PE at inclusion (56). Douketis *et al*. reported the outcome of 602 patients with symptomatic PE, with or without associated DVT, who were enrolled in one clinical trial and in one cohort study (57). Patients in both cohorts were followed after the cessation of oral anticoagulant treatment and the rate of subsequent fatal recurrences of PE was assessed. The 602 patients were followed for a total of 2437 person-years; the frequency of fatal PE was 0.57 per 100 person-years of follow-up and the frequency of definite or probable fatal PE was 0.20 per 100 person-years of follow-up. The case fatality rate of recurrent venous thromboembolism in patients with an initial PE was 3.9% for definite or probable PE.

Randomized controlled trials comparing different durations of anticoagulant treatment in patients with PE

The optimal duration of anticoagulant treatment in patient with PE has been assessed in five studies (51,58–61). Agnelli *et al*. carried out the only randomized clinical trial evaluating two different durations of anticoagulant therapy in patients with a first episode of PE (51). This study included 326 patients who had received 3 months of anticoagulant treatment with no recurrence or bleeding. Patients were randomized to two groups: anticoagulation therapy was stopped after the initial 3 months in one group and continued for a further 3–9 months in the other. The mean follow-up was 33.8 months and all patients were followed for several months after the end of anticoagulant treatment. The incidence of recurrent venous thromboembolism was 3.1 and 3.8% per patient-year after the cessation of anticoagulant treatment, a non significant difference (51). Kearon *et al*. compared prolonged warfarin treatment with placebo in 162 patients with venous thromboembolism who had completed 3 months of anticoagulant therapy (59). Of the 83 patients assigned to the placebo group, 22 had symptomatic PE at presentation and five (22.7%) suffered recurrent venous thromboembolism during a mean follow-up period of 9 months. Of the 79 patients given prolonged anticoagulation treatment, 19 had PE at presentation and one had recurrent venous thromboembolism (59). The small number of patients with PE in this study precludes meaningful comparisons. In addition, the patients given prolonged anticoagulant treatment were not followed beyond the end of treatment. Of the 61 patients with DVT allocated to the placebo group, 12 (16.9%) presented recurrent venous thromboembolism during follow-up (Table 23.2). In another

Table 23.2 Recurrences in patients with PE and patients with DVT after the cessation of anticoagulant treatment.

Study	DVT (*n*)	PE (*n*)	Overall VTE recurrence rate (%)[a]	
			Patients with initial DVT	Patients with initial PE
Kearon (59)	61	22	20.3	27.2
Schulman (61)	790	107	6.4	10
Eichinger (54)	274	162	3.8	6.9
van Gogh (58)	337	304	6.4	8.6

[a]Recurrence rate are given as events per 100 patient-years.

study, 897 patients with venous thromboembolism were allocated to groups receiving 6 weeks or 6 months of anticoagulant therapy and were followed for 2 years (61). PE was present at inclusion in 107 of these patients and 22 patients (20.5%) had recurrent venous thromboembolism during the follow-up period (corresponding to a recurrence rate of 10.2% per patient-year), with most recurrences occurring after the cessation of anticoagulant therapy (61). In the same study, the overall recurrence rate was 12.8% in the 790 patients who had initially had a DVT. The recurrence rate was 26.8% in the 56 patients with PE allocated to the 6 week treatment group and 7% in the 51 patients with PE who received 6 months of anticoagulant treatment (OR, 2.3; 95% CI, 0.9 to 6.2) (61). In the van Gogh extension study, 1215 patients with venous thromboembolism who had completed 6 months of anticoagulant treatment were allocated to groups receiving idraparinux or placebo for a further period of 6 months (58). In total, 587 patients initially had a PE; 283 of these patients received idraparinux, three of whom had a recurrent event (1.1%). By contrast, 13 of the 304 patients with PE who were given placebo presented recurrent venous thromboembolism during the 6 month treatment period (4.3%, corresponding to an 8.6% per patient-year recurrence rate). In the same study, patients with an initial DVT given idraparinux had a 1% recurrence rate, whereas patients receiving placebo had a 3.2% recurrence rate (Table 23.2) (58).

In another study reporting on the long-term recurrence rate after PE, warfarin treatment was continued in 738 randomly selected patients who had completed 3 or more months of treatment, with a target INR of 2.0–3.0 or 1.5–1.9; these patients were followed for an average of 2.4 years (62). This study included 259 patients with PE: 142 were allocated to the conventional-intensity treatment group, two of whom suffered recurrent venous thromboembolism (0.6% per patient-year); 117 were allocated to the low-intensity therapy group, seven of whom had a recurrent event (2.6% per patient-year) (62). These data suggest that the rate of recurrent thromboembolism is higher in patients receiving a short treatment of six weeks to 6 months than in patients given more prolonged treatment (58,59,61). However, in most studies, the patients treated for longer periods were not followed after cessation of the treatment and the number of patients with PE studied was generally small. These studies also suggest that the rate of recurrent venous thromboembolism after the cessation of anticoagulant treatment, is higher in patients who had initially had PE than in those who had initially had DVT (Table 23.2).

CONCLUSION

There is now a large body of evidence from large randomized comparisons that unfractionated heparin, low molecular weight heparin and fondaparinux are all safe and effective options for the initial anticoagulant treatment of clinically stable patients with PE. Low molecular weight heparin and fondaparinux are easier to administer, but recent data have suggested that the use of a fixed dose of unfractionated heparin may give similar results in selected patients. In patients with impaired renal function, unfractionated heparin remains the safest option. Following the cessation of anticoagulant treatment after 3–6 months, the rate of recurrent venous thromboembolism appears to be higher in patients who initially had PE than in those who initially had DVT, as shown by both cohort studies and most randomized controlled trials (54,59,61). However, the rate of fatal PE remains low after the cessation of anticoagulant treatment and does not appear to be higher than the risk of fatal bleeding during prolonged anticoagulant treatment (57,63). In randomized controlled trials, the rate of recurrent thromboembolism is generally higher in patients receiving a short treatment of 6 weeks to 6 months than in patients given more prolonged treatment (58,59,61). However, in most studies, the patients treated for longer periods were not followed after cessation of the treatment and the number of patients with PE studied was generally small. It remains unclear whether prolonged anticoagulant treatment reduces the overall long-term rate of recurrent venous thromboembolism or simply delays subsequent thromboembolic events. The available data do not support a policy of treating PE patients with anticoagulants for longer than patients with DVT. According to the ACCP guidelines, patients with a reversible risk factor should be treated for at least 3 months and those with idiopathic PE should receive at least 6 months of anticoagulant treatment (27). Decisions concerning longer periods of treatment should be taken on a case-by-case basis, according to the risks of recurrence and bleeding specific to each patient.

REFERENCES

1. Azarian R, Wartski M, Collignon MA, Parent F, Herve P, Sors H, et al. Lung perfusion scans and hemodynamics in acute and chronic pulmonary embolism. *J Nucl Med* 1997; **38**:980–3.
2. Goldhaber SZ, Visani L, De Rosa M. Acute pulmonary embolism: clinical outcomes in the International Cooperative Pulmonary Embolism Registry (ICOPER). *Lancet* 1999; **353**:1386–9.
3. Kasper W, Konstantinides S, Geibel A, Olschewski M, Heinrich F, Grosser KD, et al. Management strategies and determinants of outcome in acute major pulmonary embolism: results of a multicenter registry. *J Am Coll Cardiol* 1997; **30**:1165–71.
4. Alpert JS, Smith R, Carlson J, Ockene IS, Dexter L, Dalen JE. Mortality in patients treated for pulmonary embolism. *JAMA* 1976; **236**:1477–80.
5. Grifoni S, Olivotto I, Cecchini P, Pieralli F, Camaiti A, Santoro G, et al. Short-term clinical outcome of patients with acute pulmonary embolism, normal blood pressure and echocardiographic right ventricular dysfunction. *Circulation* 2000; **101**:2817–22.
6. Vieillard-Baron A, Page B, Augarde R, Prin S, Qanadli S, Beauchet A, et al. Acute cor pulmonale in massive pulmonary embolism: incidence, echocardiographic pattern, clinical implications and recovery rate. *Intensive Care Med* 2001; **27**:1481–6.
7. Task Force on Pulmonary Embolism, European Society of Cardiology. Guidelines on diagnosis and management of acute pulmonary embolism. *Eur Heart J* 2000; **21**:1301–36.
8. Quinlan DJ, McQuillan A, Eikelboom JW. Low-molecular-weight heparin compared with intravenous unfractionated heparin for treatment of pulmonary embolism: a meta-analysis of randomized, controlled trials. *Ann Intern Med* 2004; **140**:175–83.
9. Büller HR, Cohen AT, Davidson B, Decousus H, Gallus AS, Gent M, et al. Idraparinux versus standard therapy for venous thromboembolic disease. *N Engl J Med* 2007; **357**:1094–104.
10. Ribeiro A, Lindmarker P, Juhlin-Dannfelt A, Johnsson H, Jorfeldt L. Echocardiography Doppler in pulmonary embolism: right ventricular dysfunction as a predictor of mortality rate. *Am Heart J* 1997; **134**:479–87.
11. Kucher N, Rossi E, De Rosa M, Goldhaber SZ. Prognostic role of echocardiography among patients with acute pulmonary embolism and a systolic arterial pressure of 90mmHg or higher. *Arch Intern Med* 2005; **165**:1777–81.
12. Kostrubiec M, Pruszczyk P, Bochowicz A, Pacho R, Szulc M, Kaczynska A, et al. Biomarker-based risk assessment model in acute pulmonary embolism. *Eur Heart J* 2005; **26**:2166–72.

13. Kucher N, Printzen G, Goldhaber SZ. Prognostic role of brain natriuretic peptide in acute pulmonary embolism. *Circulation* 2003; **107**:2545–7.

14. Pieralli F, Olivotto I, Vanni S, Conti A, Camaiti A, Targioni G, *et al*. Usefulness of bedside testing for brain natriuretic peptide to identify right ventricular dysfunction and outcome in normotensive patients with acute pulmonary embolism. *Am J Cardiol* 2006; **97**:1386–90.

15. Konstantinides S, Geibel A, Olschewski M, Heinrich F, Grosser K, Rauber K, *et al*. Association between thrombolytic treatment and the prognosis of hemodynamically stable patients with major pulmonary embolism: results of a multicenter registry. *Circulation* 1997; **96**:882–8.

16. Scridon T, Scridon C, Skali H, Alvarez A, Goldhaber SZ, Solomon SD. Prognostic significance of troponin elevation and right ventricular enlargement in acute pulmonary embolism. *Am J Cardiol* 2005; **96**:303–5.

17. Hamel E, Pacouret G, Vincentelli D, Forissier JF, Peycher P, Pottier JM, *et al*. Thrombolysis or heparin therapy in massive pulmonary embolism with right ventricular dilation: results from a 128-patient monocenter registry. *Chest* 2001; **120**:120–5.

18. Pruszczyk P, Bochowicz A, Torbicki A, Szulc M, Kurzyna M, Fijalkowska A, *et al*. Cardiac troponin T monitoring identifies high-risk group of normotensive patients with acute pulmonary embolism. *Chest* 2003; **123**:1947–52.

19. Pruszczyk P, Kostrubiec M, Bochowicz A, Styczynski G, Szulc M, Kurzyna M, *et al*. N-terminal pro-brain natriuretic peptide in patients with acute pulmonary embolism. *Eur Respir J* 2003; **22**:649–53.

20. Aujesky D, Perrier A, Roy PM, Stone RA, Cornuz J, Meyer G, *et al*. Validation of a clinical prognostic model to identify low-risk patients with pulmonary embolism. *J Intern Med* 2007; **261**:597–604.

21. Aujesky D, Obrosky DS, Stone RA, Auble TE, Perrier A, Cornuz J, *et al*. Derivation and validation of a prognostic model for pulmonary embolism. *Am J Respir Crit Care Med* 2005; **172**:1041–6.

22. Aujesky D, Obrosky DS, Stone RA, Auble TE, Perrier A, Cornuz J, *et al*. A prediction rule to identify low-risk patients with pulmonary embolism. *Arch Intern Med* 2006; **166**:169–75.

23. Aujesky D, Roy PM, Le Manach CP, Verschuren F, Meyer G, Obrosky DS, *et al*. Validation of a model to predict adverse outcomes in patients with pulmonary embolism. *Eur Heart J* 2006; **27**:476–81.

24. Douketis JD, Kearon C, Bates S, Duku EK, Ginsberg JS. Risk of fatal pulmonary embolism in patients with treated venous thromboembolism. *JAMA* 1998; **279**:458–62.

25. Büller HR, Davidson BL, Decousus H, Gallus A, Gent M, Piovella F, *et al*. Subcutaneous fondaparinux versus intravenous unfractionated heparin in the initial treatment of pulmonary embolism. *N Engl J Med* 2003; **349**:1695–702.

26. Barritt DW, Jordan SC. Anticoagulant drugs in the treatment of pulmonary embolism: a controlled trial. *Lancet* 1960; **i**:1309–12.

27. Büller HR, Agnelli G, Hull RD, Hyers TM, Prins MH, Raskob GE. Antithrombotic therapy for venous thromboembolic disease: the Seventh ACCP Conference on Antithrombotic and Thrombolytic Therapy. *Chest* 2004; **126**:401S–428S.

28. Heit JA, Silverstein MD, Mohr DN, Petterson TM, O'Fallon WM, Melton LJ III. Predictors of survival after deep vein thrombosis and pulmonary embolism: a population-based, cohort study. *Arch Intern Med* 1999; **159**:445–53.

29. Kearon C, Ginsberg JS, Julian JA, Douketis J, Solymoss S, Ockelford P, *et al*. Comparison of fixed-dose weight-adjusted unfractionated heparin and low molecular-weight heparin for acute treatment of venous thromboembolism. *JAMA* 2006; **296**:935–42.

30. Martel N, Lee J, Wells PS. Risk for heparin-induced thrombocytopenia with unfractionated and low molecular-weight heparin thromboprophylaxis: a meta-analysis. *Blood* 2005; **106**:2710–5.

31. Simonneau G, Sors H, Charbonnier B, Page Y, Laaban JP, Azarian R, *et al*. A comparison of low molecular-weight heparin with unfractionated heparin for acute pulmonary embolism. The THESEE Study Group. Tinzaparine ou Heparine Standard: Evaluations dans l'Embolie Pulmonaire. *N Engl J Med*. 1997; **337**:663–9.

32. Gouin-Thibault I, Pautas E, Siguret V. Safety profile of different low molecular weight heparins used at therapeutic dose. *Drug Saf* 2005; **28**:333–49.

33. Prandoni P, Siragusa S, Girolami B, Fabris F. The incidence of heparin-induced thrombocytopenia in medical patients treated with low molecular-weight heparin: a prospective cohort study. *Blood* 2005; **106**:3049–54.

34. Warkentin TE, Greinacher A. Heparin-induced thrombocytopenia: recognition, treatment and prevention: the Seventh ACCP Conference on Antithrombotic and Thrombolytic Therapy. *Chest* 2004; **126**:311S–37S.

35. Layish DT, Tapson VF. Pharmacologic hemodynamic support in massive pulmonary embolism. *Chest* 1997; **111**:218–24.

36. Mercat A, Diehl JL, Meyer G, Teboul JL, Sors H. Hemodynamic effects of fluid loading in acute massive pulmonary embolism. *Crit Care Med* 1999; **27**:540–4.

37. McDonald IG, Hirsh J, Hale GS, Cade JF, McCarthy RA. Isoproterenol in massive pulmonary embolism: haemodynamic and clinical effects. *Med J Aust* 1968; **2**:201–5.

38. Boulain T, Lanotte R, Legras A, Perrotin D. Efficacy of epinephrine therapy in shock complicating pulmonary embolism. *Chest* 1993; **104**:300–2.

39. Hopf HB, Flossdorf T, Breulmann M. [Recombinant tissue-type plasminogen activator for the emergency treatment of perioperative life-threatening pulmonary embolism (stage IV). Results in 7 patients]. *Anaesthesist* 1991; **40**:309–14.

40. Scheeren TW, Hopf HB, Peters J. [Intraoperative thrombolysis with rt-PA in massive pulmonary embolism during venous thrombectomy]. *Anasthesiol Intensivmed Notfallmed Schmerzther* 1994; **29**:440–5.

41. Igarashi A, Amagasa S, Yokoo N. [Case of postoperative pulmonary embolism after tonsillectomy in a healthy young woman]. *Masui* 2007; **56**:1085–7.

42. Mathru M, Venus B, Smith RA, Shirakawa Y, Sugiura A. Treatment of low cardiac output complicating acute pulmonary hypertension in normovolemic goats. *Crit Care Med* 1986; **14**:120–4.

43. Jardin F, Genevray B, Brun-Ney D, Margairaz A. Dobutamine: a hemodynamic evaluation in pulmonary embolism shock. *Crit Care Med* 1985; **13**:1009–12.

44. Manier G, Castaing Y. Influence of cardiac output on oxygen exchange in acute pulmonary embolism. *Am Rev Respir Dis* 1992; **145**:130–6.

45. Capellier G, Jacques T, Balvay P, Blasco G, Belle E, Barale F. Inhaled nitric oxide in patients with pulmonary embolism. *Intensive Care Med* 1997; **23**:1089–92.

46. surEstagnasie P G, Le Bourdelles L, Mier F, Coste D, Dreyfuss. Use of inhaled nitric oxide to reverse flow through a patent foramen ovale during pulmonary embolism. *Ann Intern Med* 1994; **120**:757–9.

47. Koopman MM, Prandoni P, Piovella F, Ockelford PA, Brandjes DP, van der Meer J, *et al*. Treatment of venous thrombosis with intravenous unfractionated heparin administered in the hospital as compared with subcutaneous low molecular-weight heparin administered at home. The Tasman Study Group. *N Engl J Med* 1996; **334**:682–7.

48. Levine M, Gent M, Hirsh J, Leclerc J, Anderson D, Weitz J, *et al*. A comparison of low molecular-weight heparin administered primarily at home with unfractionated heparin administered in the hospital for proximal deep-vein thrombosis. *N Engl J Med* 1996; **334**:677–81.

49. Kovacs MJ, Anderson D, Morrow B, Gray L, Touchie D, Wells PS. Outpatient treatment of pulmonary embolism with dalteparin. *Thromb Haemost* 2000; **83**:209–11.

50. Wells PS, Kovacs MJ, Bormanis J, Forgie MA, Goudie D, Morrow B, *et al*. Expanding eligibility for outpatient treatment of deep venous thrombosis and pulmonary embolism with low molecular-weight heparin: a comparison of patient self-injection with homecare injection. *Arch Intern Med* 1998; **158**:1809–12.

51. Agnelli G, Prandoni P, Becattini C, Silingardi M, Taliani MR, Miccio M, *et al*. Extended oral anticoagulant therapy after a first episode of pulmonary embolism. *Ann Intern Med* 2003; **139**:19–25.

52. Murin S, Romano PS, White RH. Comparison of outcomes after hospitalization for deep venous thrombosis or pulmonary embolism. *Thromb Haemost* 2002; **88**:407–14.

53. Büller HR, Davidson BL, Decousus H, Gallus A, Gent M, Piovella F, *et al*. Fondaparinux or enoxaparin for the initial treatment of symptomatic deep venous thrombosis: a randomized trial. *Ann Intern Med* 2004; **140**:867–73.

54. Eichinger S, Weltermann A, Minar E, Stain M, Schonauer V, Schneider B, *et al*. Symptomatic pulmonary embolism and the risk of recurrent venous thromboembolism. *Arch Intern Med* 2004; **164**:92–6.

55. Pengo V, Lensing AW, Prins MH, Marchiori A, Davidson BL, Tiozzo F, *et al*. Incidence of chronic thromboembolic pulmonary hypertension after pulmonary embolism. *N Engl J Med* 2004; **350**:2257–64.

56. Schulman S, Lindmarker P, Holmstrom M, Larfars G, Carlsson A, Nicol P, *et al*. Post-thrombotic syndrome, recurrence and death 10 years after the first episode of venous thromboembolism treated with warfarin for 6 weeks or 6 months. *J Thromb Haemost* 2006; **4**:734–42.

57. Douketis JD, Gu CS, Schulman S, Ghirarduzzi A, Pengo V, Prandoni P. The risk for fatal pulmonary embolism after discontinuing anticoagulant therapy for venous thromboembolism. *Ann Intern Med* 2007; **147**:766–74.

58. Büller HR, Cohen AT, Davidson B, Decousus H, Gallus AS, Gent M, *et al*. Extended prophylaxis of venous thromboembolism with idraparinux. *N Engl J Med* 2007; **357**:1105–12.

59. Kearon C, Gent M, Hirsh J, Weitz J, Kovacs MJ, Anderson DR, *et al*. A comparison of three months of anticoagulation with extended anticoagulation for a first episode of idiopathic venous thromboembolism. *N Engl J Med* 1999; **340**:901–7.

60. Wells PS, Anderson DR, Rodger M, Ginsberg JS, Kearon C, Gent M, *et al*. Derivation of a simple clinical model to categorize patients probability of pulmonary embolism: increasing the models utility with the SimpliRED D-dimer. *Thromb Haemost* 2000; **83**:416–20.

61. Schulman S, Rhedin AS, Lindmarker P, Carlsson A, Larfars G, Nicol P, *et al*. A comparison of six weeks with six months of oral anticoagulant therapy after a first episode of venous thromboembolism. Duration of Anticoagulation Trial Study Group. *N Engl J Med* 1995; **332**:1661–5.

62. Kearon C, Ginsberg JS, Kovacs MJ, Anderson DR, Wells P, Julian JA, *et al*. Comparison of low-intensity warfarin therapy with conventional-intensity warfarin therapy for long-term prevention of recurrent venous thromboembolism. *N Engl J Med* 2003; **349**:631–9.

63. Palareti G, Leali N, Coccheri S, Poggi M, Manotti C, D'Angelo A, *et al*. Bleeding complications of oral anticoagulant treatment: an inception-cohort, prospective collaborative study (ISCOAT). Italian Study on Complications of Oral Anticoagulant Therapy. *Lancet* 1996; **348**:423–8.

CHAPTER 24

Thrombolysis for the Treatment of Pulmonary Embolism

Giancarlo Agnelli and Cecilia Becattini

Internal and Cardiovascular Medicine, University of Perugia, Perugia, Italy

RATIONALE

Anticoagulant therapy is the mainstay of the management of patients with acute pulmonary embolism (PE). Given the high mortality seen in patients with acute PE despite anticoagulant treatment, the use of more aggressive treatments, such as thrombolytic agents, has been suggested for selected patients. Indeed, recurrent PE was the cause of death in 91, 45 and 10% of the cases at 30 days, 90 days and at 1 year in three studies in patients who were followed after a proven PE event (1–3). These data indicate that mortality due to PE is high during the first 2 weeks after hospital admission and then declines over time. Mortality due to PE is mainly due to the abrupt onset of pulmonary hypertension leading to right heart overload (4). Hence it is conceivable that a rapid decrease in pulmonary hypertension obtained with a rapid lysis of the emboli can result in a rapid improvement in haemodynamics and reduce mortality in these patients. In the ICOPER registry, the 2 week mortality rate was 11.4% and the incidence of recurrence was 7.9% at 3 months despite anticoagulant treatment (2). The incidence of major bleeding in this registry was 10.5%. Therefore, the potential clinical benefit of more aggressive therapies, such as thrombolytic therapy, need to be balanced with the risk of major bleeding. As a result, patients should be selected for thrombolytic therapy based on their risk of death at the time of diagnosis and during the subsequent initial period after diagnosis.

CLINICAL SEVERITY OF PULMONARY EMBOLISM

Mortality in patients with acute PE varies among the different studies and between randomized trials and registries (5). This variability is mainly due to different inclusion criteria leading to the selection of different study populations.

Haemodynamic status is currently the main determinant of short-term mortality. The ICOPER registry reported a 2 week mortality of 58% in haemodynamically unstable patients with acute PE, whereas mortality was 15% in haemodynamically stable patients (2). These data confirmed previous observations of a higher 30 day mortality in patients with hypotension (12.3% versus 7.3%, $p = 0.021$) (1). The low rate of mortality (near 1%) observed in some randomized studies suggests that haemodynamically stable patients with PE can be further stratified according to the risk for short-term mortality.

The role of other clinical features as prognostic factors (heart rate, respiratory rate, temperature and pulse oximetry), clinical signs (distended jugular veins, systolic murmur of tricuspid regurgitation or an accentuated P2) or ECG abnormalities (right bundle branch block, $S_I Q_{III} T_{III}$ and T wave inversion in leads V1–V4) has been evaluated in observational studies. Different combinations of individual features have been included in algorithms for risk assessment.

An Italian cohort study in 209 patients with haemodynamically stable acute PE showed that echocardiography can be used to differentiate those patients who have a 5% in-hospital mortality from patients who have a 10% incidence of in-hospital mortality or clinical deterioration (6). This finding was confirmed in a number of studies and in a subgroup analysis of the ICOPER study (7). Currently, right ventricle dilation is the more extensively evaluated measure for right ventricle dysfunction in acute PE (8). However, the definition of right ventricle dysfunction varies among the studies. More recently, right to left ventricle end-diastolic dimension ratio over 0.9 and over 1.0 has been consistently shown to be associated with an increased likelihood for death and clinical deterioration in patients with PE and normal blood pressure.

Serum levels of brain natriuretic peptide (BNP) have been shown to have a high negative predictive value (99–100%) in patients with acute PE (9). Thus, BNP levels can be used to identify those patients with PE who are more likely to experience a favourable outcome.

Evidence exists that serum levels of troponin, a marker of myocardial injury, can be used to identify those patients with PE at higher risk for death and clinical deterioration (10). Promising evidence exists that a new marker of myocardial injury, heart-type fatty acid binding peptide, can identify patients with acute PE at risk for death and clinical deterioration within 30 days from diagnosis (11).

In conclusion, three classes of patients with acute PE can be identified with respect to short-term prognosis (12):

- high risk: haemodynamically unstable patients
- intermediate risk: haemodynamically stable patients with right ventricle dysfunction or injury
- low risk: haemodynamically stable patients without right ventricle dysfunction or injury.

THROMBOLYTIC AGENTS FOR PULMONARY EMBOLISM

All thrombolytic agents act as exogenous plasminogen activators. Streptokinase is the first thrombolytic agent which underwent clinical development (13). Streptokinase is a compound derived from beta haemolytic streptococci that maintain an antigenic effect. Streptokinase has a half-life of 4–30 min. Thus, therapeutic regimens for PE require a prolonged (24–48 h) continuous intravenous infusion in the order of 250 000–750 000 IU over 30 min, followed by an infusion of 100 000 IU/h for one or more days. Short-infusion regimens of streptokinase were found to be associated with hypotension and this limited their use in the setting of acute PE. After the assessment of its efficacy in the setting of myocardial infarction, streptokinase was nearly abandoned due to the high incidence of systemic allergic reactions.

Urokinase was first isolated from human urine and then obtained from renal cell cultures (14). Urokinase is a direct activator of plasminogen with a half-life similar to that of streptokinase (4 min). Urokinase is not associated with systemic allergic reactions, thereby allowing repeated administrations and reducing the incidence of side-effects. Two regimens are currently approved for the treatment of PE with urokinase: a 24 h infusion regimen consisting of 4000 IU/kg over 10 min followed by 4000 IU/kg/h for 12–24 h and a short-infusion regimen consisting of 10^6 IU in 10 min followed by 2×10^6 IU over 110 min.

Recombinant tissue plasminogen activator (rtPA) is the first of the so-called second-generation thrombolytic agents, which can be produced through cloned cell cultures (15). This class of agents has the advantage of a more selective lytic effect. More specifically, they act on fibrin-bound plasminogen and are only marginally active on free plasminogen. It is this property that has been implicated as the basis for its reduced association with bleeding complications. The half-life of rtPA is about 30 min. Different regimens of rtPA have been evaluated in patients with acute myocardial infarction. Regimens for patients with acute PE are derived from those adopted in acute myocardial infarction. A 2 h infusion regimen is commonly used for PE, consisting of 15 mg bolus, followed by 50 mg in the first 30 min and a further 35 mg in the next 60 min.

Synthetic thrombolytics mainly derived from rtPA are identified as third-generation thrombolytic compounds. These agents are characterized by a longer half-life and a better specificity. Only a minority of these agents have been studied in clinical studies.

Tenecteplase is a triple-combination mutant of alteplase developed to avoid some of the limitations of second-generation thrombolytic agents. Tenecteplase has a longer plasma half-life (20 versus 4 min) and higher resistance to inhibition by plasminogen-activator inhibitor-1 than alteplase. Because of the ease of administration, bolus fibrinolysis facilitates rapid administration, allowing treatment before admission to hospital in selected patients with acute myocardial infarction, and may reduce the rate of medication errors. Efficacy for clot lysis of single bolus administration of tenecteplase was studied in patients with myocardial infarction (16). Multiple studies have since confirmed that a body weight-adjusted single bolus of 0.50–0.55 mg/kg tenecteplase would be equivalent to a 90 min regimen of alteplase regarding efficacy and safety.

Stafilokinase is a thrombolytic agent derived from staphylococci. This drug has never been evaluated in patients with PE.

HAEMODYNAMIC EFFECTS OF THROMBOLYSIS

The efficacy of thrombolytic therapy in obtaining a rapid resolution of thromboembolic obstruction and an improvement in haemodynamic parameters has been consistently shown in randomized trials.

In the UPET study, 160 patients with angiographically proven pulmonary embolism were randomly assigned to receive heparin or urokinase (a bolus infusion of 4400 IU/kg followed by a continuous 24 h administration of 4400 IU/kg/h) (17). At 24 h, a 23% reduction in mean pulmonary artery pressure was observed in patients randomized to urokinase as compared with no change in patients randomized to heparin. No effect of urokinase was observed in other haemodynamic parameters.

In a randomized trial in 25 patients, repeated pulmonary angiography showed an 80% increase in cardiac index and a 40% decrease in pulmonary artery pressure after 72 h of treatment with streptokinase (18).

In an open cohort study, 47 patients with PE were treated with 50 mg rtPA given in 2 h (19). Angiography was repeated at the end of the infusion. Patients with residual emboli were given an additional 40 mg rtPA. Overall, 83% of the patients had a moderate or major resolution of embolism load. However, this study also showed an increased risk of bleeding in patients undergoing prolonged rtPA infusion. Therefore, a short infusion regimen was adopted for the use of rtPA in patients with acute PE in the following studies. A 57% increase in pulmonary perfusion as assessed by perfusion lung scan was observed at 24 h from rtPA in 19 patients (20).

In the PAIMS-2 study, 36 patients with PE were randomized to receive heparin or 100 mg rtPA given by a 2 h infusion (21). A 12% decrease in vascular obstruction as assessed by follow-up angiograms was observed at the end of the 2 h infusion period in patients randomized to rtPA. No change was observed in patients receiving heparin. Moreover, rtPA induced a 30% reduction in mean pulmonary artery pressure and a 15% increase in cardiac index.

Direct comparisons between different thrombolytic agents have also been performed. In one trial, a faster reduction of total pulmonary resistance (ratio between mean pulmonary artery pressure and cardiac index) was observed at 2 h in patients randomized to receive 100 mg rtPA as compared with patients randomized to receive a weight-adjusted 12 h infusion of urokinase (22). This difference was no longer observed after 6 h. In a study with a similar experimental design, 45 patients were randomized to receive a 2 h infusion of 100 mg rtPA or 24 h weight-adjusted urokinase (23). Thrombus resolution was observed at 2 h in 82% of the patients randomized to rtPA as compared with 48% of the patients randomized to urokinase. Consistent with previous results, this difference was no longer present at perfusion lung scan performed after 24 h.

In order to improve the effects of urokinase, an accelerated regimen (3×10^6 IU given in 2 h) was compared with the 2 h infusion regimen of rtPA (24). No difference in effectiveness was shown between the two regimens, despite a higher incidence of adverse reactions among patients receiving urokinase, mainly due to allergic reactions.

Similarly, the 2 h infusion of rtPA appeared to be superior over a 12 h infusion of streptokinase (at 100 000 IU/h), but no difference was observed when the same streptokinase dosage was given over 2 h (25).

The 2 h regimen of rtPA 100 mg was compared with a short infusion regimen (over 15 min) of rtPA 0.6 mg/kg in two trials. Similar reperfusion rates (26) and similar reductions in total pulmonary resistance (27) were observed with the two rtPA regimens. However, a trend towards a higher incidence of bleeding complications was observed with the short infusion regimen in both studies.

No additional advantage was obtained by direct infusion of rtPA via a catheter in the pulmonary artery relative to systemic intravenous thrombolysis (28). Nevertheless, a combination of local delivery of thrombolytic agents and catheter fragmentation or thrombus evacuation may have additional value, as discussed in Chapter 26.

In conclusion, thrombolytic therapy results in faster lysis of emboli as evidenced by more rapid resolution of perfusion scan abnormalities, decreased embolism load as demonstrated by angiography and a reduction in pulmonary artery pressures. No substantial difference in efficacy was observed between different thrombolytic regimens, whereas an advantage in terms of a reduced incidence of adverse reaction was observed with rtPA. Therefore, at present rtPA is the preferred choice for treatment of high-risk, significant PE.

EFFECTS OF THROMBOLYSIS ON THE RIGHT VENTRICLE

The efficacy of rtPA in reducing right ventricle hypokinesis and right ventricle dilation as assessed at echocardiography was evaluated in a study in 101 haemodynamically stable patients with acute PE (29). Overall, 46 patients were randomized to rtPA (100 mg over 2 h) plus heparin and 55 to heparin alone. Abnormal echocardiography was found in about half of the patients at randomization. A significant reduction in mean right ventricle end diastolic area on echocardiography was found at 3 h after treatment with rtPA. Repeated echocardiography showed an improvement in right ventricle hypokinesis in 39% of the patients randomized to receive rtPA as compared with 17% of patients receiving heparin alone. Echocardiography performed at 24 h showed a rate of worsening of right ventricle hypokinesis of 2.4% in patients randomized to rtPA as compared with

17% in patients randomized to heparin alone. The reduction in right ventricle end-diastolic area observed at 24 h was statistically significantly higher in patients randomized to rtPA as compared with patients randomized to heparin alone.

The efficacy of tenecteplase in reducing right ventricle dysfunction with respect to heparin has recently been shown in haemodynamically stable patients with PE (30).

EFFECTS OF THROMBOLYSIS ON CLINICAL OUTCOME

Given the small number of patients currently randomized in trials in PE, the clinical benefit of thrombolysis for this indication remains controversial. Overall, fewer than 800 patients have been enrolled in randomized trials of thrombolysis plus anticoagulation versus anticoagulation alone for the treatment of PE.

The efficacy of thrombolysis was first shown in a randomized trial of reduced sample size in patients with acute PE and clinically overt haemodynamic instability (31). This trial was interrupted after the inclusion of the first eight patients as all the four patients randomized to heparin alone died. Hence, due to the high risk of mortality in patients with acute PE who suffer from significant circulatory impairment, consensus exists that thrombolysis should be used as a life-saving treatment.

The efficacy of urokinase given as a 12 or 24 h infusion was compared with that of streptokinase given as a 24 h infusion in 167 patients with PE (32). This randomized study showed an equal incidence of death and non fatal recurrent embolic events with the three treatment regimens.

In the MAPPET-3 study, 256 haemodynamically stable patients were randomized to receive thrombolytic therapy with rtPA or heparin alone. Patients were included in the study provided that they had evidence of right ventricular dysfunction at either echocardiography or ECG (33). Tissue plasminogen activator, compared with placebo, reduced the incidence of in-hospital death or escalation of therapy (need for catecholamine infusion, mechanical ventilation, cardiopulmonary resuscitation or open-label thrombolysis) by approximately 50%. No effect was observed in overall mortality (about 3% in both groups) and no increase in major bleeding was encountered in patients receiving rtPA.

The results of randomized trials on thrombolysis for the treatment of PE have been summarized in three meta-analyses. One of these analyses showed the efficacy of thrombolysis in reducing the incidence of death or recurrent PE [relative risk (RR), 0.55; 95% confidence interval (CI), 0.33 to 0.96)] (34). This analysis also showed that the increased incidence of major bleeding observed with thrombolysis relative to heparin was mainly accounted for by studies requiring invasive procedures for the diagnosis and the evaluation of study outcomes. Therefore, the authors hypothesized that safer thrombolytic regimens (short infusion rtPA) given in the absence of invasive procedures could be as safe as thrombolytic treatment in the setting of acute myocardial infarction. In a different analysis, thrombolysis was associated with a trend toward a reduction in mortality [6.2 vs 12.7%; odds ratio (OR), 0.47; 95% CI, 0.20 to 1.10] in the five trials (total of 254 patients) that focused on patients with more severe PE (35).

In our recent analysis, thrombolysis was effective in reducing death due to PE (OR, 0.21; 95% CI, 0.21 to 0.95) (Table 24.1) (34).

BLEEDING COMPLICATIONS

A considerable risk of major bleeding complications has been described in clinical trials applying thrombolytic therapy. In the ICOPER, which enrolled 2454 patients with acute PE, intracranial

Table 24.1   Deaths due to PE in patients with acute PE randomized to thrombolysis or heparin (34)

	No. of studies	No. of patients	Deaths (%)		OR (95% CI)
			Lysis	Heparin	
Streptokinase vs heparin	3	94	2.2	16.7	0.21 (0.05 to 0.92)
Urokinase vs heparin	2	190	2.0	4.5	0.46 (0.08 to 2.60)
rtPA vs heparin	5	464	1.4	2.1	0.69 (0.20 to 2.37)
Overall	10	748	1.7	4.7	0.42 (0.19 to 0.95)

bleeding occurred in 3.0% of the patients who received thrombolytic therapy compared with 0.3% of the non-thrombolysis-treated patients (2). In the MAPPET registry, the incidence of major bleeding episodes was 11.1% (1). The rate of major bleeding was significantly higher among the patients receiving thrombolysis than in patients receiving heparin alone (21.9 versus 7.8%). In this study, cerebral haemorrhage was rare, occurring in two patients in each group (1.2 and 0.4%, respectively).

Overall, data from randomized trials report a 13% cumulative rate of major bleeding in patients with PE receiving thrombolytic treatment. The estimated OR for major bleeding in patients with PE treated with thrombolysis is 1.4 (95% CI, 0.8 to. 5).

The incidence of intracranial haemorrhage observed in studies in patients with acute PE treated with rtPA is about 2%. This incidence is higher than that observed in studies of thrombolysis in patients with acute myocardial infarction (0.5–0.74%) (36,37).

However, more recent trials report lower incidence rates of major bleeding complications (Table 24.2). This could be the result of the use of safer thrombolytic regimens with shorter infusion times and possibly safer agents compared with first-generation thrombolytic drugs. An additional explanation is the reduced use of invasive strategies for diagnosis and monitoring of patients with PE, with non-invasive tools such as echocardiography and CT pulmonary angiography replacing the old-fashioned pulmonary angiogram. In fact, a number of major bleeding complication in initial studies were directly related to invasive procedures, occurring during and immediately after the procedure had been performed.

Table 24.2   Incidence of major bleeding and intracranial haemorrhage in clinical trials comparing rtPA and heparin and in recent registries in patients with acute PE[a]

	Clinical status	Invasive procedures	Major bleeding (%)		ICH (%)	
			rtPA	Heparin	rtPA	Heparin
Clinical trials						
PIOPED(40)	HD stable	AGF time 0 and 2 h	0	0	0	0
Levine(39)	HD stable	No	9.1	12.0	0	0
PAIMS-2(21)	HD stable	AGF	25.6	14.1	5.0	0
Goldhaber(29)	HD stable	AGF in a minority	6.5	3.6	2.1	0
Konstantinides(33)	HD stable	No	0.8	3.6	0	0
Registries						
MAPPET(1)	HD stable	No	21.9	7.8	1.2	0.4
ICOPER(2)	HD stable and unstable	No	21.7	8.8	3.0	0.3

[a]ICH, intracranial haemorrhage; HD, haemodynamically; AGF, angiography.

INDICATIONS FOR THROMBOLYTIC TREATMENT IN PATIENTS WITH PULMONARY EMBOLISM

Consensus exists that thrombolytic therapy should be used to treat PE associated with haemodynamic compromise. If one were to select haemodynamically stable patients with PE to receive thrombolytic therapy, this would require rapid and accurate risk stratification of the competing risks of death from PE versus those due to bleeding complications.

Overall, six studies have been performed, which randomized haemodynamically stable patients with PE to receive thrombolysis plus heparin or heparin alone. None of these studies provide definitive data on the net clinical benefit of thrombolytic treatment in this setting. Hence further studies are needed to determine the risk and benefits of thrombolytic therapy in haemodynamically stable patients with PE and signs of right ventricle dysfunction and/or injury.

A European multicentre, double-blind trial is currently ongoing aimed at assessing the clinical value of tenecteplase in haemodynamically stable patients with PE and signs of right ventricle dysfunction and/or injury. It is hoped that this study will cast some light on the feasibility of stratification of a subgroup of patients without overt haemodynamic instability, who may benefit from more aggressive therapy.

THROMBOLYTIC AGENTS AND REGIMENS FOR PULMONARY EMBOLISM

The approved thrombolytic regimens of streptokinase, urokinase and rtPA are shown in Table 24.3. Preliminary data appear to support the efficacy and safety of tenecteplase in acute pulmonary embolism when given at the same weight-adjusted doses currently used in patients with myocardial infarction.

Intravenous unfractionated heparin has been used in conjunction with thrombolytic therapy in the trials that have evaluated thrombolysis for PE. No data are currently available on the use of low molecular weight heparin in association with thrombolysis in this setting. Thus, initial anti-coagulation with intravenous heparin is recommended if thrombolytic therapy is being considered (38). Before thrombolytic therapy is started, unfractionated heparin should be given in full therapeutic doses. No direct comparison exists between the two strategies to either continue or suspend the infusion of unfractionated heparin during administration of thrombolytic therapy. In accordance with current guidelines, heparin should not be infused during the infusion of streptokinase or urokinase, while it can be given during rtPA administration. These indications are aimed at reducing bleeding complications and are not uniform across the world. More specifically, US regulatory bodies recommend suspension of unfractionated heparin during the 2 h infusion of 100 mg of rtPA, whereas unfractionated heparin is continued during the rtPA infusion in many other countries. After administration of thrombolytic therapy, the infusion of unfractionated heparin should

Table 24.3 Approved thrombolytic regimens for PE

Treatment	Regimen
Streptokinase	250 000 IU as a loading dose over 30 min, followed by 100 000 IU/h over 12–24 h
	Accelerated regimen: 1.5×10^6 IU over 2 h
Urokinase	4400 IU/kg as a loading dose over 10 min, followed by 4400 IU/kg/h over 12–24 h
	Accelerated regimen: 3×10^6 IU over 2 h
rtPA	100 mg over 2 h
	Accelerated regimen: 0.6 mg/kg over 15 min

Table 24.4 Conditions which increase the bleeding risk associated with thrombolytic therapy

Recent surgery, trauma, bleeding episode or cerebrovascular event:
- Cardiopulmonary resuscitation; major surgery, delivery, organ biopsy, puncture of non-compressible vessels; acute gastrointestinal bleeding
- Major trauma
- Neurosurgery or ophthalmologic surgery
- Ischaemic stroke

Concomitant medical conditions at risk for haemorrhage:
Uncontrolled severe hypertension (systolic pressure >180 mmHg; diastolic pressure>110 mmHg)
Platelet count <100 000/mm^3; prothrombin time <50%
Pregnancy
Bacterial endocarditis
Diabetic haemorrhagic retinopathy

be restarted or continued. If unfractionated heparin has not been suspended, the infusion is continued at the same rate with ongoing adjustment according to activated partial prothrombin time results. The risk for bleeding complications has to be carefully evaluated in all patients candidates for thrombolytic treatment (Table 24.4).

CONCLUSIONS

In patients with acute PE, thrombolytic therapy should be used in the presence of overt haemodynamic instability or sustained hypotension.

In haemodynamically stable patients, the decision to use thrombolysis should be based on the evaluation of markers of myocardial injury and dysfunction and based on the individual's risk of bleeding.

REFERENCES

1. Konstantinides S, Geibel A, Olschewski M, *et al*. Association between thrombolytic treatment and the prognosis of hemodynamically stable patients with major pulmonary embolism. *Circulation* 1997; **96**:882–886.
2. Goldhaber SZ, Visani L, De Rosa M. Acute pulmonary embolism: clinical outcomes in the International Cooperative Pulmonary Embolism Registry. *Lancet* 1999; **353**:1386–9.
3. Carson JL, Kelley MA, Duff A, *et al*. The clinical course of pulmonary embolism. *N Engl J Med* 1992; **326**:1240–5.
4. Wood KE. Major pulmonary embolism: review of a pathophysiologic approach to the golden hour of hemodynamically significant pulmonary embolism. *Chest* 2002; **121**:877–905.
5. Becattini C, Agnelli G. Acute pulmonary embolism: risk stratification in the emergency department. *Intern Emerg Med*. 2007; **2**:119–29.
6. Grifoni S, Olivotto I, Cecchini P, *et al*. Short term clinical outcome of patients with pulmonary embolism, normal blood pressure and echocardiographycal right ventricular dysfunction. *Circulation* 2000; **101**:2817–22.
7. Kucher N, Rossi E, De Rosa M, Goldhaber SZ. Prognostic role of echocardiography among patients with acute pulmonary embolism and a systolic arterial pressure of 90mmHg or higher. *Arch Intern Med* 2005; **165**:1777–81.
8. Goldhaber SZ. Echocardiography in the management of pulmonary embolism *Ann Intern Med* 2002; **136**:691–700.
9. Kucher N, Printzen G, Doernhoefer T, Windecker S, Meier B, Hess OM. Low pro-brain natriuretic peptide levels predict benign clinical outcome in acute pulmonary embolism. *Circulation* 2003; **107**:1576–8.

10. Becattini C, Vedovati MC, Agnelli G. Prognostic value of troponins in acute pulmonary embolism. A meta-analysis. *Circulation* 2007; **116**:427–33.

11. Kaczynska A, Pelsers M, Bochowicz A, Kostrubiec M, Glatz J, Pruszcyk P. Plasma heart-type fatty acid binding protein is superior to troponin and myoglobin for rapid risk stratification in acute pulmonary embolism. *Clin Chim Acta* 2006; **371**:117–23.

12. Torbicki A, Perrier A, Konstantinides S, *et al*. Guidelines in the diagnosis and management of acute pulmonary embolism: the task force for the diagnosis and management of acute pulmonary embolism of the European Society of Cardiology. *Eur Heart J* 2008; **29**:2276–315.

13. Tillet WS, Garner RL. The fibrinolytic activity of haemolytic streptococci. *J Exp Med* 1933; **68**:485–502.

14. MacFarlane RG, Pilling J. Fibrinolytic activity in normal urine. *Nature* 1947; **159**:779.

15. Pennica D, Holmes WE, Kohr WH, *et al*. Cloning and expression of human tissue-type plasminogen activator cDNA in *E. coli*. *Nature* 1983; **301**:214–221.

16. Assessment and Efficacy of a New Thrombolytic (ASSENT-2) Investigators. Single-bolus tenecteplase compared with front-loaded alteplase in acute myocardial infarction: the ASSENT-2 double-blind randomised trial. *Lancet* 1999; **28**:716–22.

17. Urokinase Pulmonary Embolism Trial Study Group. Urokinase pulmonary embolism trial: phase I results. *JAMA* 1970; **214**:2163–72.

18. Ly B, Arnesen H, Eie H, *et al*. A controlled clinical trial of streptokinase and heparin in the treatment of major pulmonary embolism. *Acta Med Scand* 1978; **203**:465–70.

19. Goldhaber SZ, Vaughan DE, Markis JE, *et al*. Acute pulmonary embolism treated with tissue plasminogen activator. *Lancet* 1986; **ii**:886–9.

20. Parker JA, Markis JE, Palla A, *et al*. Early improvement in pulmonary perfusion after rtPA therapy for acute pulmonary embolism: segmental perfusion scan analysis. *Radiology* 1988; **166**:441–5.

21. Dalla-Volta S, Palla A. PAIMS 2-alteplase combined with heparin versus heparin in the treatment of acute pulmonary embolism: Plasminogen Activator Italian Multicenter Study 2. *J Am Coll Cardiol* 1992; **20**:520–6.

22. Meyer G, Sors H, Charbonnier E, *et al*. Effects of intravenous urokinase versus alteplase on total ulmonary resistace in acute massive pulmonary embolism. A European, multicenter, double-blind trial. *J Am Coll Cardiol* 1992; **19**:239–45.

23. Goldhaber SZ, Kessler CM, Heit J, *et al*. A randomized, controlled trial of recombinant tissue plasminogen activator versus urokinase in the treatment of acute pulmonary embolism. *Lancet* 1988; **ii**:293–8.

24. Goldhaber SZ, Kessler Cm, Heit J *et al*. recombinant tissue plasminogen activator versus a novel dosing-regimen of urokinase in acute pulmonary embolism: a randomized, controlled, multicenter trial. *J Am Coll Cardiol* 1992; **20**:24–30.

25. Meneveau N, Schiele F, Vuillemenot A, *et al*. Streptokinase vs alteplase in massive pulmonary embolism. A randomized trial assessing right heart haemodynamics and pulmonary vascular obstruction. *Eur Heart J* 1997; **18**:1141–8.

26. Goldhaber SZ, Agnelli G, Levine MN. Reduced dose bolus alteplase vs conventional alteplase infusion for pulmonary embolism thrombolysis. An international multicenter randomized trial. The Bolus Alteplase Pulmonary Embolism Group. *Chest* 1994; **106**:718–24.

27. Sors H, Pacouret G, Azarian R, Meyer G, Charbonnier B, Simonneau G. Hemodynamic effects of bolus vs 2-h infusion of alteplase in acute massive pulmonary embolism. A randomized controlled multicenter trial. *Chest* 1994; **106**:712–7.

28. Verstraete M, Miller GA, Bounameaux H, *et al*. Intravenous and intrapulmonary recombinant tissue-type plasminogen activator in the treatment of acute massive pulmonary embolism. *Circulation* 1988; **77**:353–60.

29. Goldhaber SZ, Haire WD, Feldstein ML, *et al*. Alteplase versus heparin in acute pulmonary embolism: randomised trial assessing right-ventricular function and pulmonary perfusion. *Lancet* 1993; **341**:507–511.

30. Becattini C, Agnelli G, Salvi A, *et al*. Effect of bolus tenecteplase (TNK) on right ventricular dysfunction in normotensive patients with pulmonary embolism: a randomized, double-blind, placebo-controlled study. Abstracts ISTH 2008.

31. Jerjes-Sanchez C, Ramirez-Rivera A, de Lourdes Garcia M, *et al*. Streprokinase and heparin versus heparin alone in massive pulmonary embolism: a randomized controlled trial. *J Thromb Thrombolysis* 1995; **2**:227–9.

32. Gore JM, Sloan M, Price TR, *et al*. Urokinase–streptokinase embolism trial. Phase 2 result. *JAMA* 1974; **229**:1606–13.

33. Konstantinides S, Geibel A, Heusel G, Heinrich F, Kasper W. Heparin plus alteplase compared with heparin alone in patients with submassive pulmonary embolism. *N Engl J Med* 2002; **347**:1143–50.

34. Agnelli G, Becattini C, Kirschstein T. Thrombolysis vs heparin in the treatment of pulmonary embolism: a clinical outcome-based meta-analysis. *Arch Intern Med* 2002; **162**:2537–41.

35. Wan S, Quinlan DJ, Agnelli G, *et al*. Thrombolysis compared with heparin for the initial treatment of pulmonary embolism: a meta-analysis of the randomized controlled trials. *Circulation* 2004; **110**:744–9.

36. Gore JM, Sloan M, Price TM, *et al*. Intracerebral hemorrhage, cerebral infarction and subdural hematoma after acute myocardial infarction and thrombolytic therapy in the thrombolysis in myocardial infarction Phase iI, pilot and clinical trial. *Circulation* 1991; **83**:448–59.

37. Aylward PE, Wilcox RG, Horgan JH, *et al*. Relation of increased blood pressure to mortality and stroke in the context of contemporary thrombolytic therapy for acute myocardial infarction. *Ann Intern Med* 1996; **125**:891–900.

38. Kearon C, Kahn SR, Agnelli G, *et al*. Antithrombotic therapy for venous thromboembolic disease. *Chest* 2008; **133**:454S–545S.

39. Levine M, Hirsh J, Weitz J, *et al*. A randomized trial of a single bolus dosage regimen of recombinant tissue plasminogen activator in patients with acute pulmonary embolism. *Chest*. 1990; **98**:1473–9.

40. The PIOPED investigators. Tissue plasminogen activator for the treatment of acute pulmonary embolism. *Chest* 1990; **97**:528–33.

CHAPTER 25

Surgical Intervention in the Treatment of Pulmonary Embolism and Chronic Thromboembolic Pulmonary Hypertension

Michael M. Madani and Stuart W. Jamieson

Division of Cardiothoracic Surgery, University of California at San Diego
Medical Center, San Diego, CA, USA

OPERATIVE MANAGEMENT OF ACUTE PULMONARY EMBOLISM

Pulmonary embolism (PE) remains a significant cause of morbidity and mortality in the USA and worldwide. The estimated incidence of acute pulmonary embolism is approximately 63 per 100 000 patients in the USA based on clinical and radiographic data (1) and is related to approximately 235 000 deaths per year based on autopsy data. It is believed that acute PE is the third most common cause of death (after heart disease and cancer). The annual prevalence of deep vein thrombosis (DVT) in the USA has been estimated at approximately 2 million cases (2). Although the exact incidence of PE remains unknown, there are some valid estimates.

Approximately 75% of autopsy-proven PEs are not detected clinically. Dalen and Alpert (2) calculated that PE results in 630 000 symptomatic episodes in the USA yearly, making it about half as common as acute myocardial infarction and three times as common as cerebrovascular accidents. This is, however, a low estimate, since pre-mortem diagnosis was completely unsuspected in 70–80% of the patients with PE as the primary cause of death (3,4). The disease is particularly common in hospitalized elderly patients. Of all hospitalized patients who develop PE, 12–21% will die in the hospital and another 24–39% will die within 12 months (5–7). Thus, approximately 36–60% of the patients who survive the initial episode live beyond 12 months and may present later in life with a wide variety of symptoms. More than 90% of clinically detected PEs are associated with lower extremity DVT, but in two-thirds of patients with DVT and PE, the DVT is asymptomatic (8,9). Greenfield estimates that approximately 2.5 million Americans develop DVT each year (10).

At the present time, three treatment modalities that may be beneficial in this subgroup are available: thrombolysis (see Chapter 24), catheter embolectomy or dispersion (see Chapter 26) and operative embolectomy. The first two interventions are discussed in depth elsewhere in this volume; the initial portion of this chapter will focus on the third.

In 1908, Trendelenberg reported his initial experience with operative management of acute PE (11). Although none of his three patients survived, the important concept of immediate restitution of pulmonary blood flow gained rapid acceptance. However, even though the technical aspects of embolectomy were readily mastered, clinical diagnosis was infrequent prior to circulatory collapse and, in the absence of suitable resuscitation techniques, hypoxic brain injury was almost certain. Long-term survival with complete functional recovery was therefore not reported until 1924 (12). In 1960, Allison *et al*. successfully used total body hypothermia and circulatory arrest for this operation, (13), although the advantages of this technique were rapidly superseded by those afforded by cardiopulmonary bypass (14). Even within the past decade, however, embolectomy with inflow occlusion has been advocated as a life-saving alternative when extracorporeal support is not readily available (15).

Despite the feasibility of embolectomy, its role in the management of acute PE has long been contested and we are unaware of persuasive new data that might permit resolution of this debate. Suffice it to say that so long as patients die of acute PE, the method will justifiably have advocates. For the most part, DVT and acute PE are managed medically. Cardiac surgeons rarely become involved in the management of acute PE, unless it is in a hospitalized patient who survives a massive embolus that causes life-threatening acute right heart failure with low cardiac output, with a large clot burden.

Massive PE is truly life-threatening and is defined as a PE that causes haemodynamic instability. It is sometimes associated with occlusion of more than 50% of the pulmonary vasculature, but may occur with much smaller occlusions, particularly in patients with pre-existing cardiac or pulmonary disease. The diagnosis is clinical, not anatomical. Patients develop acute dyspnea, tachypnea, tachycardia and diaphoresis, and sometimes may lose consciousness. Both hypotension and low cardiac output (index <1.8 L/m^2/ min) are present. Cardiac arrest may occur. Neck veins are distended; central venous pressure is elevated and a right ventricular impulse may be present. Room air blood gases show severe hypoxia (PaO_2 <50 Torr), hypocarbia ($PaCO_2$ <30 Torr) and sometimes acidosis. Urine output falls and peripheral pulses and perfusion are poor.

Management of acute massive embolism

If the circulation cannot be stabilized at survival levels within several minutes or if cardiac arrest occurs after a massive PE, time becomes of paramount importance. Most deaths from acute PE occur before effective treatment is instituted, often as a result of failure of diagnosis. About 11% of patients with fatal PE die within the first hour, 43–80% within 2 h and 85% within 6 h (16). To a great extent, circumstances and the timely availability of necessary equipment and personnel determine therapeutic options. Mitigating factors such as advanced age, irreversible underlying health problems and the likelihood of brain damage also enter decision-making. A decision to treat medically in an effort to stabilize the circulation at a survival level may pre-empt life-saving surgery, but also may make surgery unnecessary.

For many reasons, retrospective studies are of limited relevance for this decision. Sometimes surgical treatment is not available immediately; at other times deteriorating patients are referred to surgery too late after failing medical therapy. The relative infrequency of treatment opportunities in massive PE, mitigating factors and the lack of clear criteria for prescribing medical or surgical therapy leave the management of massive PE unsettled.

Better understanding of the condition and newer technology offer a reasonable, if untried, algorithm for dealing with 'probable massive PE with life-threatening haemodynamic instability' in hospitalized patients. In otherwise healthy patients in whom surgery poses little risk or morbidity, emergency thromboembolectomy with preoperative confirmation of the diagnosis in the operating room by transoesophageal echocardiography offers the best chance of survival, even though an occasional patient may undergo an unnecessary general anaesthesia or even less likely an operation. When surgery is not immediately available or in patients who may not be surgical candidates or in whom an alternate diagnosis seems more likely, emergency extracorporeal life support (ECLS) using peripheral cannulation is an attractive alternative (17,18). In prepared institutions, ECLS can be instituted rapidly outside the operating room. ECLS compensates for acute cor pulmonale and hypoxia and sustains the circulation until the clot partially lyses, pulmonary vascular resistance falls and pulmonary blood flow becomes adequate.

Operative technique

Emergency pulmonary thromboembolectomy is indicated for suitable patients with life-threatening circulatory insufficiency as discussed earlier, but should not be done without a definitive diagnosis. In those patients not already sustained by extracorporeal support, circulatory stability is precarious. Under such circumstances, the hazards implicit in any delay in operation must be balanced by the advantages that might accrue with the provision of additional invasive monitoring prior to induction. However, at the minimum, the surface electrocardiogram, cutaneous oximetry and arterial pressure should be monitored.

It is worthwhile mentioning that a clinical diagnosis of PE is often wrong (16,19–21). If a patient has been taken directly to the operating room without a definitive diagnosis, transoesophageal echocardiography and colour Doppler mapping can confirm or refute the diagnosis in the operating room. Transoesophageal echocardiography permits good assessment of right ventricular volume, contractility and tricuspid regurgitation, which are strongly associated with massive PE and acute cor pulmonale. Echocardiographic detection of a large clot trapped within the right atrium or ventricle in a haemodynamically compromised patient with massive acute PE is another indication for emergency pulmonary thromboembolectomy (22–24).

A midline sternotomy incision is used. The ascending aorta and both cavae are cannulated after full heparinization and cardiopulmonary bypass is initiated. The heart may be electrically fibrillated or arrested with cold cardioplegic solution. Significant hypothermia may not be necessary since only a short period of complete bypass is needed. The main pulmonary artery is then opened 1–2 cm downstream of the valve and the incision is extended into the proximal left pulmonary artery. Forceps and suction catheters remove the clot from the left pulmonary artery and behind the aorta to the right pulmonary artery. Unless operation has been delayed for several days, the embolic material is not adherent and can be easily extracted. Because some fragmentation may have occurred, either preoperatively or during the evacuation, it is essential to inspect the distal vessels to ensure patency. Extracorporeal flow can be transiently reduced or interrupted to facilitate this examination. Any thrombotic material encountered can generally be removed with forceps or suction; gentle, manual inflation of the lungs may dislodge more distal fragments and propel them centrally to allow easy retrieval.

The right pulmonary artery can also be exposed and opened between the aorta and superior vena cava to allow better exposure in the distal segments, if necessary. If a sterile paediatric bronchoscope is available, the surgeon can use this instrument to locate and remove thrombi in tertiary and quaternary pulmonary vessels. Alternatively, pleural spaces are entered and each lung is gently compressed to dislodge small clots into larger vessels and suctioned out. The pulmonary arteriotomy is then closed with a fine running suture (e.g., 6-0 polypropylene). After restarting the heart, the patient is weaned from bypass, decannulated and closed.

Extracorporeal life support (ECLS)

The wider availability of long-term ECLS using peripheral vessel cannulation to stabilize the circulation offers a compromise position since most massive PEs will dissolve in time. ECLS can be implemented outside the operating room, but extensive preparations must be made before ECLS is available for emergency therapy. An emergency team must be assembled and trained and needed equipment and supplies must be collected. ECLS can be implemented within 15–30 min by an equipped team of trained personnel.

The femoral vein and artery are rapidly cannulated under sterile conditions using local anaesthesia. If the circulation is reasonably stable, both vessels can be cannulated over guide wires inserted via No. 16 angiographic needle punctures. A small skin incision is made to accommodate the cannulae and, after giving a bolus of heparin (1 mg/kg), first dilators and then cannulae are inserted. Alternatively, surgical cut-down and then cannulation using guide wires under direct vision can expose both femoral vessels. If pulses are absent or weak, a cut-down is usually faster; however, since patients need heparin and possibly fibrinolytic drugs, a minimal wound is preferred. The tip of the venous catheter is advanced into the right atrium to obtain flow rates of 2.5–4 L/min using an emergency pump–oxygenator circuit primed with crystalloid. The perfusion circuit consists of a small venous reservoir with intravenous access tubes, a centrifugal pump and membrane oxygenator. An arterial filter is not needed; an electromagnetic flow-meter is usually placed on the arterial line. During ECLS, heparin is infused to maintain activated clotting times between 180 and 200 s. Activated clotting times are measured every 30 min initially and every hour thereafter.

Although the groin wound is minimal, some bleeding occurs. Usually the amount of bleeding is small, but it is often persistent. Theoretically, the addition of thrombolytic drugs accelerates clot lysis and may decrease the duration of ECLS; however, these drugs are likely to increase bleeding complications and may not be needed once the circulation is stabilized. An alternative is to give low-dose fibrinolytic therapy directly into the thrombus via a pulmonary arterial catheter (see Chapter 26). ECLS should not be needed beyond a few hours or 1–2 days since clot lysis proceeds rapidly. Once pulmonary vascular resistance is adequately reduced and the patient achieves more stable haemodynamics, ECLS should be removed. The circuit and femoral cannulae should be discontinued in the operating room, since vessels will need to be sutured closed because of the need for heparin and long- term anticoagulation.

Postoperative care

Postoperative care is very similar to that for other patients who require open cardiac surgery. Cardiac output is maintained by pharmacological means and is usually adequate if the patient can be weaned from cardiopulmonary bypass and has not suffered irreversible myocardial injury. Reperfusion pulmonary oedema is not a problem, but renal failure and ischaemic brain damage from preoperative periods of inadequate circulation may become apparent. Antibiotics are required, particularly if sterile conditions were compromised in the resuscitation effort.

Results

Mortality rates for emergency pulmonary thromboembolectomy vary widely between 10 and 92% (16,22–44) Results are best if cardiopulmonary bypass is used to support the circulation during pulmonary arteriotomy. Not unexpectedly, perioperative mortality following embolectomy for acute PE is related to the severity of preoperative disability and to a lesser extent on the operative technique. The eventual outcome depends largely upon the preoperative condition and circulatory status of the patient. If cardiac arrest occurs and external massage cannot be stopped (without ECLS), mortality ranges between 45 and 75% and without cardiac arrest mortality ranges between 8 and 36% (22,24,25) Relatively few patients (26%) withstand normothermic arrest with inflow occlusion when the operation follows a preoperative arrest, although in experienced hands this same technique affords excellent survival (97%) when undertaken in patients with lesser degrees of impairment (26).

Late evaluation of survivors indicates the initial haemodynamic improvements are generally sustained and functional impairment is rare in the absence of recurrent embolization. Concurrent disease, primarily malignancy, is the most important determinant of late survival (39,44,45).

CHRONIC THROMBOEMBOLIC PULMONARY HYPERTENSION

Epidemiology and natural history

The incidence of pulmonary hypertension caused by chronic PE is even more difficult to determine than that of acute PE. There are more than 500 000 survivors per year of acute symptomatic episodes of acute PE (46,47). The incidence of chronic thrombotic occlusion in the population depends on what percentage of patients fail to resolve acute embolic material. It is estimated that chronic thromboembolic disease develops in only 0.5–3.8% of patients with a clinically recognized acute PE (46–48). If these figures are correct and counting only patients with symptomatic acute PE, a minimum of 2500 and as many as 19 000 individuals would progress to chronic thromboembolic pulmonary hypertension (CTEPH) in the USA each year. However, because most patients diagnosed with CTEPH have no antecedent history of acute embolism, the true incidence of this disorder is probably much higher.

Regardless of the exact incidence or the circumstances, it is clear that acute embolism and its chronic relation, fixed chronic thromboembolic occlusive disease, are both much more common than generally appreciated and are seriously underdiagnosed. Houk *et al*. (49) in 1963 reviewed the literature of 240 reported cases of chronic thromboembolic obstruction of major pulmonary arteries and found that only six cases had been diagnosed correctly before death. Calculations extrapolated from mortality rates and the random incidence of major thrombotic occlusion found at autopsy would support a postulate that more than 100 000 people in the USA currently have pulmonary hypertension that could be relieved by operation.

Although most individuals with CTEPH are unaware of a past thromboembolic event and give no history of DVT, the origin of most cases of unresolved PE are from acute embolic episodes. Why some patients have unresolved emboli is not certain, but a variety of factors must play a role, alone or in combination. The volume of acute embolic material may simply overwhelm the lytic mechanisms. The total occlusion of a major arterial branch may prevent lytic material from reaching, and therefore dissolving, the embolus completely. Repetitive emboli may not be able to be resolved. The emboli may be made of substances that cannot be resolved by normal mechanisms (already well-organized fibrous thrombus, fat or tumour). The lytic mechanisms themselves may be abnormal or some patients may actually have a propensity for thrombus or a hypercoaguable state. After the clot becomes wedged in the pulmonary artery, one of two processes occurs (50): (1) the organization of the clot proceeds to canalization, producing multiple small endothelialized channels separated by fibrous septa (i.e., bands and webs) or (2) complete fibrous organization of the fibrin clot without canalization may result, leading to a solid mass of dense fibrous connective tissue totally obstructing the arterial lumen.

In addition, there are other special circumstances. Chronic indwelling central venous catheters and pacemaker leads are sometimes associated with PE. Rarer causes include tumour emboli. Tumour fragments from stomach, breast and kidney malignancies have been demonstrated to cause chronic pulmonary arterial occlusion. Right atrial myxomas may also fragment and embolize.

As previously described and discussed, in addition to the embolic material, a propensity for thrombosis or a hypercoaguable state may be present in a few patients. This abnormality may result in spontaneous thrombosis within the pulmonary vascular bed, encourage embolization or be responsible for proximal propagation of thrombus after an embolus. However, whatever the predisposing factors to residual thrombus within the vessels, the final genesis of the resultant pulmonary vascular hypertension may be complex. With the passage of time, the increased pressure and flow as a result of redirected pulmonary blood flow in the previously normal pulmonary vascular bed can create a vasculopathy in the small pre-capillary blood vessels similar to the Eisenmenger syndrome.

Factors other than the simple haemodynamic consequences of redirected blood flow are probably also involved in this process. For example, after a pneumonectomy, 100% of the right ventricular output flows to one lung, yet little increase in pulmonary pressure occurs, even with follow-up to 11 years (51). In patients with thromboembolic disease, however, we frequently detect pulmonary hypertension even when less than 50% of the vascular bed is occluded by thrombus. It therefore appears that sympathetic neural connections, hormonal changes or both might initiate pulmonary hypertension in the initially unaffected pulmonary vascular bed. This process can occur with the initial occlusion either being in the same or the contralateral lung.

Regardless of the cause, the evolution of pulmonary hypertension as a result of changes in the previously unobstructed bed is serious, because this process may lead to an inoperable situation. Consequently, with our accumulating experience in patients with thrombotic pulmonary hypertension, we have increasingly been inclined towards early operation so as to avoid these changes. In the absence of operation, the prognosis for patients with chronic thromboembolic disease and pulmonary hypertension is poor. Survival is inversely related to the severity of pulmonary hypertension at diagnosis; fewer than 10% survive 5 years when the pulmonary artery pressure exceeds 50 mmHg (52).

The natural history of CTEPH is dismal and nearly all patients die of progressive right heart failure (52). Because of the insidious onset, the diagnosis is usually made relatively late in the progression of the disease when dyspnea and/or early symptoms of right heart failure develop and pulmonary hypertension is severe (>40 mmHg mean). In Riedel et al.'s series of 13 patients, nine died a mean of 28 months after the diagnosis of right heart failure (52). Seven of the 13 had recurrent episodes of fresh emboli demonstrated by new perfusion defects or by autopsy. The severity of pulmonary hypertension at the time of diagnosis inversely correlates with duration of survival.

Chronic anticoagulation represents the mainstay of the medical regimen. Although anticoagulation is primarily employed to forestall future embolic episodes, it also serves to limit the development of thrombus in regions of low flow within the pulmonary vasculature. Inferior vena caval filters are routinely employed to prevent recurrent embolization. If caval filtration and anticoagulation fail to prevent recurrent emboli, immediate thrombolysis may prove useful, but it must be noted that lytic agents are incapable of altering the chronic component of the disease.

The symptomatic manifestations of right ventricular failure are conventionally treated with diuretics and vasodilators and, while improvement may ensue, the effect is generally transient unless the fundamental pathophysiological process is addressed.

Clinical evaluation

CTEPH is an uncommon and frequently under-recognized, but treatable, cause of pulmonary hypertension. The condition forms part of the larger group of diseases with pulmonary hypertension and is more extensively discussed in Chapter 18. There are no signs or symptoms specific for chronic thromboembolism. The most common symptom associated with CTEPH, as with all other causes of pulmonary hypertension, is exertional dyspnea. This dyspnea is out of proportion to any abnormalities found on clinical examination. Like complaints of easy fatiguability, dyspnea that initially occurs only with exertion is often attributed to anxiety or being 'out of shape'. Syncope or presyncope (light-headedness during exertion) is another common symptom in pulmonary hypertension. Generally, it occurs in patients with more advanced disease and higher pulmonary arterial pressures.

Non-specific chest pains or tightness occur in approximately 50% of patients with more severe pulmonary hypertension. Haemoptysis can occur in all forms of pulmonary hypertension and probably results from abnormally dilated vessels distended by increased intravascular pressures. Peripheral oedema, early satiety and epigastric or right upper quadrant fullness or discomfort may develop as the right heart fails (cor pulmonale). Some patients with chronic pulmonary thromboembolic disease present after a small acute pulmonary embolus that may produce acute symptoms of right heart failure. A careful history brings out symptoms of dyspnea on minimal exertion, easy fatiguability, diminishing activities and episodes or angina-like pain or light-headedness. Further examination reveals the signs of pulmonary hypertension.

The physical signs of pulmonary hypertension are the same no matter what the underlying pathophysiology. Initially the jugular venous pulse is characterized by a large A-wave. As the right heart fails, the V-wave becomes predominant. The right ventricle is usually palpable near the lower left sternal border and pulmonary valve closure may be audible in the second intercostal space. Occasional patients with advanced disease are hypoxic and slightly cyanotic. Clubbing is an uncommon finding.

The second heart sound is often narrowly split and varies normally with respiration; P2 is accentuated. A sharp systolic ejection click may be heard over the pulmonary artery. As the right heart fails, a right atrial gallop usually is present and tricuspid insufficiency develops. Because of the large pressure gradient across the tricuspid valve in pulmonary hypertension, the murmur is high pitched and may not exhibit respiratory variation. These findings are quite different from those usually observed in tricuspid valvular disease. A murmur of pulmonic regurgitation may also be detected.

Pulmonary function tests reveal minimal changes in lung volume and ventilation; patients generally have normal or slightly restricted pulmonary mechanics. Diffusing capacity (DLCO) is often reduced and may be the only abnormality on pulmonary function testing. Pulmonary arterial pressures are elevated and supra-systemic pulmonary pressures are not uncommon. Resting cardiac outputs are lower than the normal range and pulmonary arterial oxygen saturations are reduced. Most patients are hypoxic; room air arterial oxygen tension ranges between 50 and 83 Torr, the average being 65 Torr (53). CO_2 tension is slightly reduced and is compensated by reduced bicarbonate. Dead space ventilation is increased. Ventilation–perfusion studies show moderate mismatch with some heterogeneity among various respirator units within the lung and correlate poorly with the degree of pulmonary obstruction (54).

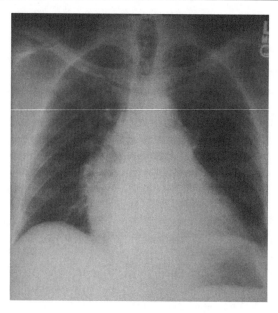

Figure 25.1   Chest radiographs reveals severe cardiomegaly with right ventricular enlargement. Note the enlarged right atrium, right ventricle, pulmonary arteries and the hypoperfusion in several areas of the lung fields.

Diagnosis

To ensure diagnosis in patients with CTEPH, a standardized evaluation is recommended for all patients who present with unexplained pulmonary hypertension. This workup includes a chest radiograph, which may show either apparent vessel cutoffs of the lobar or segmental pulmonary arteries or regions or oligaemia suggesting vascular occlusion. Central pulmonary arteries are enlarged and the right ventricle may also be enlarged without enlargement or the left atrium or ventricle (Figure 25.1). However, one should keep in mind that despite these classic findings, a large number of patients might present with a relatively normal chest radiograph, even in the setting of high degrees of pulmonary hypertension. The electrocardiogram demonstrates findings of right ventricular hypertrophy (right axis deviation, dominant R-wave in V1). Pulmonary function tests are necessary to exclude obstructive or restrictive intrinsic pulmonary parenchymal disease as the cause of pulmonary hypertension.

The ventilation–perfusion lung scan is the essential test for establishing the diagnosis of unresolved pulmonary thromboembolism. An entirely normal lung scan excludes the diagnosis of both acute or chronic, unresolved thromboembolism. The usual lung scan pattern in most patients with pulmonary hypertension either is relatively normal or shows a diffuse non-uniform perfusion (53–56). When subsegmental or larger perfusion defects are noted on the scan, even when matched with ventilatory defects, pulmonary angiography is appropriate to confirm or rule out thromboembolic disease.

In recent years, computed tomographic (CT) pulmonary angiography and magnetic resonance imaging (MRI) have been advocated as screening techniques for the diagnosis of CTEPH. These modalities are described in more detail in Chapters 7 and 9. Thrombus within the central pulmonary arteries is much better demonstrated by these newer generation CT scanners than either conventional CT or MRI, although the absence of thrombus proximal to the segmental pulmonary arteries is not a valid exclusionary criteria, nor does its presence exclude other pulmonary hypertensive disorders. In addition, CT scans may also demonstrate enlarged bronchial arteries or a pattern of mosaic oligaemia; the latter appears to be a relatively specific marker for chronic thromboembolic disease. The adjunct visualization of other thoracic structures with either method may suggest other causes of pulmonary hypertension, including mediastinal fibrosis and neoplasia. CT pulmonary angiography provides visualization of the thromboembolic material while also providing a clear picture of the vascular lumen and the degree of patency. However, in our opinion, at the present time neither MRI nor CT has sufficient accuracy to provide the ultimate information to proceed with or abandon an operation in CTEPH patients, although the advance of multidetector row CT and newer MR perfusion techniques is rapid and, with newer and faster systems, this is likely to change in the future. For this reason, neither one of these tests is currently routinely used at our institution, although their use is becoming increasingly more popular and mainstream. We continue to rely on pulmonary angiography and V/Q scanning for final assessment of our patients.

Currently, pulmonary angiography still remains the gold standard for the diagnosis of CTEPH. Organized thromboembolic lesions do not have the appearance of the intravascular filling defects seen with acute pulmonary emboli and experience is essential for the proper interpretation of pulmonary angiograms in patients with unresolved, chronic embolic disease. Organized thrombi appear as unusual filling defects, webs or bands or completely thrombosed vessels that may resemble congenital absence of the vessel (56) (Figure 25.2). Organized material along a vascular wall of a recanalized vessel produces a scalloped or serrated lumenal edge. Because of both vessel-wall thickening and dilatation of proximal vessels, the contrast-filled lumen may appear relatively normal in diameter. Distal vessels demonstrate the rapid tapering and pruning characteristic of pulmonary hypertension (Figure 25.2).

Although some risk remains, the benefit of establishing the presence of a treatable cause of the hypertension far outweighs the small risk; and pulmonary angiography should be performed whenever there is a possibility that chronic thromboembolism is the aetiology of pulmonary hypertension. Historically, angiography in those with pulmonary hypertension has been thought to carry disproportionate risk. We have found that not to be the case and at our institution pulmonary

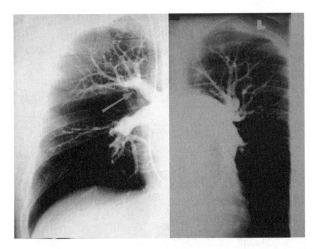

Figure 25.2 Right and left pulmonary angiograms demonstrate markedly diminished flow to lower lobes, with abrupt cut-offs, webs and multiple pouches. Preservation of perfusion to the upper lobes can be appreciated. Arrow points to the angiographic appearance of a web or band.

angiographies are performed daily in these patients with minimal associated risks. Several thousand angiograms in pulmonary hypertensive patients have now been performed at our institution without mortality or any significant morbidity.

In addition to pulmonary angiography, patients over 40 years old undergo coronary arteriography and other cardiac investigation as necessary. If significant disease is found, additional cardiac surgery is performed at the time of pulmonary thromboendarterectomy.

In approximately 15% of cases, the differential diagnosis between primary pulmonary hypertension and distal and small vessel pulmonary thromboembolic disease remains unclear and hard to establish. In these patients, pulmonary angioscopy is often helpful. The pulmonary angioscope is a fibre-optic telescope that is placed through a central line into the pulmonary artery. The tip contains a balloon that is then filled with saline and pushed against the vessel wall. A bloodless field can thus be obtained to view the pulmonary artery wall. The classic appearance of chronic pulmonary thromboembolic disease by angioscopy consists of intimal thickening, with intimal irregularity and scarring and webs across small vessels. These webs are thought to be the residue of resolved occluding thrombi of small vessels, but are important diagnostic findings. The presence of embolic disease, occlusion of vessels or the presence of thrombotic material is diagnostic.

Medical treatment

Chronic anticoagulation represents the mainstay of the medical regimen. Anticoagulation is primarily used to prevent future embolic episodes, but it also serves to limit the development of thrombus in regions of low flow within the pulmonary vasculature. Inferior vena caval filters are used routinely to prevent recurrent embolization. If caval filtration and anticoagulation fail to prevent recurrent emboli, immediate thrombolysis may be beneficial, but lytic agents are incapable of altering the chronic component of the disease.

Right ventricular failure is treated with diuretics and vasodilators and, although some improvement may result, the effect is generally transient because the failure is due to a mechanical obstruction and will not resolve until the obstruction is removed. Similarly, the prognosis is unaffected by medical therapy (57,58), which should be regarded as only supportive. Because of the bronchial circulation, PE seldom results in tissue necrosis. Therefore, surgical endarterectomy will allow distal pulmonary tissue to be used once more in gas exchange.

The only other surgical option for these patients is transplantation. However, we consider transplantation not to be appropriate for this disease because of the mortality and morbidity rates of patients on the waiting list, the higher risk of the operation and the contrasted survival rate (approximately 80% at 1 year at experienced centres for transplantation versus. 95% for pulmonary thromboendarterectomy). Furthermore, pulmonary thromboendarterectomy appears to be permanently curative and the issues of a continuing risk of rejection and immunosuppression are not present.

Operative management of chronic thromboembolic pulmonary hypertension

Holister and Cull first proposed thromboebdarterctomy for CTEPH in 1956 (59). Although there were previous attempts, Allison et al. (13) did the first successful pulmonary 'thromboendarterectomy' through a sternotomy using surface hypothermia, but only fresh clots were removed. The operation was performed 12 days after a thigh injury that led to PE and there was no endarterectomy component in this case. Since then, there have been many occasional surgical reports of the surgical treatment of CTEPH (60–64), but most of the surgical experience in pulmonary endarterectomy has been reported from the UCSD Medical Center. Braunwald commenced the UCSD experience with this operation in 1970, which now totals more than 2300 cases. The operation described below, using deep hypothermia and circulatory arrest, is the standard procedure.

Indications

When the diagnosis of CTEPH has been firmly established, the decision for operation is made based on the severity of symptoms and the general condition of the patient. Early in the pulmonary endarterectomy experience, Moser *et al*. (61) pointed out that there were three major reasons for considering thromboendarterectomy: haemodynamic, alveolo-respiratory and prophylactic. The haemodynamic goal is to prevent or ameliorate right ventricular compromise caused by pulmonary hypertension. The respiratory objective is to improve respiratory function by the removal of a large ventilated but unperfused physiological dead space, regardless of the severity of pulmonary hypertension. The prophylactic goal is to prevent progressive right ventricular dysfunction or retrograde extension of the obstruction, which might result in further cardio-respiratory deterioration or death (61). Our subsequent experience has added another prophylactic goal: the prevention of secondary arteriopathic changes in the remaining patent vessels.

Most patients who undergo operation are within New York Heart Association (NYHA) class III or class IV. The ages of the patients in our series have ranged from 7 to 85 years. A typical patient will have a severely elevated pulmonary vascular resistance (PVR) level at rest, the absence of significant co-morbid disease unrelated to right heart failure and the appearances of chronic thrombi on angiogram that appear to be relatively in balance with the measured PVR level. Of course, some exceptions to this general rule do occur.

Although most patients have a PVR level in the region of 800 dyn/s/cm^5 and pulmonary artery pressures less than systemic, the hypertrophy of the right ventricle that occurs over time makes pulmonary hypertension to suprasystemic levels possible. Therefore, many patients (approximately 20% in our practice) have a level of PVR in excess of 1000 dyn/s/cm^5 and suprasystemic pulmonary artery pressures. There is no upper limit of PVR level, pulmonary artery pressure or degree of right ventricular dysfunction that excludes patients from operation.

We have become increasingly aware of the changes that can occur in the remaining patent (unaffected by clot) pulmonary vascular bed subjected to the higher pressures and flow that result from obstruction in other areas. Therefore, with the increasing experience and safety of the operation, we now tend to offer surgery to symptomatic patients whenever the angiogram demonstrates CTEPH. A rare patient might have a PVR level that is normal at rest, although elevated with minimal exercise. This is usually a young patient with total unilateral pulmonary artery occlusion and unacceptable exertional dyspnea because of an elevation in dead space ventilation. Operation in this circumstance is performed not only to reperfuse lung tissue, but also to re-establish a more normal ventilation perfusion relationship (thereby reducing minute ventilatory requirements during rest and exercise) and also to preserve the integrity of the contralateral circulation and prevent chronic arterial changes associated with long-term exposure to pulmonary hypertension. If not previously implanted, an inferior vena caval filter is routinely placed several days in advance of the operation.

The criteria defining operative accessibility encompass both anatomy and operative experience. We are confident in our ability to recognize the various endovascular manifestations of this disease and can readily initiate a plane of dissection within the individual segmental pulmonary arteries, if necessary. Hence it is our feeling that pulmonary hypertension as a result of emboli is always operable. However, it can be arduous to discriminate between chronic thrombo-obliterative disease and chronic, atheromatous changes that develop secondary to long-standing pulmonary hypertension, particularly when the pathological changes are encountered at relatively distal levels. It is worth emphasizing that at whatever level the obstruction begins, success can be assured only if the more distal tendrils of the propagated thrombus are removed. Operation is almost inevitably lethal whenever a significant improvement in pulmonary flow is not achieved in those patients with very high preoperative pulmonary vascular resistance.

Our screening evaluation comprises the assessment previously elaborated, in addition to any additional studies necessary to assess risk fully in an individual destined to undergo a major operation. Advanced chronological age is not considered a barrier and we have successfully operated on individuals well within their eighth decade.

Operative technique

There are several guiding principles for the operation. Surgical treatment and endarterectomy must be bilateral, because this is a bilateral disease in most of our patients. Furthermore, for pulmonary hypertension to be a major factor, both pulmonary vasculatures are typically involved. The only reasonable approach to both pulmonary arteries is through a median sternotomy incision. Historically, there were many reports of unilateral operation and occasionally this is still performed, in inexperienced centres, through a thoracotomy. However, the unilateral approach ignores the disease on the contralateral side, subjects the patient to haemodynamic jeopardy during the clamping of the pulmonary artery, does not allow good visibility because of the continued presence of bronchial blood flow and exposes the patient to a repeat operation on the contralateral side. In addition, collateral channels develop in chronic thrombotic hypertension not only through the bronchial arteries but also from diaphragmatic, intercostal and pleural vessels. The dissection of the lung in the pleural space via a thoracotomy incision can therefore be extremely bloody. The median sternotomy incision, apart from providing bilateral access, avoids entry into the pleural cavities and allows the ready institution of cardiopulmonary bypass.

Cardiopulmonary bypass is essential to ensure cardiovascular stability when the operation is performed and to cool the patient to allow circulatory arrest. Excellent visibility is required, in a bloodless field, to define an adequate endarterectomy plane and to then follow the pulmonary endarterectomy specimen deep into the subsegmental vessels. Because of the copious bronchial blood flow usually present in these cases, periods of circulatory arrest are necessary to ensure perfect visibility. Again, there have been sporadic reports of the performance of this operation without circulatory arrest. However, it should be emphasized that although endarterectomy is possible without circulatory arrest, a complete endarterectomy is not. We always initiate the procedure without circulatory arrest and a variable amount of dissection, but never complete dissection, is possible before the circulation is stopped. The circulatory arrest periods are limited to 20 min, with restoration of flow between each arrest. With experience, the endarterectomy usually can be performed with a single period of circulatory arrest on each side.

A true endarterectomy in the plane of the media must be accomplished. It is essential to appreciate that the removal of visible thrombus is largely incidental to this operation. Indeed, in most patients, no free thrombus is present, and on initial direct examination, the pulmonary vascular bed may appear normal. The early literature on this procedure indicates that thrombectomy was often performed without endarterectomy and in these cases the pulmonary artery pressures did not improve, often with the resultant death of the patient.

Following induction and intubation and prior to incision, monitoring is supplemented by the addition of capnography, transoesophageal echocardiography, electro-encephalography and cerebral oxymetry. Because gradient frequently develops between central and peripheral arterial pressure during cooling and rewarming periods, an additional arterial pressure line is routinely used in the femoral artery. Body temperature is assessed using thermostats incorporated in the pulmonary artery, bladder catheter and rectal temperature probe. Left atrial pressure is not regularly determined. If the patient maintains permissive haemodynamics following the induction of anaesthesia, up to 500 mL of autologous full blood is withdrawn for later use in the volume deficit replaced with crystalloid.

After a median sternotomy incision is made, the pericardium is incised longitudinally and attached to the wound edges. Typically the right heart is enlarged, with a tense right atrium and a variable degree of tricuspid regurgitation. There is usually severe right ventricular hypertrophy and, with critical degrees of obstruction, the patient's condition may become unstable with the manipulation of the heart.

Anticoagulation is achieved with the use of beef-lung heparin sodium (400 units/kg, intravenously) administered to prolong the activated clotting time beyond 400 s. Full cardiopulmonary bypass is instituted with high ascending aortic cannulation and two caval cannulae. These cannulae must be inserted into the superior and inferior vena cavae sufficiently to allow subsequent opening of the right atrium. The heart is emptied on bypass and a temporary pulmonary artery vent is placed in the midline of the main pulmonary artery 1 cm distal to the pulmonary valve. This will mark the beginning of the left pulmonary arteriotomy.

When cardiopulmonary bypass is initiated, surface cooling with both the head jacket and the cooling blanket is begun. The blood is cooled with the pump–oxygenator. During cooling, a 10 °C gradient between arterial blood and bladder or rectal temperature is maintained (62). Cooling generally takes 45–60 min. When ventricular fibrillation occurs, an additional vent is placed in the left atrium through the right superior pulmonary vein. This prevents atrial and ventricular distension from the large amount of bronchial arterial blood flow that is common with these patients.

It is most convenient for the primary surgeon to stand initially on the patient's left side. During the cooling period, some preliminary dissection can be performed, with full mobilization of the right pulmonary artery from the ascending aorta. The superior vena cava is also fully mobilized. The approach to the right pulmonary artery is made medial, not lateral, to the superior vena cava. All dissection of the pulmonary arteries takes place intra-pericardially and neither pleural cavity should be entered. An incision is then made in the right pulmonary artery from beneath the ascending aorta out under the superior vena cava and entering the lower lobe branch of the pulmonary artery just after the take-off of the middle lobe artery. It is important that the incision stays in the centre of the vessel and continues into the lower, rather than the middle, lobe artery.

Any loose thrombus, if present, is now removed. This is necessary to obtain good visualization. It is most important to recognize, however, that first, an embolectomy without subsequent endarterectomy is ineffective, and second, in most patients with CTEPH, direct examination of the pulmonary vascular bed at operation generally shows no obvious embolic material. Therefore, to the inexperienced or cursory glance, the pulmonary vascular bed may well appear normal even in patients with severe CTEPH.

If the bronchial circulation is not excessive, the endarterectomy plane can be found during this early dissection. However, although a small amount of dissection can be performed before the initiation of circulatory arrest, it is unwise to proceed unless perfect visibility is obtained because the development of a correct plane is essential.

There are four broad types of pulmonary occlusive disease related to thrombus that can be appreciated and we use the following classification (56, 94). Type I disease (approximately 20–25% of cases of CTEPH; Figure 25.3) refers to the situation in which major vessel clot is present and readily visible on the opening of the pulmonary arteries. As mentioned earlier, all central thrombotic material has to be completely removed before the endarterectomy. In type II disease

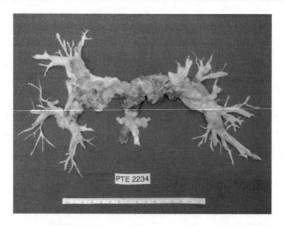

Figure 25.3 Surgical specimen removed from a patient with type I disease. The specimen is arrayed in anatomical position. Large amount of proximal thromboembolic material is noted in the main and both right and left pulmonary arteries. The thickened fibrous material seen in the distal vessels is characteristic of remodelled thrombus. Note that simple removal of large proximal thromboembolic material, without a complete endarterectomy, will leave a significant amount of distal disease behind and will result in the patient's demise. A full colour version of this image appears in the plate section of this book.

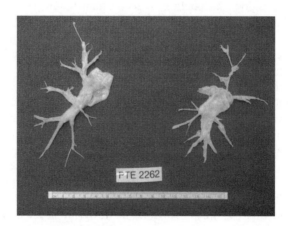

Figure 25.4 Surgical specimen removed from a patient with type II disease. Both pulmonary arteries have evidence of chronic thromboembolic material, but there is no evidence of fresh thromboembolic material. Note the distal tails of the specimen in each branch. Full resolution of pulmonary hypertension is dependent on complete removal of all the distal tails A full colour version of this image appears in the plate section of this book.

(approximately 45–50% of cases; Figure 25.4), no major vessel thrombus can be appreciated. In these cases, only thickened intima can be seen, occasionally with webs, and the endarterectomy plane is raised in the main, lobar or segmental vessels. Type III disease (approximately 25–30% of cases; Figure 25.5) presents the most challenging surgical situation. The disease is very distal and confined to the segmental and subsegmental branches. No occlusion of vessels can be seen initially. The endarterectomy plane must be carefully and painstakingly raised in each segmental and subsegmental branch. Type III disease is most often associated with presumed repetitive thrombi from indwelling catheters (such as pacemaker wires) or ventriculoatrial shunts. Type IV

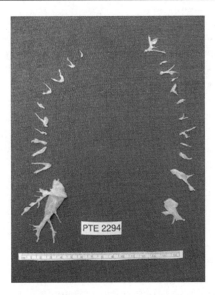

Figure 25.5 Surgical specimen removed from a patient with type III disease. Note that in this group of patients the disease is more distal and the plane of dissection has to be raised individually at each segmental level. A full colour version of this image appears in the plate section of this book.

disease does not represent primary thromboembolic pulmonary hypertension and is inoperable. In this entity there is intrinsic small vessel disease, although secondary thrombus may occur as a result of stasis. Small-vessel disease may be unrelated to thromboembolic events ('primary' pulmonary hypertension) or occur in relation to thromboembolic hypertension as a result of a high flow or high pressure state in previously unaffected vessels similar to the generation of Eisenmenger's syndrome. We believe that there may also be sympathetic 'cross-talk' from an affected contralateral side or stenotic areas in the same lung.

When the patient's temperature reaches 20 °C, the aorta is cross-clamped and a single dose of cold cardioplegic solution (1 L) is administered. Additional myocardial protection is obtained by the use of a cooling jacket. The entire procedure is now performed with a single aortic cross-clamp period with no further administration of cardioplegic solution.

A modified cerebellar retractor is placed between the aorta and superior vena cava. When blood obscures direct vision of the pulmonary vascular bed, thiopental is administered (0.5–1 g) until the electroencephalogram becomes isoelectric. Circulatory arrest is then initiated and the patient undergoes exsanguination. All monitoring lines to the patient are turned off to prevent the aspiration of air. Snares are tightened around the cannulae in the superior and inferior vena cavae. It is rare that one 20 min period for each side is exceeded. Although retrograde cerebral perfusion has been advocated for total circulatory arrest in other procedures, it is not helpful in this operation because it does not allow a completely bloodless field and, with the short arrest times that can be achieved with experience, it is not necessary.

Any residual loose, thrombotic debris encountered is removed. Then, a microtome knife is used to develop the endarterectomy plane posteriorly, because any inadvertent egress in this site could be repaired readily or simply left alone. Dissection in the correct plane is critical because if the plane is too deep the pulmonary artery may perforate, with fatal results, and if the dissection plane is not deep enough inadequate amounts of the chronically thromboembolic material will be removed.

When the proper plane is entered, the layer will strip easily and the material left with the outer layers of the pulmonary artery will appear somewhat yellow. The ideal layer is marked with a pearly white plane, which strips easily. There should be no residual yellow plaque. If the dissection is too deep, a reddish or pinkish colour indicates that the adventitia has been reached. A more superficial plane should be sought immediately.

Once the plane is correctly developed, a full-thickness layer is left in the region of the incision to ease subsequent repair. The endarterectomy is then performed with an eversion technique. Because the vessel is everted and subsegmental branches are being worked on, a perforation here will become completely inaccessible and invisible later. This is why the absolute visualization in a completely bloodless field provided by circulatory arrest is essential. It is important that each subsegmental branch is followed and freed individually until it ends in a 'tail', beyond which there is no further obstruction. Residual material should never be cut free; the entire specimen should 'tail off' and come free spontaneously.

Once the right-sided endarterectomy is completed, circulation is re-started and the arteriotomy is repaired with a continuous 6-0 polypropylene suture. The haemostatic nature of this closure is aided by the nature of the initial dissection, with the full thickness of the pulmonary artery being preserved immediately adjacent to the incision.

After the completion of the repair of the right arteriotomy, the surgeon moves to the patient's right side. The pulmonary vent catheter is withdrawn and an arteriotomy is made from the site of the pulmonary vent hole laterally to the pericardial reflection, avoiding entry into the left pleural space. Additional lateral dissection does not enhance intraluminal visibility, may endanger the left phrenic nerve and makes subsequent repair of the left pulmonary artery more difficult.

The left-sided dissection is virtually analogous in all respects to that accomplished on the right. The duration of circulatory arrest intervals during the performance of the left-sided dissection is subject to the same restriction as the right.

After the completion of the endarterectomy, cardiopulmonary bypass is reinstituted and warming is commenced. Methylprednisolone (500 mg, intravenously) and mannitol (12.5 g, intravenously) are administered and during warming a $10\,°C$ temperature gradient is maintained between the perfusate and body temperature, with a maximum perfusate temperature of $37\,°C$. If the systemic vascular resistance level is high, nitroprusside is administered to promote vasodilatation and warming. The rewarming period is generally approximately 90–120 min but varies according to the body mass of the patient.

When the left pulmonary arteriotomy has been repaired, the pulmonary artery vent is replaced at the top of the incision. The heart is retracted upwards and to the left and a posterior pericardial window is made, between the aorta and the left phrenic nerve. Alternatively, prior to closure, a posterior pericardial drain can be placed and removed once drainage has substantially decreased.

The right atrium is then opened and examined. Any intra-atrial communication is closed. Although tricuspid valve regurgitation is invariable in these patients and is often severe, tricuspid valve repair is not performed. Right ventricular remodelling occurs within a few days, with the return of tricuspid competence. If other cardiac procedures are required, such as coronary artery or mitral or aortic valve surgery, these are conveniently performed during the systemic rewarming period. Myocardial cooling is discontinued once all cardiac procedures have been concluded. The left atrial vent is removed and the vent site is repaired. All air is removed from the heart and the aortic cross-clamp is removed.

When the patient has rewarmed, cardiopulmonary bypass is discontinued. Dopamine hydrochloride is routinely administered at renal doses and other inotropic agents and vasodilators are titrated as necessary to sustain acceptable haemodynamics. The cardiac output is generally high, with a low systemic vascular resistance. Temporary atrial and ventricular epicardial pacing wires are placed.

Despite the duration of extracorporeal circulation, haemostasis is readily achieved and the administration of platelets or coagulation factors is generally unnecessary. Wound closure is routine. A vigorous diuresis is usual for the next few hours, also a result of the previous systemic hypothermia.

Postoperative care

Meticulous postoperative management is essential to the success of this operation. All patients are mechanically ventilated for at least 24 h and all patients are subjected to a maintained diuresis with the goal of reaching the patient's preoperative weight within 24 h. Although much of the postoperative care is common to more ordinary open-heart surgery patients, there are some important differences.

The electrocardiogram, systemic and pulmonary arterial and central venous pressures, temperature, urine output, arterial oxygen saturation, chest tube drainage and fluid balance are monitored. A pulse oxymeter is used to monitor continuously peripheral oxygen saturation. Management of cardiac arrhythmias and output and treatment of wound bleeding are identical with those in other open heart operations. In addition, a higher minute ventilation is often required early after the operation to compensate for the temporary metabolic acidosis that develops after the long period of circulatory arrest, hypothermia and cardiopulmonary bypass. Tidal volumes higher than those normally recommended after cardiac surgery are therefore generally used to obtain optimal gas exchange. The maximum inspiratory pressure is maintained below 30 cm of water if possible.

Although we used to believe that prolonged sedation and ventilation were beneficial and led to less pulmonary oedema, subsequent experience has shown this not to be so. Extubation should be performed on the first postoperative day, whenever possible.

Patients have a considerable positive fluid balance after operation. After hypothermic circulatory arrest, patients initiate an early spontaneous aggressive diuresis for unknown reasons, but this may be related, in part, to the increased cardiac output related to a now lower pulmonary vascular resistance (PVR) level and improved right ventricular function. This should be augmented with diuretics, however, with the aim of returning the patient to the preoperative fluid balance within 24 h of operation. Because of the increased cardiac output, some degree of systemic hypotension is readily tolerated. Fluid administration is minimized and the patient's haematocrit level should be maintained above 30% to increase oxygen-carrying capacity and mitigate against the pulmonary reperfusion phenomenon.

The development of atrial arrhythmias, at approximately 10%, is no more common than that encountered in patients who undergo other types of non-valvular heart surgery. The small, inferior atrial incision, away from the conduction system of the atrium or its blood supply may be helpful in the reduction of the incidence of these arrhythmias.

Despite the requirement for the maintenance of an adequate haematocrit level, with careful blood conservation techniques used during operation, transfusion is required in only a few patients.

A Greenfield filter is usually inserted before operation, to minimize recurrent PE after pulmonary endarterectomy. However, if this is not possible, it can also be inserted at the time of operation. If the device is to be placed at operation, radiopaque markers should be placed over the spine that correspond to the location of the renal veins to allow correct positioning. Postoperative venous thrombosis prophylaxis with intermittent pneumatic compression devices is used and the use of subcutaneous heparin is begun on the evening of surgery. Anticoagulation with warfarin is begun as soon as the pacing wires and mediastinal drainage tubes are removed, with a target international normalized ratio of ratio 2.5:3.

Patients are subject to all the complications associated with open heart and major lung surgery (arrhythmias, atelectasis, wound infection, pneumonia, mediastinal bleeding, etc.), but also may develop complications specific to this operation. These include persistent pulmonary hypertension, reperfusion pulmonary response and neurological disorders related to deep hypothermia.

Persistent pulmonary hypertension

The decrease in PVR level usually results in an immediate and sustained restoration of pulmonary artery pressures to normal levels, with a marked increase in cardiac output. In a few patients, an immediately normal pulmonary vascular tone is not achieved, but an additional substantial reduction may occur over the next few days because of the subsequent relaxation of small vessels and the resolution of intraoperative factors such as pulmonary oedema. In such patients, it is usual to see a large pulmonary artery pulse pressure, the low diastolic pressure indicating good runoff, yet persistent pulmonary arterial inflexibility still resulting in a high systolic pressure.

There are a few patients in whom the pulmonary artery pressures do not resolve substantially. We do operate on some patients with severe pulmonary hypertension but equivocal embolic disease. Despite the considerable risk of attempted endarterectomy in these patients, since transplantation is the only other avenue of therapy there may be a point when it is unlikely that a patient will survive until a donor is found. In our most recent 500 patients, more than one-third of perioperative deaths were directly attributable to the problem of inadequate relief of pulmonary artery hypertension. This was a diagnostic rather than an operative technical problem. Attempts at pharmacological manipulation of high residual PVR levels with sodium nitroprusside, epoprostenol sodium or inhaled nitric oxide are generally not effective. Because the residual hypertensive defect is fixed, it is not appropriate to use mechanical circulatory support or extracorporeal membrane oxygenation in these patients if they deteriorate subsequently.

The 'reperfusion response'

A specific complication that occurs in most patients to some degree is localized pulmonary oedema or the 'reperfusion response'. Reperfusion response or reperfusion injury is defined as a radiological opacity seen in the lungs within 72 h of pulmonary endarterectomy (Figure 25.6). This unfortunately loose definition may therefore encompass many causes, such as fluid overload and infection.

True reperfusion injury that directly adversely impacts the clinical course of the patient now occurs in approximately 10% of patients. In its most dramatic form, it occurs soon after operation (within a few hours) and is associated with profound desaturation. Oedema-like fluid, sometimes with a bloody tinge, is suctioned from the endotracheal tube (64). Frank blood from the endotracheal tube, however, signifies a mechanical violation of the blood airway barrier that has occurred at operation and stems from a technical error. This complication should be managed, if possible, by identification of the affected area by bronchoscopy and balloon occlusion of the affected lobe until coagulation can be normalized.

One common cause of the reperfusion pulmonary oedema is persistent high pulmonary artery pressures after operation when a thorough endarterectomy has been performed in certain areas, but there remains a large part of the pulmonary vascular bed affected by type IV change. However, the reperfusion phenomenon is often encountered in patients after a seemingly technically perfect operation with complete resolution of high pulmonary artery pressures. In these cases, the response may be one of reactive hyperaemia, after the revascularization of segments of the pulmonary arterial bed that have long experienced no flow. Other contributing factors may include perioperative pulmonary ischaemia and conditions associated with high permeability lung injury in the area of the now denuded endothelium. Fortunately, the incidence of this complication is

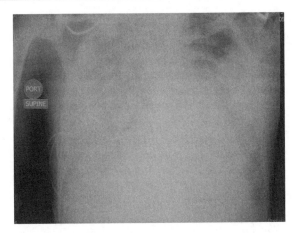

Figure 25.6 Chest radiograph of a patient with severe bilateral postoperative reperfusion response developed on postoperative day 3 after PTE. Note that haziness and opacification, although non-specific, are characteristic of this complication.

much less common now in our series, probably as a result of the more complete and expeditious removal of the endarterectomy specimen that has come with the large experience over the last decade.

Results

Although pulmonary endarterectomy is now performed at several major cardiovascular centres throughout the world, the majority of experience with this operation has been at the University of California, San Diego (UCSD), where the technique of this operation was pioneered and refined. More than 2300 pulmonary endarterectomy operations have been performed at UCSD since 1970; while the entire reported world's literature on this operation (exclusive of UCSD) is approximately 1500 cases, 1300 cases have been completed at UCSD since 1997 (65). The mean patient age in the last 10 years was 51.6 years, with a range of 8.9–84.8 years. There is a slight male predominance, reflecting either disease predilection, surgical bias or both. In 40% of cases, at least one additional cardiac procedure was performed at the time of operation. Most commonly, the adjunct procedure was closure of a persistent foramen ovale or atrial septal defect (18.9%) or coronary artery bypass grafting (7.9%) (66).

With this operation, a reduction in pulmonary pressures and resistance to normal levels and corresponding improvement in pulmonary blood flow and cardiac output are generally immediate and sustained (67,68). These changes are permanent (69). Table 25.1 lists the most current statistics for the last 1100 patients who underwent pulmonary endarterectomy at UCSD with respect to haemodynamic improvement. Whereas before the operation more than 78.7% of the patients were in NYHA functional class III or IV in this series, at 1 year after operation 97% of patients were reclassified as NYHA functional class I or II. In addition, echocardiographic studies have demonstrated that, with the elimination of chronic pressure overload, right ventricular geometry rapidly reverts toward normal (70). Right atrial and right ventricular hypertrophy and dilatation regresses. Tricuspid valve function returns to normal within a few days as a result of restoration of tricuspid annular geometry after the remodelling of the right ventricle, therefore tricuspid valve repair is not performed with this operation (71).

Table 25.1 Haemodynamic results for pulmonary thromboendarterectomy based on thromboembolic disease classification[a]

Parameter	Type I (n = 415, 37.7%)	Type II (n = 469, 42.6%)	Type III (n = 192, 17.5%)	Type IV (n = 24, 2.2%)	All patients (n = 1100, 100%)
Cardiac output (L/min)	3.7±1.4	4.1 ± 1.3	4.0 ± 1.5	3.8 ± 1.2	3.9 ± 1.3
	5.5 ± 1.5	5.5 ± 1.5	5.2 ± 1.4	4.5 ± 1.1	5.4 ± 1.5
Systolic PA pressure (mmHg)	76.8 ± 18.7	75.0 ± 19.5	75.8 ± 16.4	78.4 ± 15.6	75.9 ± 18.6
	44.4 ± 15.1	44.5 ± 15.0	52.7 ± 17.1	73.8 ± 32.1	46.4 ± 16.6
Mean PA pressure (mmHg)	47.0 ± 11.4	45.2 ± 11.6	46.5 ± 10.3	50.2 ± 10.5	46.2 ± 11.3
	27.2 ± 8.7	27.5 ± 9.1	31.8 ± 10.1	42.4 ± 15.5	28.4 ± 9.6
PVR (dyn/s/cm^5)	924.2 ± 450.4	799 ± 417.2	863.2 ± 454.6	884.6 ± 412.3	859.4 ± 439.5
	269.8 ± 176.6	270 ± 191.3	350.8 ± 183.3	595.2 ± 360.2	290.4 ± 195.7
Mortality (%)	16 (3.9)	22 (4.7)	12 (6.3)	4 (16.7)	52 (4.7)

[a]Data are shown as means ± standard deviations or as absolute numbers (percentage). The top rows of numbers are representative of the measured values preoperatively and the lower rows are postoperative measurements just prior to removal of Swan–Ganz catheter. PA, pulmonary artery; PVR, pulmonary vascular resistance.

Severe reperfusion injury is the single most frequent complication after pulmonary endarterectomy, historically occurring in approximately 15% of patients, but now in a much smaller percentage of our patients (about 5%).

A survey of surviving patients who underwent pulmonary endarterectomy between 1970 and 1995 at UCSD has formally evaluated long-term outcome from this operation (72). Questionnaires were mailed to 420 patients who were more than 1 year after operation and responses were obtained from 308. Survival, functional status, quality of life and the subsequent use of medical assistance were assessed. Survival after pulmonary endarterectomy was found to be 75% at 6 years or more. This survival exceeds single or double lung transplant survival for CTEPH. Some 93% of the patients were found to be in NYHA class I or II, compared with about 95% of the patients being in NYHA class III or IV preoperatively. Of the working population, 62% of patients who were unemployed before operation returned to work. Patients who had undergone pulmonary endarterectomy scored several quality of life components slightly lower than normal individuals, but significantly higher than the patients before operation. Only 10% of patients used oxygen after surgery. In response to the question, 'How do you feel about the quality of your life since your surgery?', 77% replied much improved and 20% replied improved. These data appear to confirm that pulmonary endarterectomy offers substantial improvement in survival, function and quality of life.

Future challenges

In the majority of patients, the development of CTEPH signifies a medical failure, initially in the prophylaxis and management of venous thrombosis and secondarily in the recognition, treatment and follow-up surveillance of those patients developing an acute PE. The appropriate remedies are elaborated elsewhere in this book. Those observations notwithstanding, acute embolism is clinically occult in a significant proportion of patients diagnosed with chronic thromboembolic disease and in an even greater proportion of individuals, the disorder altogether eludes diagnosis during life. It can be assumed that within the latter population, chronic CTEPH caused significant disability and contributed to premature death, even though an effective surgical therapy was available. Increased awareness of the prevalence of this disease and its many manifestations should reduce the likelihood that this disorder escapes ante-mortem detection, even in an era in which economic constraints increasingly influence clinical practice. However, even when the full array of methods currently available are employed by an experienced group, some residual diagnostic uncertainty persists in between 10 and 20% of patients, and in most such instances 'operative accessibility' of the disease is the usual basis for concern.

It is our opinion that all thromboembolic disease is reachable at operation; however, there may be other factors (such as irreversible small vessel pulmonary hypertensive changes) which are inoperable. At this time, the sole therapeutic alternative to pulmonary thromboendarterectomy is pulmonary transplantation. Because many of the patients in whom the wisdom of operation is deemed equivocal are by virtue of age or other restrictions ineligible for transplantation, it is inevitable that we will continue to offer operation at an assumed higher risk to some patients for whom this judgment is in retrospect erroneous. The less palatable alternative is to exclude all such patients from consideration, even while recognizing that many might benefit from the operation. Based on our present experience, we anticipate that in the future this hazard will continue to account for an operative mortality of between 2 and 4%.

The successive improvements in technique developed over the last four to five decades since the initial operative attempts allow pulmonary thromboendarterectomy to be offered now to patients with an acceptable mortality and excellent anticipation of clinical improvement. Over this same period, substantial improvements in anaesthetic management, perioperative monitoring and the methods of extracorporeal circulatory assistance have effected a significant overall reduction in the risk of open cardiac procedures. Former patients have benefited from these developments and we will continue to incorporate important new refinements.

CONCLUSION

It is increasingly apparent that pulmonary hypertension caused by chronic PE is a condition which is under-recognized and carries a poor prognosis. Medical therapy is ineffective in prolonging life and only transiently improves the symptoms. The only therapeutic alternative to pulmonary thromboendarterectomy is lung transplantation. The advantages of thromboendarterectomy include a lower operative mortality and excellent long-term results without the risks associated with chronic immunosuppression and chronic allograft rejection. The mortality for thromboendarterectomy at our institution is now in the region of 4.5%, with sustained benefit. These results are clearly superior to those for transplantation both in the short and long term.

Although pulmonary thromboendarterectomy is technically demanding for the surgeon and requires careful dissection of the pulmonary artery planes and the use of circulatory arrest, excellent short- and long-term results can be achieved. It is the successive improvements in operative technique developed over the last four decades which now allow pulmonary endarterectomy to be offered to patients with an acceptable mortality rate and excellent anticipation of clinical improvement. With this growing experience, it has also become clear that unilateral operation is obsolete and that circulatory arrest is essential.

The primary problem remains that this is an under-recognized condition. Increased awareness of both the prevalence of this condition and the possibility of a surgical cure should avail more patients of the opportunity for relief from this debilitating and ultimately fatal disease.

REFERENCES

1. DeMonaco NA, Dang Q, Kapoor WN, *et al*. Pulmonary embolism incidence is increasing with use of spiral computed tomography. *Am J Med* 2008; **121**:611–617.
2. Dalen JE, Alpert JS. Natural history of pulmonary embolism. *Prog Cardiovasc Dis* 1975; **17**:257–270.
3. Goldhaber SZ, Hennekens CH, Evens DA, *et al*. Factors associated with correct antemortem diagnosis of major pulmonary embolism. *Am J Med* 1982; **73**:822–826.
4. Rubinstein1, Murray D, Hoffstein V. Fatal pulmonary emboli in hospitalized patients: an autopsy study. *Arch Intern Med* 1988; **148**:1425–1426.
5. Kniffin WD Jr, Baron JA, Barrett J, *et al*. The epidemiology of diagnosed pulmonary embolism and deep venous thrombosis in the elderly. *Arch Intern Med* 1994; **154**:861.
6. Martin M:PHLECO. A multicenter study of the fate of 1647 hospital patients treated conservatively without fibrinolysis and surgery. *Clin Invest* 1993; **71**:471.
7. Carson JL, Kelley MA, Duff A, *et al*. The clinical course of pulmonary embolism. *N Engl J Med* 1992; **326**:1240.
8. Clagett GP, Anderson FA Jr, Levine MN, *et al*. Prevention of venous thromboembolism. *Chest* 1992; **102**:391S.
9. Anderson FA Jr, Wheeler HB. Venous thromboembolism; risk factors and prophylaxis. In Tapson VF, Fulkkerson WJ, Saltzman HA (eds), *Clinics in Chest Medicine, Venous Thromboembolism*, Vol **16**. WB Saunders, Philadelphia, 1995, p. 235.
10. Greenfield LJ. Venous thrombosis and pulmonary thromboembolism. In Schwartz SI (ed), *Principals of Surgery*, 6th edn, McGraw-Hill, New York, 1994, p. 989.
11. Trendelenburg F. Über die operative Behandlung der Embolie der Lungenarterie. *Arch Klin Chir* 1908; **86**:686–700.

12. Kirschner M. Ein durch die Trendelenburgsche Operation genheilter Fall von Embolie der Arterien Pulmonalis. *Arch Klin Chir* 1924; **133**:312.
13. Allison PR, Dunnill MS, Marshall R. Pulmonary embolism. *Thorax* 1960; **15**:273–283.
14. Sharp EH. Pulmonary embolectomy: successful removal of a massive pulmonary embolus with the support of cardiopulmonary bypass: a case report. *Ann Surg* 1962; **156**:161.
15. Clarke DB, Abrams LD. Pulmonary embolectomy: a 25 year experience. *J Thorac Cardiovasc Surg* 1986; **92**:442–445.
16. Mattox KL, Feldtman RW, Beall AC, De Bakey ME. Pulmonary embolectomy for acute massive pulmonary embolism. *Ann Surg* 1982; **195**:726.
17. Anderson HL III, Delius RE, Sinard JM, *et al*. Early experience with adult extracorporeal membrane oxygenataion in the modern era. *Ann Thorac Surg* 1992; **53**:553.
18. Wenger R, Bavaria JB, Ratcliff MB, Edmunds LH Jr. Flow dynamics of peripheral venous catheters during extracorporeal membrane oxygenator (ECMO) with a centrifuge pump. *J Thorac Cardiovasc Surg* 1988; **96**:478.
19. Tow De, Wagner HN. Recovery of pulmonary arterial blood flow in patients with pulmonary embolism. *N Engl J Med* 1967; **276**:1053.
20. Goldhaber SZ, Haire WD, Feldstein ML, *et al*. Alteplase versus heparin in acute PE; randomized trial assessing right ventricular function and pulmonary perfusion. *Lancet* 1993; **341**:507.
21. Boulafendis D, Bastounis E, Panayiotopoulos YP, Papalambros EL. Pulmonary embolectomy: answered and unanswered questions. *Int J Angiol* 1991; **10**:187.
22. Gray HH, Morgan JM, Miller GAH. Pulmonary embolectomy for acute massive pulmonary embolism; an analysis of 71 cases. *Br Heart J* 1988; **60**:196.
23. Del Campo C. Pulmonary embolectomy: a review. *Can J Surg* 1985; **28**: 111.
24. Clark DB. Pulmonary embolectomy has a well-defined and valuable place. *Br J Hosp Med* 1989; **41**:468.
25. Schmid C, Zietlow S, Wagner TOF, *et al*. Fulminant pulmonary embolism: symptoms, diagnostics, operative technique and results. *Ann Thorac Surg* 1991; **52**:1102.
26. Clarke DB, Abrams LD. Pulmonary embolectomy: a 25 year experience. *J Thorac Cardiovasc Surg* 1986; **92**:442–445.
27. Jaumin P, Moriau M, el Gariani A, *et al*. Pulmonary embolectomy, clinical experience. *Acta Chir Belg* 1986; **86**:123–125.
28. Stalpaert G, Suy R, Daenen W, *et al*. Surgical treatment of acute massive pulmonary embolism. Results and follow-up. *Acta Chir Belg* 1986; **86**:118–122.
29. Lund O, Nielsen TT, Schifter S, *et al*. Treatment of pulmonary embolism with full-dose heparin, streptokinase or embolectomy – results and indications. *Thorac Cardiovasc Surg* 1986; **34**:240–246.
30. Gray HH, Morgan JM, Paneth M, *et al*. Pulmonary embolectomy for acute massive pulmonary embolism: an analysis of 71 cases. *Br Heart J* 1988; **60**:196–200.
31. Meyer G, Tamisier D, Sors H, *et al*. Pulmonary embolectomy: a 20-year experience at one center. *Ann Thorac Surg* 1991; **51**:232–236.
32. Kieny R, Charpentier A, Kieny MT. What is the place of pulmonary embolectomy today? *J Cardiovasc Surg* 1991; **32**:549–554.
33. Schmid C, Zietlow S, Wagner TO, *et al*. Fulminant pulmonary embolism: symptoms, diagnostics, operative technique and results. *Ann Thorac Surg* 1991; **52**:1102–1105.
34. Bauer EP, Laske A, von Segesser LK, *et al*. Early and late results after surgery for massive pulmonary embolism. *Thorac Cardiovasc Surg* 1991; **39**:353–356.
35. Meyns B, Sergeant P, Flameng W, *et al*. Surgery for massive pulmonary embolism. *Acta Cardiol* 1992; **47**:487–493.
36. Laas J, Schmid C, Albes JM, *et al*. Surgical aspects of fulminant pulmonary embolism. *Z Kardiol* 1993; **82**:25–28.
37. Stulz P, Schlapfer R, feer R, *et al*. Decision making in the surgical treatment of massive pulmonary embolism. *Eur J Cardiothorac Surg* 1994; **8**:188–193.
38. Jakob H, Vahl C, Lange R, *et al*. Modified surgical concept for fulminant pulmonary embolism. *Eur J Cardiothorac Surg* 1995; **9**:557–560.
39. Doerge HC, Schoendube FA, Loeser H, *et al*. Pulmonary embolectomy: review of a 15-year experience and role in the age of thrombolytic therapy. *Eur J Cardiothorac Surg* 1996; **10**:952–957.
40. Doerge HC, Schoendube FA, Voss M, *et al*. Surgical therapy of fulminant pulmonary embolism: early and late results. *Thorac Cardiovasc Surg* 1999; **47**:9–13.

41. Ullmann M, Hemmer W, Hannekum A. The urgent pulmonary embolectomy: mechanical resuscitation in the operating theatre determines the outcome. *Thorac Cardiovasc Surg* 1999; **47**:5–8.
42. Aklog L, Williams CS, Byrne JG, *et al*. Acute pulmonary embolectomy: a contemporary approach. *Circulation* 2002; **105**:1416–1419.
43. Digonnet A, Moya-Plana A, Aubert S, *et al*. Acute pulmonary embolism: a current surgical approach. *Int Cardiovasc Thorac Surg* 2007; **6**:27–29.
44. Glassford DM, Alford WC, Burrus GR, Stoney WS, Thomas CS. Pulmonary embolectomy. *Ann Thorac Surg* 1981; **32**:28–32.
45. Lund O, Nielsen TT, Ronne K, Schifter S. Pulmonary embolism: long-term follow-up after treatment with full-dose heparin, streptokinase or embolectomy. *Acta Med Scand* 1987; **221**:61–71.
46. Benotti JR, Ockene IS, Alpert JS, Dalen JE. The clinical profile of unresolved pulmonary embolism. *Chest* 1983; **84**:669–678.
47. Moser KM, Auger WF, Fedullo PF. Chronic major-vessel thromboembolic pulmonary hypertension. *Circulation* 1990; **81**:1735–1743.
48. Pengo V, Lensing AW, Prins MH, *et al*. Incidence of chronic thromboembolic pulmonary hypertension after pulmonary embolism. *N Engl J Med* 2004; **350**:2257–2264.
49. Houk VN, Hufnnagel CA, McClenathan JE, Moser KM. Chronic thrombosis obstruction of major pulmonary arteries: report of a case successfully treated by thromboendarterectomy and review of the literature. *Am J Med* 1963; **35**:269–282.
50. Dibble JH. Organization and canalization in arterial thrombosis. *J Pathol Bacteriol* 1958; **75**:1–4.
51. Cournad A, Rilev RL, Himmelstein A, Austrian R. Pulmonary circulation in the alveolar ventilation perfusion relationship after pneumonectomy. *J Thorac Surg* 1950; **19**:80–116.
52. Riedel M, Stanek V, Widimsky J, Prerovsky I. Long term follow up of patients with pulmonary embolism: late prognosis and evolution of hemodynamic and respiratory data. *Chest* 1982; **81**:151.
53. Kapitan KS, Buchbinder M, Wagner PD, Moser KM. Mechanisms of hypoxemia in chronic pulmonary hypertension. *Am Rev Respir Dis* 1989; **139**:1149.
54. Moser KM, Daily PO, Peterson K, *et al*. Thromboendarterectomy for chronic, major vessel thromboembolic pulmonary hypertension: immediate and longterm results in 42 patients. *Ann Int Med* 1987; **107**:560.
55. Moser KM. Pulmonary vascular obstruction due to embolism and thrombosis. In Moser KM (ed), *Pulmonary Vascular Disease*, Marcel Dekker, New York, 1979, p. 341.
56. Jamieson SW, Kapalanski DP. Pulmonary endarterectomy. *Curr Probl Surg* 2000; **37**(3):165–252.
57. Dantzker DR, Bower JS. Partial reversibility of chronic pulmonary hypertension caused by pulmonary thromboembolic disease. *Am Rev Respir Dis* 1981; **124**:129–131.
58. Dash H, Ballentine N, Zelis R. Vasodilators ineffective in secondary pulmonary hypertension. *N Engl J Med* 1980; **303**:1062–1063.
59. Hollister LE, Cull VL. The syndrome of chronic thromboembolism of the major pulmonary arteries. *Am J Med* 1956; **21**:312–320.
60. Simonneau G, Azarian R, Bernot F, *et al*. Surgical management of unresolved pulmonary embolism: a personal series of 72 patients [abstract]. *Chest* 1995; **107**:52S.
61. Moser KM, Houk VN, Jones RC, Hufnagel CC. Chronic, massive thrombotic obstruction of the pulmonary arteries: analysis of four operated cases. *Circulation* 1965; **32**:377–385.
62. Winkler MH Rohrer CH, Ratty SC, *et al*. Perfusion techniques of profound hypothermia and circulatory arrest for pulmonary thromboendarterectomy. *J Extracorp Technol* 1990; **22**:57–60.
63. Jamieson SW. Pulmonary thromboendarterectomy. In Franco KL, Putnam JB (eds), *Advanced Therapy in Thoracic Surgery*, BC Decker, Hamilton, ON, 1998, pp. 310–318.
64. Levinson RM, Shure D, Moser KM. Reperfusion pulmonary edema after pulmonary artery thromboendarterectomy. *Am Rev Respir Dis* 1986; **134**:1241–1245.
65. Jamieson SW. Historical perspective: surgery for chronic thromboembolic disease. *Semin Thorac Cardiovasc Surg* 2006; **18**:218–222.
66. Thistlethwaite PA, Auger WR, Madani MM, *et al*. Pulmonary thromboendarterectomy combined with other cardiac operations: indications, surgical approach and outcome. *Ann Thorac Surg* 2001; **72**:13–17.
67. Menzel T, Kramm T, Mohr-Kahaly S, *et al*. Assessment of cardiac performance using Tei indices in patients undergoing pulmonary thromboendarterectomy. *Ann Thorac Surg* 2002; **73**:762–766.
68. Thistlethwaite PA, Madani MM, Jamieson SW: Outcomes of pulmonary endarterectomy surgery. *Semin Thorac Cardiovasc Surg* 2006; **18**:257–264.
69. Corsico AG, D'Armini AM, Cerveri I, *et al*. Long-term outcome after pulmonary endarterectomy. *Am J Respir Crit Care Med* 2008 June 12 (epub ahead of print).

70. Ilino M, Dymarkowski S, Chaothawee L, *et al*. Time course of reversed remodeling after pulmonary endarterectomy in patients with chronic pulmonary thromboembolism. *Eur Radiol* 2008; **18**:792–9.

71. Thistlethwaite PA, Jamieson SW. Tricuspid valvular disease in the patient with chronic pulmonary thromboembolic disease. *Curr Opin Cardiol* 2003; **18**:111–16.

72. Archibald CJ, Auger WR, Fedullo PF, *et al*. Long-term outcome after pulmonary thromboendarterectomy. *Am J Respir Crit Care Med* 1999; **160**:523–28.

CHAPTER 26

Interventional Techniques for Venous Thrombosis

Jim A. Reekers[1] and Edwin J.R. van Beek[2]

[1]Department of Radiology, Academic Medical Center, Amsterdam,
The Netherlands
[2]Department of Radiology, Carver College of Medicine, Iowa City, USA

INTRODUCTION

In most instances, acute treatment of venous thrombosis is less mandatory compared with arterial thrombosis. However, there are special circumstances where an acute intervention is indicated and may be life saving.

Interventional techniques for venous thrombosis are performed either by local administration of thrombolytic agents, mechanical thrombectomy or surgery. The aims of treatment of venous thrombosis are different for specific locations. In massive pulmonary embolism (PE), with haemo-dynamic impairment, rapid restoration of flow is important to prevent death or late sequelae such as pulmonary hypertension. On the other hand, catheter-related thrombosis is treated to preserve line patency if possible and (more importantly) to preserve the venous anatomy and access site for future therapy. The aim of treating deep vein thrombosis (DVT) with local lytic drugs is to prevent late complications such as venous insufficiency or to treat a possible underlying lesion, such as May–Turner syndrome.

PERCUTANEOUS INTERVENTIONS IN PULMONARY EMBOLISM

Immediate mortality due to PE is about 10%. and mortality is correlated with larger and more extensive embolic obstruction and with the presence of underlying cardiopulmonary disease. The main consequence of such life-threatening situations is the compromised haemodynamics as a result of the increased right ventricular afterload. In these patients, rapid restoration of pulmonary blood flow and reduction of the thrombus bulk can be live saving.

Intravenous thrombolysis

Systemic thrombolysis by injection of the lytic drug into a peripheral vein is often used (for a more complete discussion, see Chapter 24). Fibrinolytic therapy can still be successfully applied within

Deep Vein Thrombosis and Pulmonary Embolism   Edited by Edwin J.R. van Beek, Harry R. Büller and Matthijs Oudkerk
© 2009 John Wiley & Sons, Ltd

14 days after the onset of symptoms (1). It has been shown that with peripheral lytic therapy there is an improvement in perfusion of lung scans compared with heparin alone (2,3). This therapy can be lifesaving in patients with massive PE, cardiogenic shock or haemodynamic instability (4). A potential risk with this technique is the time delay between the onset of therapy and the actual clot lysis. There is also an increase in bleeding complications with systemic lysis. The most used intravenous thrombolytic regiments are (1) urokinase 2000 IU/lb loading dose over 10 min followed by 2000 IU/lb/h for 12–24 h and (2) 100 mg recombinant tissue plasminogen activator (rtPA) as a continuous infusion over 2 h (5). Contraindications to systemic thrombolysis include stroke, recent major surgery, intracranial neoplasm and abdominal or gastrointestinal bleeding.

Catheter-directed Thrombolysis

With this technique, the thrombolytic drug is infused directly into the pulmonary artery, which can take place immediately after diagnostic angiography has confirmed the seriousness of PE. There is some discussion as to whether the tip of the catheter should be in the main pulmonary artery or should be embedded into the thrombus. The most commonly used drugs are urokinase and rtPA. After puncture of a femoral vein, the catheter tip is positioned in or near the clot, followed by a bolus of 250 000 IU urokinase. This is followed by an infusion of 100.000 IU/h for 12–24 h. The patient is also heparinized to maintain a pulmonary transit time (PTT) at 1.5–2.5 times the normal limits. For rtPA, a bolus of 10 mg is followed by 20 mg/h over 2 h.

Although haemorrhagic complications may be fewer with low-dose catheter-directed thrombolysis due to a decreased systemic concentration of fibrinolytic agent, there are no data that conclusively show that this technique has fewer complications. One study, which used rtPA, did not show any significant benefit of local intrapulmonary infusion over the intravenous route (6). In the UPET study, the rate of major bleeding complications was 6% for rtPA and 12–27% for urokinase (7). In spite of local infusion of fibrinolytic agents, clot lysis remains a time-consuming process and when pulmonary blood flow is not restored quickly the outcome may still be fatal.

Additional mechanical clot fragmentation with a catheter, a balloon catheter or other devices may increase the velocity of thrombolysis. An increase in the clot surface area and thus enhanced exposure to the lytic drug due to the larger surface area is probably the mechanism of improved lysis. The effectiveness of combined clot fragmentation and local thrombolysis has been demonstrated in several studies (8–11). Although it is reasonable to assume that early clot lysis and reperfusion will give a better early and long-term outcome concerning survival, there are no randomized studies to prove this, and the overall number of described cases remains small.

Thromboembolectomy

In the last decade, a variety of devices have been developed for local embolectomy or thrombectomy. Recently, many of these devices have been withdrawn from the market, not because of poor performance, but due to registration regulations and profitability. Owing to new European market regulations that govern product registration, regular renewal has become mandatory. The administrative burden and costs of this process are often not matched by the actual profits, because these products do not have a sufficiently high turnover.

Some of these devices will retrieve clots whereas others use mechanical fragmentation, sometimes in combination with aspiration. Although there is almost never a total removal of thrombus, debulking in combination with fragmentation can be very beneficial. The rationale for this is that the volume of the peripheral pulmonary circulation is twice that of the central pulmonary arteries. Fragmentation and redistribution of central clot into the peripheral pulmonary arteries may improve pulmonary blood flow and thus prevent right heart failure.

Whether mechanical thrombectomy can work as a stand-alone technique in massive PE or if a combination with local lysis is superior remains to be proven. A theoretical advantage of not using lytic drugs is the reduction in haemorrhagic complications.

THROMBOEMBOLECTOMY DEVICES

There are devices that are specially dedicated to the treatment of PE. All the other currently available devices are designed for thromboembolectomy in any vascular environment.

Dedicated thromboembolectomy devices

The greenfield embolectomy device (no longer on the market)

This device, which was specially designed for the treatment of PE, worked with suction alone for soft and non-wall-adherent thrombus recovery. The device required a venotomy or a 24 French (Fr) sheath for its introduction into the venous system (12). Only limited results were obtained and the device did not gain widespread acceptance (13).

Impeller basket device (no longer on the market)

This device was designed for the treatment of PE. It consisted of a flexible wire shaft inside a 7 Fr catheter with a small impeller mounted on the wire and in the centre of a metallic self-expandable basket. The impeller was connected through the wire to an external electric motor which could rotate at 100 000 rpm. The impeller created a vortex inside the vessel lumen and pulled the thrombus into the basket, causing fragmentation. The basket protected the vessel wall from the rotational impeller (14). The device had limited steerability and was relatively stiff and difficult to position. A modified impeller device was also developed (15). However, other than experimental animal data, only limited human experience exists and it is highly doubtful that this device would play a significant role in the treatment of PE (16).

Rotatable pigtail catheter (no longer on the market)

The rotatable pigtail catheter is modelled on a custom-made high-torque pigtail catheter with a diameter of 5 Fr, a length of 110 cm, 10 side ports and a radiopaque tip. With a straightened stiff wire, through the oval side hole in the pigtail curve, the catheter is connected to an electric motor (maximum 500 rpm). During rotation the pigtail can be advanced or withdrawn over the wire as a guide rail (17). In dogs this device seems to work, but no human data are available.

Reekers PE hydrolyser catheter (no longer on the market)

A 90 cm long, 7 Fr hydrolyser catheter (for a description see the section General thrombectomy devices, below) with a fixed pigtail tip was developed to allow for stability in the large pulmonary artery. The wire cannot enter this pigtail tip, which is essentially glued on to the end of the catheter. The catheter was introduced through a 9 Fr guiding catheter into the main pulmonary artery (Figures 26.1 and 26.2).

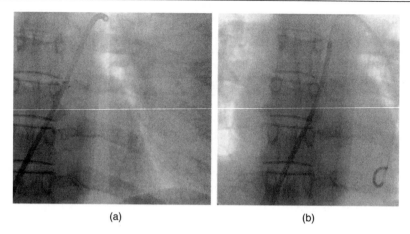

(a)   (b)

Figure 26.1 Example of the Reekers PE hydrolyser catheter, demonstrating positioning and deployment into the left main and lower lobe pulmonary artery.

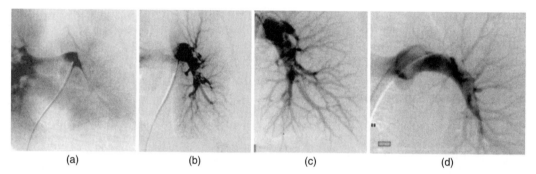

(a)   (b)   (c)   (d)

Figure 26.2 A 42-year-old female with progressive dyspnoe over a period of 5 days. No haemodynamic problems. The V/Q scan showed no perfusion over the left lung. (a) Pulmonary angiography with catheter tip in pulmonary trunk. Occlusion of the left main pulmonary artery. (b) Reekers PE hydrolyser catheter introduced through a long 9 Fr sheath at the origin of the left pulmonary artery. (c) After three runs with the device there was no further angiographic improvement. Major debulking of thrombus in the left pulmonary artery. There was an instant improvement both clinically and regarding the O_2 demand. Treatment was continued with systemic low -molecular heparin for 1 week followed by coumarin. (d) Control angiography at 6 months shows further improvement, but part of the lingula branch is still missing. The patient is symptom free.

General thrombectomy devices

There are two different, more or less evaluated, types of mechanical thrombectomy devices available on the market today: devices which have a mechanical, external motor-driven, rotating action for fragmentation of the clot and devices whose functioning is based on a modified water pump whereby the principal action is thrombosuction.

Rotating devices

The two commercially available and FDA-approved rotating devices are the Amplatz Clot Buster and the Arrow-Trerotola device. The main action of both of these devices is fragmentation of thrombus, which can in some instances be followed by aspiration. There is one successful case report of the use of the Arrow-Trerotola device in a patient with massive PE (18). Furthermore, there are only some animal work data available (19). One literature review could find only minimal experience with these devices, albeit with high success rates (20). Based on these minimal data, it is not possible to give advice concerning the use of these devices in massive PE.

The Amplatz Thrombectomy Device (Microvena, White Bear Lake, MN, USA)

This device was first reported in 1989 (21). It is an 8 Fr rapidly spinning helical screw propeller which is housed in an 8 Fr short metal protective capsule. The metal capsule has several side ports allowing for recirculation and maceration of thrombotic material. The capsule is attached to a 100 cm long catheter. Torque to the helix is transmitted by a cable driven by an air motor at approximately 100 000 rpm. Liquefaction of the clot produces particles ranging in size from 13 to $1000 \mu m$ (22). The device was studied for a possible haemolytic effect, which was shown to be transiently present and related to the activation time (23). This device is approved by the FDA only for thrombosed dialysis fistulae. There are two publications on pulmonary application of this device for massive PE in critically ill patients, but the series that is published is too small to draw any definite conclusions on clinical efficacy (24,25). The main disadvantages of this device are the catheter size (8 Fr) and the lack of guide wire operability. Some of this was updated and a 6 Fr device (still without guide wire option) is currently available. To date there is no information regarding possible vessel wall damage.

Hydrodynamic devices

The two commercially available hydrodynamic devices are the Hydrolyser and the Angiojet. The main action of these devices is the mobilization of fresh clot and its subsequent removal by suction.

The Hydrolyser (CORDIS, Roden, The Netherlands)

The Hydrolyser is a 6 or 7 Fr double lumen catheter with a small injection lumen and a larger exhaust lumen. The exhaust lumen is connected to a collection bag. The device is activated with a standard contrast injection pump filled with saline. For the 7 Fr device a flow of 4 mL/s at 750 psi through the injection lumen is required (26). The device, which is available in different lengths, can be guided over a 0.025 in wire through the exhaust lumen. The latest version of the 6 Fr device is a flexible triple lumen catheter with a separate 0.020 in guide wire lumen and can be applied safely in vessels between 3 and 8 mm. It has been shown in vivo that the Hydrolyser does not give rise to vessel wall damage (27). The main disadvantage of this catheter, as is the case for all hydrodynamic systems, is that it only works effectively in fresh clot, which means an arterial clot no older than about 10 days. The great advantage of the Hydrolyser system is that no investment is required for an extra pump or other hardware, it is simply a catheter. There is growing clinical experience with this device in PE which reports good results (28–32). A special PE hydrolyser was designed with a fixed pigtail at the tip to offer increased stability in the relatively large pulmonary artery lumen. This device seems to be a good, effective and safe alternative to local lysis or surgery.

The Angiojet Catheter (Possis Medical, Minneapolis, MN, USA)

This device consists of a 4–6 Fr dual lumen tubing catheter, with a small injection lumen and a larger exhaust lumen. At the catheter tip there are three holes through which water jets exit perpendicularly, with a pressure of about 1–2 psi. Additionally, three water jets with a pressure of 1000 psi are directed into the catheter lumen to remove fragmented thrombus with the aid of the Venturi effect. To work this device, a special pump is necessary which can provide a pressure of 10 000–15 000 psi to the catheter. The catheter can be guided over a wire. There is increasing evidence for the clinical effectiveness of this device for the treatment of acute massive PE (33–35). Severe arrhythmia has been a safety concern with the use of this device in the pulmonary arteries and it has been postulated that this is related to potassium release from clot destruction. To be prepared for such an event, an external pacemaker system should always be available when using this device in the pulmonary arteries.

STENTS FOR MASSIVE PULMONARY EMBOLISM

There have been two reports concerning stent placement in critically ill patients with massive, therapy-resistant wall-adherent PE (36,37). In both reports this treatment was used as a final emergency option after all other available techniques had been used. The stents were placed in the main pulmonary artery, thus compressing the massive thrombus and allowing for rapid reperfusion with immediate relieve of complaint. In one of the studies the patient was symptom free at 8 months (36). Although there is a lot of experience with stents at other arterial and venous locations, with the currently available data this technique can only be advised as a last resort.

PERCUTANEOUS INTERVENTIONS FOR SUBCLAVIAN VEIN THROMBOSIS

Subclavian vein thrombosis

It is generally believed that subclavian thrombosis does not produce long-term disability due to good collateral circulation. Nevertheless, a post-thrombotic arm syndrome can be recognized in up to 70% of patients with a subclavian vein thrombosis (38). Data which prove the need for more invasive therapy for all subclavian thrombosis, such as local thrombolysis or percutaneous thrombectomy, are not available. However, there seem to be indications for treatment of subclavian vein thrombosis which have literature support. Early clot removal for active, healthy patients with a need to use the limb in sport and work is favoured by a panel of experts of American vascular surgeons, who promote catheter-directed thrombolysis as initial therapy (39).

Subclavian vein effort thrombosis

Thrombosis of the subclavian vein is often seen in combination with a costoclavicular compression syndrome. Compression of the vein at the thoracic outlet is the aetiology for this problem. In the acute phase, with a history of thrombosis shorter than 2 weeks, local catheter-directed thrombolytic therapy followed by surgical removal of the first rib is the first choice of management (40,41). The aim of lytic therapy is to prevent chronic fibrous obliteration of the subclavian vein. The outcome for patients with spontaneous subclavian vein thrombosis, treated with heparin and oral anticoagulants alone is inferior to lytic therapy, for both recanalization and symptom resolution (42). Mechanical thrombectomy with the Angiojet device can be very successful in removing the clot. This therapy has to be followed by 6 months anticoagulant therapy with vitamin K antagonists.

Subclavian vein thrombosis with indwelling lines

Indwelling subclavian lines for dialysis, chemotherapy and nutrition have a high risk for thrombosis. It is likely that this is related to a combination of flow obstruction and underlying thrombotic states in patients who require lines, such as cancer. The primary treatment target is not so much the prevention of post-thrombotic problems, rather is aimed at preservation of the line and/or venous access for future use, particularly as many patients require multiple line insertions in prolonged disease states. Catheter-directed thrombolysis or percutaneous thrombectomy devices can both be useful in clinical practice. The thrombectomy devices have a shorter treatment time, reduced hospitalization time and lack the potential adverse effects of systemic thrombolytic drugs (Figure 26.3).

CATHETER-DIRECTED THROMBOLYSIS FOR LOWER EXTREMITY DEEP VEIN THROMBOSIS

Introduction

The therapeutic goals for treating the patient with acute DVT include preventing PE, restoration of unobstructed blood flow through the thrombosed segment, prevention of recurrent thrombosis and preservation of venous valve function. Success in achieving these goals will minimize the morbidity and mortality of PE and will also diminish the sequelae of the post-thrombotic syndrome (PTS). As shown by Johnson et al., it is the combination of reflux and obstruction that correlates with the severity of PTS, as opposed to either of these factors in isolation (43). Up to two-thirds of the patients with iliofemoral DVT will develop oedema and pain, with 5% developing ulcers in spite of adequate anticoagulation (44).

The standard of care at present includes systemic anticoagulation with heparin followed by oral anticoagulants (see Chapter 22) (45). Such a regimen, however, does not promote lysis to reduce the thrombus load, nor does it contribute to restoration of venous valvular function. Anticoagulation alone, therefore, does not protect the limb from PTS, which can occur months to years following the acute thrombotic event (44).

Thrombolysis is a potentially attractive form of therapy since it provides the opportunity for promptly restoring venous patency and preserving venous valve function. This therapy provides the potential for preventing the long-term sequelae of DVT. There is published evidence that thrombolytic agents, even administered systemically, are superior to standard anticoagulation therapy in achieving early lysis of thrombus. In a pooled analysis of 13 randomized studies, Comerota and Aldridge found that only 4% of patients treated with heparin had significant or complete lysis compared with 45% of patients randomized to systemic streptokinase therapy (46). Similarly, in reviewing pooled data from six trials judged to have proper randomization, systemic thrombolysis was 3.7 times more effective in producing some degree of lysis than heparin (47). In spite of these results, progress was hindered, probably because of the trade-off between haemorrhagic complications and the use of systemic administration, where the drug does not reach the thrombus in sufficient concentration to provide optimal results.

In 1994, a report by Semba and Dake provided the first insight into the potential role of catheter-directed thrombolytic (CDT) techniques (48). They reported complete lysis in 72% of the patients with concomitant resolution of symptoms. Only one patient suffered a bleeding complication of haem-positive stools. After the drug was discontinued, there were no significant adverse sequelae. Delivering the thrombolytic agent directly into the thrombus offers significant advantages over systemic therapy, which may fail to reach and penetrate an occluded venous segment.

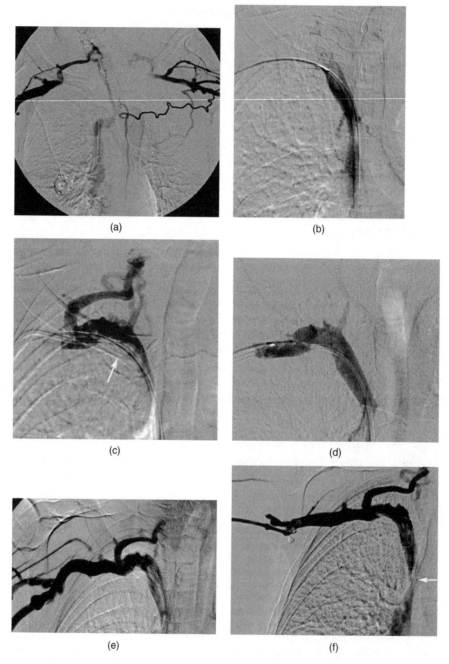

(a)   (b)

(c)   (d)

(e)   (f)

Figure 26.3   Patient with a catheter-related bilateral subclavian vein thrombosis, requiring dialysis access. Current symptoms were acute right arm and neck swelling. (a) Thrombosis of the bilateral subclavian and brachiocephalic veins. (b) The thrombus is passed with the catheter. Venogram demonstrates acute thrombus. (c) After mechanical thrombectomy with a 7 Fr hydrolyser, through the right basilic vein. Total removal of thrombus and re-functioning of the line. (d) End result after thrombectomy day 1. (e) Control study at 48 h shows vessels remain patent. (f) At 8 months, minor change in symptoms. Venogram reveals re-stenosis at the superior vena cava, but still patency of the vessels. Therefore, catheter access was maintained in this patient.

Because thrombolytic agents activate plasminogen within the thrombus, delivery of the drug to that site enhances its effectiveness. In addition, higher concentrations can be delivered, improving lysis rates and reducing treatment duration and the risk of complications. The progress of CDT can be monitored by direct imaging techniques and lesions potentially contributing to the thrombosis can be identified. These defects, such as stenosis of the common iliac vein, can be treated by balloon angioplasty with or without the placement of endovascular stents (Figure 26.3).

Technique of catheter-directed lysis

With the patient prone on the angiographic table, we prefer the ipsilateral popliteal venous approach because it is often difficult to penetrate an occluded superficial femoral vein from the internal jugular vein or the contralateral common femoral vein, due to venous valves that may prevent safe catheter and guide wire manipulations. The popliteal vein should be accessed under ultrasound guidance with a small-gauge echogenic needle to avoid inadvertent puncture of the popliteal artery. A 5 Fr short sheath is then introduced, via which all subsequent catheters can be exchanged. Following baseline venography obtained via the popliteal sheath, the occluded venous is crossed with a straight-tip 5 Fr catheter and a 0.035 in curved-tip glide wire. Venography is then repeated to confirm intraluminal passage of the catheter, which is then exchanged for a 5 Fr infusing coaxial system, consisting of a proximal multi-sidehole catheter and a distal infusing wire. It is critical to position the system directly into the thrombus, to maximize plasminogen activation at the site of obstruction. Urokinase therapy is initiated at 150 000–200 000 IU/h, evenly split between the infusing ports. As a general rule, we rarely employ a total urokinase dose of greater than 200 000 IU/h regardless of the thrombus burden. Intravenous heparin is concomitantly administered via the popliteal sheath at a rate of 500–1000 IU/h following a 5000 IU bolus of heparin. Patients are monitored in the ICU or a step-down unit, similar to those receiving thombolytic treatment for acute PE or an arterial occlusion. Because the duration of therapy may be in excess of 48 h, it is not necessary to assess the progress of lysis frequently. The frequency of follow-up venograms should be every 12 h, primarily to reposition the infusion devices into the remaining thrombus. Gentle thrombus maceration with a 6 mm balloon angioplasty catheter may be helpful, particularly in the superficial femoral vein, where focal stenosis may be encountered, probably representing sites of organized thrombus. Typically, unless a complication were to dictate otherwise, lytic therapy should be continued until complete lysis is achieved, unless no discernible progress is demonstrated venographically from the previous venogram obtained 12 h earlier. Since the grade of thrombolysis has been shown in the registry to be a strong predictor of continued patency, it is critical that a complete lysis venogram be achieved (49). Lesions uncovered in the iliac venous segments should probably be treated with stents, although the long-term benefits of such devices are not known. However, if left untreated, there appears to be a significant risk of early rethrombosis.

The early results of local lysis

Clearly, the initial report by Semba and Dake suggested that CDT can be effective in achieving significant lysis of thrombus and may be associated with low complication rates. This experience stimulated the development of a multicentre registry. The conclusions of the registry were published almost a decade ago (49). The purpose of the registry was to evaluate catheter-directed thrombolysis for treatment of symptomatic lower extremity DVT. In the registry there were 473 patients with symptomatic lower limb DVT, results of 312 urokinase infusions in 303 limbs of 287 patients (137 male and 150 female patients, mean age 47.5 years) were analysed. DVT symptoms were acute (⩽

10 days) in 188 (66%) patients, chronic (>10 days) in 45 (16%) and acute and chronic in 54 (19%). A history of DVT existed in 90 (31%). Lysis grades were calculated by using venographic results. Iliofemoral DVT [$n = 221$ (71%)] and femoral–popliteal DVT [$n = 79$ (25%)] were treated with urokinase infusions (mean 7.8×10^6 IU) for a mean of 53.4 h. After thrombolysis, 99 iliac and five femoral vein lesions were treated with stents. Grade III (complete) lysis was achieved in 96 (31%) infusions, grade II (50–99% lysis) in 162 (52%) and grade I (<50% lysis) in 54 (17%). For acute thrombosis, grade III lysis occurred in 34% of cases of acute and in 19% of cases of chronic DVT ($p < 0.01$). Major bleeding complications occurred in 54 patients (11%), most often at the puncture site. Six patients (1%) developed pulmonary emboli. Two deaths (<1%) were attributed to PE and intracranial haemorrhage. At 1 year, the primary patency rate was 60%. Lysis grade was predictive of 1 year patency rate (grade III, 79%; grade II, 58%; grade I, 32%; $p < 0.001$). The conclusion from this registry was that catheter-directed thrombolysis is safe and effective in dissolving thrombus from the deep veins of identifiable groups of patients with symptomatic lower limb DVT (49). The best results can be expected in patients with acute symptoms without a prior history of DVT, who are treated with CDT without systemic infusion. The long-term benefits of this form of therapy are not yet known and cannot be conclusively derived from this registry.

New treatment dombinations for DVT

Recently, rheolytic percutaneous mechanical thrombectomy (PMT) in combination with catheter lysis for upper and lower extremity DVT has been shown to be a promising alternative, which is as effective as catheter lysis alone (50–52). The basic idea is that after removal of the bulk of the thrombus with mechanical thrombectomy, the remaining thrombus is removed with catheter lysis, but this requires a significantly shorter treatment duration and lower lytic doses. All of these studies have been performed with the Angiojet catheter (Figure 26.4). However, before we

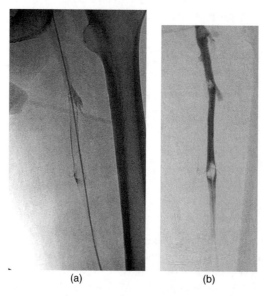

(a)   (b)

Figure 26.4   Patient with severe leg swelling and DVT. (a) Demonstrates guidewire through the thrombus from popliteal vein to femoral vein. (b) After use of an Angiojet catheter, there is restoration of venous patency. Images courtesy of Dr Kong-Ten Tan, University of Toronto, Canada.

can draw any conclusions on the more pro-active treatment of DVT compared with the systemic treatment, we need to have better evidence and long term-follow-up. A randomized controlled trial comparing systemic anticoagulation with mechanical thrombectomy and subsequent local lysis is still not available.

REFERENCES

1. Daniels LB, Parker JA, Patel SR, Grodstein F, Goldhaber SZ. Relation of duration of symptoms with response to thrombolytic therapy in pulmonary embolism. *Am J Cardiol* 1997; **80**:184–8.
2. Tow DE, Wagner HN. Urokinase pulmonary embolism trial: phase I results. *JAMA* 1970; **214**: 2163–72.
3. Urokinase–Streptokinase Pulmonary Embolism Trial: phase 2 results. *JAMA* 1974; **229**:1606–13.
4. Jerjes-Sanchez C, Ramirez-Rivera A, Garcia M, *et al*. Streptokinase and heparin versus heparin alone in massive pulmonary embolism: a randomized controlled trial. *J Thromb Thrombol* 1995; **2**:227–9.
5. Goldhaber SZ. Thrombolytic therapy for pulmonary embolism. *Semin Vasc Surg* 1992; **5**:69–75.
6. Verstraete M, Miller GAH, Bounameux H, *et al*. Intravenous and intrpulmonary recombinant tissue-type plasminogen activator in the treatment of acute massive pulmonary embolism. *Circulation* 1988; **77**:353–60.
7. The Urokinase Pulmonary Embolism Trial: a national cooperative study. *Circulation* 1973; **47**:1–108.
8. Brady AJ, Crake T, Oakley CM. Percutaneous catheter fragmentation and distal dispersion of proximal pulmonary embolus. *Lancet* 1991; **338**:1186–9.
9. Essop MR, Middlemost S, Skoularigis J, Sareli P. Simultaneous mechanical clot fragmentation and pharmacologic thrombolysis in acute massive pulmonary embolism. *Am J Cardiol* 1992; **70**: 427–30.
10. Fava M, Loyola S, Flores P, Huete I. Mechanical fragmentation and pharmacologic thrombolysis in massive pulmonary embolism. *J Vasc Interv Radiol* 1997; **8**:261–6.
11. Stock KW, Jacob AL, Schnabel KJ, Bongartz G, Steinbrich W. Massive pulmonary embolism: treatment with thrombus fragmentation and local fibrinolysis with recombinant human-tissue plasminogen activator. *Cardiovasc Intervent Radiol* 1997; **20**:364–8.
12. Greenfield LJ, Kimmel D, McCurdy WC. Transvenous removal of pulmonary emboli by vacuum-cup transcatheter technique. *J Surg Res* 1969; **9**:347–52.
13. Greenfield LJ, Proctor MC, Williams DM, Wakefield TW. Long-term experience with transvenous catheter pulmonary embolectomy. *J Vasc Surg* 1993; **18**:450–6.
14. Schmitz-Rode T, Vorwerk D, Guenther RW, *et al*. Percutaneous fragmentation of pulmonary emboli in dogs with the impeller basket catheter. *Cardiovasc Interv Radiol* 1993; **16**:234–42.
15. Schmitz-Rode T, Adam G, Kilbingr M, *et al*. Fragmentation of pulmonary emboli: in vivo experimental evaluation of 2 high-speed rotating catheters. *Cardiovasc Interv Radiol* 1996; **19**:165–9.
16. Schmitz-Rode T, Guenther RW. New device for percutaneous fragmentation of pulmonary emboli. *Radiology* 1991; **180**:135–7.
17. Schmitz-Rode T, Guenther RW, Pfeffer JG, *et al*. Acute massive pulmonary embolism: use of a rotatable pigtail catheter for diagnosis and fragmentation therapy. *Radiology* 1995; **197**:157–62.
18. Rocek M, Peregrin J, Velimsky T. Mechanical thrombectomy of massive pulmonary embolism using an Arrow-Trerotola percutaneous thrombolytic device. *Eur Radiol* 1998; **8**:1683–5.
19. Brown DB, Cardella JF, Wilson RP, Singh H, Waybill PN. Evaluation of a modified arrow-trerotola percutaneous thrombolytic device for treatment of acute pulmonary embolus in a canine model. *J Vasc Interv Radiol* 1999; **10**:733–40.
20. Skaf E, Beemath A, Siddiqui T, Janjua M, Patel NR, Stein PD. Catheter-tip embolectomy in the management of acute massive pulmonary embolism. *Am J Cardiol* 2007; **99**:415–20.
21. Bildsoe MC, Moradian GP, Hunter DW, *et al*. Mechanical clot dissolution: new concept. *Radiology* 1989; **171**:231–3.
22. Yasui K, Qian Z, Nazarian GK, *et al*. Recirculation-type Amplatz clot macerator: determination of particle size and distribution. *J Vasc Intervent Radiol* 1993; **4**:275–8.
23. Nazarian GK, Qian Z, Coleman CC, *et al*. Haemolytic effect of the Amplatz thrombectomy device. *J Vasc Interv Radiol* 1994; **5**:155–60.
24. Uflacker R, Strange C, Vujic I. Massive pulmonary embolism: preliminary results of treatment with the Amplatz thrombectomy device. *J Vasc Intervent Radiol* 1996; **7**:19–28.

25. Müller-Hülsbeck S, Brossmann J, Jahnke T, *et al*. Mechanical thrombectomy of major and massive pulmonary embolism with use of the Amplatz thrombectomy device. *Invest Radiol* 2001; **36**: 317–22.

26. Reekers JA, Kromhout JG, van der Waal K. Catheter for percutaneous thrombectomy: first clinical experience. *Radiology* 1993; **188**:871–74.

27. van Ommen V, van der Veen FH, Daemen MJ, *et al*. In vivo evaluation of the Hydrolyser hydrodynamic thrombectomy catheter. *J Vasc Intervent Radiol* 1994; **5**:823–6.

28. Henry M, Amor M, Henry I, Tricoche O, Allaoui M. The Hydrolyser thrombectomy catheter: a single center experience. *J Endovasc Surg* 1998; **5**:24–31.

29. Michalis LK, Tsetis DK, Rees MR. Percutaneous removal of pulmonary artery thrombus in a patient with massive pulmonary embolism using the Hydrolyser catheter: the first human experience. *Clin Radiol* 1997; **52**:158–61.

30. Koning R, Cribier A, Gerber L, *et al*. A new treatment for severe pulmonary embolism: percutaneous rheolytic thrombectomy. *Circulation* 1997; **96**:2498–500.

31. Fava M, Loyola S, Huete I. Massive pulmonary embolism: treatment with the Hydrolyser thrombectomy catheter. *J Vasc Intervent Radiol* 2000; **11**:1159–64.

32. Reekers JA, Baarslag HJ, Koolen MG, van Delden O, van Beek EJ. Mechanical thrombectomy for early treatment of massive pulmonary embolism. *Cardiovasc Intervent Radiol* 2003; **26**:246–50.

33. Zeni PT Jr, Blank BG, Peeler DW. Use of rheolytic thrombectomy in treatment of acute massive pulmonary embolism. *J Vasc Interv Radiol*. 2003; **14**:1511–15.

34. Chauhan MS, Kawamura A. Percutaneous rheolytic thrombectomy for large pulmonary embolism: a promising treatment option. *Catheter Cardiovasc Intervent* 2007; **70**:121–8.

35. Margheri M, Vittori G, Vecchio S, *et al*. Early and long-term clinical results of AngioJet rheolytic thrombectomy in patients with acute pulmonary embolism. *Am J Cardiol* 2008; **101**:252–8.

36. Haskal ZJ, Soulen MC, Huettl EA, Palevsky HI, Cope C. Life-threatening pulmonary emboli and cor pulmonale:Treatment with percutaneous pulmonary artery stent placement. *Radiology* 1994; **191**: 473–5.

37. Koizumi J, Kusano S, Akima T, *et al*. Emergent Z stent placement for treatment of cor pulmonale due to pulmonary emboli after failed lytic treatment:Technical considerations. *Cardiovasc Intervent Radiol* 1998; **21**:254–7.

38. Rochester JR, Beard JD. Acute management of subclavian vein thrombosis. *Br J Surg* 1995; **82**: 433–4.

39. Rutherford RB, Hurlbert SN. Primary subclavian-axillary vein thrombosis: consensus and commentary. *Cardiovasc Surg* 1996; **4**:420–3.

40. Molina JE. Need for emergency treatment in subclavian vein effort thrombosis. *J Am Coll Surg* 1995; **181**:414–20.

41. Sheeran SR, Hallisey MJ, Murphy TP, *et al*. Local thrombolytic therapy as part of a multidisciplinary approach to acute axillosubclavian vein thrombosis (Paget–Schroetter syndrome). *J Vasc Intervent Radiol* 1997; **8**:253–60.

42. AbuRahma AF, Short YS, White JF III, Boland JP. Treatment alternatives for axillary subclavian vein thrombosis: long-term follow up. *Cardiovasc Surg* 1996; **4**:783–7.

43. Johnson BF, Manzo RA, Bergelin RO, Srandness DE Jr. Relationship between changes in the deep venous system and the development of the post-thrombotic syndrome after an acute episode of lower limb deep venous thrombosis: a one-to-six year follow-up. *J Vasc Surg* 1995; **21**:307.

44. Strandness DE, Langlois Y, Cramer M, Randkett A, *et al*. Long-term sequelae of acute venous thrombosis. *JAMA* 1983; **250**:1289–92.

45. Hull RD, Raskob GE, Rosenbloom D, Panju AA, Brill-Edwards P, Ginsberg JF, Hirsch J, Martin GJ, Green D. Heparin for 5 days as compared with 10 days in the initial treatment of proximal venous thrombosis. *N Engl J Med* 1990; **322**:1260–4.

46. Comerota A, Aldridge SC. Thrombolytic therapy for deep venous thrombosis: a clinical review. *Can J Surg* 1993; **36**:359–64.

47. Goldhaber SZ, Buring JE, Lipnick RJ, *et al*. Pooled analysis of randomized trials of streptokinase and heparin in phlebographically documented acute deep venous thrombosis. *Am J Med* 1984; **76**: 393–7.

48. Semba CP, Dake MD. Catheter directed thrombolysis for iliofemoral venous thrombosis. *Radiology* 1994; **191**:487–94.

49. Mewissen MW, Seabrook GR, Meissner MH, *et al*. Catheter-directed thrombolysis for lower extremity deep venous thrombosis: report of a national multicenter registry. *Radiology* 1999; **211**: 39–49.

50. Bush RL, Lin PH, Bates JT, *et al*. Pharmacomechanical thrombectomy for treatment of symptomatic lower extremity deep venous thrombosis: safety and feasibility study. *J Vasc Surg* 2004;**40**: 965–70.
51. Kim HS, Patra A, Paxton BE, Khan J, Streiff MB. Catheter-directed thrombolysis with percutaneous rheolytic thrombectomy versus thrombolysis alone in upper and lower extremity deep vein thrombosis. *Cardiovasc Intervent Radiol* 2006; **29**:1003–7.
52. Lin PH, Zhou W, Dardik A. Catheter-direct thrombolysis versus pharmacomechanical thrombectomy for treatment of symptomatic lower extremity deep venous thrombosis. *Am J Surg* 2006; **192**: 782–8.

Index

Notes: Page references in *italics* refer to Figures; those in **bold** refer to Tables
DVT = deep vein thrombosis; PE = pulmonary embolism; VTE = venous thromboembolism